D1479418

**CLARK'S**

SPECIAL PROCEDURES IN

# DIAGNOSTIC IMAGING

# CLARK'S



# SPECIAL PROCEDURES IN DIAGNOSTIC IMAGING

**A. Stewart Whitley** HDCR FCR TDCR

District Radiographer and
Radiology Business Manager
Radiology Directorate
Blackpool Victoria Hospital NHS Trust
Blackpool Lancashire UK

**Chrissie W. Alsop** DCR

Superintendent Radiographer
Department of Diagnostic Radiology
University of Manchester and
Manchester Royal Infirmary UK

**Adrian D. Moore** MA TDCR HDCR FCR

Professor of Health Sciences
Anglia Polytechnic University
Cambridge UK

with contributions from

**Michael J. Wright**

Formerly Superintendant Radiographer
Derby Royal Infirmary

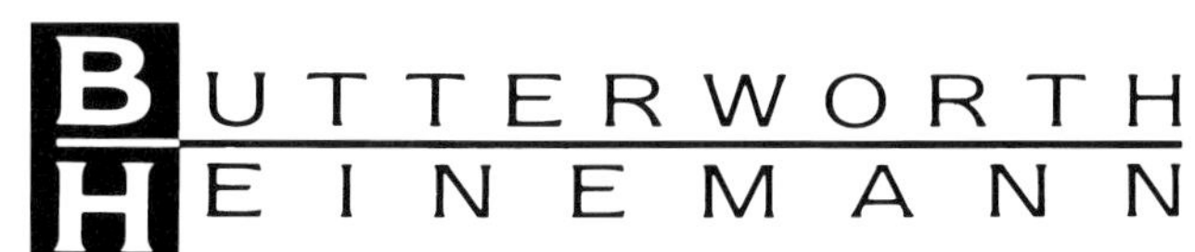


OXFORD AUCKLAND BOSTON JOHANNESBURG MELBOURNE NEW DELHI

Butterworth-Heinemann
Linacre House, Jordan Hill, Oxford OX2 8DP
225 Wildwood Avenue, Woburn, MA 01801-2041
A division of Reed Educational and Professional Publishing Ltd

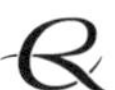 A member of the Reed Elsevier plc group

First published 1999



**British Library Cataloguing in Publication Data**
Whitley, A. S.
Clark's special procedures in diagnostic imaging
1. Diagnostic imaging
I. Title II. Alsop, Chrissie W. III. Moore, Adrian D.
616'.0754

**Library of Congress Cataloguing in Publication Data**
Whitley, A. Stewart.
Clark's special procedures in diagnostic imaging/A. Stewart Whitley, Chrissie W. Alsop, Adrian D. Moore.
p. cm.
Companion v. to: Clark's positioning in radiography.
Includes bibliographical; references and index.
ISBN 0 7506 1715 2
1. Diagnostic imaging. I. Alsop, Chrissie W. II. Moore, Adrian D. III. Clark, Kathleen C. (Kathleen Clara). Clark's positioning in radiography. IV. Title.
[DNLM: 1. Diagnostic Imaging – methods. 2. Technology, Radiologic – methods. WN 180 W613c]
RC78.7.D53W48 98–20552
616.07'54 – dc21 CIP

ISBN 0 7506 1715 2

Composition by Genesis Typesetting, Laser Quay, Rochester, Kent
Printed and bound in Great Britain by The University Press, Cambridge

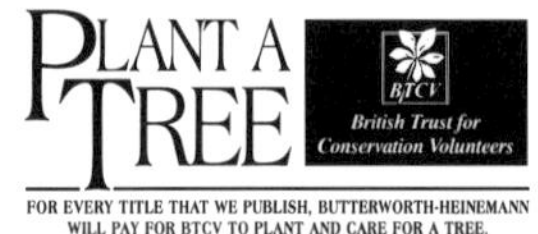

# CONTENTS

# FOREWORD

It is a great pleasure to write the Foreword to what will become a 'Bible' of radiography. To prepare a single volume which encompasses all possible special procedures is a mammoth task and the authors deserve hearty congratulations. At least their names will become even better known, as this volume will be an essential item within every imaging department. One of its great strengths is that it is so very comprehensive. It is exactly the book that everyone will turn to when they have to perform an occasional specialised investigation. Hence the book seems set for an illustrious career which will match others in the long and distinguished history of radiography textbooks. Just look what Kitty Clark started!

So far I have emphasised the value of this book as a reference manual. It is no less useful as a teaching resource. Many students of radiography, whether studying for basic or higher degree courses, will need this book for the wealth of data it contains. Radiologists in training (and those supposedly trained!) would benefit from its contents too.

This book has made a serious stride into the twenty-first century with considerable reference to the increasing role of magnetic resonance imaging. Of course, any book such as this can only reflect current practice in a rapidly evolving field. Nevertheless the authors have made every attempt to allude to clinical situations where practice is likely to change. For example, they include a comment about the current research role of MR cholangiopancreatography, a technique which has been advanced at Cambridge. This will become a standard investigation during the lifetime of this book. So too will breath hold MR imaging.

There are very few things here that anyone can take exception to. A personal and idiosyncratic grouse is that the word 'scan' is slightly overused! I never quite know what it means. Is it one image or a whole investigation? What is a liver scan? Wherever possible the precise term – ultrasound, computed tomography, etc. – should be used. Even if we use the word freely with our patients.

This book promises to be a major player in imaging over the next few years. I much enjoyed reading it. I am sure that you will too. I can guarantee that you do not know all that it contains.

Adrian K. Dixon MD FRCR FRCP

Honorary Consultant and
Professor of Radiology
Addenbrooke's Hospital and
the University of Cambridge

# PREFACE

This book has been written as a companion volume to *Clark's Positioning in Radiography*, currently in its eleventh edition, the history of which is detailed below.

The aim of this book is to provide coverage of the many special diagnostic and interventional procedures used in the modern imaging department. It is believed that such a book is long overdue, since those techniques have only been given minimal coverage in previous editions of *Positioning in Radiography.*

The authors acknowledge that because of the many techniques which are rapidly changing it has been difficult to give a comprehensive in-depth account of certain procedures. For example, in the area of magnetic resonance imaging which is under continuous research and development, the basic principles of physics and imaging are described but more complex techniques such as diffusion, perfusion and function are still under clinical development and are not included in this edition. From the text it is hoped that the student will gain the core of knowledge of many special imaging procedures found in diagnostic imaging departments.

We are indebted to the editors and the many radiographers and radiologists, who, over the years, have contributed to the work of 'Kitty Clark'. Their dedication and foresight has laid the foundation to this new book. We trust we have not failed in maintaining their high standards.

The authors are particularly grateful for the support and encouragement of their respective spouses: Eunice Whitley, Graham Alsop and Gill Moore. Without their patient endurance this book would never have been concluded.

We would also like to acknowledge the valuable contributions of Michael Wright and especially his wife, Margaret, for her kind hospitality at their home in Derby which acted as an important meeting point.

We are particularly indebted to the Health Imaging Division of Kodak Limited UK for their sponsorship towards the production of the photographs and images which appear in this book. This assistance was invaluable and was greatly appreciated by the authors.

We are also indebted to E. Merck Pharmaceuticals (Merck Radiology) for their sponsorship for the production of the many anatomical illustrations.

We gratefully acknowledge the help and advice given by the staff and students of Radiodiagnostic Departments Blackpool Victoria Hospital NHS Trust, the Department of Diagnostic Radiology University of Manchester and the School of Applied Sciences, Anglia Polytechnic University; Manchester Royal Infirmary; Royal Preston Hospitals NHS Trust; Sharoe Green Hospital, Preston; Christie Hospital NHS Trust; South Manchester University Hospitals NHS Trust, Withington Hospital; Centre for Magnetic Resonance Investigations, Hull Royal Infirmary; Bristol Royal Infirmary; Bristol M.R.I. Centre; The Oxford Radcliffe Hospital – The John Radcliffe; Papworth Hospital, Cambridge; Department of Radiology and Imaging Sciences, University College St Martin's; Belfast City Hospital and Addenbrooke's Hospital NHS Trust, Cambridge.

We are particularly indebted for advice, illustrations and images to the following: Dr P. Fielden, Dr D.P. Montgomery, Dr G.M. Hoadley, Dr T. Kane, Dr R.W. Bury, Dr P.K. Bowyer, Dr L. Morris, Dr C. Walshaw, Dr L. Hacking, Mr D. Dewitt, Mrs K. Hughes, Mrs V Mountain, Ms C. Hurst, Mrs S. Mohindra, Miss N. Whiteside, Mrs L.A. Stanney, Miss S. Taylor, Mrs K. Walsh, Mrs S. Kaminiski, Mrs K Brute, Mrs B Mingham, Radiology Department, and Mrs L. V. Stanley and Mrs G. Fallows, Cardiology Department, Blackpool Victoria Hospital NHS Trust; Professor J.E. Adams, Professor I. Isherwood, Dr C. Hutchinson, Miss Y. Watson, Mrs I. Hodgkinson, Mr S. Capener, Department of Diagnostic Radiology, University of Manchester; Dr P.M. Taylor, Dr J. Gillespie, Miss K. O'Neill, Mr J. Yates and Mrs J. Johnson, Manchester Royal Infirmary; Dr S. Rimmer and Mrs R. Lee, Radiology Department, St Mary's Hospital, Manchester; Dr J. Hill, Dr W.J. Gunawardena, Mrs L. Parkinson, Mrs J. Jackson, Mr S. Denton, Mr P. Bowker, Mrs D. Hall, Mrs D. Wilson and Mrs T. Tomlinson, Royal Preston Hospital; Mrs C. Barnes and Mrs M. Clenton, Sharoe Green Hospital, Preston; Miss P. Nuttall, Mr D. McHugh, Miss S. Owens, Mr S. P. Jeans and Mr B. Murby, North Western Medical Physics Department, Christie Hospital NHS Trust; Dr S. Glenn, Coulter Pharmaceutical, INC.; Dr P. Sambrook, Mr L. Readman, Mrs A. M. Hibbert and Mr C. McCullough, Department of Radiology, South Manchester University Hospitals NHS Trust, Withington Hospital; Professor A. Horsman and Mr R. Devlin, Centre for Magnetic Resonance Investigations, Hull Royal Infirmary; Mrs D. Pressdee, Bristol Royal Infirmary; Mrs A. Case, Bristol M.R.I. Centre; Dr D. Nolan and Mrs I. Miller, Department of Radiology, The Oxford Radcliffe Hospital – The John Radcliffe; Dr R. Coulden, Papworth Hospital, Cambridge; Mrs J. Marshall, Department of Radiology and Imaging Sciences, University College St Martin's; Mr R. Herbert, Department of Radiology, Belfast City Hospital; Miss A. Zuydam, Speech Therapy Department, Walton Hospital, Liverpool; Dr L. Chitty, Fetal Medicine Unit, Obstetric Hospital University College Hospital and Mr D. Altman, Centre for Statistics in Medicine, Institute of Health Sciences and Blackwell Science for charts quoted in the *British Journal of Obstetrics & Gynaecology*; Dr J. McIvor and P.F. Evans, Department of Radiology, A. Perry, Speech Therapy and A.D. Cheesman, Ear Nose and Throat Surgery, Charing Cross Hospital; Dr S. Field, Department of Diagnostic Radiology, Kent and Canterbury Hospitals NHS Trust; Professor D. Longmore, Magnetic Resonance Unit, Royal Brompton Hospital; Peri Gretton G.E. Medical Systems Europe; Dr R. Pulvertaft, Newmarket Hospital; Mrs C. Price,

Morriston Hospital, Swansea; Mrs C. Sims and Dr A. Freeman, Radiology Department, Addenbrooke's Hospital, Cambridge; Mrs I. Kendall, Wolfson Brain Imaging Centre, Cambridge University; Miss J. Birks, librarian, and Mrs H. Taylor, School of Applied Sciences, Anglia Polytechnic University; Liz Jennings A.T.L; Mrs G. Moore, BUPA Cambridge Lea Hospital; Dr J. Giles and Mr D. Forrest for use of SVC material; Justin Boag and Amanda Bowen, Amersham Health Care, for support and co-ordinating RNI images from the Nuclear Medicine and Radiology Departments of the Royal United Hospital, Bath; Ninewells Hospital, Dundee; Hammersmith Hospital; Middlesex Hospital; North Tees General Hospital, Stockton; Hope Hospital, Salford; Mount Vernon Hospital and the Freeman Hospital, Newcastle.

Our thanks are also extended to many students at Blackpool Victoria Hospital, the Royal Preston Hospital and Manchester Royal Infirmary all of whom patiently endured long hours of modelling for the positioning illustrations.

The Radiological Imaging Trade gave valuable support in the form of advice, photographic illustrations, diagrams and charts and we would therefore like to thank: G.E. Medical Systems Europe; A.T.L; Sonotron; Philips Medical Systems; Picker International Limited; Siemens plc Medical Engineering; Lunar Corporation; Hologic, Inc; Schering Health Care Limited; E-Z-EM Limited; Schneider UK; Bard; Amersham Healthcare; Cordis and Coulter Pharmaceutical, Inc.

The book contains a vast number of new positioning illustrations and images representative of the many imaging procedures described in the manuscript. We are indebted to the Medical Illustration Department, Royal Preston Hospital, and the Department of Diagnostic Radiology, University of Manchester, and the Medical Illustrations Department Blackpool Victoria Hospital, particularly the photographic skills of Simon Hills, David Ellard and Robert Drobny.

We also wish to thank the many secretaries at the various institutions for their valuable typing and administration support. We would particularly like to thank Mrs A. Russell, Miss C. Yeo and Mrs D. Cleary.

## K. C. Clark and the origins of *Clark's Positioning in Radiography*

Miss K.C. Clark was Principal of the Ilford Department of Radiography and Medical Photography at Tavistock House, from 1935 to 1958. She had an intense interest in the teaching and development of radiographic positioning and procedures, which resulted in an invitation by Ilford Limited to produce the classic text, *Positioning in Radiography* (first published in 1938), which was to be used by generations of students and practising radiographers. Her enthusiasm in all matters pertaining to this subject was infectious. Ably assisted by her colleagues she was responsible for many innovations in radiography, playing a notable part in the development of mass miniature radiography. Her ability and ever active endeavour to cement teamwork between radiologist and radiographer gained her worldwide respect.

At the conclusion of her term of office as the President of the Society of Radiographers in 1936 she was elected to Honorary Fellowship. In 1959 she was elected to Honorary Membership of the Faculty of Radiologists and Honorary Fellowship of the Australasian Institute of Radiography.

Miss Clark died in 1968 and the Kathleen Memorial Library was established by the Society of Radiographers and originally housed at their premises in Upper Wimpole Street as a tribute to her contribution to Radiography. The Society and College of Radiographers have now transferred this material to the library at the British Institute of Radiology 36 Portland Place, London.

The ninth edition was published in two volumes, edited and revised by James McInnes FSR, TE, FRPS, whose involvement with *Positioning in Radiography* began in 1946 when he joined Miss Clark's team at Tavistock House. He originated many techniques in radiography and in 1958 became Principal of Lecture and Technical Services at Tavistock House which enabled him to travel as lecturer to the Radiographic Societies of Britain, Canada, America, South and West Africa.

The tenth edition, also published in two volumes, was revised and edited by Louis Kreel MD, FRCP, FRCR, a radiologist of international repute and wide experience of new imaging technologies.

The eleventh edition, published in one volume, was revised and edited by Alan Swallow FCR, TE, Principal of the Nottinghamshire School of Radiodiagnosis, Nottingham and Eric Naylor FCR, TE, Principal of the Bradford School of Radiography together with assistance from Stewart Whitley FCR, HDCR, TDCR, District Radiographer at the Blackpool Victoria Hospital and Dr E.J. Roebuck MB, BS DMRD, FRCR. Consultant Radiologist at the University Hospital, Nottingham. Eric Naylor, in November 1986, was the first person to be awarded the College of Radiographers Silver medal for outstanding services to Radiography.

# 1

# INTRODUCTION

## CONTENTS

# 1 Introduction

## General Information

This book is dedicated to special imaging procedures, using different imaging modalities, and contrast media studies which feature in the modern imaging department alongside established plain film radiography examinations which are described in the 11th edition of Clark's *Positioning in Radiography*. Both conventional and cross-sectional imaging are represented as well as reference to the use of computers in post data image reconstruction and image manipulation.

The type of imaging modality selected either for static or dynamic imaging is based on the ability of the system to provide optimum diagnostic information for the disease process under investigation. The modalities will include ultrasound, computed tomography (CT), magnetic resonance imaging (MRI), radionuclide imaging (RNI) and conventional radiography or fluorographic equipment.

Chapter 1, by way of introduction, describes patient and equipment positioning terminology as well as focusing on important parameters which affect image production and image quality for each of the imaging modalities mentioned in the book. This chapter also provides a broad overview to patient preparation and after-care, including equipment and safety considerations, for many of the procedures described. Chapter 2 is dedicated to contrast enhancement agents and radiopharmaceuticals. Chapters 3–11 are dedicated to a separate anatomical system, while Chapter 12 brings together various miscellaneous procedures.

Imaging procedures are described using standard subheadings; however it is important to note that the description given may vary from hospital to hospital in terms of the imaging parameters and contrast media recommended, equipment used, individual radiologists' preferences and the patient's condition, and therefore such information quoted in the text is meant only as a guide. For MRI, the imaging parameters quoted, except where otherwise indicated, are based on a 0.5 tesla system.

Rapid advances in imaging technology will also mean that some of the CT and MRI procedures described will become outdated.

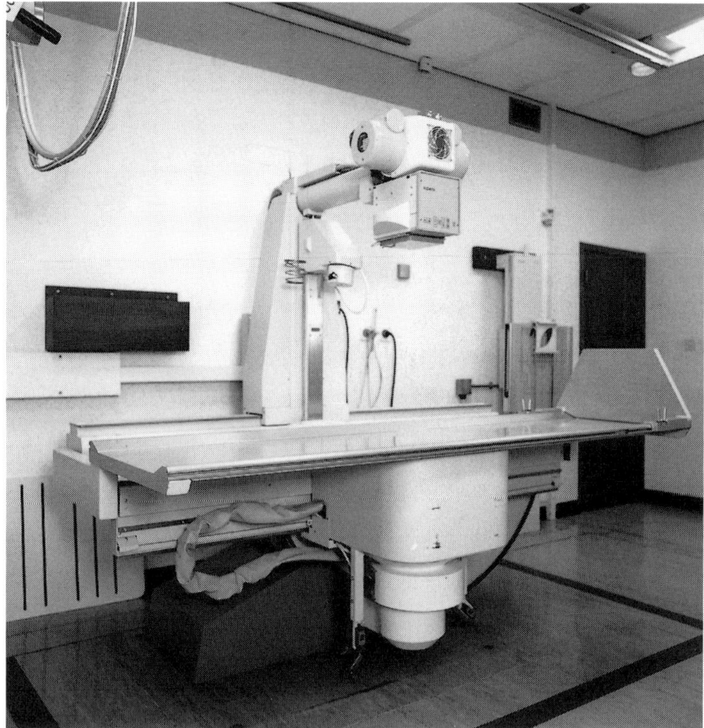

**Figure 1.1a** Remote control fluoroscopy unit

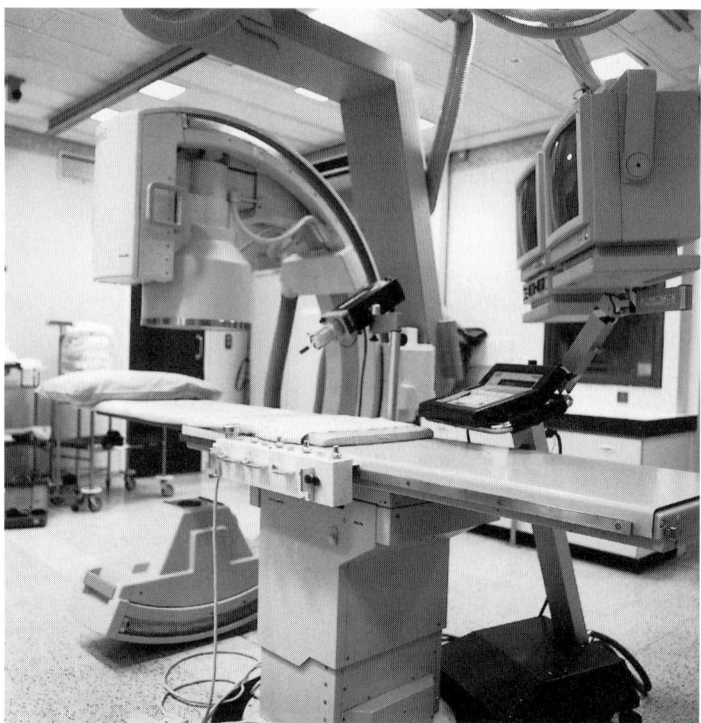

**Figure 1.1b** Angiography equipment with C-arm image intensifier

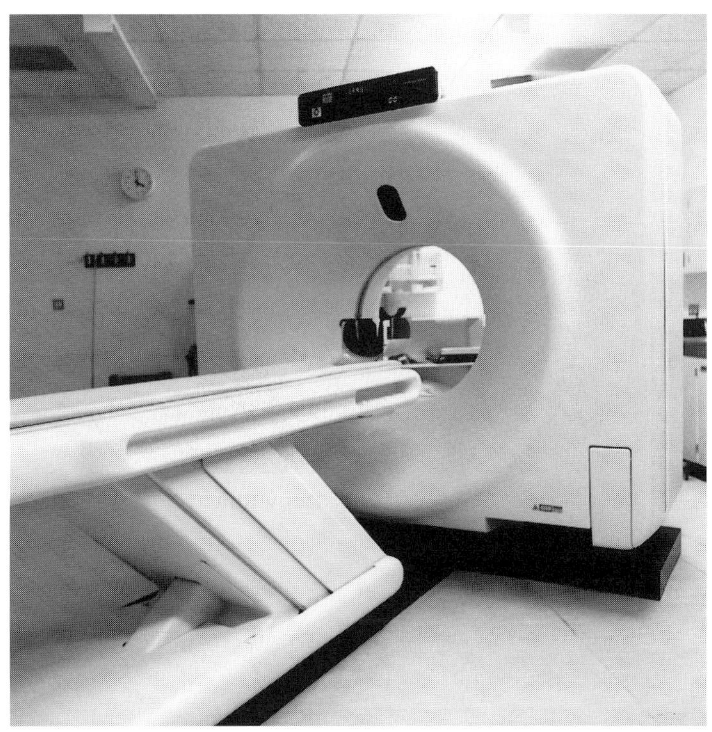
Figure 1.2a Computed tomography equipment

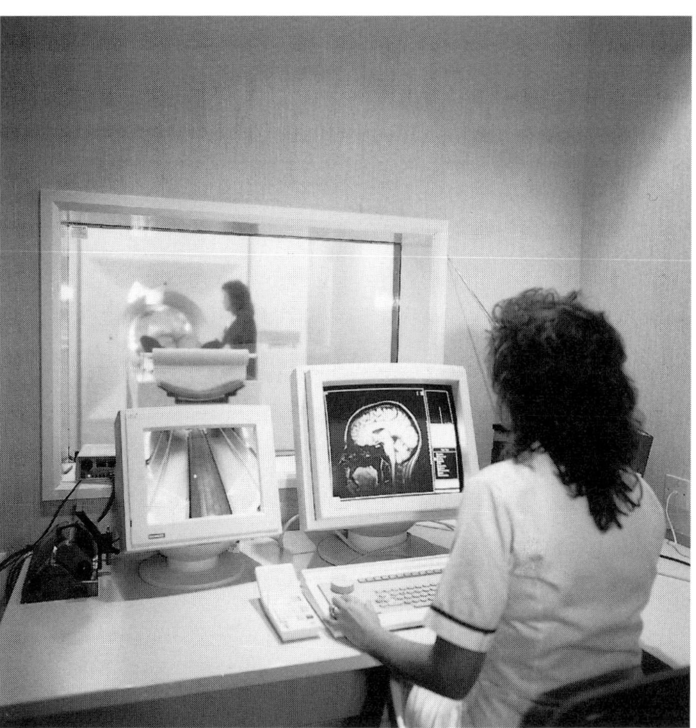
Figure 1.2c Magnetic resonance imaging equipment

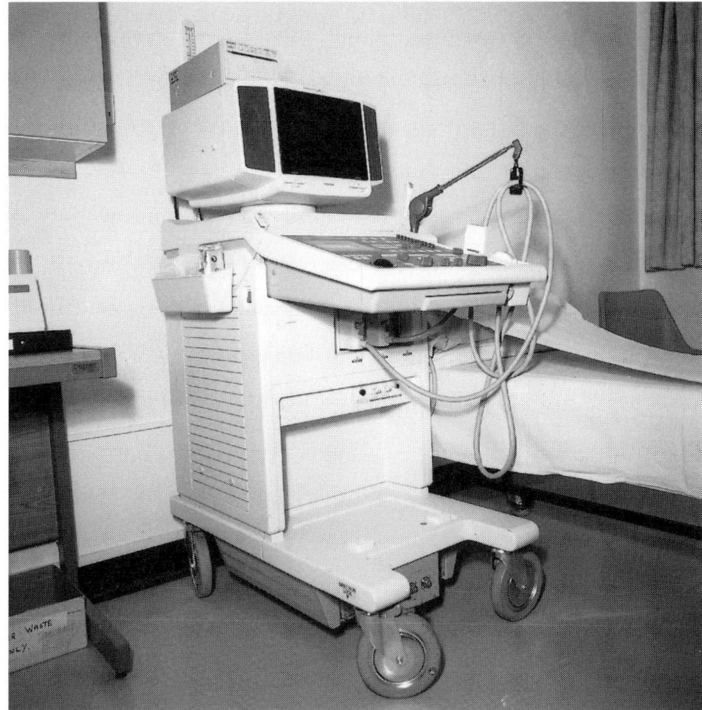
Figure 1.2b Ultrasound unit

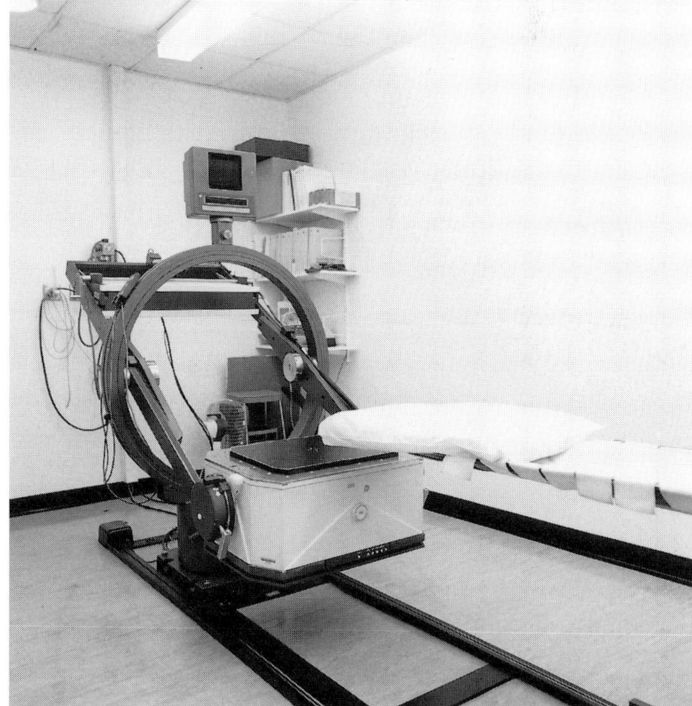
Figure 1.2d Radionuclide imaging equipment

# Introduction

## Anatomical Terminology

### Patient aspect

The anterior aspect is that observed when viewing the patient from the front, while the posterior aspect is that seen when viewing the patient from the back. The lateral aspect refers to the view of the patient from the side. Cranial describes towards the head and caudal describes towards the feet.

### Planes of the body

Three planes, known collectively as the orthogonal planes, divide the body into anatomical sections and are used to describe which aspect of the body anatomy is being imaged and viewed. These planes are mutually at right angles to each other and are known as the sagittal, coronal and transverse planes.

The **median sagittal plane** is a plane which divides the body into right and left halves. Planes parallel to this plane are known as sagittal or parasagittal planes.

A **coronal plane** divides the body into an anterior and posterior part.

A **transverse plane** (transaxial plane) divides the body into a superior and an inferior part.

**Oblique planes** or compound oblique planes lying at different angles relative to the median sagittal, coronal and transverse planes are employed to show a body structure at a different and more useful perspective. Oblique planes may be acquired directly, e.g. using ultrasound or reconstructed from image data as part of a post data processing package which allows the operator to freely demonstrate any plane relative to the orthogonal planes.

#### Organ planes

Organs which are the subject of routine investigations, such as the heart and kidneys, are in fixed positions relative to the orthogonal planes and can be described as having **short-axis** and **long-axis planes** which are at right angles to each other. Images may therefore be described as being acquired relative to either the long axis or short axis of the organ. For example, for the heart, ultrasound images may be acquired parallel to the vertical or horizontal component of the long axis of the heart.

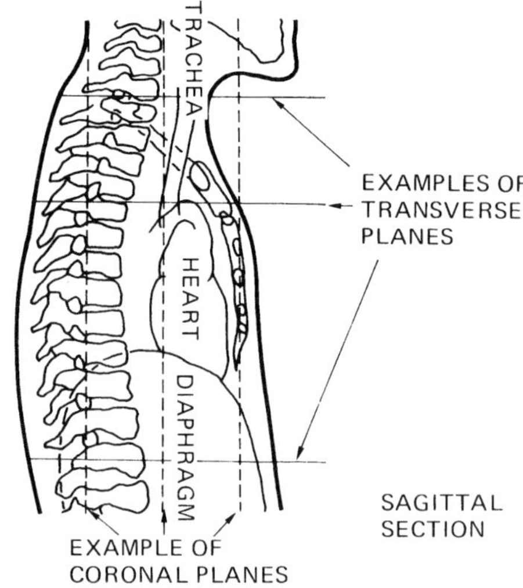


**Figure 1.3a** Sagittal section through the thorax

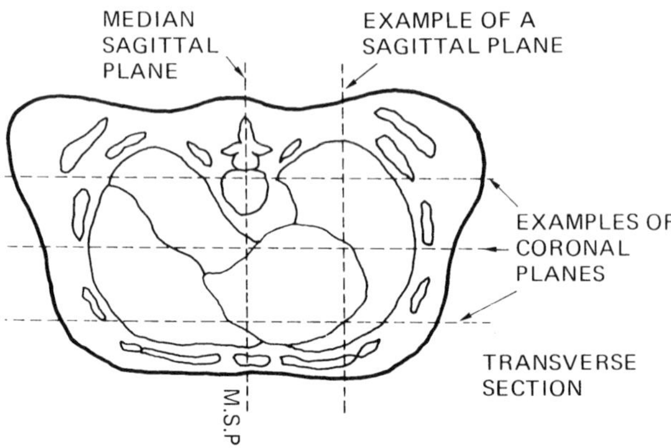


**Figure 1.3b** Transverse section through the thorax

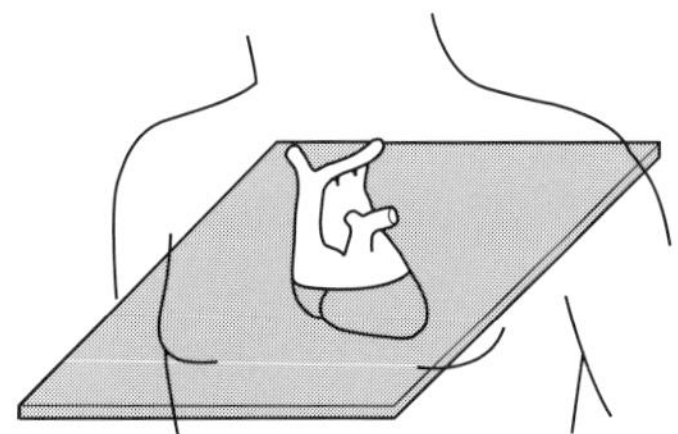

**Figure 1.4a** Transaxial plane shown through the heart

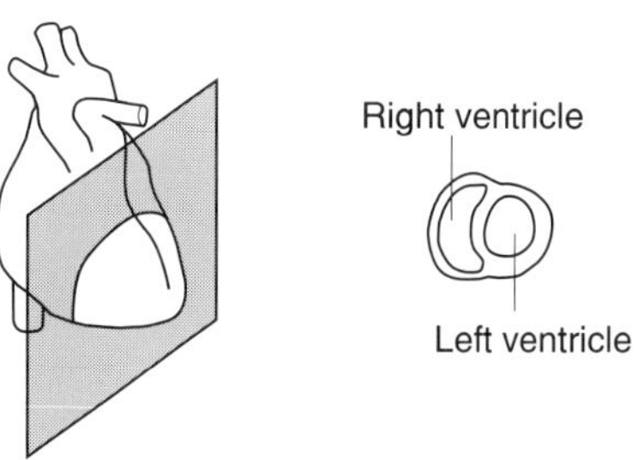


**Figure 1.4d** Short-axis plane of the heart

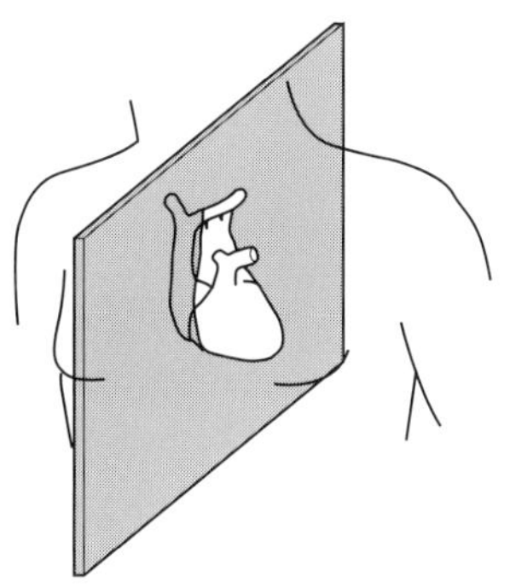

**Figure 1.4b** Sagittal plane shown through the heart

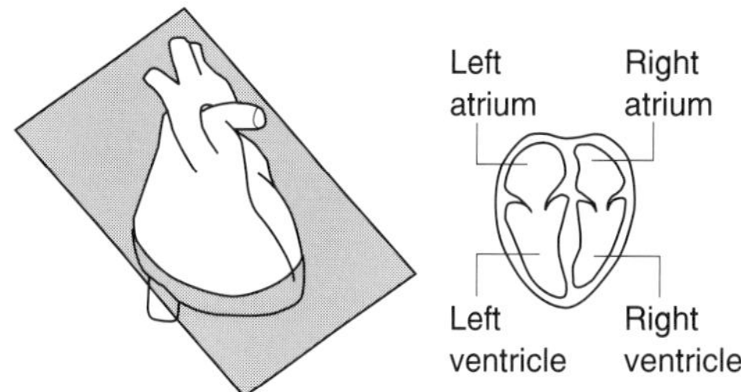


**Figure 1.4e** Long-axis (horizontal) plane of the heart

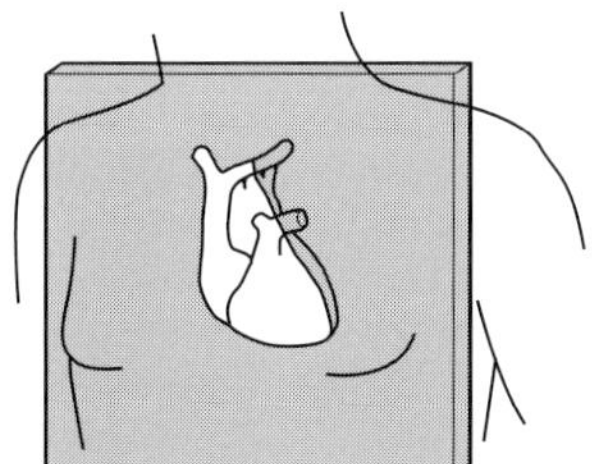

**Figure 1.4c** Coronal plane shown through the heart

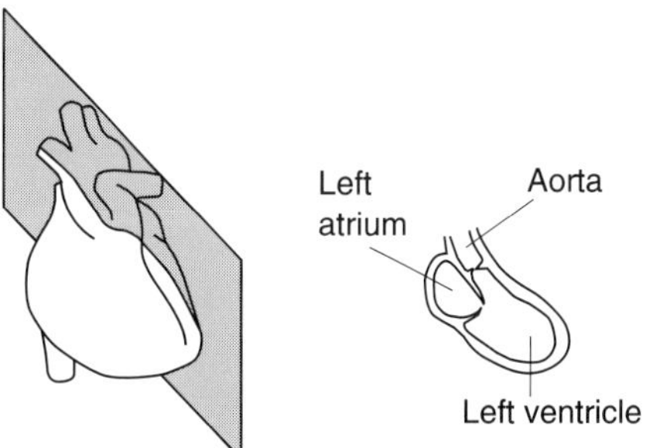


**Figure 1.4f** Long-axis (vertical) plane of the heart

# 1 Introduction

## Anatomical Terminology

### The skull

For imaging procedures of the skull, terminology adopted by the Commission of Neuroradiology of Milan (1961) is used.

**Landmarks**

**Outer canthus of the eye** indicates where the upper and lower eyelids meet laterally.

**Infra-orbital point** describes the lowest point on the inferior orbital margin.

**Nasion** describes the frontonasal articulation.

**Glabella** is the bony prominence just above the nasion.

**Vertex** describes the highest point of the skull in the median sagittal plane.

**External occipital protuberance (inion)** is the bony protuberance on the occipital bone.

**External auditory meatus** is the opening into the external auditory canal.

**Lines**

The **interorbital (interpupillary) line** extends between the centre of the two orbits (or the centre of the two pupils) and is at right angles to the median sagittal plane.

The **infra-orbital line** joins the two infra-orbital points.

Two baselines in general use which meet at an angle of 10°:

- The **anthropological baseline** (ABL) extends from the infra-orbital margin to the upper border of the external auditory meatus.
- The **orbitomeatal baseline** (OMBL) extends from the outer canthus of the eye to the central point of the external auditory meatus (EAM) and is often known as the *radiographic baseline*. This line is about 10° to the anthropological baseline.

The **auricular line** crosses the anthropological line at right angles and passes through the external auditory meatus.

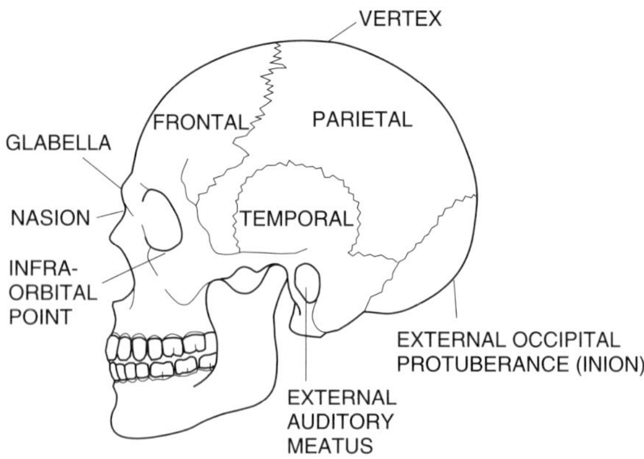


**Figure 1.5a** Lateral aspect of skull demonstrating major landmarks

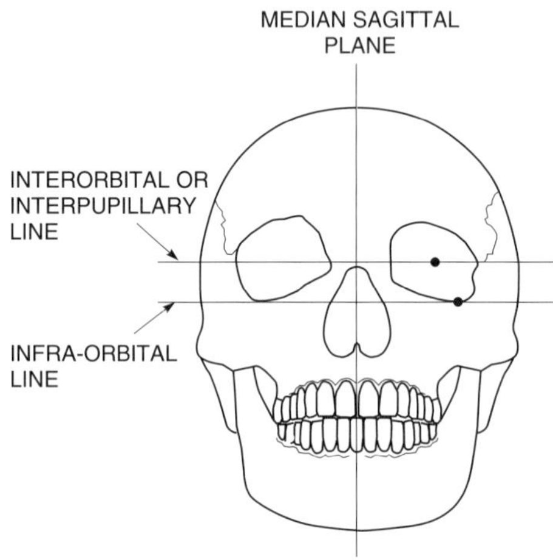


**Figure 1.5b** Frontal aspect of skull showing major lines

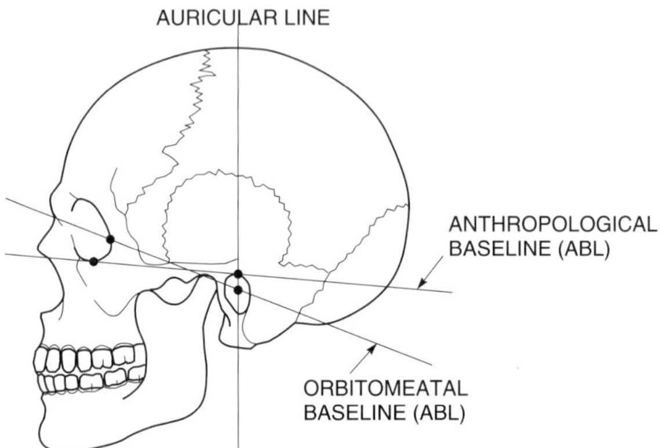


**Figure 1.5c** Lateral aspect of skull showing major lines

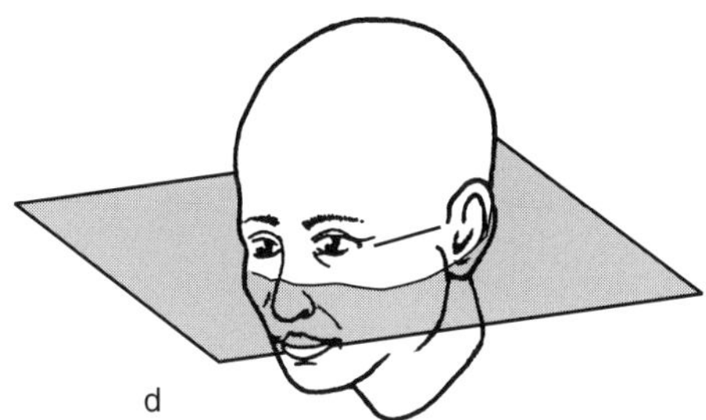

**Figure 1.6** (a) Median sagittal plane, (b) Coronal plane, (c) Anthropological plane, (d) Orbitomeatal plane

**Planes**

The **median sagittal plane** divides the skull into right and left halves.

The **anthropological plane** is a horizontal plane containing the two anthropological baselines and the infra-orbital line. Transaxial images of the skull are parallel to this plane.

The **orbitomeatal plane** contains the two orbitomeatal basal lines and is at an angle of 10° to the anthropological plane.

The **coronal planes** are at right angles to the median sagittal plane and divide the skull into anterior and posterior parts.

The **auricular plane** is perpendicular to the anthropological plane and passes through the centre of the two external auditory meati and corresponds to one of the coronal planes.

The median sagittal, anthropological and coronal planes are mutually at right angles.

# 1 Introduction

## Projection and Cross-sectional Imaging

### Projection terminology

In conventional radiography an 'X-ray image' or 'radiographic projection' is obtained of structures within the body. This is a result of the projection of those structures by the X-ray beam onto film or other image receptor, e.g. image intensifier. The shape or form of each structure recorded is dependent on the relationship of the structure relative to the central X-ray beam and the image receptor.

A true representation of a structure is produced if its long axis is parallel to the image receptor, with the central ray also at right angles to the long axis. The appearance will therefore vary as the angle of the central ray and the planes of the body are modified.

As the body is a three-dimensional structure, the resultant two-dimensional image is made up of many superimposed structures within the X-ray beam.

**Anteroposterior (AP)** indicates that the central ray is incident on the anterior aspect, passes through a transverse plane and along or parallel to the median sagittal plane and emerges from the posterior aspect.

**Postero-anterior (PA)** indicates that the central ray is incident on the posterior aspect, passes through a transverse plane and along or parallel to the median sagittal plane and emerges from the anterior aspect.

**Lateral** indicates that the central ray passes from one side of the body to the other along a coronal and a transverse plane. A projection is called a right lateral if the central ray passes from the left side to the right side and a left lateral if the central ray passes from the right to the left side.

These projections can be modified by directing the central ray at an angle to a transverse plane, i.e. either caudal or cranial (cephalic) angulation.

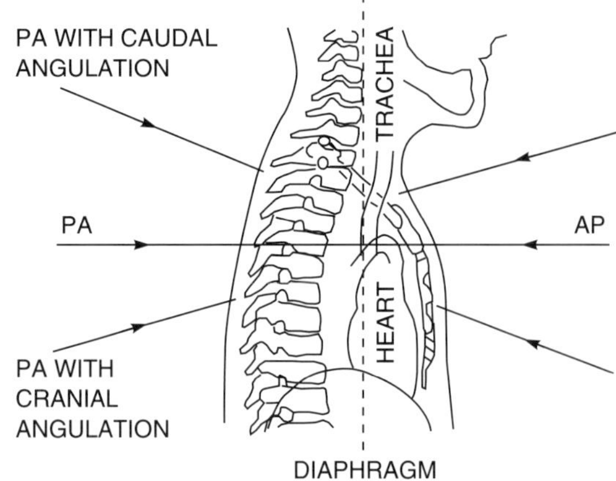


**Figure 1.7b** Anterior and posterior projections

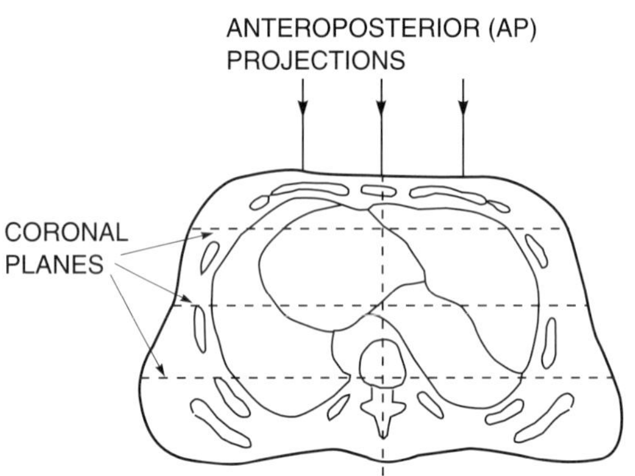


**Figure 1.7c** Anteroposterior projection

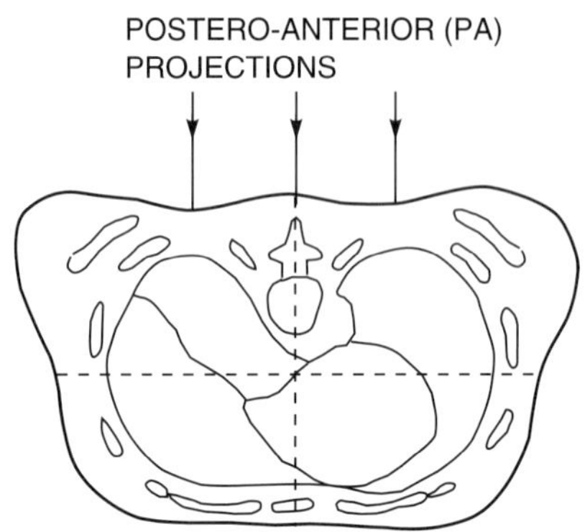


**Figure 1.7d** Postero-anterior projection

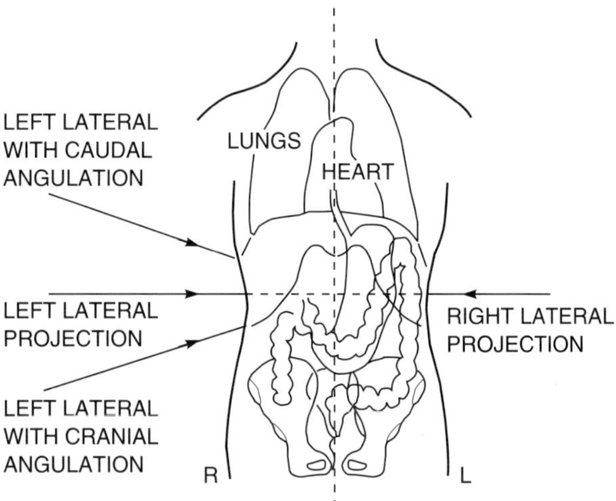


 **Figure 1.7a** Lateral projections

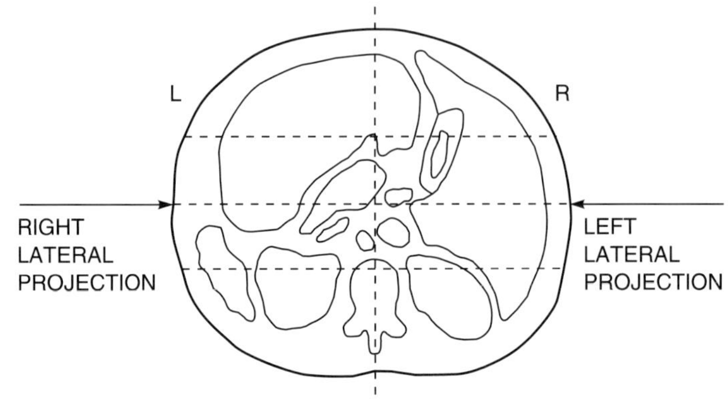


**Figure 1.7e** Right and left lateral projections

## Projection and Cross-sectional Imaging

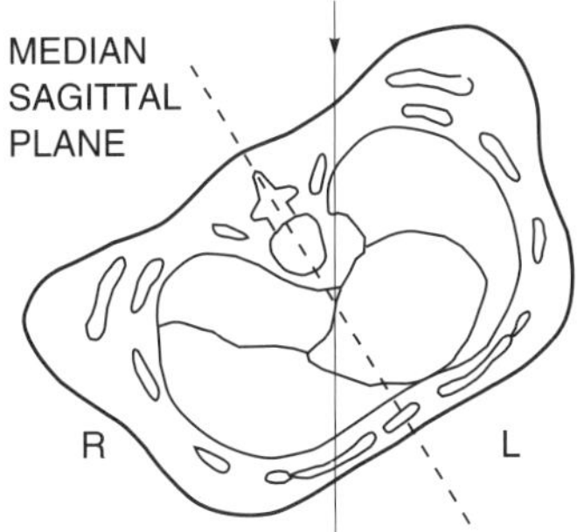


**Figure 1.8a** Right anterior oblique

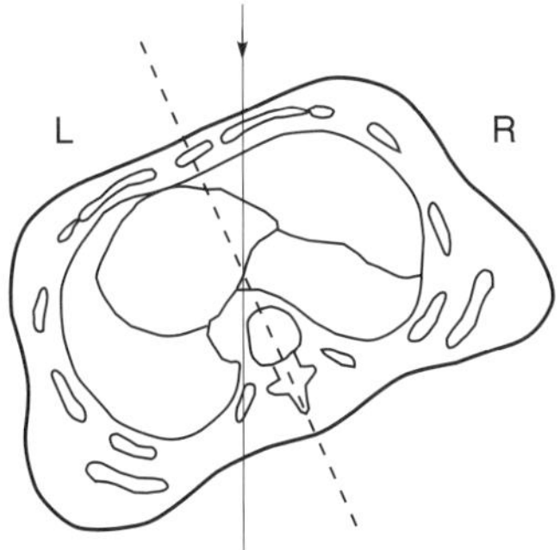


**Figure 1.8b** Left posterior oblique

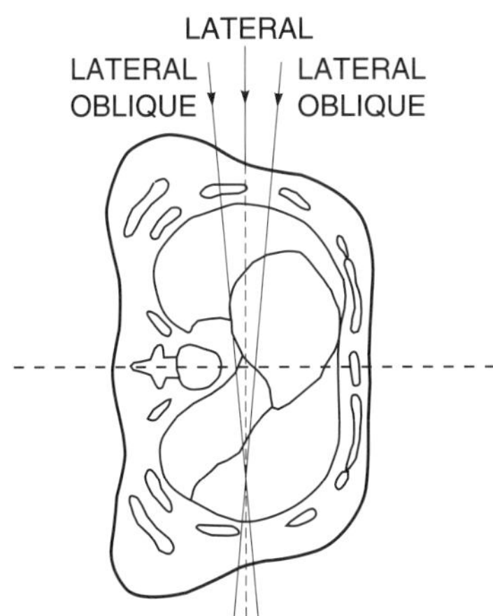


**Figure 1.8c** Lateral obliques

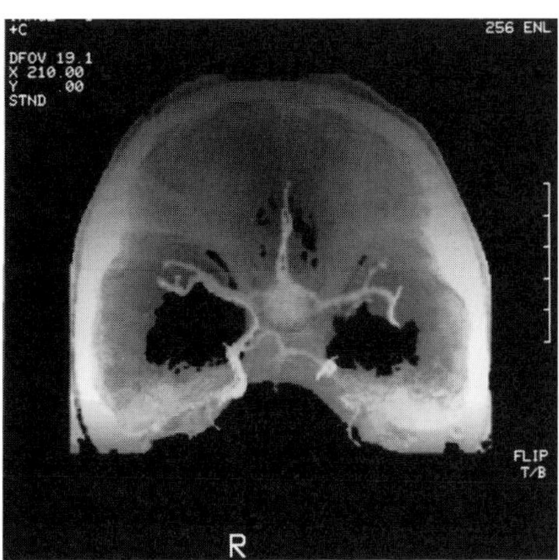


**Figure 1.8d** Three-dimensional CT image showing circle of Willis and pituitary tumour

**Oblique projections**

Oblique projections are taken with the central ray passing through the body along a transverse plane at a specific angle between the median sagittal and coronal planes. For this projection the patient is usually positioned with the median sagittal plane at a specific angle between 0° and 90° to the film and the central ray at right angles to the film or image intensifier. If the patient is positioned with the median sagittal plane at right angles to or parallel to the film or image intensifier, the projection is obtained by directing the central ray at a specific angle to the median sagittal plane.

**Anterior oblique** indicates that the central ray enters the posterior aspect, passes along a transverse plane at a specific angle to the median sagittal plane and emerges from the anterior aspect.

With the patient prone and the median sagittal plane at right angles to the film, right and left anterior oblique projections are obtained by angling the central ray to the median sagittal plane.

**Posterior oblique** indicates that the central ray enters the anterior aspect, passes along a transverse plane and emerges from the posterior aspect.

**Lateral oblique** indicates that the central ray enters one lateral aspect, passes along a transverse plane at a specific angle to the coronal plane and emerges from the opposite aspect. With the coronal plane at right angles to the film or image intensifier, lateral oblique projections are obtained by angling the central ray to the coronal plane.

### Cross-sectional imaging

With the exception of conventional radiography and the majority of radionuclide imaging procedures, scans of the body can be directly acquired using MRI, CT and ultrasound which record the shape, nature and relationship of structures within a specific scan width. These images, of a chosen scan plane, will correspond to one of the orthogonal planes.

Three-dimensional imaging using MR and CT which is an optional feature on many machines facilitates post-image manipulation and manual selection of the optimum cross-sectional image in any of the body planes.

## Positioning Terminology

### The patient

This describes patient positioning for the imaging procedure. The patient may decubitus (lying down), erect (siting or standing) or semi-recumbent or rotated in the decubitus or erect position.

If **decubitus** the patient may be:

(a) Supine (dorsal decubitus) – lying on the back.
(b) Prone (ventral decubitus) – lying face down.
(c) Lateral decubitus – lying on the side. Right lateral decubitus – lying on the right side. Left lateral decubitus – lying on the left side.

The above positioning is more precisely described by reference to the appropriate orthogonal planes, e.g. transverse plane is at right angles to the imaging couch or sagittal plane is perpendicular to the gamma camera face.

When **erect** the patient may be sitting or standing with:

(a) The posterior aspect against the imaging device.
(b) The anterior aspect against the imaging device.
(c) The right or left side against the imaging device.

The above positioning is more precisely described by reference to the appropriate orthogonal planes, e.g. coronal plane parallel to the imaging couch or sagittal plane perpendicular to the gamma camera face.

When the patient is **rotated** the following stages are described:

(a) Starting position, e.g. supine or erect with posterior aspect in contact with the image intensifier.
(b) Direction of rotation, e.g. the left side is raised or the left side moved away from the image intensifier.
(c) Degree of rotation of the relative orthogonal planes, e.g. the patient is supine and then the right side raised to bring the coronal plane at an angle of 30° to the image intensifier.

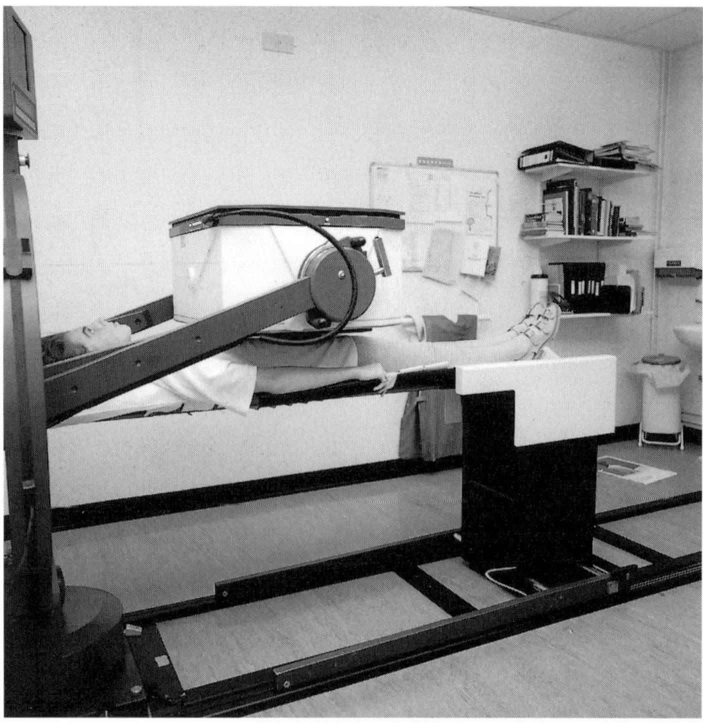

**Figure 1.9a** Supine: median sagittal plane is at right angles and coronal plane parallel to the gamma camera

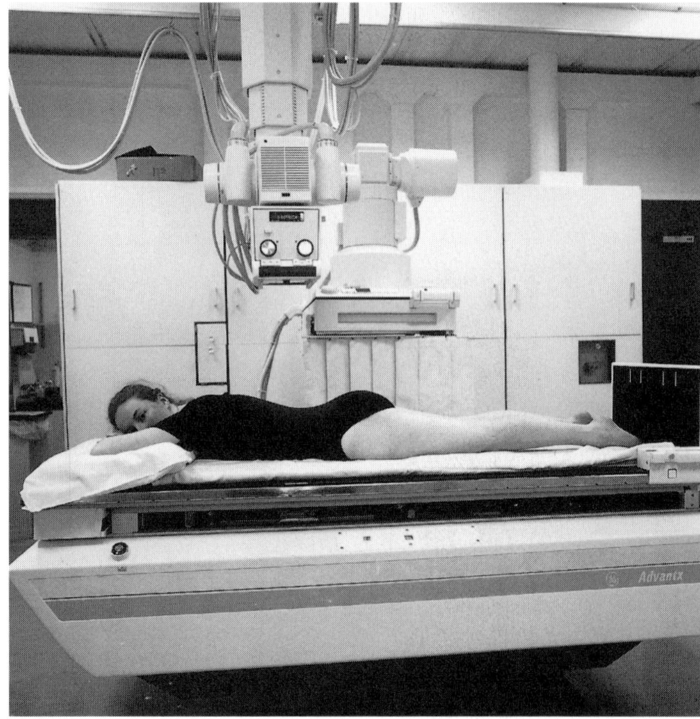


**Figure 1.9b** Prone: median sagittal plane is at right angles and coronal plane parallel to the image intensifier

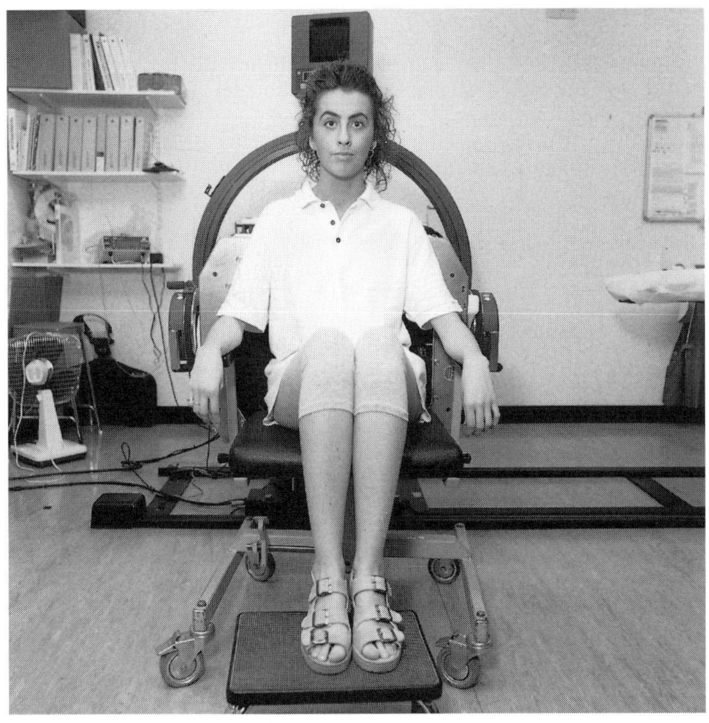

**Figure 1.10a** Erect: patient erect with the posterior aspect of the trunk against the gamma camera and coronal plane parallel to camera face

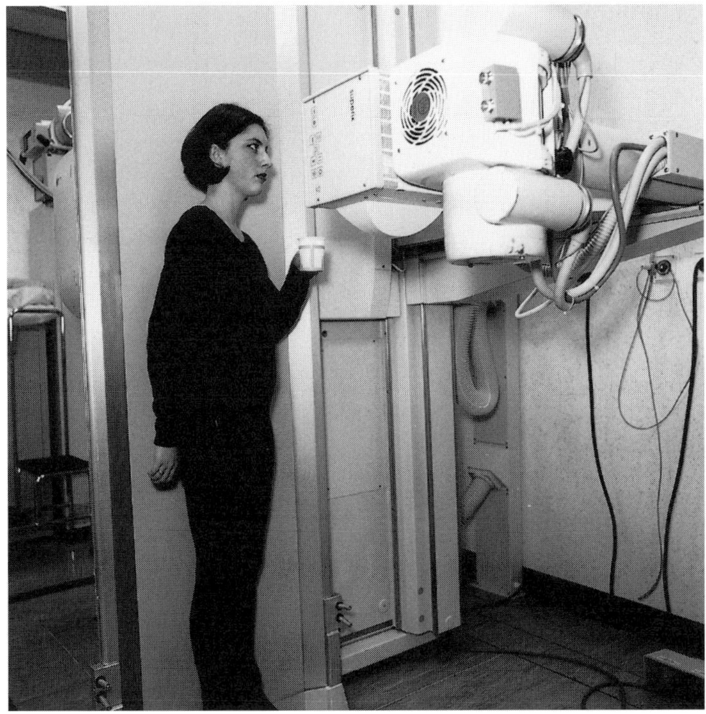

**Figure 1.10b** Left posterior oblique, intensifier posterior to table: patient stands with posterior aspect against the table top, right side raised away from the table until the median sagittal plane is at an angle of 45° to the image receptor

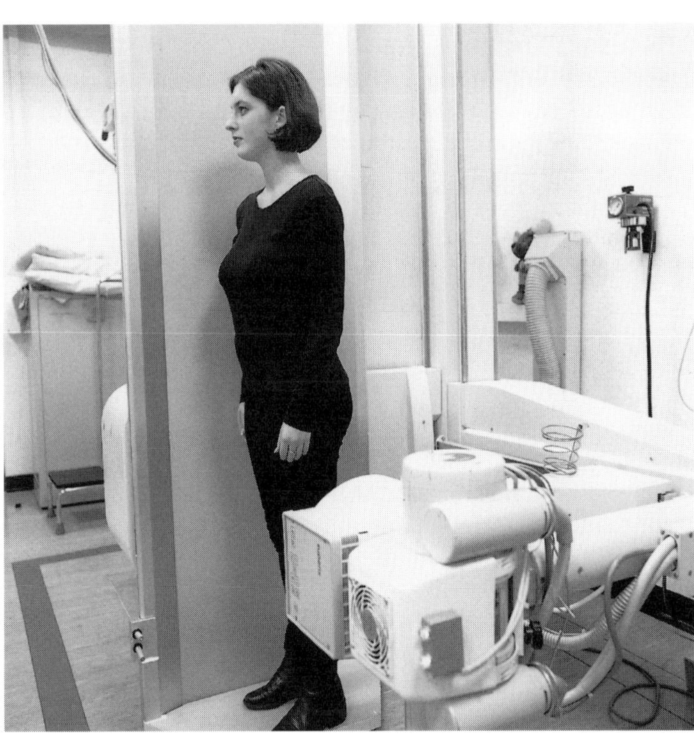

**Figure 1.10c** Lateral erect: standing with right side against the table; median sagittal plane parallel to the image intensifier and table top

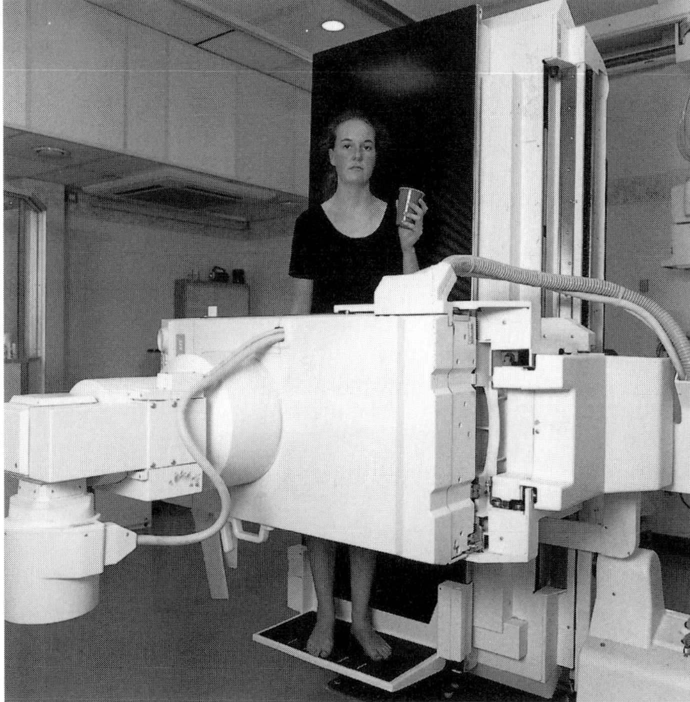

**Figure 1.10d** Right anterior oblique, intensifier anterior to table: patient stands with posterior aspect against the table top, right side raised away from the table until the median sagittal plane is at an angle of 45° to the image receptor

# 1 Introduction

## Positioning Terminology

### Imaging modality

This refers to the imaging modality being used and includes ultrasound, computed tomography (CT), magnetic resonance imaging (MRI), radionuclide imaging (RNI) and conventional or digital radiography or fluorographic equipment.

Guidance is given on how the imaging equipment is positioned and aligned relative to the patient by reference to aspects of the body and orthogonal planes.

For conventional radiography aspects of the body are referred to as **centring points**, whereas in CT and MR cross-sectional imaging these same aspects are referred to as **reference points**.

#### X-ray equipment

Description is given of the direction and centring of the X-ray beam relative to aspects and planes of the body. Reference may also be made to the position of an image intensifier input field or cassette front relative to the surface of the patient.

The central ray may be vertical or horizontal in direction. The specific degree of angulation required for certain projections is achieved by rotating the X-ray tube in either a caudal (towards the feet), cranial (towards the head) direction or across the body.

#### Computed tomography

In CT the table height and the relationship of the gantry, containing the X-ray tube and image receptor system, relative to the patient is described. For initial scan projection radiographs the length of couch travel is quoted. For cross-sectional images the section width and table increments are given.

#### Magnetic resonance imaging

For MRI, the position of the anatomical part and the receiving coil selected relative to the isocentre of the magnet is described.

The normal routine will involve positioning the anatomical part to the receiving coil selected which is then moved to the isocentre of the magnet.

Localiser images are quoted from which the scan series are prescribed. Examples are given of imaging parameters and preferred anatomical planes.

The acquisition plane and location of images are controlled electronically.

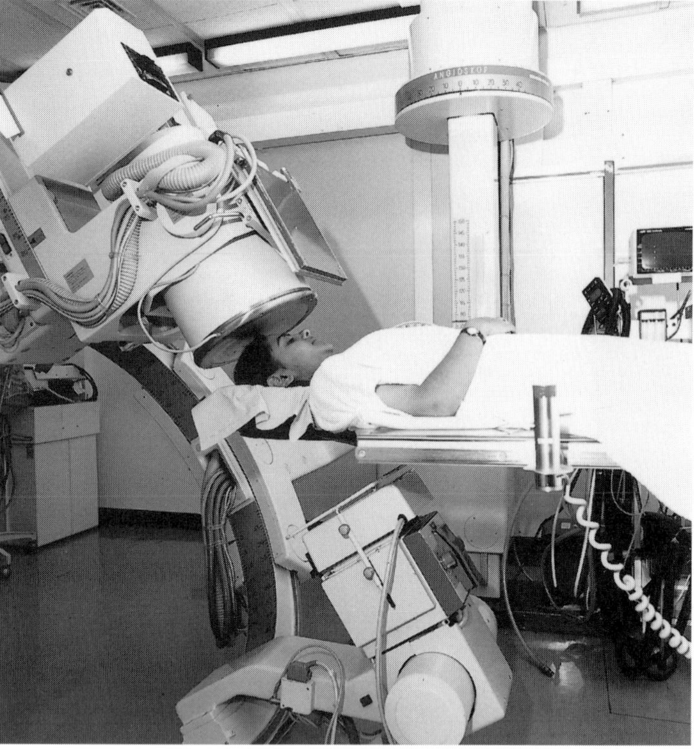

**Figure 1.11a** Cerebral angiography – occipitofrontal 30° cephalad. The central ray is angled cranially so that it makes an angle of 30° to the anthropological plane

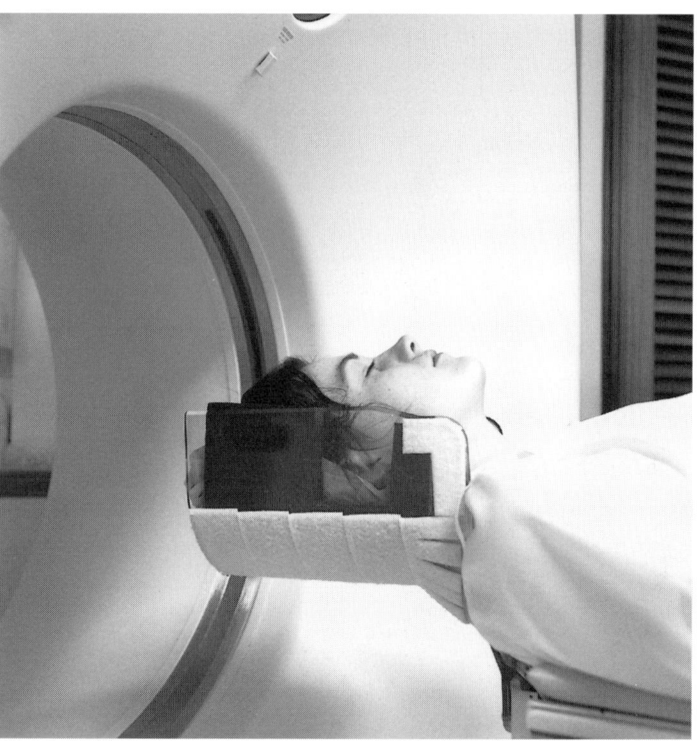

**Figure 1.11b** Computed tomography – standard brain protocol. The orbitomeatal baseline is parallel to and the median sagittal plane perpendicular to the scan plane

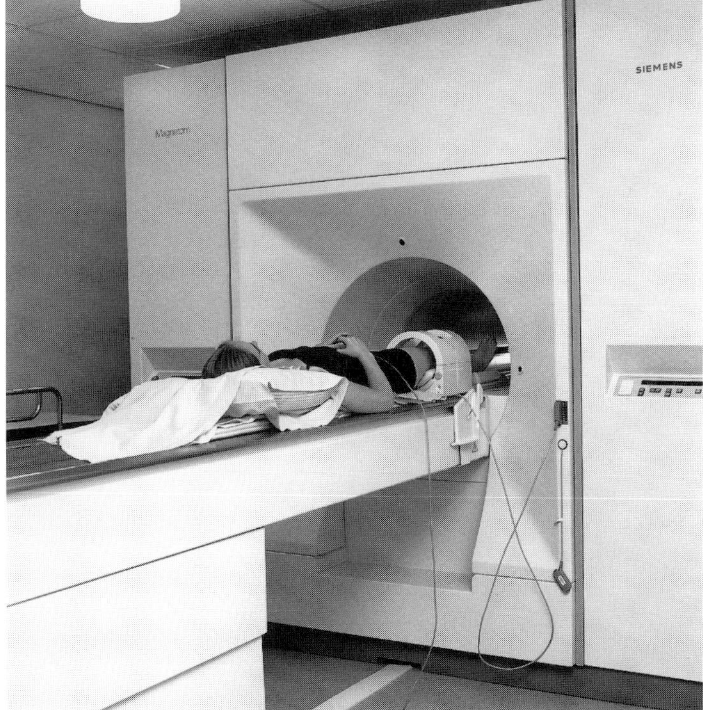


**Figure 1.12a** Magnetic resonance imaging of the knee. Patient lies supine with knee joint positioned in the centre of the receiver coil. The centre of the coil is aligned to the external reference point

### Ultrasound

In ultrasound the position, direction and movement of the hand-held transducer (probe) relative to the body is described. Techniques are also described using endorectal and endovaginal transducers.

### Radionuclide imaging

For RNI, the position of the gamma camera face relative to the patient is described.

The gamma camera may be used in different positions around the imaging couch, or with the face vertical for the patient to sit or stand against.

In SPECT imaging, the gamma camera will be rotated in a circular or elliptical movement around the couch. In some instances cameras can only perform circular movements, but can generate elliptical tomography as the result of controlled side-to-side movement of the couch. This is known as profile body contouring.

Total body scanning is performed by controlled longitudinal movement of the couch or gamma camera.

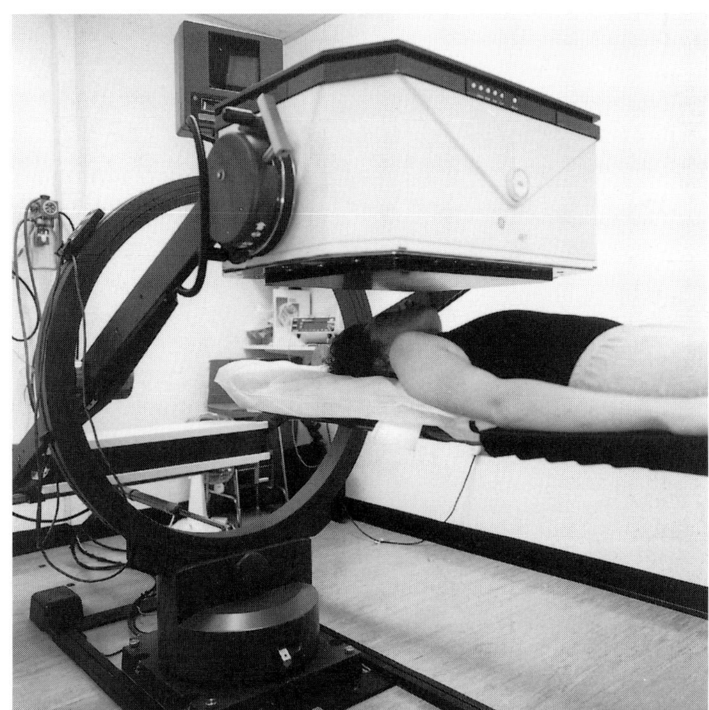

**Figure 1.12b** Radionuclide imaging – cerebral blood flow using SPECT. The gamma camera is position for the initial 360° circular tomogram of the brain

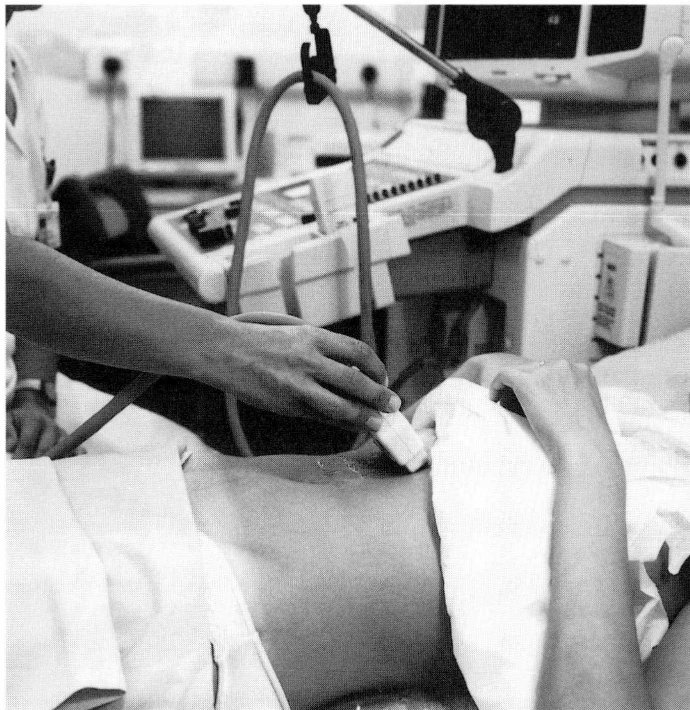

**Figure 1.12c** Ultrasound of the pancreas. The transducer is held transversely, in direct contact with the skin surface, and angled to produce a long-axis view of the pancreas

# 1 Introduction

## Alignment and Orientation

### Imaging modality

**Conventional radiography**
Positioning the patient and the film/screen combination or image intensifier system using overcouch radiography is assisted by the use of the light beam diaphragm attached to the X-ray tube. This is used also to restrict the radiation field to the size required. Using specialised angiographic equipment the angulation of the C-arm relative to the patient is displayed numerically either on the equipment or the television monitor.

**Computed tomography**
In CT, external alignment lights attached to the scanning gantry equipment enable the patient to be positioned to the desired anatomical reference point and also highlight the three orthogonal body planes.

The table height is adjusted to bring the patient into the centre of the scan plane by using coronal alignment light. The patient is positioned on the scanning couch so that the sagittal alignment light lies along the midline of the body. The table is adjusted until the anatomical reference point coincides with the transverse alignment light. From this point the table is then moved the fixed distance into the centre of the scan field.

The gantry angle selected will be displayed on the equipment and the television monitor.

**Magnetic resonance imaging**
External alignment lights, similar to that used in CT, are attached to the magnet housing. The sagittal alignment ensures that the patient is positioned centrally on the scanning table. The patient and the appropriate receiver coil are moved until the transverse alignment light coincides with either the desired anatomical reference point or the centre of the coil. From this position the patient and coil are moved the fixed distance into the isocentre of the magnet. The table height is fixed and therefore the coronal lights are not used in positioning.

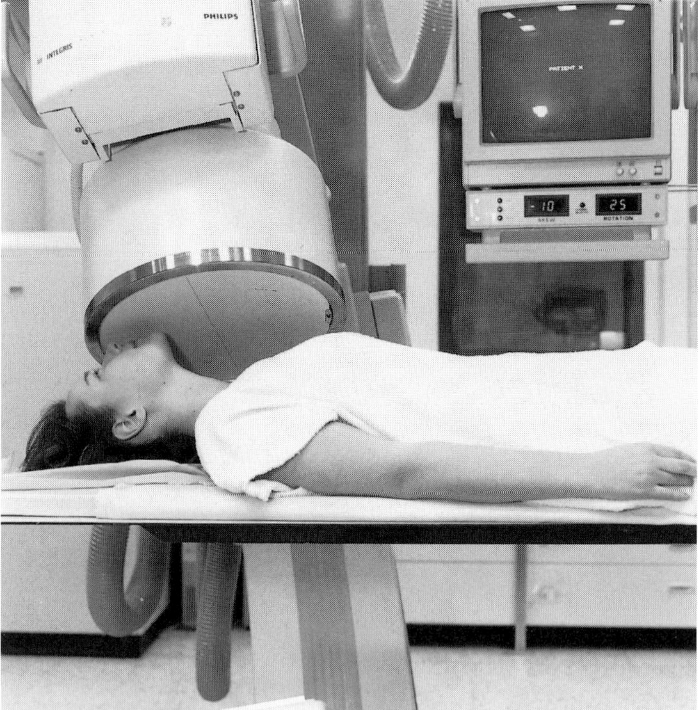


**Figure 1.13a** Angiographic C-arm system showing angulation indicator (below TV monitor)

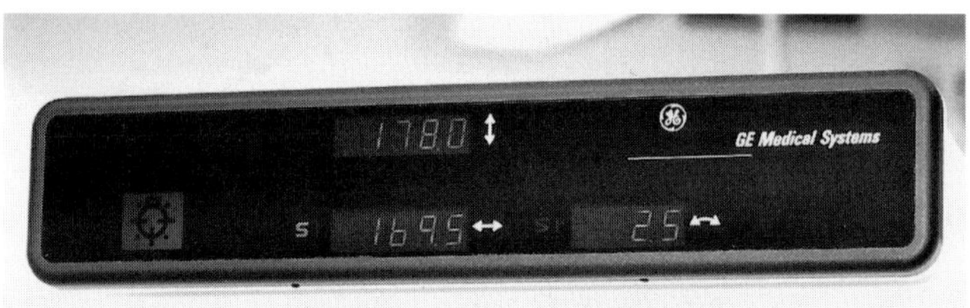


**Figure 1.13b** CT system showing gantry angulation indicator

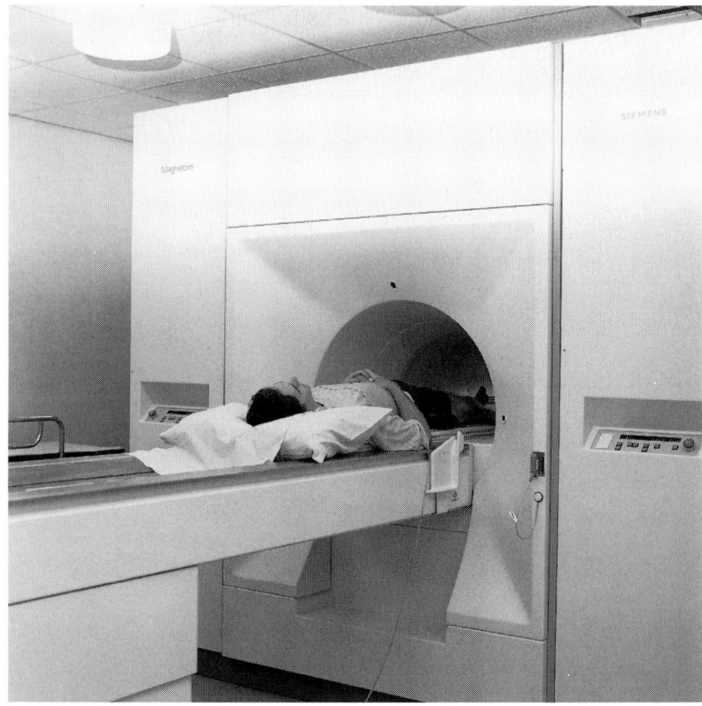

**Figure 1.13c** MR system showing alignment lights

## Alignment and Orientation

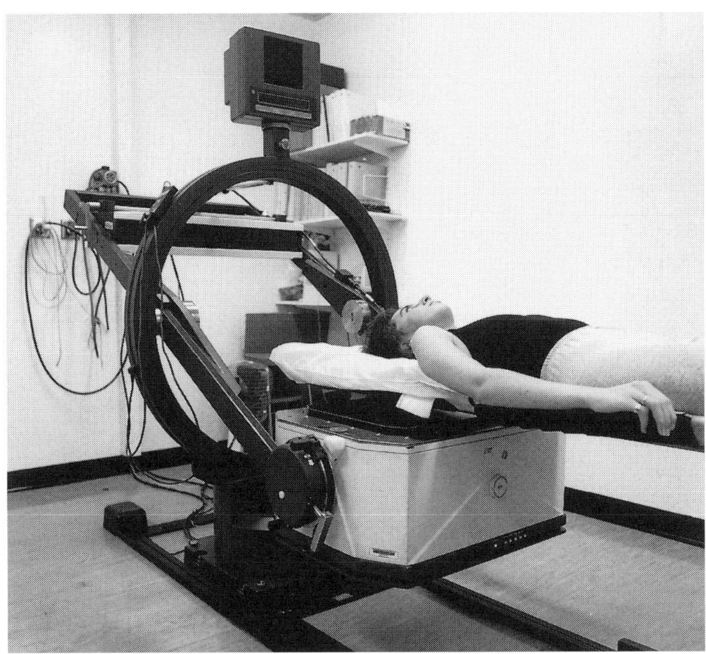

**Figure 1.14a** RNI equipment showing persistence scope attached to circular arm

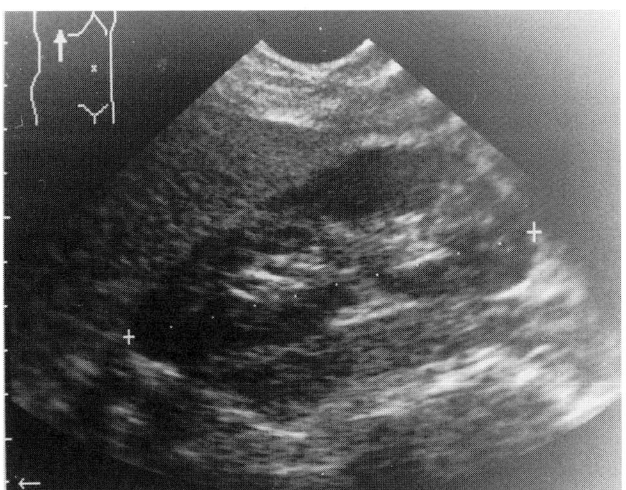

**Figure 1.14b** Ultrasound image showing body orientation marker

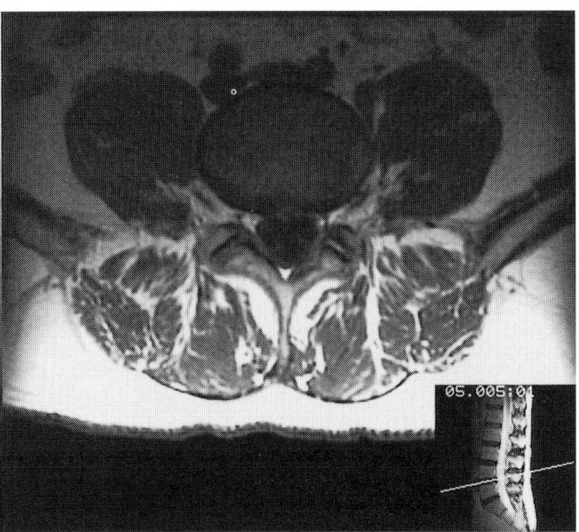

**Figure 1.14c** Transverse MR image showing inset indicating orientation of image plane selected

**Radionuclide imaging**

In RNI, positioning of the patient relative to the centre of the gamma camera is assisted by the use of a short persistence scope monitor which allows the operator to position the patient, following injection of a radionuclide, into the ideal position before data acquisition begins.

Cobalt ($^{57}$Co)-sources are used to identify the left or right side of the body. Lead surface markers such as lead strips, which absorb gamma rays, are also used to identify anatomical structures.

**Ultrasound imaging**

For ultrasound procedures the transducer (probe) is held directly against the patient's skin over the region under investigation in the desired plane. The scan plane selected, however, can be recorded on the image by selecting an appropriate orientation body marker (if available) to assist those observing the image at a future date.

### Acquisition and viewing principles

It is important that images are acquired with correct patient identification details, together with relevant body orientation information and specific details of which part of a dynamic sequence the image was taken. Each hospital will have individual standard routines for different types of procedures which must be adhered to strictly to avoid any confusion.

Orientation will include identification of the patient's right and left side, and when cross-sectional imaging is involved may include additional identification of anterior or posterior aspects of the body. When three-dimensional protocols are employed, any display of an imaging plane, e.g. oblique, coronal, sagittal or transverse, will usually be accompanied by a small image of the body part, alongside the main image, showing with the aid of a line the location and angle of the image plane relevant to the orthogonal planes.

Included on CT and MR cross-sectional images will also be details of the thickness of the scan section and the location of the scan with reference to the scan reference point from which body location imaging commenced.

Transaxial images of the head are normally viewed bottom up (inferior to superior), with the rest of the body viewed top to bottom (superior to inferior).

# 1 Introduction

## The Digital Image

In conventional radiography the information held in the emergent X-ray beam is recorded on X-ray film as a continuous range of densities. Similarly, in conventional fluoroscopy a dynamic image derived from an analogue signal is displayed on a television monitor (cathode ray tube).

Each of these processes fails to display much of the information available, since the recorded image cannot display the entire range of absorption values as a single grey scale nor can the human eye distinguish between subtle differences. Neither process offers the opportunity for manipulation of the image once it has been recorded.

Digital imaging systems use electronic methods to record and store information. This information is recorded in the form of 'bits' (binary digits). These bits are electrical signals which have only one of two possible values (zero or one).

Digital radiography uses storage phosphors to record information in the emergent X-ray beam. This information can later be retrieved and processed using a photomultiplier and analogue-to-digital converter to produce binary values for each point on the screen.

In each of the other modalities which use digital imaging the values recorded represent the different characteristics which produce the image. For example, in digital fluoroscopy the recorded value represents X-ray intensity, in ultrasound the strength of the reflected wave reaching the transducer, and in MRI the strength of the signal detected by the radiofrequency coils.

### Image matrix, pixels and voxels

The digital image itself is recorded and displayed as a matrix made up of many individual picture elements or **pixels**. In practice each pixel represents a given volume element or **voxel** in a patient (see Figure 1.15b).

Each pixel or voxel will have a value assigned to it which is proportional to the signal produced by the imaging process.

The resolution of the image depends on the number of pixels within the matrix. High-resolution images are typically 1024 × 1024 pixels, while 256 × 256 and 512 × 512 combinations are also available. Greater computer storage is demanded with the 1024 × 1024 matrix size.

### Image manipulation

Digital images can be manipulated and displayed in a variety of ways to provide access to all the information received by the detector (e.g. subtraction or edge enhancement). Pixels which are made up of 12 bits can have any value between 0 and 4096 ($2^{12}$). Since the human eye can only differentiate a limited number of shades of grey, a 'look-up' table is used to map each pixel value to one of 256 shades of grey.

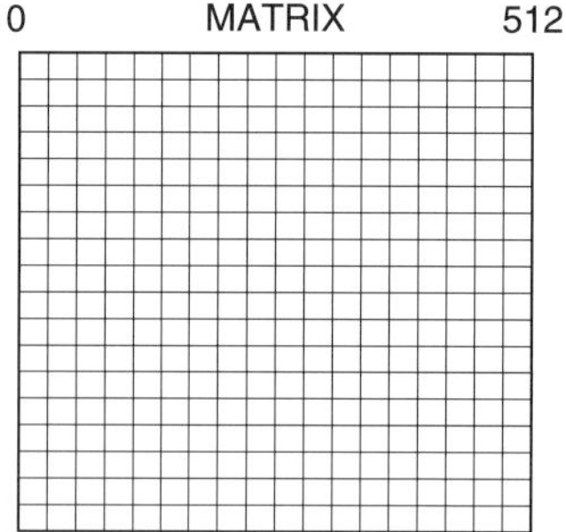


**Figure 1.15a** Example of 512 × 512 matrix containing 262 144 pixels

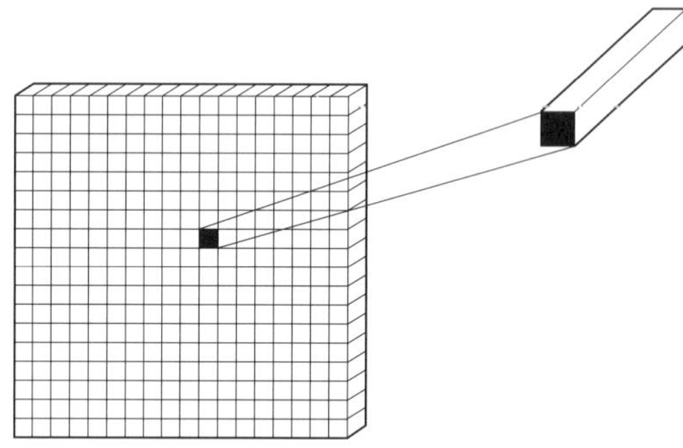

**Figure 1.15b** Matrix showing volume element 'voxel'

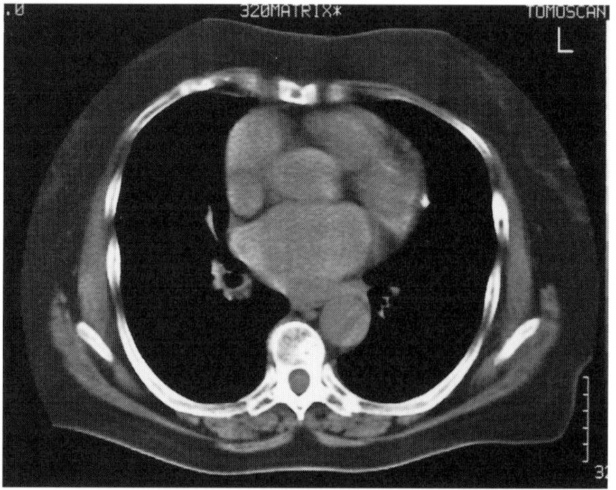


**Figure 1.15c** CT image of thorax – 320 matrix

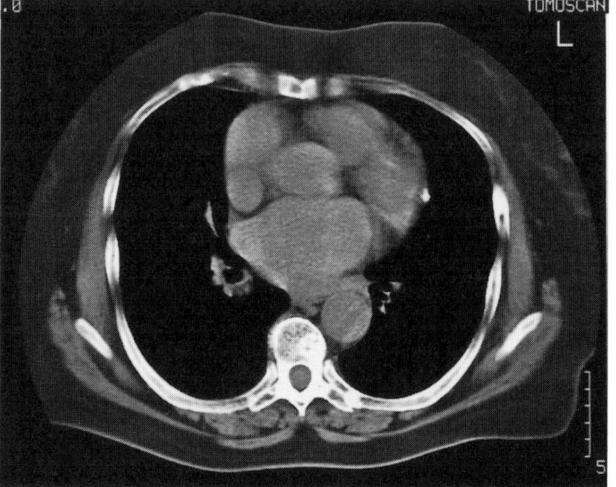


**Figure 1.15d** CT image of thorax – 512 matrix

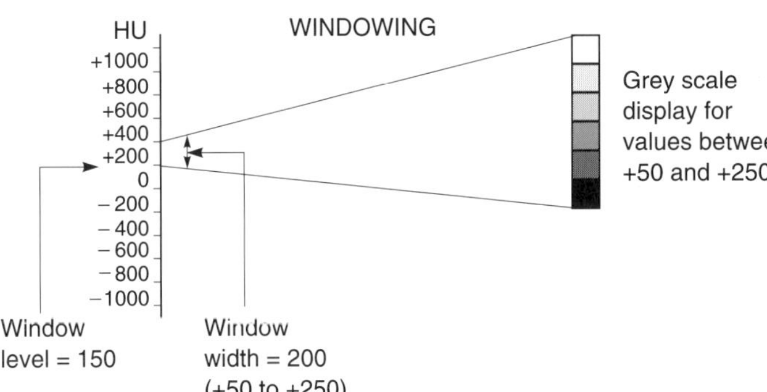


**Figure 1.16a** Windowing principle

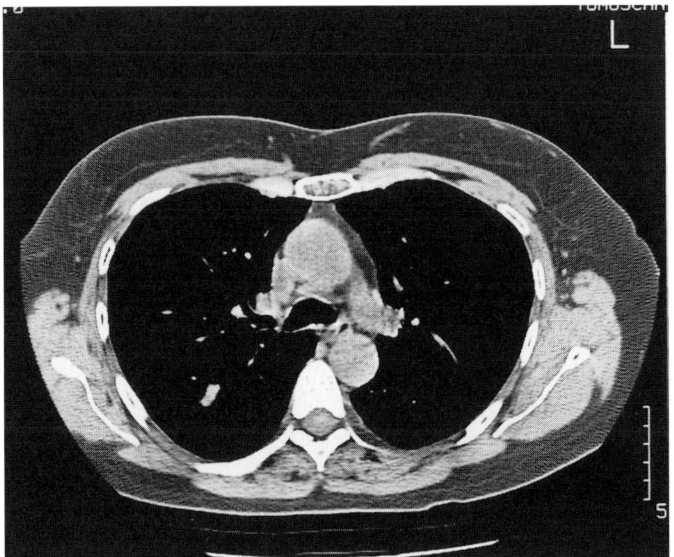


**Figure 1.16b** CT image of thorax at soft tissue setting

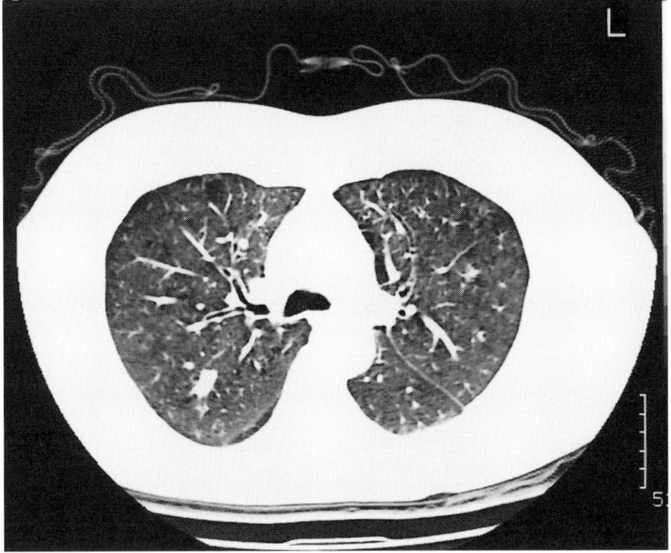


**Figure 1.16c** CT image of thorax at lung tissue setting

## Windowing

Since the digital image has a much greater dynamic range a technique known as windowing is used on the image display. A selected range of densities, rather than the whole image, is viewed. The range and the display contrast can be varied using window width and window level controls.

In some equipment, such as that used in digital fluoroscopy, window values are preset to optimum values by the manufacturer within given organ programmes.

## Window width

Window width is used to select a range of absorption values which are displayed as a grey scale, e.g. 200 units (see Figure 1.16a). Attenuation values below this range will appear as black, whereas attenuation values above this range will appear as white.

## Window level

Window level is used to select the centre point of the window. For example, Figure 1.16a shows a window level of 150 and a window width of 200. This would result in values between +50 and +250 as a grey scale. Values less than 50 appear as black and values greater than 250 as white.

The values selected depend on the type of examination and suspected pathology.

## Image viewing

The resultant image may be viewed in either positive or negative modes.

Subtraction can easily be carried out on digital images by superimposing positive and negative mode images. Electronic subtraction of the two images results in the display of information which appeared in only one of the images (e.g. contrast media).

## Applications

Computed tomography and MRI rely on digitisation to produce the image. Dedicated digital fluoroscopy and digital subtraction angiography equipment are now commonplace. Similarly ultrasound and RNI equipment employ digital techniques in image processing and reconstruction.

With improvements in resolution, digital radiography systems are now increasingly replacing conventional film/screen systems.

Images generated digitally may be stored in digital format or selectively downloaded to hard copy using a laser imager.

## Computed Tomography

Since the introduction of CT in 1972 major developments have occurred in gantry design and computing power, resulting in improvements in both image acquisition times and data processing.

The first two designs or 'generations' of CT scanners used an X-ray tube with a narrow fan-shaped X-ray beam with a number of detectors mounted opposite. This was mounted on a gantry which moved around the patient in a translate–rotate movement. Both generations required relatively long scan times, typically 20 s to 4 min. Third-generation machines usc a rotatc–rotate principle, using an arc of detectors coupled to an X-ray tube. The whole system rotates through 360° around the patient. This has reduced scan times to 1–3 s.

Fourth-generation scanners use a circular array of detectors and an X-ray tube rotating within the array.

Spiral scanning (helical) is the latest development in CT which enables rapid acquisition of data with the patient travelling through a continuously rotating beam of X-rays, effectively giving a volume scan. Typically a patient/table travel of 30 cm can be imaged in 20 s. The data can be reconstructed to produce high-resolution narrow sections with image overlap.

All gantries have the facility for cranial and caudal angulation. Detection systems are either gas or solid state.

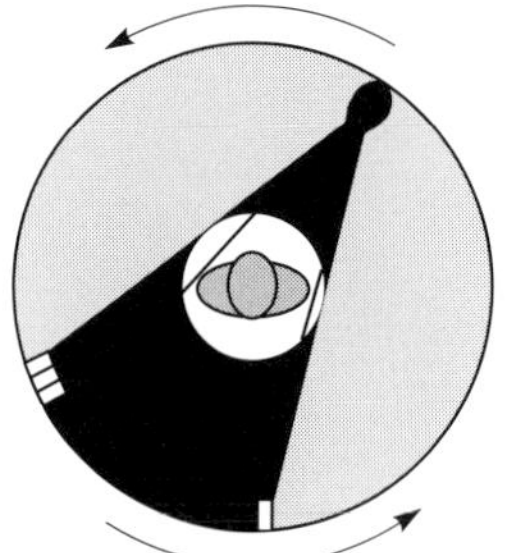

**Figure 1.17a** Third generation – diagram of a rotate system showing the arc of detectors coupled to the X-ray tube, rotating through 360°

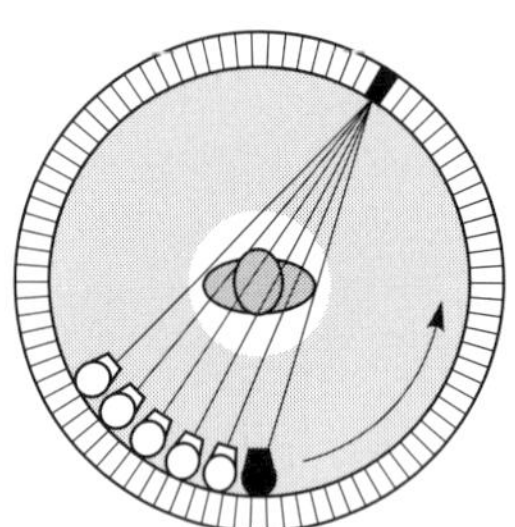

**Figure 1.17b** Fourth generation – diagram showing the circular array of detectors and the X-ray tube rotating within the array

### Windowing

CT scanners were the first imaging modality to use digitised image data. Early first-generation scanners used the EMI range of attenuation values but these were soon replaced by Hounsfield units with a range of –1000 (air) to +3000 (dense bone) with a baseline of zero for pure water. Examples of the range of attenuation values are shown opposite. The principle of windowing is described in the previous section on The Digital Image. Dual windowing, where two window levels are displayed simultaneously can be used. One application of this technique is used to visualise the mediastinum and lungs on the same image.

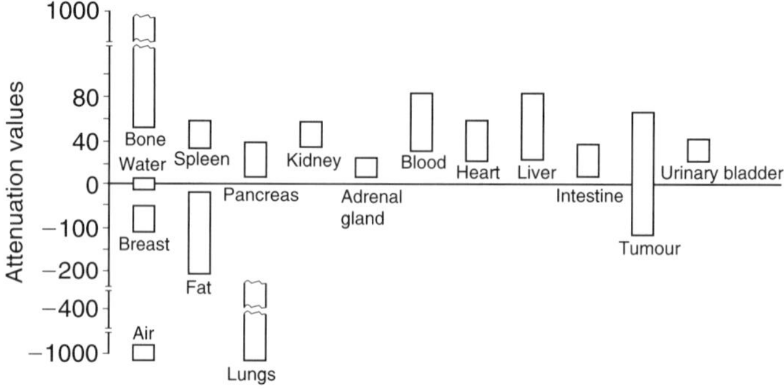


**Figure 1.17c** CT attenuation values for human tissues

### Slice width and spacing

Beam collimation is controlled primarily at the tube output port, offering slice thickness in the range of 1–10 mm, with spacing determined in axial scanning by selection of different couch increments. By decreasing slice width the spatial resolution is increased, but the radiation factors (mAs) have to be increased to compensate for increased image noise.

Incremental scanning is performed routinely, i.e. a section is obtained, the table moves the preselected distance and another section acquired until the anatomical area has been imaged.

Sequential scanning involves a series of scans at one anatomical position without table movement.

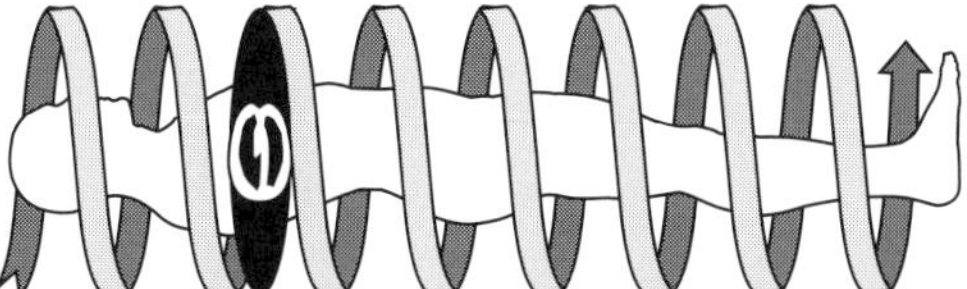

**Figure 1.18a** Diagram demonstrating volume acquisition

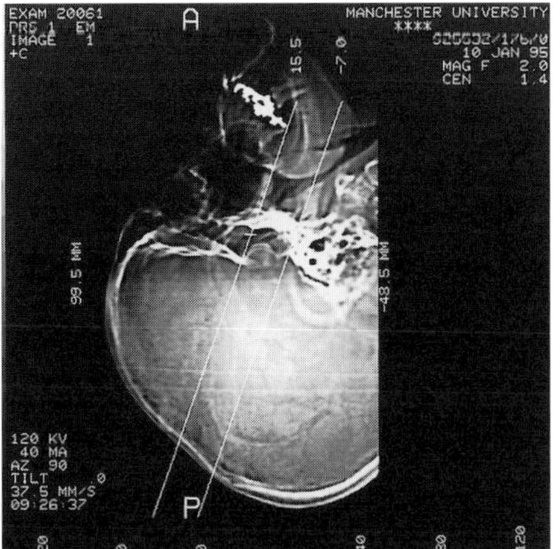


**Figure 1.18b** Lateral scan projection radiograph of skull

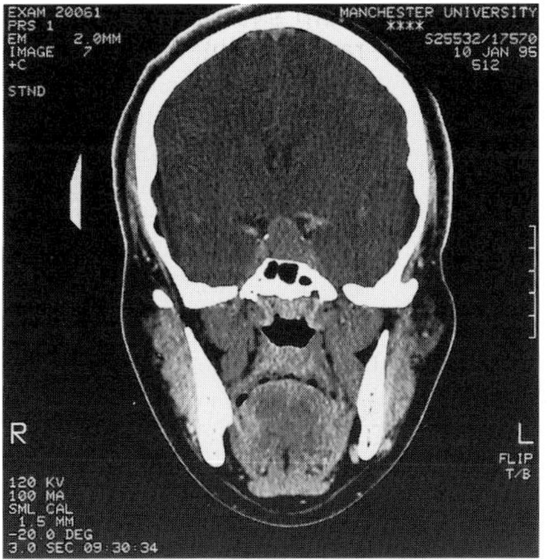


**Figure 1.18c** High-resolution CT image (1.5 mm slice width)

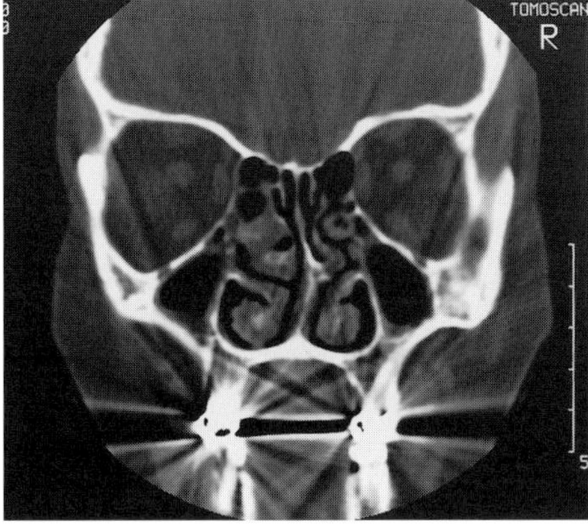


**Figure 1.18d** Degraded CT image with artefacts from dental fillings

## Volume acquisition

In volume scanning the patient is moved continuously through the gantry while the X-ray tube and detector system rotates continuously. Thus the delay inherent in incremental scanning to allow the table to move into the next position is eliminated. As a result the actual scanning time is dramatically reduced, thus allowing a complete volume to be acquired in a single breath hold and eliminating any misregistration of anatomy associated with arrested respiration techniques used in conventional incremental scanning.

Data acquired during spiral scanning are processed to produce either contiguous sections or overlapping sections. The overlapping sections can be reformatted to give high-resolution images in coronal, sagittal, transaxial and oblique anatomical planes, including 3D.

## Scan projection radiograph

All CT scanners offer the facility of a scan projection radiograph. This is normally undertaken prior to the commencement of scanning and is similar to a plain radiograph. It is produced when the patient is first positioned in the scanner by moving the patient through the scanner while the X-ray tube is exposed in a stationary position (lateral or AP/PA). It enables precise location of the scan plane and angulation of the gantry to be prescribed.

## Image quality

Image quality may be considered as the ability of the system to image small structures (spatial resolution) and its ability to discriminate between small differences in absorption in tissues (sensitivity). Many factors affect spatial resolution, including slice thickness, matrix size, gantry geometry and scanning speed. Sensitivity is determined by beam quality, noise and data processing algorithms.

The resolution and sensitivity of any system also depends on the radiation dose reaching the detectors. High-resolution images with narrow slice widths and fine matrices significantly increase patient dose. However, image quality also depends on the CT numbers of adjacent structures. In abdominal scanning, for instance, good visualisation of structures is dependent on the presence of abdominal fat with its inherent low CT number. The absence of fat makes it difficult to differentiate between organs and structures.

## Artefacts

The image reconstruction process is susceptible to artefact formation, e.g. streak artefact from dense material such as dental fillings and partial volume effects, where part of a structure only partially fills a voxel in adjacent sections.

# 1 Introduction

## Magnetic Resonance Imaging

The principle of nuclear magnetic resonance imaging has been known to scientists since the 1950s who used the technique for spectroscopy of small samples. It is only in the past 15 years, however, that technology has permitted the development of whole body imaging using the same physical principles. The equipment required for MRI and the physical principles underlying the phenomenon are complex. The description below is intended only to illustrate the principles of this imaging modality, as detailed consideration of both the system components and physics principles are beyond the scope of this book.

### Basic instrumentation

A powerful magnet is used to provide a static uniform magnetic field. Different types of magnet are used, including superconducting, resistive and permanent magnets, offering field strengths between 0.15 and 2.0 tesla (T).

Small gradient coils are used to superimpose an additional field along each of the three main axes. These coils are used to vary the field strength locally to provide spatial localisation.

The Gz (z gradient field) is used to define the image plane. The Gx (x gradient field) and Gy (y gradient field) are used to spatially locate each signal within the selected scan plane. This is done by varying the frequency within the Gx field and changing the phase of the processing protons within the Gy field in a carefully controlled way. The number of times the radiofrequency (RF) pulse and the gradient fields are turned on and off is equal to the acquisition matrix multiplied by the number of excitations. Increasing the matrix or the number of excitations will increase the acquisition (scan) time of the selected imaging sequence.

### Radiofrequency coils

The main RF coil is situated within the bore of the magnet. Its function is to transmit RF pulses to excite nuclei within a selected volume of the patient. For large areas of the body this coil also acts as a receiver coil for the imaging signal. For smaller or more superficial areas, both the signal-to-noise ratio and the spatial resolution can be improved by using a surface coil placed in close proximity to the area under examination. The body coils act as an RF transmitter and the surface coil used as a receiver. Signal drop-off occurs at a distance greater than the circumference of the coil and at a depth greater than the radius of the coil.

Phased array coils are now widely available and consist of a number of small coils linked together, to give a greater combined signal and increased anatomical coverage.

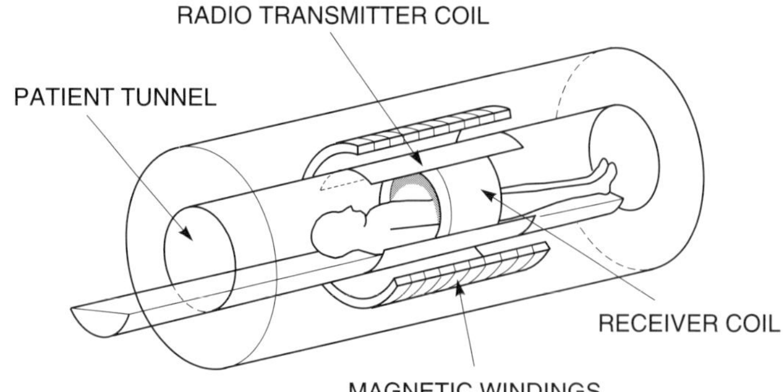


**Figure 1.19a** Diagram of MR system

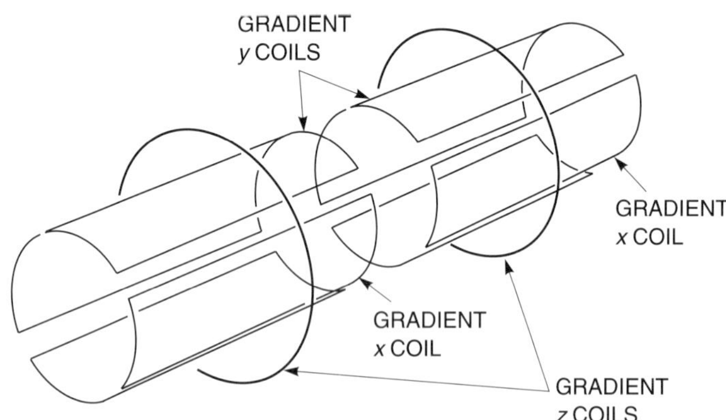


**Figure 1.19b** Diagram showing gradient coils

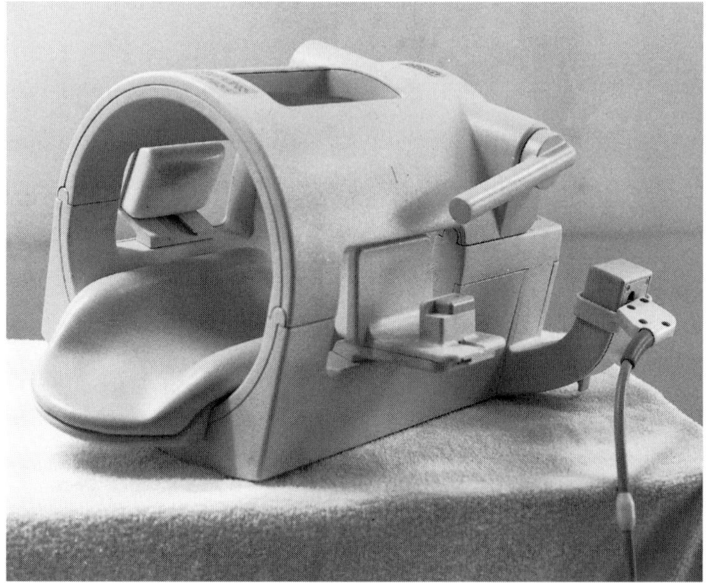

**Figure 1.19c** Typical MR head coil

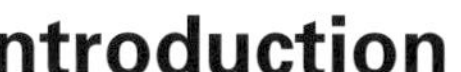

## Magnetic Resonance Imaging

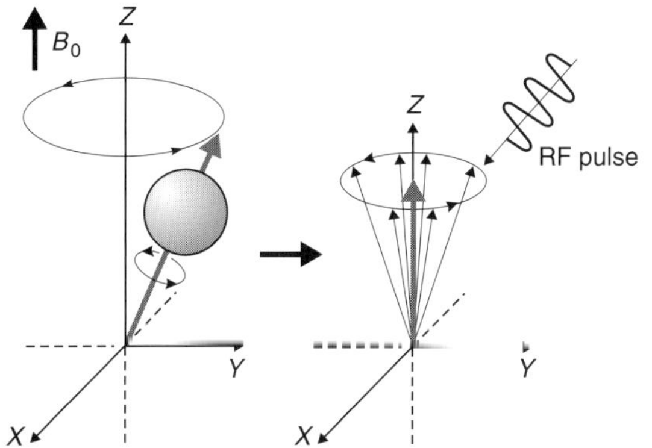


**Figure 1.20a** Spinning proton in magnetic field ($B_0$)

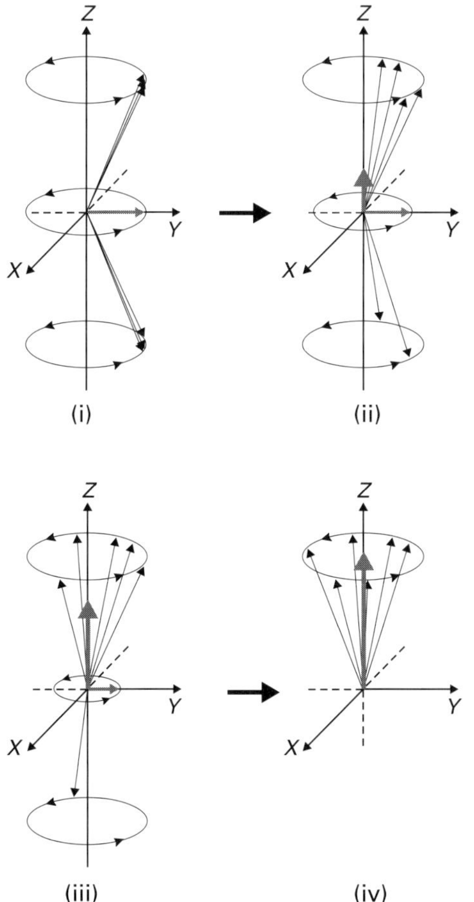


**Figure 1.20b** Immediately after RF pulse: (i) showing 90° flip angle with zero longitudinal magnetisation ($z$) and maximum transverse magnetisation ($y$); (ii)–(iv) longitudinal magnetisation ($z$) recovers and transverse magnetisation ($y$) decays

### Basic principles

Nuclei which contain an odd number of protons and neutrons in the nucleus possess the property to spin. This spin gives rise to a magnetic dipole moment associated with the atom. Examples of such nuclei include $^{1}H$, $^{31}P$ and $^{23}Na$. Hydrogen (the nucleus of which contains a single photon) is the element chosen for MRI, since it is found in great abundance in the body.

If a static magnetic field ($B_0$) is applied to a volume containing hydrogen atoms, the hydrogen nuclei will tend to align themselves along the magnetic field (high-energy nuclei will align themselves anti-parallel to the field). Slightly more of the nuclei align themselves parallel to the field, resulting in a net magnetisation ($M_0$) which is the sum of the individual magnetic moments.

The protons do not, however, align themselves precisely with the field. The spin component creates an additional force which results in a movement known as precession. This occurs around the longitudinal axis of the magnetic field ($B_0$). This movement is often compared to that of a child's spinning-top under the influence of the earth's gravitational field. The frequency of precession depends solely on the strength of the applied magnetic field ($B_0$), increasing field strength resulting in higher precessional frequencies.

The precessional frequency (or Larmor frequency) is given by the equation $w = B_0 \times \lambda$ where $B_0$ is the strength of the external magnetic field and $\lambda$ is the gyromagnetic ratio (a constant for a specific nucleus). In the case of hydrogen, the gyrometric ratio is 42.57 MHz/T.

Thus the precessional frequency of hydrogen in a 1 T field is 42.57 MHz or 21.28 MHz in a 0.5 T field.

The nuclei of other elements have different gyroscope ratios and hence different precessional frequencies. This allows hydrogen to be imaged in isolation from other elements.

### Resonance

If the nuclei are subjected to a second magnetic field generated by a radiowave at the precessional frequency and at right angles to the applied magnetic field ($B_0$), the nuclei will acquire energy and can be deflected through an angle of 90° (flip angle). The phenomenon is known as resonance. The magnitude of the flip angle depends on the amplitude and duration of the RF pulse.

Resonance results not only in a change in direction of the net magnetisation from the longitudinal axis to the transverse axis but also causes the nuclei to precess 'in phase' with each other. A receiver coil placed in the transverse plane will have voltage (signal) induced in it. This signal is the MR signal, its magnitude being dependent on the net magnetisation in the transverse plane. Once the RF pulse is removed the nuclei will gradually return to their alignment with the applied external magnetic field ($B_0$). This process is known as relaxation.

# 1 Introduction

## Magnetic Resonance Imaging

### Signal decay

The decrease in the signal recorded in the transverse plane during the relaxation process is known as **free induction decay** and its value permits measurement of the proton density in the volume being imaged.

This decrease in transverse magnetism is caused by a process known as $T_2$ decay (spin–spin relaxation or transverse relaxation time). This occurs as the phase coherence between adjacent nuclei is lost. This process is the first process to occur and results in a marked reduction in the signal strength. $T_2$ relaxation time is defined as the time taken for the transverse magnetisation to reduce to 63% of its original value.

The recovery and resultant increase in longitudinal magnetisation is caused by a process known as $T_1$ recovery (spin–lattice relaxation). This occurs as the nuclei give up their energy to the surrounding environment and it is defined as the time taken for the longitudinal value of the magnetisation to recover to 63% of its former value.

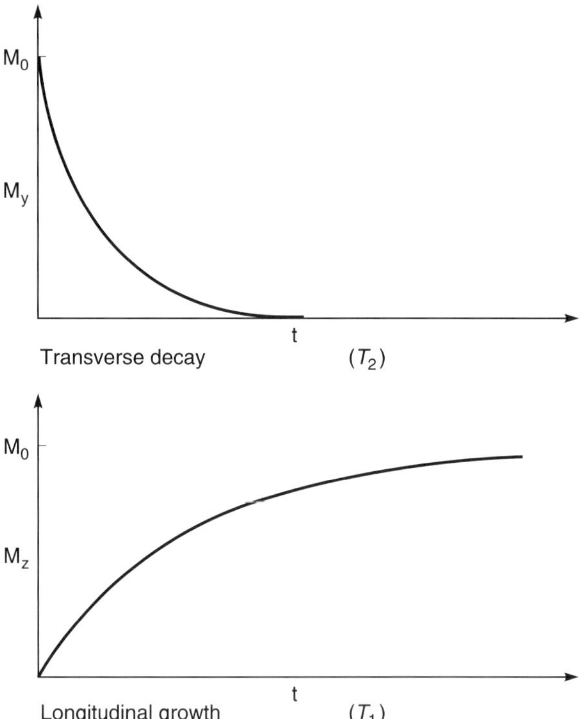


**Figure 1.21**

### Pulse sequences

Pulse sequences (Tables 1.1–1.3) are a combination of applied RF pulses, signal acquisitions and recovery times. A typical sequence will include repeated application of RF at given intervals where the time in milliseconds between application is known as TR (time to repeat). The time between applications of RF and this signal peak in the receiving coil is known as TE (echo time). Each TR gives a single line of image data (phase encoding) and needs to be reapplied to each data line to acquire the full image. $T_1$ and $T_2$ relaxation times occur simultaneously and the choice is made to image either one or the other. By altering the parameters which make up the pulse sequences, different weighting can be achieved to produce either predominantly $T_1$ or $T_2$. For example, a spin-echo sequence with a TR time of 500 ms and a TE time of 20 ms will result in a $T_1$ weighted image. A TR time of 2000 ms and a TE time of 80 ms will result in a $T_2$ weighted image. These sequences, however, have the penalty of longer scan times (typically 5–15 min). This has led to the development of faster sequences, but these may carry the penalties of reduced contrast and/or signal-to-noise ratio (SNR). An example of such a sequence is the gradient echo (typical scan time 7 s to 5 min). Because of the short scan time, 3D volume imaging can be used to improve the SNR. Specialised sequences can be used to enhance differences between tissues; for example, fat suppression and blood flow imaging.

**Table 1.1 Spin-echo sequences**

| *Weighting* | *TR* | *TE* | *Flip angle* |
|---|---|---|---|
| $T_1$ | short | short | 90° |
| $T_2$ | long | long | 90° |
| PD | long | short | 90° |

**Table 1.2 Gradient echo sequences**

| *Weighting* | *TR* | *TE* | *Flip angle* |
|---|---|---|---|
| $T_1$ | short | short | long |
| $T_2$ | short | long | small |
| PD | short | short | small |

**Table 1.3 Image contrast**

| | *$T_1$ weighted* | *$T_2$ weighted* |
|---|---|---|
| Fat | high signal intensity | high signal intensity |
| Water | low signal intensity | high signal intensity |

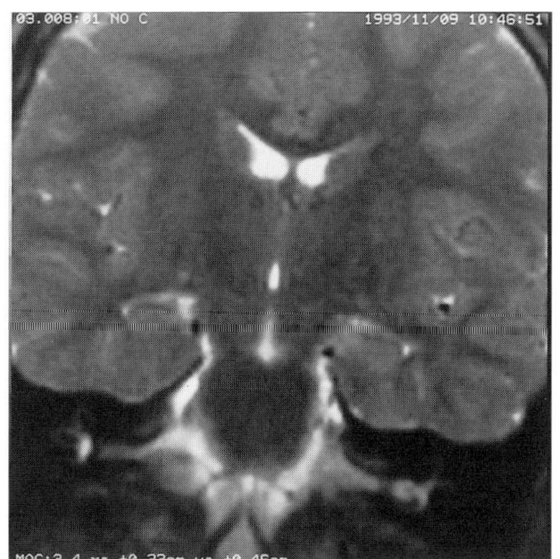


**Figure 1.22a** MR coronal image through the brain

**Imaging parameters**

| FOV | Matrix | No. of NEX | Pixel size |
|---|---|---|---|
| 25 cm | 192/256 | 3 | 1 mm |

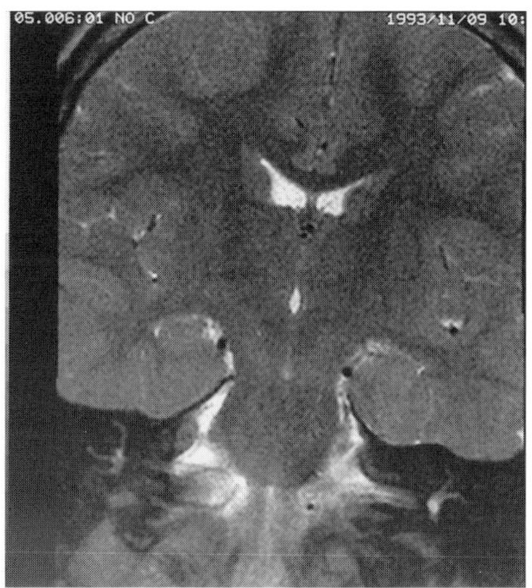


**Figure 1.22b** MR image showing improved resolution by altering image parameters

**Imaging parameters**

| FOV | Matrix | No. of NEX | Pixel size |
|---|---|---|---|
| 20 cm | 160/320 | 6 | 0.6 mm |

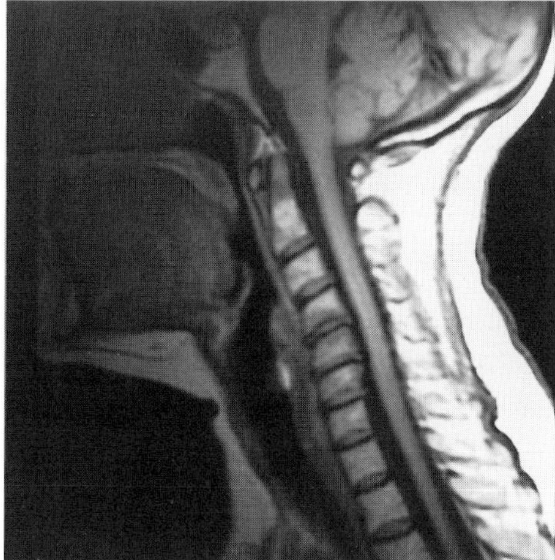

**Figure 1.22c** Standard image of neck showing signal drop-off anteriorly

## Factors affecting image quality, voxel size and spatial resolution

The image matrix defines the number of pixels used to construct an image for a given field of view (FOV). The actual volume of each voxel is determined by the FOV, matrix size and the slice thickness selected. Spatial resolution is the ability of the imaging system to resolve closely spaced anatomical structures. The larger the voxel size, the poorer is the resolution.

For a given FOV, high spatial resolution images can be obtained by increasing the number of pixels/voxels within the image matrix and reducing the slice thickness. However, total imaging time is longer, increasing the risk of patient movement which reduces spatial resolution by blurring image detail and producing ghost-like artefacts.

## Signal-to-noise ratio

In MRI, the presence of background noise limits the detection of weak signal. The signal-to-noise ratio can be defined as the ratio of the amplitude of the signal received to the average amplitude of the noise. Voxel size, signal averaging, pulse sequence timing, magnetic field strength and RF coils can affect the SNR. Reducing the volume of the voxel will reduce the signal intensity but has no effect on background noise. Therefore, decreasing the slice width and/or increasing the matrix size will increase spatial resolution but reduce the SNR.

## Number of signal averages (NEX)

The signals are measured more than once and the signal from the successive measurements are summed to produce a total intensity which increases as the number of signal averages increases. Increasing the NEX will improve the SNR, but significant improvements will need substantial increase in total imaging time. Increasing the NEX may reduce motion artefact. The greater the number of times the signal is averaged, the greater the possibility that the artefact may be averaged out.

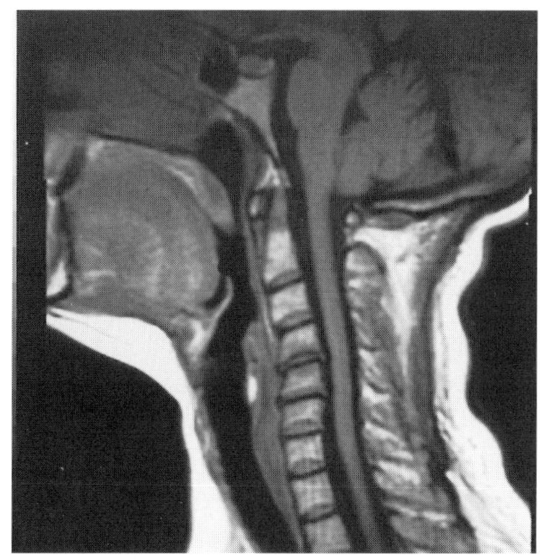

**Figure 1.22d** Improved resolution of neck using a volumetric surface coil

# 1 Introduction

## Magnetic Resonance Imaging

### Flow imaging

The imaging of fluid-filled vessels and structures within the body is made possible by the use of special pulse sequences which are designed to distinguish between the movement of fluids within vessels and that of surrounding structures where no flow is present. Such protocols enable vessels and structures to be visualised as well as providing quantitative information on the nature of the flow within the vessel.

Flow imaging is mainly used in the study of the cardiovascular system, where the technique is known as Magnetic Resonance Angiography (MRA), and in the study of cerebrospinal fluid in the central nervous system.

There are many different pulse sequences available and the student is advised to seek specific manufacturers' literature for detailed information. However, the major pulse sequences include:-

- Two-dimensional time of flight (2D TOF).
- Three-dimensional time of flight (3D TOF).
- Three-dimensional phase contrast (3D PC).
- Two-dimensional phase contrast (2D PC).
- Cardiac-gated 2D phase contrast.

It is important to realise that there are a number of factors which affect optimum demonstration of the vessels concerned. These include: blood flow direction, blood flow patterns, velocities of flow, vessel geometry and pulse sequence.

The pulse sequence selected will therefore be chosen to demonstrate best the type of abnormality being investigated. This will take into account the size, nature and location of the abnormality and vessel being investigated, as well as the direction, velocity and flow patterns of the type of vessel under investigation.

**Maximum intensity projection ray tracing**

In order to create vascular projections of vessels a ray tracing technique is employed which will interrogate the acquired data set.

This technique called maximum intensity pixel (MIP) produces a series of projection images of the vessels from different angles. The vessels can then be visualised by viewing the collection of projected images as a cine loop to give the appearance of rotation and depth, resulting in a 3D representation of the vascular structures.

### Time of flight (TOF) imaging

In TOF imaging using a gradient echo sequence, blood vessels are visualised because blood flowing into an imaging slice is fully magnetised and appears brighter than the partially saturated stationary tissues which appear much lower in signal intensity.

The acquisition protocol consists of a series of narrow slices being acquired of the region of interest to create a stack or volume containing the vascular structures. During this process, maximum flow-related enhancement will occur when blood flow is perpendicular to the imaging plane. Hence in examination of the carotid vessels, to ensure maximum visualisation of the vessels, axial scanning is employed.

Repetition times (TR) must be kept short with respect to the $T_1$ times of 'stationary tissues' to suppress the signal from such tissues and to maximise vessel contrast due to flow-related enhancement. As a result the fully relaxed blood moving into the slice remains unsaturated, and appears bright (high signal) compared to the low signal intensity stationary tissues.

Presaturation pulses are employed in this technique in order to discriminate between arteries and veins. A saturation band 'kills' the signal from the blood flow entering a slice and therefore this is applied either above or below a slice to show either arterial or venous blood. For instance, in a study of the carotid vessels, blood flowing into the imaging plane from above or below would be bright, resulting in both the carotid arteries and jugular veins being visualised. This could result in overlap of the vessels during rotation of the MIP images, hindering interpretation and complete visualisation of the carotid arteries. In a typical 2D TOF of the neck, a 3 cm wide saturation band is applied 0.5 cm superior to the acquisition slice and moves superiorly with each successive slice. The image data set will therefore be composed only of arterial structures. Similarly, the pelvic veins can be selectively imaged by applying a superior presaturation pulse to saturate arterial blood flowing into the imaging plane from above. The data should be acquired in the opposite direction to the direction of blood flow to minimise saturation of incoming blood caused by excitation during the previous slice acquisition.

### Phase contrast (PC) imaging

In PC, vessel enhancement is achieved by using a protocol that produces velocity-induced phase shifts in flowing spins and none in stationary tissue. Two acquisitions with opposite polarity of a bipolar flow-encoding gradient are subtracted to produce an image of the vessel.

The factors affecting image contrast include; velocity, aliasing, flow compensation and saturation effects.

In complicated blood flow situations, e.g. intracranial where blood flow has components in all directions, bipolar flow-encoding gradients are applied in $x$, $y$ and $z$ directions. The total flow image will therefore be constructed of individually measured and mathematically combined flow components where the pixel values are proportional to the product of the ordinary magnitude image and velocity values. To provide quantitative information, a velocity encoding (VENC) value should be selected that will encompass the highest velocities that are likely to be encountered across the vessels of interest. If flow velocities higher than the selected VENC value are encountered, they are incorrectly represented as lower velocity values flowing in the opposite direction due to the phenomenon of aliasing.

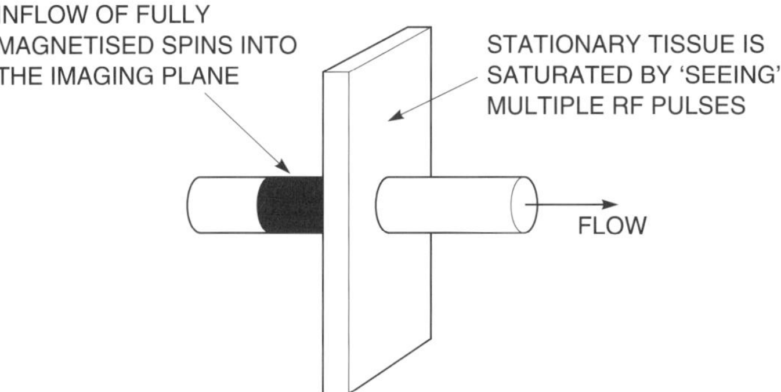


**Figure 1.23a** In 2D TOF, blood flowing into an imaging slice appears brighter than the partially saturated stationary spins

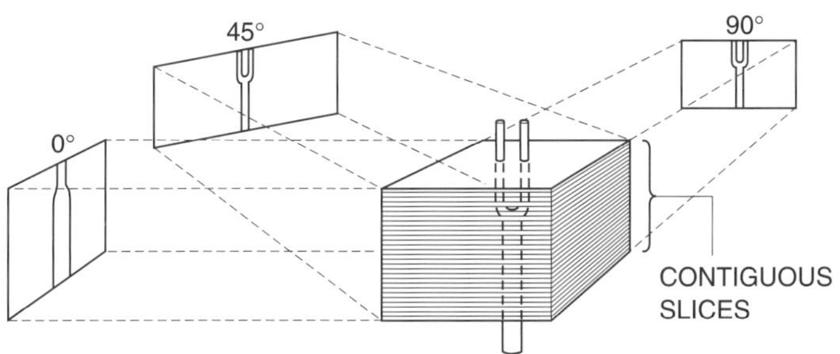


**Figure 1.23b** 2D TOF – a series of slices are acquired through the area of interest to create a volume of data. Maximum intensity pixel (MIP) tracing is applied to display the vessels

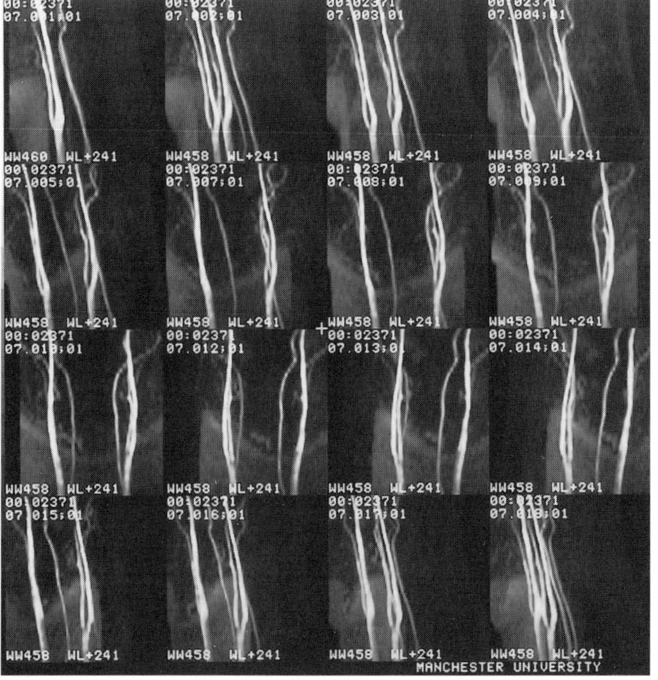


**Figure 1.23c** 2D TOF image – set of carotid arteries showing different MIP projections

Flow compensation is applied to overcome the fact that the flow velocity profile across a vessel is not constant but varies across the vessel lumen, with the velocity at almost zero near the vessel wall and increasing towards the centre. The velocity profile also becomes more complicated when flow is pulsatile and the vessel curves or bifurcates.

The phase shift induced by flowing blood in the presence of a flow-encoding gradient is directly proportional to velocity. A dispersion of velocities in a vessel will therefore result in a dispersion of phase shifts. Consequently a projection measurement of phase through a vessel with laminar flow will represent the average velocity, provided that the strength of the flow-encoding gradient is not too great. When flow becomes complex or turbulent the dispersion of velocity components along the projection may cause attenuation of the signal or even zero signal. To overcome this complication of signal loss a number of strategies are employed. The dispersion of velocities along a projection can greatly be reduced by using 3D acquisition instead of 2D. Velocity dispersion within a voxel is minimised, since a 3D voxel can be made quite small. Using 15–20° flip angles, large volumes such as the head can be imaged without serious loss of signal intensity due to saturation effects. As a result of the reduced saturation dependency, short TRs may be used, e.g. 25–28 ms, with minimal saturation of moving spins. Further reductions in saturation may be achieved by using paramagnetic intravenous contrast agents which shorten the $T_1$ of blood which will improve the signal when the velocity of blood is slow.

Three-dimensional phase contrast imaging is particularly useful for large-volume acquisition such as large intracranial aneurysms.

# 1 Introduction

## Diagnostic Ultrasound Imaging

The use of diagnostic ultrasound is widespread, with a variety of equipment available ranging from small portable imaging machines to complex computer-controlled systems offering several different imaging facilities. The majority of ultrasound machines give 2D cross-sectional images of tissue (B mode) and usually have the facility to display echo depth in one direction against time (M mode), while the more complex systems have the facility to display the Doppler spectrum or colour flow images of moving blood.

Resolution depends on parameters such as the frequency of sound, the focusing of the beam and image processing, but the final quality of the image involves factors such as the sort of tissue being scanned, the depth of interest and the skill of the operator in optimising the controls. The viewing conditions in the room and contrast and brilliance on the monitor also affect the final viewed image.

### Coupling gel

A coupling gel is essential for ensuring optimum image quality. This is applied to the patient's skin to ensure an air-free contact between the patient and the transducer face, thus ensuring optimum transmission and reception of ultrasound waves.

### Transducers

A variety of transducers, also called probes, are available for use. The type of probe selected will depend on the requirements of the examination.

**Sector probes**

Sector probes have an image with a sector format in which the lateral field of view is more restricted superficially. However, they do have a small contact area and are ideal for imaging intercostally, or scanning the neonatal brain through the anterior fontanelle. Sector probes are either 'mechanical', in which the crystal oscillates through the sector angle, or they are 'electronic phased array', in which the beam is formed from many tiny elements and steered by phasing the elements.

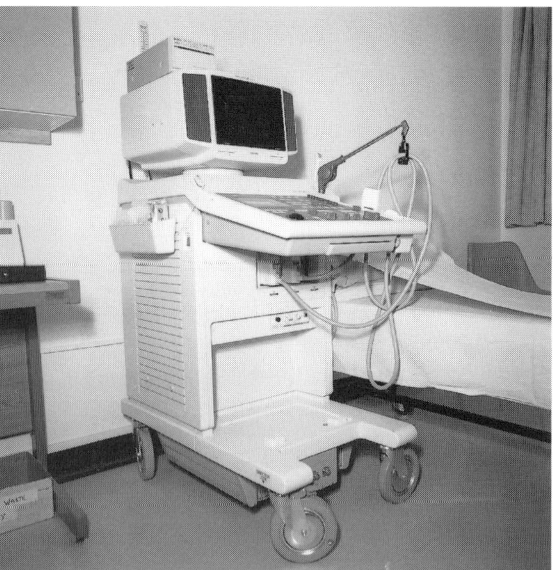

**Figure 1.24a** Typical general-purpose ultrasound system

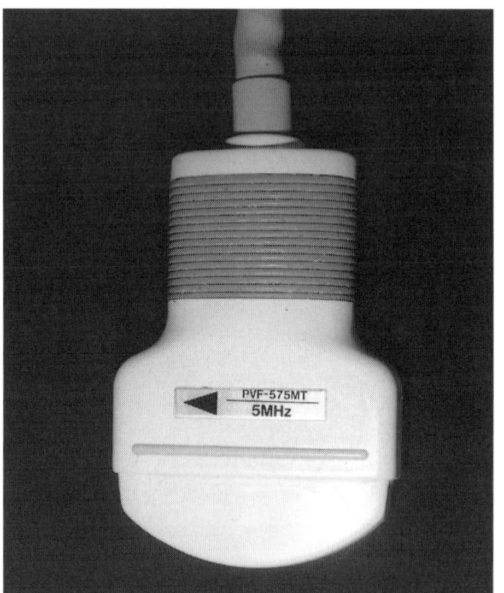


**Figure 1.24b** Electronic phased array probe

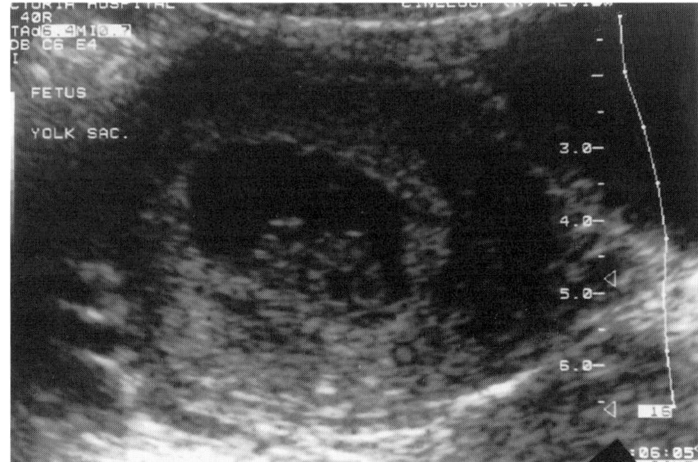


**Figure 1.24c** Image of an early but recognisable pregnancy using a curved linear array probe

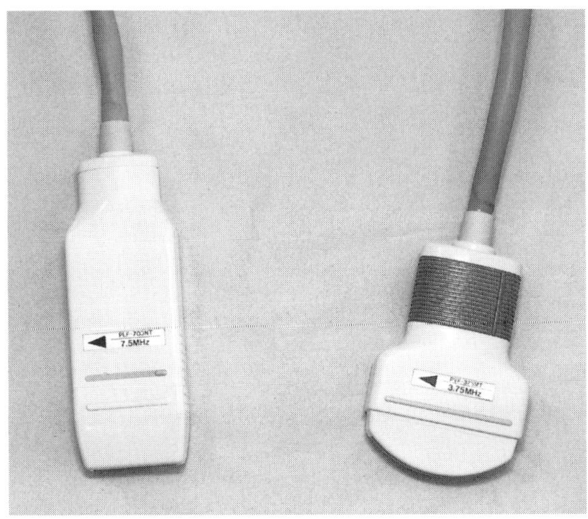

**Figure 1.25a** Straight linear and curvilinear probes (left to right)

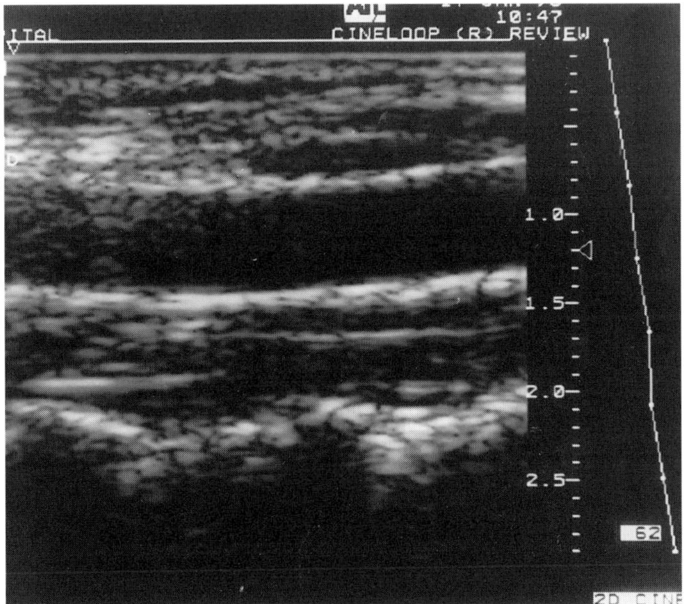


**Figure 1.25b** Image of carotid artery using a high-frequency (5 MHz) linear probe

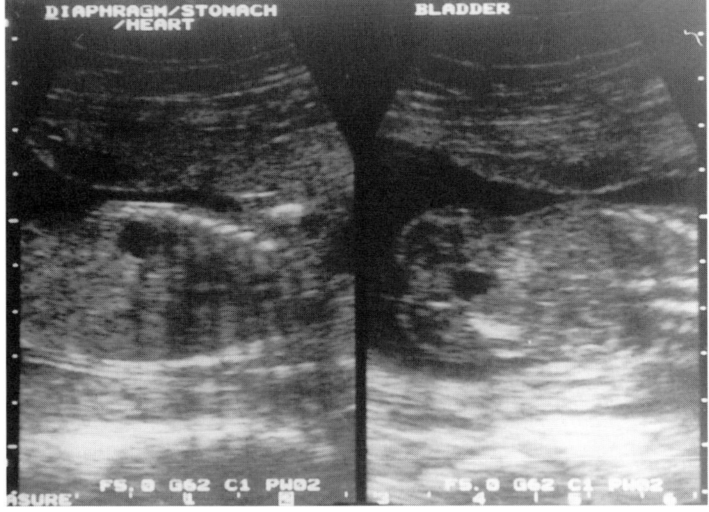


**Figure 1.25c** Image of an 18-week-old fetus using a curvilinear probe

**Electronic array probes**

An electronic linear array has a more extensive field of view superficially, but at the expense of a large contact area. There are two kinds of linear array. The first is the 'straight' linear, in which the front face is straight, giving a rectangular image format. These are most useful at higher frequencies when imaging superficial organs such as breast, thyroid or vessels. The other, more common kind is the curvilinear probe in which the front face is convex. Here the image format is an excellent compromise between sector and rectangle and is ideal for most obstetric and abdominal scanning.

## Transducer frequency

Probes of different frequencies are available which are selected for their inherent ability to scan at optimum resolution at specific tissue depths.

**3.5 MHz**

These probes provide useful penetration up to 20 cm, with optimum focus at 10–15 cm, making them suitable for posterior abdominal structures.

**5.0 MHz**

This provides adequate penetration with a short to medium focus (7–10 cm), offering superior resolution compared with the 3.5 MHz probe, making it ideal for structures such as the gallbladder and abdominal scanning in very thin adults and paediatric patients.

**7.0–7.5 MHz**

This has a short focus (2–7 cm), providing excellent resolution and good penetration of superficial structures such as the thyroid gland and testes.

**10.0 MHz**

This provides maximum resolution with minimal penetration, with the focus limited to a depth of 4 cm. This makes it ideal for structures such as the eye and the breast.

## Beam focusing

Electronic array transducers usually have the facility for the operator to control depth of focus and set it to the depth of interest. Mechanical sector transducers have a fixed focus, but a special kind of mechanical transducer, called an 'annular array', has an electronically adjustable focus.

### Depth of field

Normally the image is from the skin line to the depth set by the operator, perhaps 4–20 cm, but many systems have the facility to select a portion of the image and zoom onto it to fill the image.

### Power

This is the transmitted power and is usually indicated in decibels (dB). This should be kept as low as possible to reduce the dose to the patient. To increase the echo strength in the image, the overall gain should be increased rather than the power, consistent with an acceptable level of noise.

### Time gain compensation (TGC)

This is set so that echoes of equal amplitude are displayed as equal brightness on the monitor regardless of their depth in tissue. Echoes returning from anterior regions are much less attenuated by the tissue than those from deeper regions and so the signals need less amplification. The change in amplification with depth is called TGC and is adjusted by the operator.

### Overall gain

This control amplifies all echoes independently of their depth and so controls the size of the echoes displayed. If set too high the electronic noise becomes excessive.

### Frame rate

The frame rate is the number of frames or sweeps of the beam across the transducer per second to produce the ultrasound image. Although the image is usually displayed on a television monitor, in which a complete new picture is repeated 25 times per second, the ultrasound section of the image may be refreshed much less than this. At low frame rates there will not be any flicker, but the image may appear sluggish when looking at fast-moving structures. Imaging the heart obviously requires a high frame rate. Various operator controls affect the frame rate, such as depth and focusing, and these are adjusted for the particular organ under investigation.

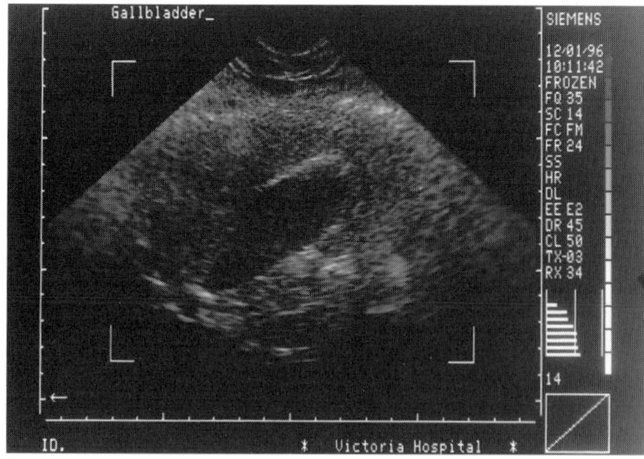


**Figure 1.26a** Image of abdomen showing gallbladder

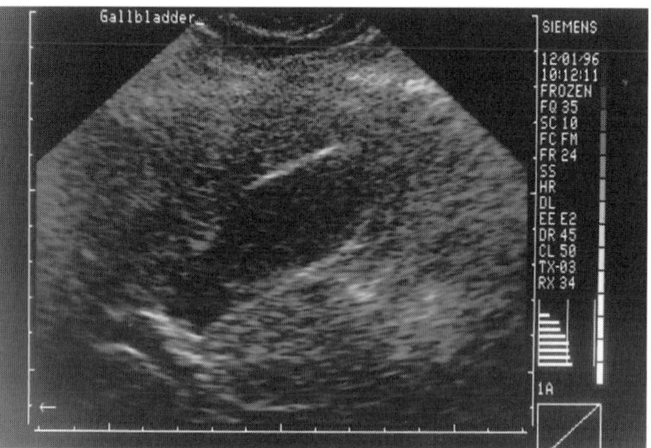


**Figure 1.26b** Zoomed image of gallbladder

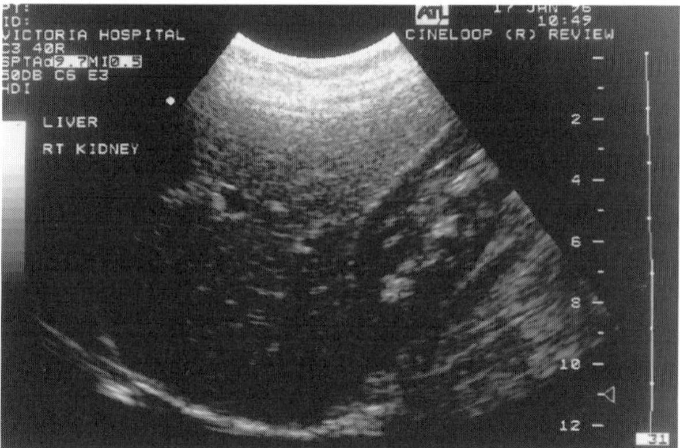


**Figure 1.26c** Image of liver showing incorrectly set time gain compensation

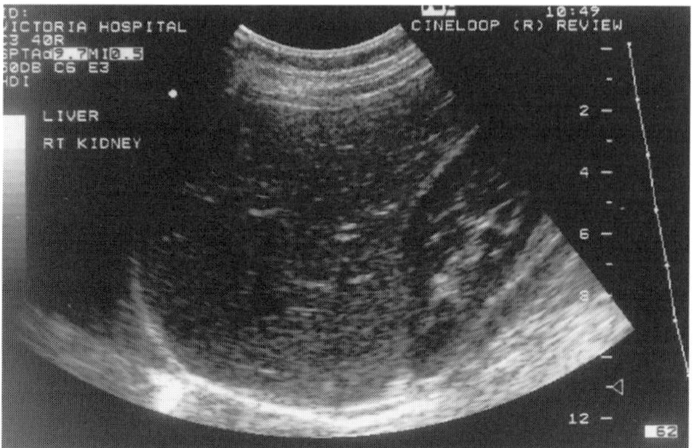


**Figure 1.26d** Image of liver showing correctly set time gain compensation (deeper tissues visualised)

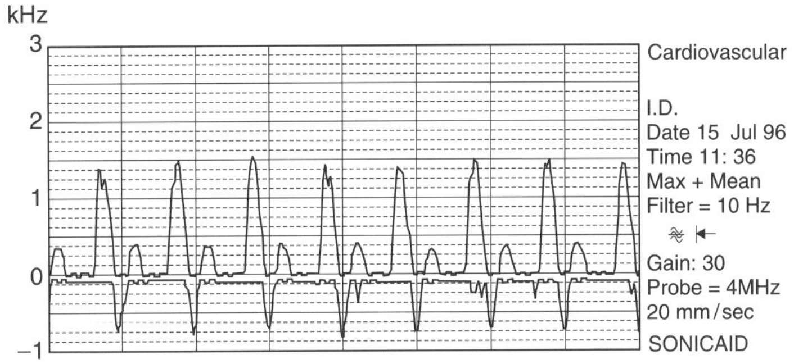

kHz
3
2
1
0
−1
Cardiovascular
I.D.
Date 15 Jul 96
Time 11: 36
Max + Mean
Filter = 10 Hz
Gain: 30
Probe = 4MHz
20 mm/sec
SONICAID

**Figure 1.27a** Typical CW spectrum of left femoral artery

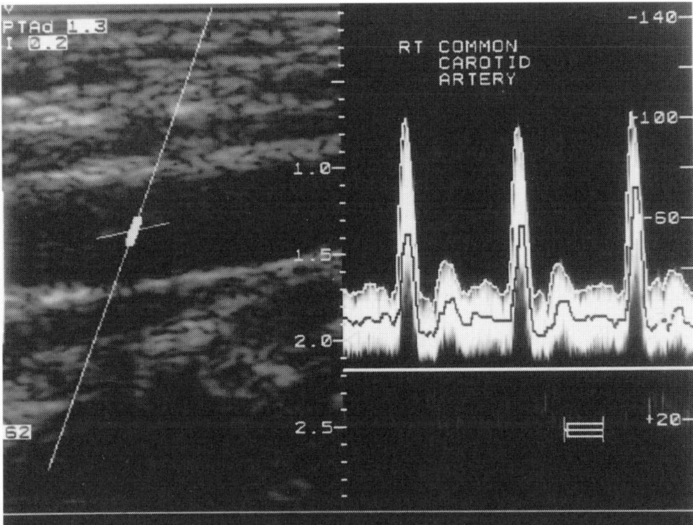


**Figure 1.27b** Ultrasound image of right common carotid artery demonstrating pulse wave Doppler spectrum

When an ultrasound beam is directed at a blood vessel, the red blood cells scatter the ultrasound. If cells are moving towards the probe, the received frequency will be higher than the transmitted frequency as a result of the Doppler effect. Conversely, for blood moving away from the probe there will be a decrease in received frequency. The difference in frequency is called the Doppler shift. This shift is proportional to the velocity of the moving blood cells, but is also dependent on the probe frequency and the angle between the probe and the vessel.

For moving blood, the Doppler shift frequency falls within the audible range, so it can be amplified and passed to a loudspeaker. It can also be displayed as a trace of the frequencies present at each instant (blood moves faster at the centre of the vessel than at the periphery) against time.

There are three different techniques based on this principle: continuous wave (CW) Doppler, pulse wave (PW) Doppler and colour flow Doppler. The probe for a CW machine usually has one crystal emitting ultrasound continuously, and another crystal acting as a receiver. As no pulsing is required, very high velocities can be measured; however, the technique has the major disadvantage of not providing any discrimination of depth in the tissues.

On the other hand, a PW machine produces a short burst of ultrasonic energy and uses the same crystal as a receiver. After an appropriate time delay the machine accepts the reflections arriving at the crystal for short durations. This corresponds to a 'sample volume' set by the operator, so that only echoes returning from this small volume of tissue are used to determine the Doppler shift. This method enables velocities in a 'sample volume' to be determined and is usually combined with 2D imaging so that the operator can see where the sample volume is in the vessel. This is a sampling method, so for higher velocities it may not be possible to pulse the probe fast enough. When this limit is reached the trace will alias and give anomalous information. Pulse wave Doppler gives flow information at only one point, i.e. in the sample volume.

A more general picture of flow can be derived using colour Doppler imaging (see Plate 1). With this method the conventional 2D image is combined with an image of moving blood generated by detecting changes in frequency from returning echoes over a section of the image (colour box). This gives a real-time image, although frame rates can be quite low. It is very useful in giving a picture of moving blood, showing direction and approximate velocity.

## Radionuclide Imaging

Gamma camera imaging can be used to show the distribution of the radioactive material in an organ or region of the body. The radiopharmaceutical used in the investigation is selected to localise in the organ of interest. A study may involve:

- **Static imaging**, where images are acquired at a time when the uptake of the radioisotope is optimal.
- **Single photon emission tomography** (SPET or SPECT), requiring the acquisition of a series of images as the gamma camera rotates around the patient. By reconstructing the planar image data after acquisition, images can be obtained in any orthogonal planes.
- **Dynamic imaging**, used to follow the changes which take place with time in the distribution of the material. Imaging usually starts immediately after the administration of the tracer and may continue for several hours.

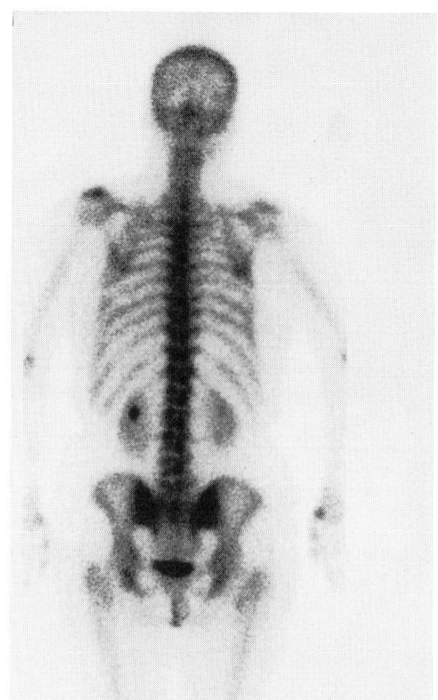

**Figure 1.28a** Example of a static image – bone scan

### Factors influencing the final image

**1. The camera collimator**

The collimator performs an essential role in the formation of the image by defining which of the gamma rays emitted from the patient reach the crystal detector. The majority of collimators have parallel holes; thus there is a 1:1 relationship between the distribution of the radioactive material in the patient and the pattern of interactions which take place in the detector.

The actual design of the collimator will depend on a number of factors including the gamma energy emitted by the radionuclide and the temporal and spatial distribution of radioactive material in the area to be imaged. A typical gamma camera system will have at least three collimators. Low-energy collimators are designed for an energy range of 80–180 keV. For applications such as bone imaging where image detail is needed, the collimators will have a high resolution (and low sensitivity). For dynamic imaging high sensitivity is necessary.

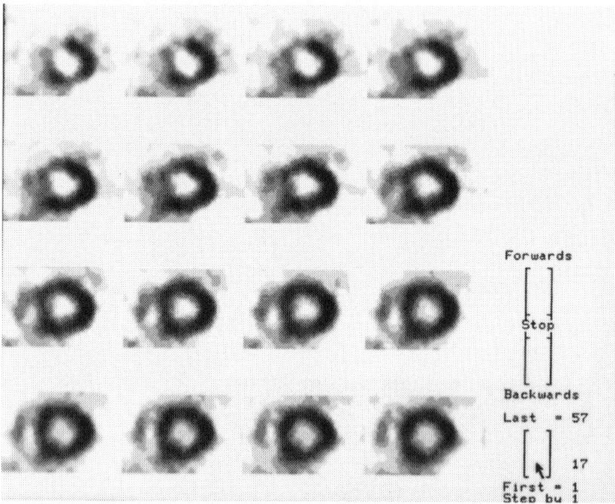


**Figure 1.28b** Example of SPECT imaging – sections along the short axis of the heart

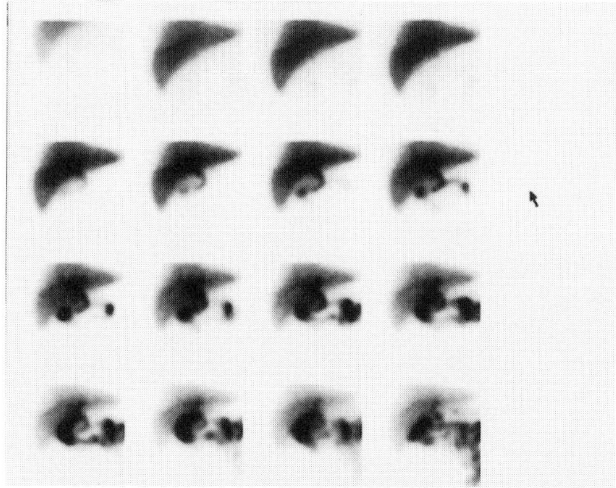

**Figure 1.28c** Example of dynamic imaging – sequential images demonstrating biliary function

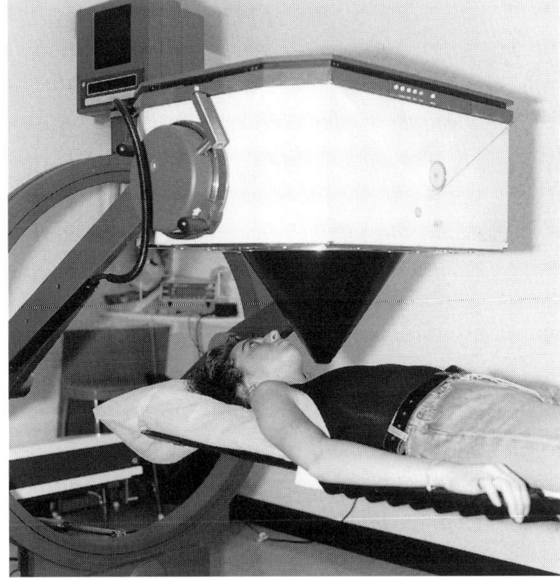

**Figure 1.29a** Typical pinhole collimator

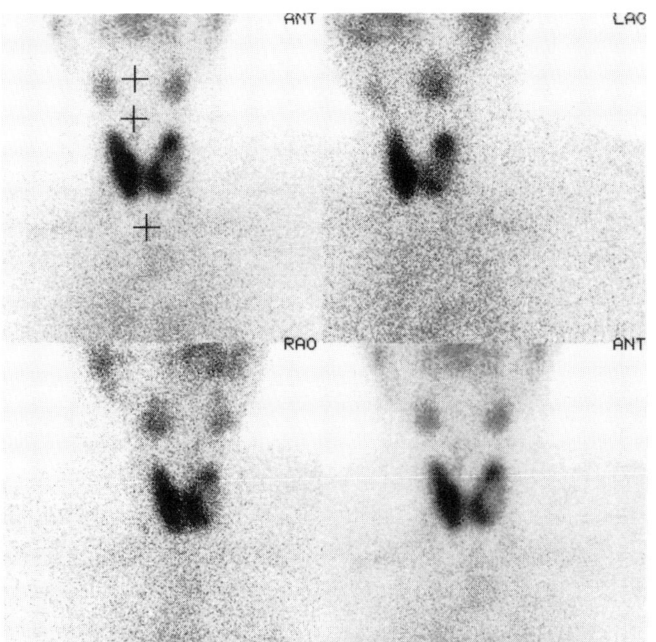


**Figure 1.29b** Normal parallel hole collimator image

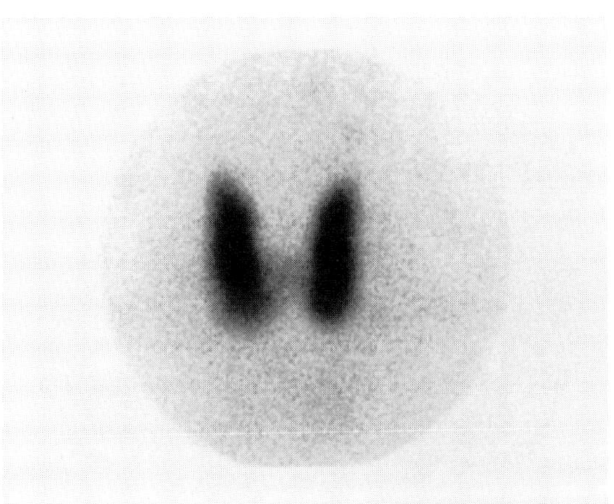

**Figure 1.29c** Pinhole collimator image

For nuclides such as In-111($^{111}$In) Ga-67 ($^{67}$Ga) and I-131 ($^{131}$I), collimators designed to work with these higher energies are needed.

Where thyroid imaging is important a special pinhole collimator is useful; in this case a hollow cone of lead with a small hole at its apex is used. This produces a high-resolution magnified image; however, the use of pinhole collimators is confined to small organs.

**2. The radiopharmaceutical used**

This topic is fully covered in Chapter 2, which explains that Tc-99m ($^{99m}$Tc) (which has a principal photon energy of 140 keV), Kr-81m ($^{81m}$Kr) and I-123 ($^{123}$I) all emit photons with energies which are efficiently detected by a gamma camera system and for which collimator design can be optimised.

A variety of compounds, suitable for different investigations, may be labelled with $^{99m}$Tc. Iodine-123 is used in thyroid studies and can also be used to label a number of different compounds. Krypton-81m may be used for ventilation lung imaging.

**3. The radiation dose to the patient**

ICRP-60, paragraph 1, suggests that we will limit the activity administered to the patient. The radiation dose depends on a number of factors, including the physical and biological half-life of the radionuclide which together form the effective half-life.

The radionuclides such as $^{99m}$Tc and $^{81m}$Kr which decay by isomeric transmission and radionuclides such as $^{123}$I which decay by the process of electron capture, give low radiation doses per MBq administered. This allows larger activities and higher counting rates to be obtained. As the time for image acquisition is limited, higher total counts can be obtained from these nuclides, raising the possibility of higher resolution in the images obtained. Strict control of use and administration of radionuclides is governed by the Administration of Radioactive Substances Committee (ARSAC) set up under the provision of the Medicines (Administration of Radioactive Substances) Regulations (as amended in 1978).

**4. Acquisition of images**

The acquisition of images can be controlled either by presetting a time of acquisition or setting the count content of the image to be acquired.

For static imaging, setting the count content enables a predetermined information content to be realised. As an example, in static imaging of the kidneys image acquisition is terminated after five hundred thousand counts (500 K/counts) have been acquired.

In dynamic imaging, a sequence of time-determined images is acquired, with frame times selected to be related to the rate of the physiological process. For example, the image acquisition protocol for a renogram investigation consists of a series of 120 images, with each image in the sequence being acquired during a 20-second time interval.

As with any other imaging process, patient movement can be a problem in terms of movement unsharpness, which will lead to a loss of definition. For longer examinations, patient immobilisation methods should be employed. For certain procedures in babies and small children, sedation may be necessary.

**5. Photopeak energy**

The pulse height analyser of a gamma camera is used to reduce the Compton scatter in an image; it is used to select photopeak events which arise from gamma photons that have been absorbed by the crystal detector without first being scattered. It is important that the analyser is correctly set on the photopeak for the radionuclide, or where the spectrum contains more than one gamma emission, the main photopeaks are appropriately set up.

*Typical photopeak energies*

Examples of photopeak energies are given in Table 1.4. below.

**Table 1.4 Some photopeak energies**

| *Radionuclide* | *Principal energy* |
|---|---|
| Technetium | 140 keV |
| Krypton | 191 keV |
| Thallium-201 | 68–91 keV (X-rays) |

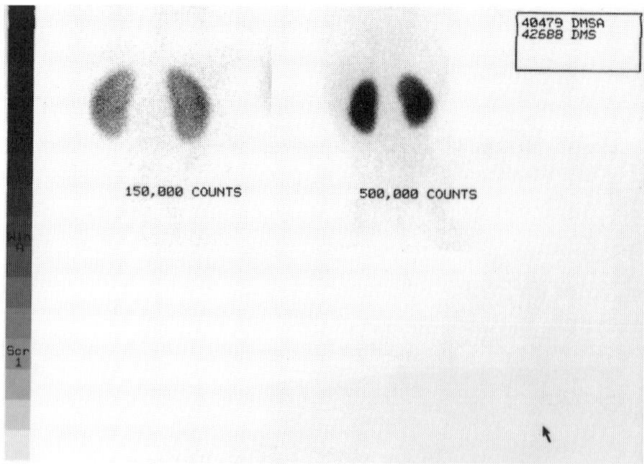


**Figure 1.30a** Dual images of a static renal scan to demonstrate effect of different count settings

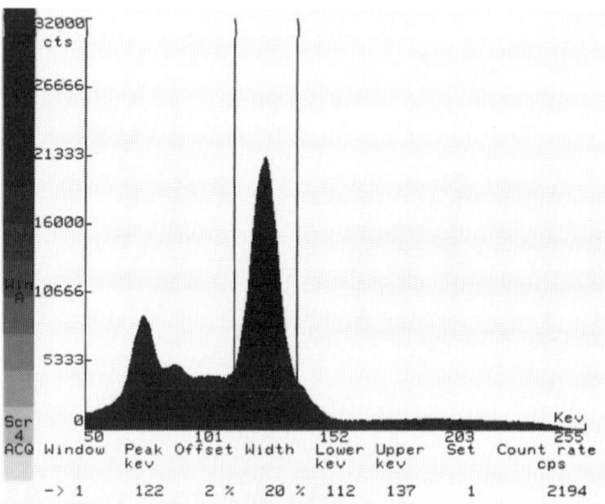


**Figure 1.30b** Image from display monitor showing photopeak and window width correctly set for technetium

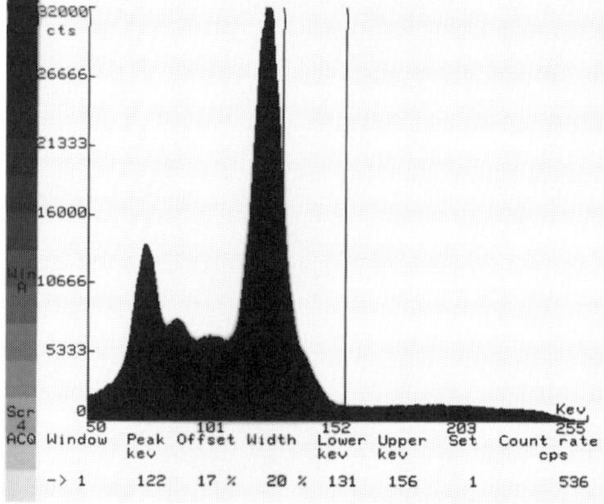


**Figure 1.30c** Image from display monitor showing photopeak incorrectly set for technetium

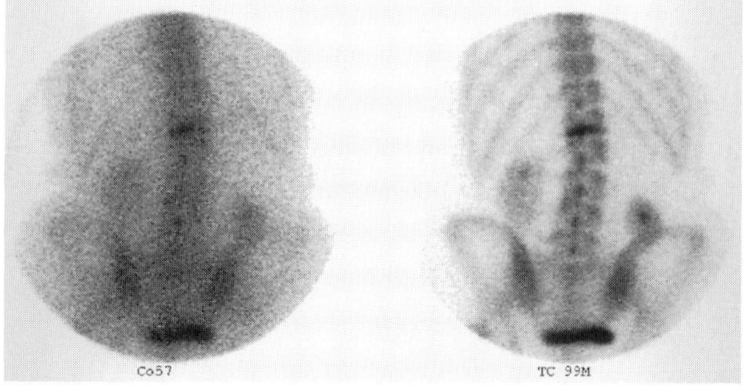


**Figure 1.30d** $^{99m}$Tc isotope scan of spine showing effect of: (i) incorrect ($^{57}$Co) photopeak energy setting; (ii) correct ($^{99m}$Tc) photopeak energy setting

32000 cts
26666
21333
16000
10666
5333
0
Kev
50 101 152 203 255
Window Peak kev Offset Width Lower kev Upper kev Set Count rate cps
-> 1 122 -14 % 40 % 81 131 1 3002

**Figure 1.31a** Image from display monitor showing window width incorrectly set for technetium

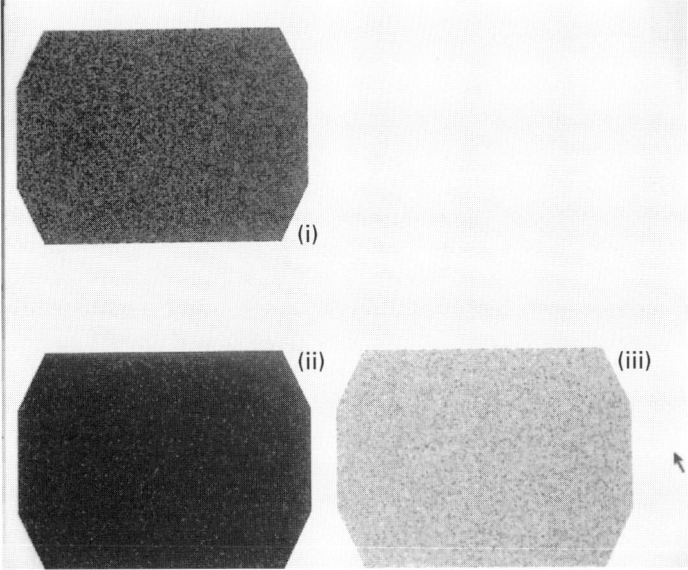


**Figure 1.31b** Images of a 'flood phantom' showing effect of different window width settings for $^{99m}$Tc. (i) 20% – optimum setting; (ii) 50% – too wide a window; (iii) 5% – too narrow a window

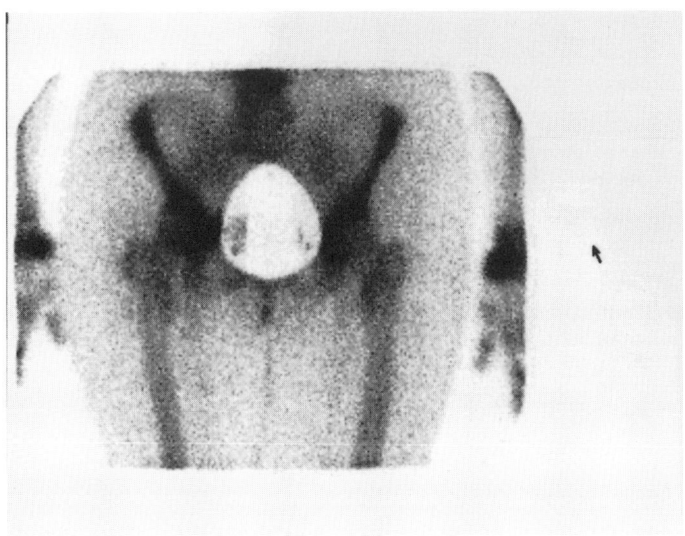

**Figure 1.31c** Image showing pelvis with bladder shielding

**6. Window width**

Window width dictates the upper and lower limits to the photon emission energies used in creating the radionuclide image. The selected value is keyed into the calibration system, prior to acquisition. For instance, using technetium a common window width of 20% is used, with the 20% window set about the principal photon energy, equidistant either side of the peak value. The window eliminates any unwanted energies which could degrade the image, i.e. Compton scatter.

A problem arises when using dual isotope techniques, where the energies within the window set for one of the radionuclides interferes or overlaps with those set for the second radionuclide. This interference is known as 'crosstalk', which creates image degradation. Smaller window widths, for each of the radionuclides used in the examination, however, can be used to help prevent this overlap.

*Accessories used in radionuclide imaging*

Lead rubber is used for a variety of reasons. In certain procedures it is used to shield the gamma camera from gamma rays which may be emitted from adjacent parts of the body which would otherwise add to the radionuclide image and reduce image resolution. For example, in conventional brain imaging for the vertex view a cape is applied around the neck to prevent a small lesion high in the cerebral hemispheres being obscured. Sheeting is also usefully employed in examinations of the bony pelvis in patients with an enlarged prostate. In this situation the concentrated source of gamma rays from a full bladder of urine labelled with technetium will obscure the adjacent bony pelvis. Using an oval-shaped piece of lead rubber which is carefully placed over the bladder, unwanted gamma rays can be absorbed, enabling the bony pelvis to be imaged free from excess radiation.

Cobalt-57 ($^{57}$Co) sources are used to enable orientation of the image to identify the right or left side of the body. This is achieved using a marker device in the shape of a pen with a $^{57}$Co source which is held against the side selected for identification. Marker sources can also be embedded into flexible rubber strips at 5 cm set points to facilitate assessment of distances and to outline borders, i.e. right costal margin in liver imaging.

Immobilisation devices, e.g. Velcro bands and foam pads, may also be used to reduce patient movement.

# 1 Introduction

## Patient care and preparation

### General considerations

The acceptance of any patient for imaging carries with it the responsibility for the patient's well-being prior to, during and immediately after the examination. This care encompasses both the physical and mental well-being of the patient, the latter having a direct effect on the success of the examination, as time spent in reassurance and explanation ensures the co-operation of the patient, thus increasing the likelihood of a successful and efficient imaging procedure. Psychological care of the patient is therefore considered to be of paramount importance.

In many procedures formal written consent requires to be obtained and this should be done in plenty of time prior to the commencement of the examination in order that in the event of refusal another patient may be scheduled and imaging time is not lost.

Confidentiality must be ensured and the relevant legal requirements observed in this respect, e.g. the Data Protection Act in the case of computer-retained records.

Preparation of the patient is of paramount importance and can only be achieved if a clear explanation is given to the patient and to other personnel involved. Valuable imaging time is frequently lost due to inadequate or erroneous patient preparation. This often arises due to assumptions being made by the imaging department. It is important, therefore, that the appropriate preparation for every procedure is given in writing and verbally explained.

The type of standard preparation prescribed will vary in nature, depending on the procedure undertaken, with the standard being modified when the patient's clinical condition warrants it. Some form of pharmaceutical intervention may be required in order to assist the imaging process, as well as some form of abdominal preparation to ensure that optimum diagnostic information is obtained.

The following text will highlight some examples of the different types of patient preparation and care which are necessary for each imaging modality and other major procedures performed in an imaging department. Where more specific information is required, this is covered in the specific imaging procedure text. These examples, however, are not meant to be prescriptive and the student is advised to follow the specific preparations laid down in their own institution.

Prevention of cross-infection is a major responsibility, in order to ensure that those attending with a known infectious disease do not spread their infection to other patients and staff. Ward patients being barrier nursed and those being reverse barrier nursed should be given the last appointment of the day to allow plenty of time for the examination and for cleaning of the equipment after the procedure.

### Radiation protection

The patient will be exposed to ionising radiation as a result of procedures associated with X-ray equipment described in this book. Such exposures must be kept as low as reasonably practicable (ALARA principle). Among those procedures contributing to the highest patient doses is CT scanning of the abdomen, but many other procedures associated with fluoroscopy, rapid sequence vascular imaging and other investigations of the urinary system and gastrointestinal tract all contribute to patient dose and therefore must be used with care. The use of radiopharmaceuticals associated with radionuclide imaging also has associated ionising radiation risks.

Guiding principles on radiation protection are found in the various documents issued by the International Commission on Radiation Protection. Many of the recommendations made in document ICRP-60, issued in 1991, are of particular importance, with these embodied in legislation in many countries. All personnel involved in the use and administration of ionising radiation have a duty to be familiar with the codes of practice, recommendations on permissible dose limits and statutory instruments of law which are connected with such activities. It is not within the scope of this book to list the individual rules and doses, but the student is referred to the appropriate national guidelines. It should also be borne in mind that legislation, codes of practice and guidelines are being updated and it is important therefore to keep up to date with such changes.

In order to reduce or indeed eliminate exposure to ionising radiation, all requests for such procedures should be carefully vetted. Such requests should only be performed in accordance with local dose reduction protocols where it has been agreed that other non-ionising procedures, e.g. ultrasound, will not provide the required diagnostic information. The radiographer has the responsibility of keeping the radiation dose within the prescribed limits and ensuring that the minimum dose is used consistent with the diagnostic information required from the procedure.

Particular care should be taken to ensure that the correct patient and region are being examined. Protocols should be written down that outline how this is done and who takes responsibility for patient identification.

To avoid irradiating a fetus, a 'pregnancy rule' should carefully be observed. If a woman is pregnant, or cannot be certain that she is not pregnant, then direct exposure of the abdomen and pelvis should be avoided. The only exception to this rule is when the radiologist or referring clinician can state the overlying clinical reasons for the requested examination to proceed. In all cases the number of exposures should be kept to a minimum and a record kept of patient dose.

## Radionuclide imaging

All patients for RNI investigations should have all previous records available, including case notes and imaging history. This can be used to assess current status, medication and ECG records when appropriate. After the investigation, note should be made in the case sheet regarding the radiopharmaceutical used, dose given and date of examination.

The possibility of pregnancy associated with the administration of radioactive material into female patients of child-bearing age is an important consideration. Application of the pregnancy rule should ensure that pregnant patients are not subjected to ionising radiation derived from radiopharmaceuticals injected into the body and concentrated, after a period of time, in urine filling the bladder. Care should also be exercised in respect to breast-feeding mothers who attend for investigation. They should be alerted to restrict breast feeding for a suitable period following the investigation to prevent the baby ingesting any milk containing traces of radioactive elements.

It is important to make the nursing staff aware that any incontinent patients due to attend for RNI investigations be catheterised prior to injection. This will reduce dose and contamination risks to staff later. However, the staff must still be made aware of how to deal with contaminated urine and bags.

As with most imaging procedures it is essential to pass all relevant information onto the patient in order to ensure their full co-operation. A general information leaflet may be sent along with a detailed appointment letter prior to the patient attending. On arrival in the department the radiographer will further explain the order of the day and answer any outstanding questions.

In paediatric cases it is necessary to change practice to cope with the difficulty and trauma of cannulation and with the necessity that the child remain still for considerable time. In infants the cannulation should be done by an experienced paediatrician and the child delayed between cannulation and the introduction of isotope so that he/she may calm down if scanning is to proceed. It may be necessary to admit children aged 3 months to 3 years as day cases so that sedation can be administered orally. If this is the case the child should be constantly monitored by pulse oximeter while asleep. For older children a small amount of EMLA (lignocaine) cream can be placed on the skin by a suitable dressing as a local anaesthetic to reduce the pain of injection. The collection of radioactive urine in young children must be considered and a U-Bag can be attached to the child to collect any urine output at the time of the test.

There are individual requirements for the various types of scans, as discussed below.

Renal scans require that patients are hydrated, so that the images will reflect the natural physiology.

Most gastrointestinal investigations require the patient be starved for 6–8 h prior to the test and that they refrain from smoking for that period. The cardiac patients also need to starve for 6 h for myocardial perfusion scans. They must be caffeine free for 24 h prior to the test and should refrain from taking beta blockers for 48 h prior to a stress test. These patients will be given a thorough explanation on arrival and a consent form must be signed in some departments. There will be full ECG and BP monitoring throughout their stress testing. As with the other imaging modalities the patient needs to remove metallic objects, e.g. jewellery, belt buckles, etc., as these will appear as artefacts on the scan. However, the patient does not need to remove clothing. In many cases it is necessary to know the weight of the patient prior to the scan. In children the dose will be adjusted according to weight and any supplementary drug injections will always be given according to weight.

## Angiography

Angiography is an invasive procedure and therefore informed consent is required from the patient before the examination may take place. A history should be taken to clarify any possible complications of the use of contrast media. Relevant pre-examination tests should be organised, e.g. a full blood count may be necessary and the patient screened for hepatitis B and other infectious diseases, the blood clotting index assessed for certain interventional procedures (PTCA) and a chest radiograph to demonstrate the aortic arch when planning the catheterisation of arteries associated with the heart and aortic arch.

The patient will normally starve for 6 h prior to the examination to ensure the stomach is empty and a full pubic shave is required for femoral catheterisation. The patient should receive sedation if it is thought necessary on the ward, and should be accompanied by the case records in order that these may be amended to record details of the procedure.

After conclusion of the procedure, pressure on the groin is maintained until haemostasis has been satisfactorily achieved. On the ward the patient must lie flat for the first 2 h, with pulse and blood pressure monitored at regular intervals. The puncture site should be observed for any potential haematoma.

The use of smaller diameter catheters has led to the practice of angiography on an outpatient basis and therefore careful explanation to the patient as to the after-care procedure to be followed on their return home is important.

## Patient Care and Preparation

### Ultrasound

Preparation for ultrasound examinations is mainly confined to general abdominal and early pregnancy investigations. All other procedures involving the infant head, neck, limbs, breast and other 'small part' investigations require only the application of coupling gel at the point of contact with the transducer. Ultrasound is thought not to carry any particular biological hazard; its use however, particularly in pregnancy, may give rise to anxiety and particular attention should be given to explanation and reassurance of the patient.

Preferably, all patients for abdominal ultrasound are prepared whenever time and clinical conditions allow. As abdominal scans will involve assessment of more than one organ, proper preparation is essential to avoid bringing the patient back for a repeat examination. For upper abdominal structures the patient is normally instructed to take nothing by mouth for at least 6 h prior to the examination. This will aid in the reduction of bowel contents and gas, providing the optimum conditions for successful imaging of the organs. The restriction of food should also have the effect of causing maximum dilatation of the gallbladder which is used as an important landmark in such investigations. When the gallbladder is the specific organ being investigated, the patient is also asked to refrain from smoking for some time before the procedure to ensure maximum dilatation of the organ.

For the pelvic organs and structures the patient is also required to drink at least half a litre of water, to be finished an hour before the examination, and not to empty their bladder until after the examination is completed. This will enable examination of the bladder and will provide an acoustic window for examination of deeper structures within the pelvis. Care must be taken that the patient is not overhydrated as this may lead to misdiagnosis of hydronephrosis. In this situation the patient is asked to micturate, following which they are re-scanned after a 10–15-minute interval. In the normal kidney, any overfilling of the kidney due to the back pressure created by a full bladder will be resolved within this time, as the kidneys are able to drain freely once the pressure has been removed.

### Barium and gastrointestinal studies

It is normal to ensure that the area of the GI tract under examination is, where possible, empty of contents so that the contrast agent will evenly coat the mucosal lining. This may be achieved by a combination of restriction of food and fluid intake, laxatives and colonic lavage. Suggested preparation and after-care specific to individual procedures will be found under the relevant examination. Specific pathologies, however, may lead to modification of these guidelines. Examples where routine preparation are modified may include diabetes or ulcerative colitis.

Diabetic patients should normally be examined first, particularly if they have a morning appointment. They are usually asked to refrain from taking their insulin if fasting, but asked to bring their insulin with them so that arrangements can be made for them to have breakfast immediately after completion of their examination.

### Computed tomography

Preparation for CT investigations is mainly confined to investigations of the abdomen where it is important to outline the normal gastrointestinal tract. Patients are also advised to have only a light meal before the examination. On arrival in the department they are given either a drink of dilute barium sulphate or a 2–5% dilute solution of Gastrografin.

For examinations involving the whole abdomen the patient is asked to drink a total volume of 900 ml of solution. This is normally administered in three stages, with the patient asked initially to drink 300 ml of solution and then asked to wait for 30 min, after which they are given a further 300 ml to drink. Again after a further 30-minute period the patient is asked to swallow the remaining 300 ml of solution. Immediately after the last drink, scanning is commenced. This three-stage approach has the effect of outlining the stomach and the remainder of the GI tract at the time of the procedure and thus stomach and loops of bowel can easily be distinguishable from surrounding organs and structures. If the pancreas or kidneys are the main organs of investigation, only 300 ml of solution is administered, following which scanning commences immediately. For pelvic investigations, 50–100 ml of dilute Gastrografin may be administered per rectum prior to scanning. For the female pelvis a tampon can be inserted into the vagina to provide a useful landmark on the resulting images. For a number of investigations, intravenous contrast media is used to enhance the vasculature of specific organs and to identify related tumours more clearly.

Comfortable padding and immobilisation devices are necessary for procedures where the patient will be required to lie still for prolonged periods. Careful rehearsing of breath-holding techniques is also important to ensure optimum imaging. For a number of procedures involving children or seriously ill patients, sedation or general anaesthetic may be necessary to ensure that the patient remains still for the procedure. In such cases all the necessary support equipment should be available, including an emergency trolley for cardiac or respiratory arrest. With patients transported by trolley and who are unable to move by themselves onto the imaging couch, suitable patient-transfer devices should be available to aid the safe transfer of patient onto the couch and back onto the trolley.

As CT is a relatively high radiation dose investigation, particularly in the abdomen, careful application of the pregnancy rule is necessary in respect of female patients of child-bearing age.

## Magnetic resonance imaging

The relatively high magnetic fields employed in MRI are such that any ferromagnetic metallic objects found near the scanner will be subject to attraction or deflection forces. It is important therefore to establish if a patient has any known metallic object or metallic implants lodged in their body. Such forces encountered may be sufficient to move or dislodge the metallic object or affect the software of implanted electromagnetic equipment.

Examples of contraindications are patients with cardiac pacemakers, implanted hearing devices, insulin and morphine implanted pumps and other electronically implanted devices. Also contraindicated are patients with known metallic aneurysm clips, certain aortic heart valves, metallic intraocular foreign bodies constructed of ferrous material and metallic shrapnel where it is lodged near vital blood vessels. Where there is any uncertainty of a metal object being lodged in the orbits or an old injury the patient should be X-rayed to ascertain the true situation.

Gone unrecognised, scanning of patients with such metallic objects in situ may have extreme implications. Before undergoing a MRI scan, therefore, the patient is asked to complete a thorough questionnaire which will hopefully alert the staff to any possible complications. An example of the content of a Patient Preparation Questionnaire is shown.

Additionally all metallic objects worn by the patient should be removed, as these may be subjected to the same magnetic field forces or alternatively cause unwanted imaging artefacts. To improve patient throughout, patients for appointments are asked to come for their scan wearing a track suit and wearing no metallic objects or carrying other personal effects such as credit cards or watches, as these too may be affected by the magnetic field forces.

The physical limitations of the scanner have to be borne in mind when consideration is given to scanning of obese patients or those with deformities which may prevent entry into narrow bore scanners. The success of the scan in respect of narrow bore type scanners will depend upon the co-operation of the patient and therefore explanation and assessment prior to scanning is of utmost importance. Gaining the confidence of the patient, particularly claustrophobic patients, is a major task for the radiographer. To help in this area, patients are frequently asked to bring a tape of their favourite music to help them relax and to distract their attention from noisy gradient switching. In high field strength scanners (1.5 T), ear protection should be worn both by the patient and those accompanying them in the scanner room.

General anaesthetic or sedation may be necessary in some patients and children, and careful planning of such sessions is necessary to overcome the special problems associated with the constraints of using standard equipment in the scanning room. The use of life support equipment in the scanner room is prohibited.

Although there are currently no recognised adverse biological effects associated with magnets up to 1.5 T, it is generally accepted that scanning in the first trimester of pregnancy is contraindicated.

**Example of Patient Preparation Questionnaire**
**(Seeking Yes/No answers)**

**Patient name** ____________________ **DOB** _______

**Address**

______________________________________

**Section A**

- Have you had a CT/MRI scan previously?
- Have you had any operations on your head?
- Have you had any operations on your spine?
- Have you had any operations on your chest or heart?
- Have you had any other operations involving the use of metallic clips or pins?

**Section B**

- Do you have a cardiac pacemaker?
- Do you have an aneurysm clip in situ?
- Is there a possibility of any metal in your eye?
- Have you ever had a shrapnel or bullet injury?
- Do you wear a false limb, calliper or brace?
- Do you wear dentures, a dental plate or hearing aid?
- Do you have any ear implants (e.g. cochlear)?

**For Females of Child-Bearing Age**

- Do you have any intrauterine contraceptive device or coil?
- Is there a possibility of you being pregnant?

**Section C**

**All metal worn or carried by the patient is to be removed.**

Pens, spectacles, keys, money, jewellery, watches, hairgrips, dentures, scissors, credit cards, hearing aids, bra, surgical supports. **YES/NO**

I understand the procedure of an MRI examination, I also understand the above questions.

I give permission for the use of an intravenous contrast agent if this is deemed necessary.

Patient's signature ____________________ Date _______

Witness's signature ____________________ Date _______

# 1 Introduction

## Instrumentation for Angiography

In order to gain access to a vessel a percutaneous puncture has to be made by an appropriate needle. The needles used for this purpose are of a general pattern, in that they consist of an inner stylet or obturator and an outer cannula. The purpose of the inner obturator is to prevent the cannula becoming occluded by tissue during insertion which could lead to the failure of blood flow from the vessel lumen, and thus the interluminal position of the needle unable to be confirmed. The inner lumen of the cannula should permit the introduction of an appropriately sized guide wire, usually 0.038 in. Recently the introduction of a plastic outer sheath to the metal cannula has become more widely used, as on removal of the inner metal components a flexible non-traumatic introducer is then available which may be advanced further into the vessel.

These introducers incorporate a one-way valve which permits the introduction of guide wires and catheters of different shapes and types during a procedure while minimising trauma to the vessel and preventing excessive blood loss. The general term applied to these introducers is a 'sheath'.

Guide wires are used to effect the introduction of catheters into vessels. They are radio-opaque and thus allow the operator to manoeuvre a wire through vessels to a specific location where the contrast medium will be delivered for maximum opacification of a vessel or organ under investigation.

Some manufacturers supply heparin-coated guide wires, though these are more costly and not widely used. The improvements in manufacturing technology has led to the ability to produce guide wires of very small diameters necessary for super-selective techniques and are of particular value in the practice of angioplasty of small vessels, e.g. coronary arteries. The construction of a guide wire consists of a central 'core' wire around which is wound an outer wire. The inner core may be fixed or movable. The wire must of necessity be atraumatic and this is achieved by the distal or leading end of the wire being 'floppy'. In the case of a movable core, this floppy end of the wire may be varied in length.

The wire may be straight or J shaped, with variable diameters for the J portion. The J wire presents a less traumatic profile and lessens the risk of subintimal entry of the wire during its passage through the vessel. A movable core J wire allows the possibility for the J portion of the wire to be straightened out, thus aiding the manoeuvrability with the vasculature.

The wire may be plain stainless steel or more usually Teflon coated. There is still a concern that Teflon is thrombogenic and on flexing of the wire Teflon particles may break away. However, the gain in lubricity of the wire by the coating of the Teflon is thought to outweigh the risk.

The various shapes available are numerous and have developed based on the experience of many workers, and it is beyond the scope of this book to discuss them in detail. The student is referred to other specialist references, including manufacturers' catalogues which contain illustrations of the catheters available, plus a description of the materials used in their manufacture.

Catheters are produced by the extrusion of the selected material under heat. This process has been further developed in order that the 'double' and 'triple' lumen catheters may be produced necessary for the incorporation of a balloon for their use in transluminal angioplasty.

The choice of the material will influence the manipulative characteristics of the catheter while in use, e.g. the flexibility and the 'torque'.

The torque capability of the catheter is the ability of the catheter to reproduce the movement (turning) of the proximal end of the catheter at the distal end in order to manipulate the catheter through the often tortuous vessels. This capability is often achieved by the incorporation of a 'braiding' in the wall of the catheter. This requirement has to be balanced against the need for flexibility of the catheter and therefore the selection of the materials is inevitably a compromise.

Other characteristics have also to be borne in mind in the construction, size of the internal and external lumen, length, 'memory' of the material of the catheter and the requirement of side holes.

The size of a catheter is usually expressed in French size, between 7F and 4F being the most common. The size of the catheter must enable the passage of contrast and other instrumentation as required by the technique and at the same time be as minimally invasive as possible. The improvements in manufacturing techniques have led to thin-walled catheters, enabling high flow rates to be achieved with smaller (5F) diameters.

The length of a catheter will be determined by its usage, since there is no point in having the catheter of an excessive length as this reduces the amount of control. Conversely, the catheter must be long enough to access the vessel or organ under examination adequately.

The memory of the material is the characteristic that allows the catheter to retain its predetermined shape during the procedure, which may require the catheter to be straightened out in order to effect its introduction into the vessel by the insertion of a guide wire. The effect of body temperature also has the potential to influence the 'plasticity' of the material.

Catheters may be produced with either a single end hole or with a number of side holes. The provision of side holes allows for the more uniform and greater distribution of contrast in a large vessel or cavity and avoids the 'jet' effect. However, in the selective catheterisation of smaller vessels it is desirable to have the single end hole, in order to visualise the distribution of the vessel and its tributaries and also for the introduction of instruments and materials, e.g. embolisation coils.

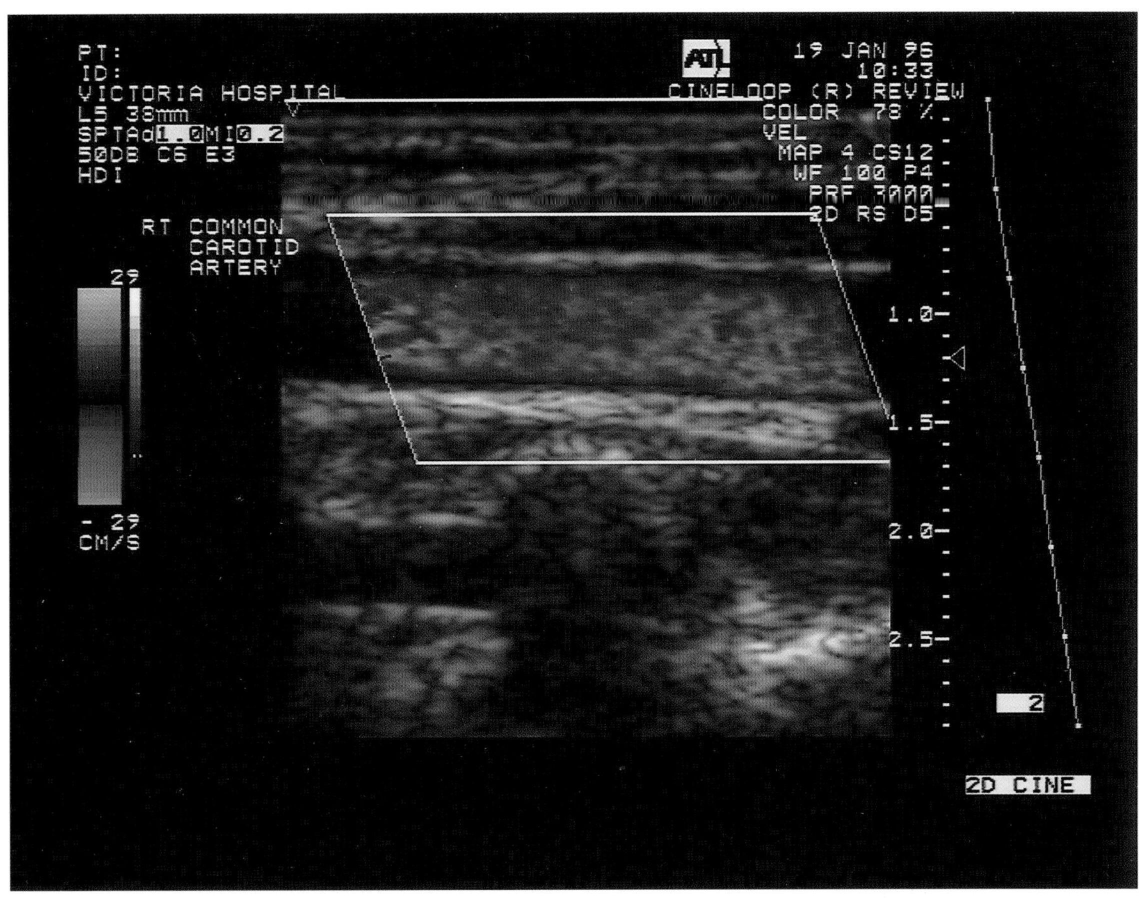


**Plate 1** Colour flow Doppler image of carotid artery (see text, page 29)

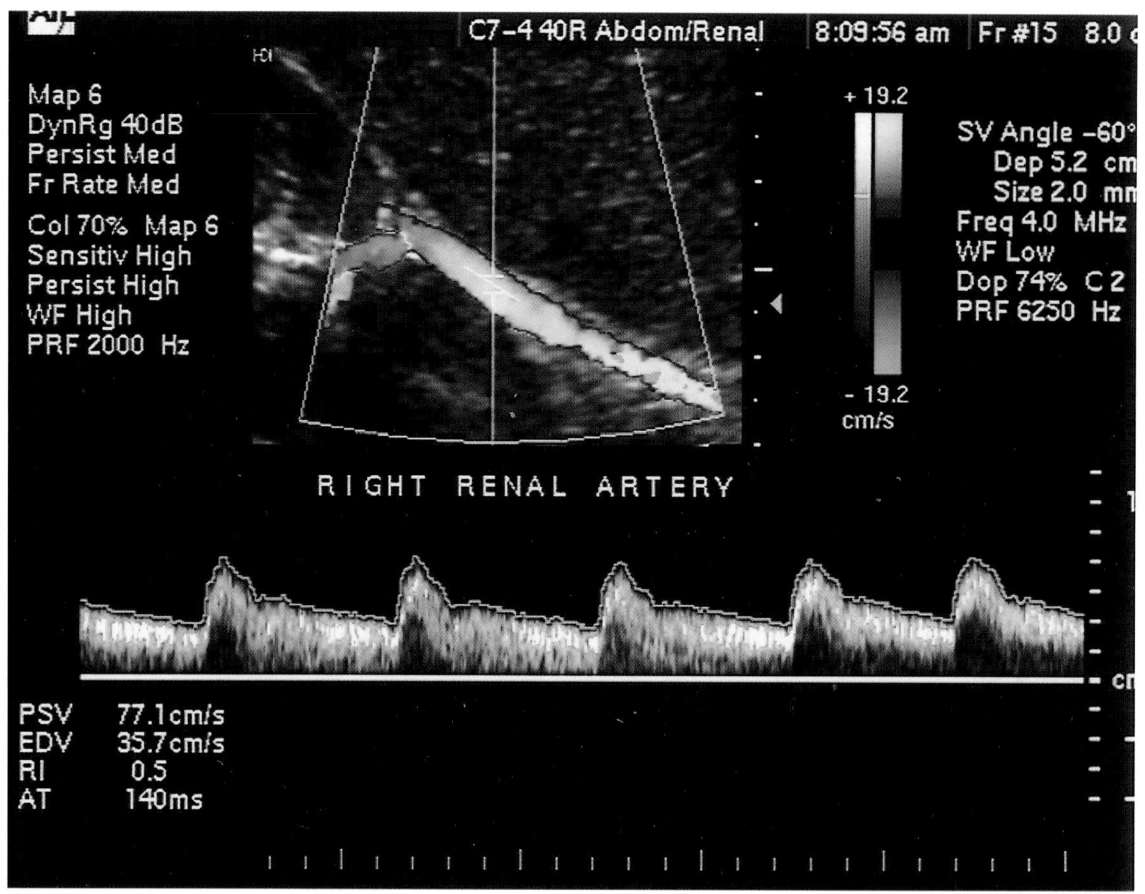


**Plate 2** Colour flow Doppler image and spectral analysis of blood flow in right renal artery (see text, page 209)

## Instrumentation for Angiography

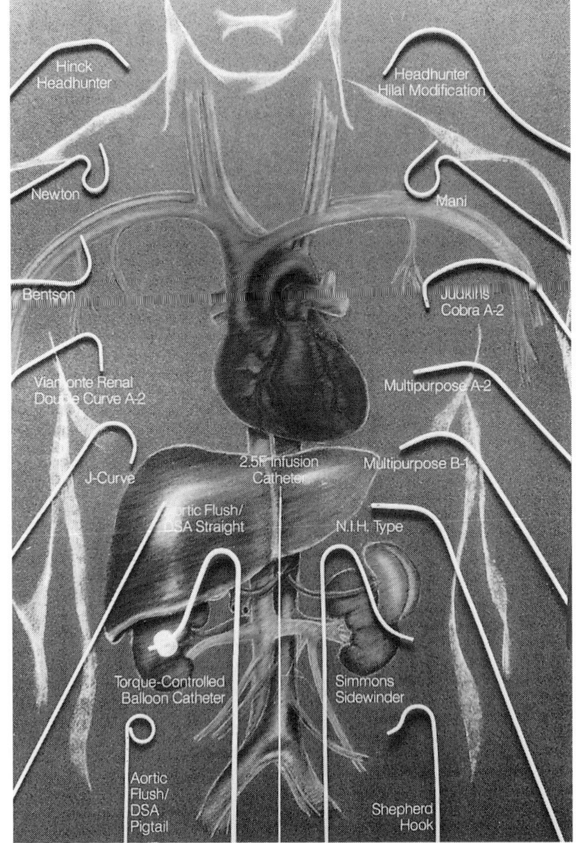


**Figure 1.32a** Chart showing typical types of angiography catheters (Courtesy of Cordis)

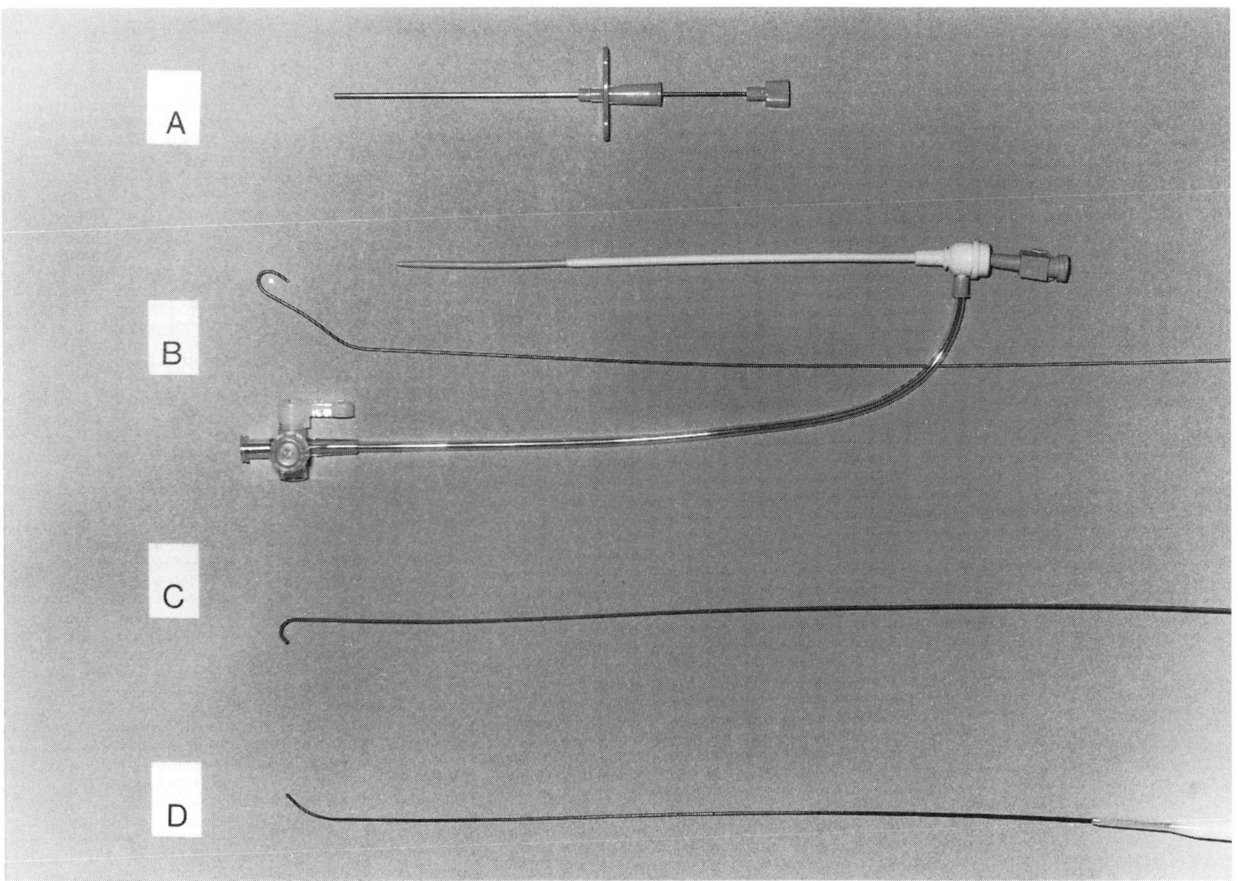


**Figure 1.32b** (A) arterial needle; (B) 6F sheath introducer system with short floppy J-tip guide wire; (C) guide wire with rigid J-shaped tip; (D) guide wire with flexible tip

## Automatic Contrast Injection Systems

The development of specialised vascular procedures has given rise to the need for controlled reproducible contrast media delivery. The availability of microprocessors has enabled systems to be developed that are extremely accurate and compact in structure. In its simplest form an injector is a pump system that will deliver a measured amount of contrast medium in a given period of time. There are of course many variables that make this simple task more complex (Table 1.5) and have given rise to the sophisticated systems that are now available. Consideration has to be given to:

- Volume of contrast medium required.
- Flow rate of contrast medium.
- Pressure limit of catheter.
- Viscosity of contrast medium.
- Time of start and duration of injection.

The volume to be injected must be accurately controlled. As it is to be delivered over a specific period of time, this will determine the flow rate necessary.

A number of external factors will affect the flow rate, including temperature and viscosity of the contrast medium, the internal diameter of the catheter (gauge) and the diameter of the vessel under examination. Modern injectors have a heating jacket, thermostat controlled, to warm and maintain the temperature of the contrast medium at body temperature for optimum viscosity and flow rates. The required flow rate will determine the pressure (psi) that will be necessary.

These considerations are computed by the injector and limitations are imposed usually based on pressure, as this is the most critical factor in the operation. For some types of injectors the maximum pressure permitted for the catheter, together with the volume and flow rate required, are selected with the injector software determining the pressure necessary to inject at the flow rate selected.

Systems are available that will provide multiple injections with delayed or advanced timing functions in relation to the image acquisition programme.

Double-headed systems are available that permit the injection of contrast to be followed by an infusion of saline. These have proved to be of particular value in CT enhancement and in digital subtraction angiography.

A mechanical safety device will be found on all injectors to prevent an accidental excess volume of contrast medium being injected should the electronic control system fail. This volume can be critical and therefore a mechanical stop device is incorporated to limit physically the injection to the set volume. When loading the syringe, it is important that the syringe and extension lines are free of air bubbles.

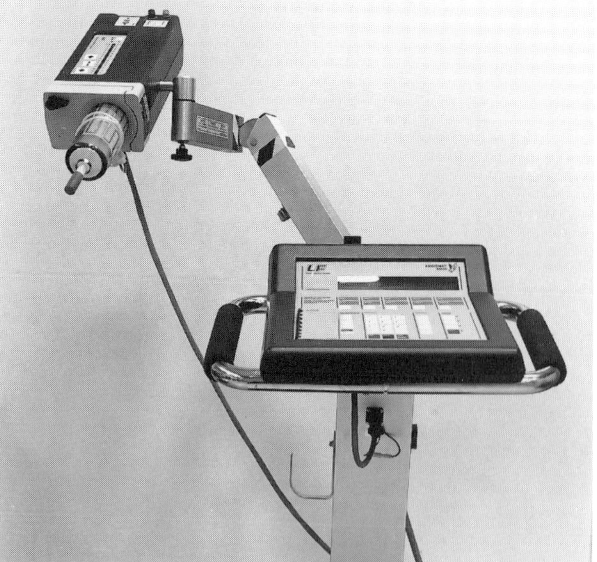

**Figure 1.33a** Typical contrast injector

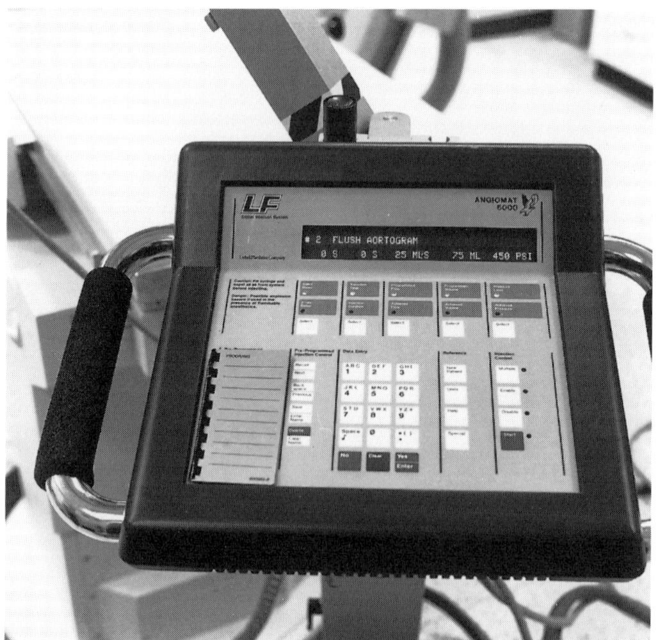


**Figure 1.33b** Control panel showing injection parameters

**Table 1.5 Typical range of injector parameters**

| *Parameter* | *Range* |
|---|---|
| Volume | 0.5–60 ml or 0.5–150 ml in increments of 0.1 ml |
| Flow rate | 0.3–50 ml/s<br>1.0–59 ml/min<br>1.0–59 ml/h |
| Linear flow rise/fall times | 0–9.9 s in 0.1 s increments |
| Catheter pressure limiting selection | 1–1400 psi |
| Injector delay | 0–99.9 s |

# 2

# CONTRAST ENHANCEMENT AGENTS

## CONTENTS

# 2 Contrast Enhancement Agents

## Introduction

The term 'contrast enhancement agents' is used in preference to the more traditional 'radiographic contrast medium'. It encompasses both radiographic contrast agents and those agents used in ultrasound and MRI and radiopharmaceuticals used in RNI.

There are two main types of radiographic contrast media, low-density (negative) and high-density (positive). In some examinations the low-density agents, e.g. air, oxygen and carbon dioxide, may be employed as a means to outline internal organs, but the use of negative agents as the sole contrast provider has been largely replaced by the other less invasive modalities, ultrasonography, CT and MRI.

Thus gynaecography, retroperitoneal pneumography, air encephalography and diagnostic pneumoperitoneum are being performed less and less frequently, if at all, while the use of high-density or positive-contrast agents containing either barium or iodine used in X-ray examinations and more specially developed 'contrast agents' in ultrasound and MRI is increasing.

There are various barium sulphate preparations used largely, if not exclusively, for the gastrointestinal tract and iodine preparations for the kidneys, gallbladder, cardiovascular system, pancreatic ducts, lymphatic system, and spinal cord. The iodine preparations are either water-soluble or fat-soluble compounds. Only the water-soluble compounds are used for intravenous or intra-arterial injections.

Preparations for ultrasound and MRI are of a specialised nature and will be discussed later.

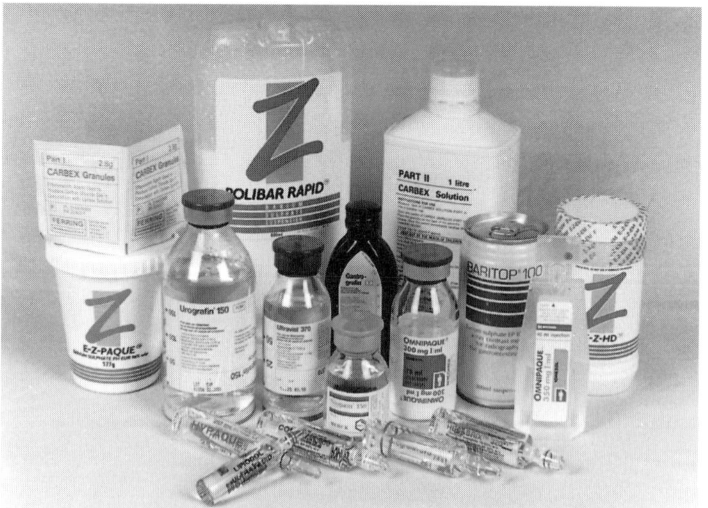


**Figure 2.1** Various types of radiographic contrast media available

**Table 2.1 Atomic numbers and densities**

| *Material* | *Effective atomic number* | *Electron density* |
|---|---|---|
| Air | 7.2 | very low |
| Soft tissue | 7.6 | ≈ 1 |
| Bone | 13.8 | ≈ 2 |
| Iodine | 53 | ≈ 2 |
| Barium | 56 | ≈ 2 |

## Physical Principles of Radiographic Contrast Media

Not all body structures can readily be demonstrated by plain radiography. This may be because their attenuation values are similar to adjacent structures or because there are overlying structures. The amount by which an X-ray beam is attenuated depends on four factors: the thickness of the material, its atomic number, density and the energy of the X-ray beam (keV). In tissues the term 'effective atomic number is sometimes used to indicate an 'average' of the atomic numbers present in their constituent proportions. It is possible however to alter the attenuation of either the structure itself or its surroundings by the introduction of so-called contrast agents.

Contrast agents are substances which contain elements that possess an atomic number or have an electron density which differs significantly from that of surrounding structures (Table 2.1).

# Physical Principles of Radiographic Contrast Media

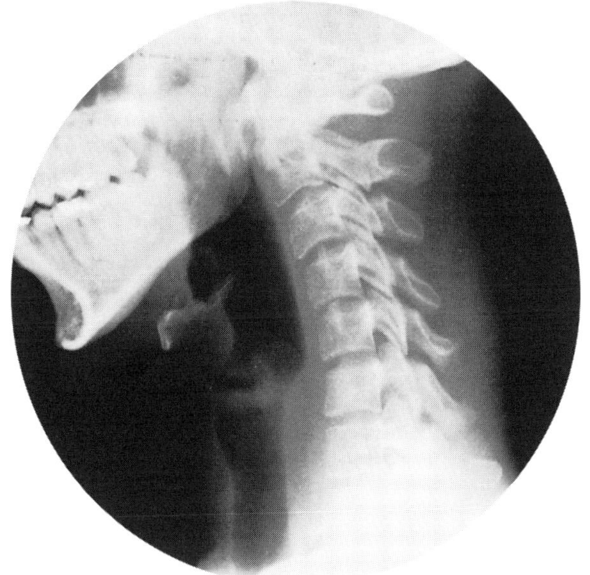

**Figure 2.2a** Use of Valsalva technique to demonstrate soft tissue structures in the neck

## Negative contrast agents

The term 'negative contrast agent' is used to indicate a substance which has lower attenuation than its surroundings. Examples are gases, including air and carbon dioxide. The reduced attenuation of the X-ray beam produces an area of increased density on the resultant radiograph or increased light intensity on the conventional fluoroscopic image.

Air can be introduced into cavities within the body, e.g. joint spaces in arthrography. It is also used in the soft tissue examination of the neck when the patient is instructed to perform the Valsalva technique to increase the volume of air in the trachea.

Air is absorbed more slowly than carbon dioxide and is used in preference to carbon dioxide when examination times are extended.

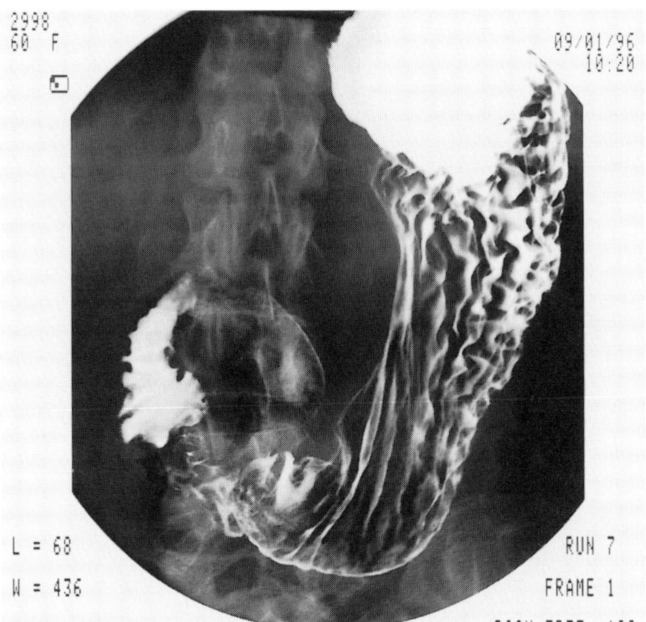


**Figure 2.2b** Image of double contrast barium meal

## Positive contrast agents

The term 'positive contrast agent' is used to indicate a substance which has relatively higher attenuation than its surroundings. Examples include iodine- and barium-based compounds. The increased attenuation of the X-ray beam results in areas of reduced density on the resultant radiograph or decreased light intensity on the conventional fluoroscopic image.

Iodine-based compounds may be introduced intravenously, intra-arterially, orally, rectally or within cavities. Barium compounds are normally introduced orally or per rectum.

Positive contrast agents are also used in CT to increase the Hounsfield number in the region of interest. This is useful in demonstrating vasculature and to distinguish between adjacent structures of similar absorption values.

Positive and negative agents may be used together to produce a double contrast technique, e.g. in the gastrointestinal tract.

# 2 Contrast Enhancement Agents

## Physical Principles of Radiographic Contrast Media

### Physical principles

X-ray attenuation is dependent on the energy of the incident beam. The degree of attenuation achieved by the use of contrast agents can therefore be increased by manipulation of the exposure factors, in particular the kilovoltage.

At lower values of kilovoltage it is the photoelectric absorption process which predominates. The relationship between the mass attenuation coefficient for photoelectric absorption and atomic number is complex. It is conventional practice in radiography, however, to accept that it is proportional to the cubed value of the atomic number of the attenuating material and inversely proportional to the cube of the energy of the X-ray beam:

$$\frac{\tau}{\rho} \propto \frac{Z^3}{E^3}$$

Positive contrast agents are normally used to increase the value of the atomic number of an anatomical structure with respect to its surroundings. Thus the use of lower values of kilovoltage will increase the attenuation of the X-ray beam by a greater degree in these structures. This produces an increased tissue differentiation on the resultant radiograph (i.e. objective contrast is increased).

As the energy of the X-ray beam increases, i.e. at higher values of kilovoltage, the relative importance of the photoelectric process of absorption reduces and the process of Compton scattering increases.

Compton scatter results in partial absorption of the energy of the X-ray beam and is dependent on electron density (rather than atomic number). Again the relationship between the mass attenuation coefficient for Compton scatter and electron density is complex. It is, however, conventional practice in radiography to accept that it is directly proportional to electron density and inversely proportional to the energy of the X-ray beam:

$$\frac{\sigma}{\rho} \propto \frac{\text{Electron density}}{E}$$

Negative contrast agents (gases) have an atomic number similar to that of soft tissue, but their electron densities are very markedly different (see Table 2.1). Thus the use of higher kilovoltages will reduce the attenuation of the X-ray beam where a negative contrast agent is present. This results in increased tissue differentiation on the resultant radiograph (i.e. objective contrast is increased).

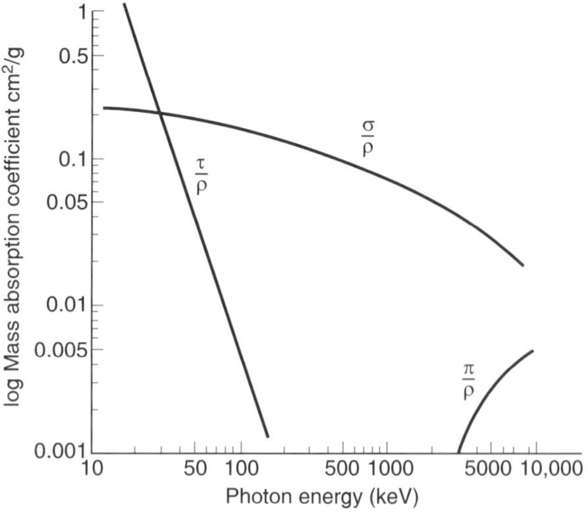


**Figure 2.3a** Variation in log mass absorption coefficient with photon energy – for water: ($\tau/\rho$, photoelectric process; $\sigma/\rho$, Compton process; $\pi/\rho$, pair production)

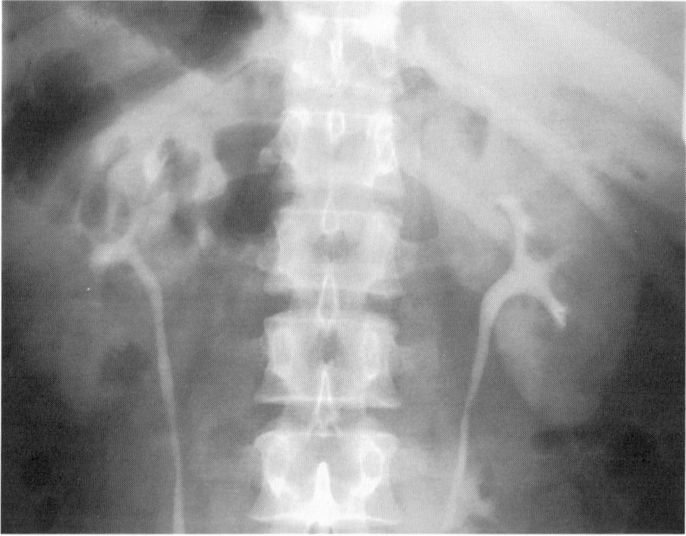

**Figure 2.3b** Image of positive contrast agent with low kVp – IVU

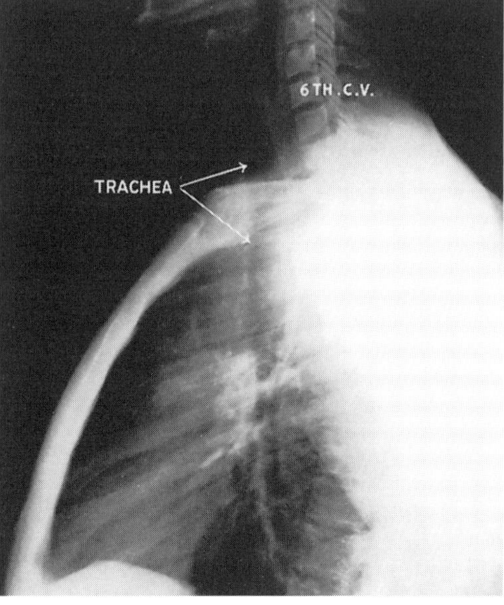


**Figure 2.3c** Image of negative contrast agent with high kVp – thoracic inlet

## Pharmacology

Pharmacology may be defined as 'the science of the nature and properties of drugs in relation to their action on the body'.

This is a vast subject and can only be dealt with briefly in this chapter. The subject however may be considered under three distinct areas:

- Pharmacodynamics – what the drug does to the body by considering the actions and effects of the drug.
- Pharmacokinetics – what the body does to the drug by considering the absorption, distribution, biotransformation and excretion of the drug.
- Toxicology – the adverse effect of drugs by considering the different mechanisms and actual side-effects which are manifested in the body.

This chapter, however, will concentrate on the toxic effects of enhancement agents and will only briefly deal with pharmacodynamic and pharmacokinetic issues.

## Toxicology

Contrast enhancement agents should ideally have no effects at all on the body except to enhance the anatomical structures or vessels under investigation from those of surrounding structures. Any pharmacological effect is unwanted and is the result of a toxic effect related to one or more mechanisms associated with contrast agents.

Toxic effects may be considered under three main headings:

- Chemotoxicity.
- Osmotoxicity.
- Electrical charge (ionicity).

Toxic effects from modern agents are rare and may be classed as being:

- Minor – with nausea, vomiting, flushing, pain at the injection site or a mild rash.
- Moderate – with severe urticaria, hypotension, bronchospasm and facial oedema.
- Severe – with laryngeal oedema, hypotensive shock, respiratory or cardiac arrest.

Osmotoxic potential effects may also be expressed as the osmotoxicity ratio (OTR) ranging as shown:

- OTR 1 – isotonic solution.
- OTR 2 – low osmolar contrast media.
- OTR 5–7 – conventional ionic high osmolar media.

### Chemotoxicity

These are effects related to the toxicity of the contrast molecule itself which differ from the other properties of the contrast media such as osmolality and electrical charge. The factors related to such events include hydrophilicity, lipophilicity, histamine release, protein binding, and the inhibition of biological function such as coagulation, etc. Most frequently, high chemotoxicity will clinically be demonstrated as high frequencies of nausea and vomiting.

Specific body toxic effects include those of nephrotoxicity which are disturbances of the renal function and of neurotoxicity which are disturbances of the nervous system.

### Hydrophilicity and lipophilicity

The hydrophilicity of a contrast agent describes its preference for aqueous solvents, whereas lipophilicity describes preference for fat-like (lipid) solvents.

Contrast agents with a relatively higher degree of lipophilicity seem to have a greater risk of toxic effects compared with those which are more hydrophilic. Ionic contrast media are relatively more lipophilic compared with non-ionic media which are considerably more hydrophilic.

The hydrophilicity of a non-ionic agent is enhanced by a more symmetrical distribution of hydrophilic hydroxyl groups and a lack of hydrophobic methyl groups associated with the molecular structure. The degree of lipophilicity is assessed by adding equal parts of water and *n*-butanol (a fat-like organic solution) to a small quantity of contrast medium. After shaking the mixture well, the solvents are allowed to separate into two layers, following which the amount of contrast medium dissolved in each solution is measured. The ratio of the amount of contrast in the *n*-butanol solution to the amount in the water layer is termed the partition coefficient. A high partition coefficient represents a solution with a high degree of lipophilicity compared to one with a low coefficient.

One of the significant moves in the direction of lower toxicity in non-ionic contrast agents has come about by the emplacement of hydroxyl groups within the molecule. These groups confer a high degree of hydrophilicity to the compound with a subsequent lowering in the lipophilicity. The resulting effect may be shown by studying the relative $LD_{50}$ values (see next page) for the non-ionic compounds.

### Histamine release

The release of histamine is characteristic of any allergic reaction and is associated with some contrast media reactions. Such an allergic-type reaction is linked to a property of mast cells located throughout the connective tissue, especially near capillaries (e.g. pulmonary system), and granulocytes in the blood. The non-ionic agents cause less allergic reactions than the ionic agents.

# 2 Physical Principles of Radiographic Contrast Media

## Pharmacology

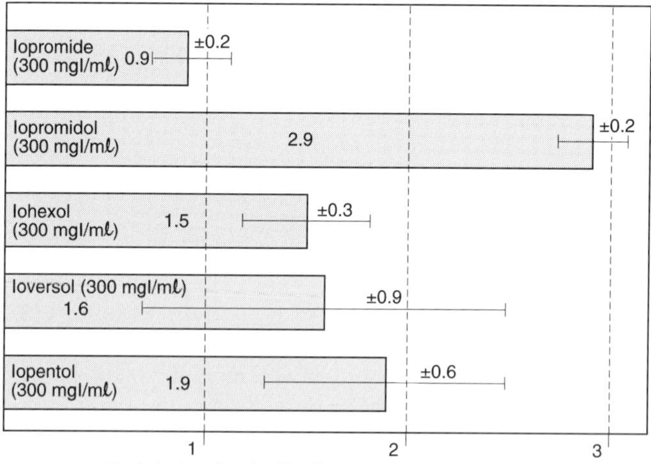


**Figure 2.4** Comparative protein binding of monomeric non-ionic contrast media (Courtesy of Schering Health Care Ltd)

### Protein binding

A certain amount of the contrast medium injected into the blood stream will become bound to the plasma protein in the blood stream. The degree of protein binding can be expressed in percentage terms and may be demonstrated graphically to compare the protein binding percentages of different contrast media. It is important to note that those agents which become protein bound will be excreted by the liver and those which are not bound will be excreted by the kidneys. Agents used for IVU and vascular examinations are formulated to be excreted by the kidneys rapidly, although it is recognised that ionic contrast media, compared with the non-ionic contrast media, have a higher protein binding percentage. Agents used to demonstrate the gallbladder and the biliary ducts are formulated to become bound to plasma proteins.

Agents with a higher degree of protein binding tend to produce a greater risk of toxic side-effects.

### $LD_{50}$

This symbolises the median lethal dose and is used to indicate the dose of a compound that results in the death of 50% of the test animals used in an experiment. Hence the higher the $LD_{50}$ value of a contrast agent, the less toxic it is. The dose of a contrast medium is usually expressed in the form of grams of iodine per kilogram of the animal's weight. For modern iodine contrast media, which are well tolerated, the value of the $LD_{50}$ will be high. $LD_{50}$ data are used to compare different types of contrast media. The lowest $LD_{50}$ data published for various non-ionic contrast media in mice studies are quoted greater than 21 g iodine/kg.

### Thyroid gland uptake

Following injection of iodinated contrast agents some iodine is extracted by the thyroid and it may take up to 20 weeks for this iodine to be eliminated. Certain radionuclide imaging procedures involving the thyroid may be affected if contrast is injected into the blood stream prior to such tests.

### Osmotoxicity

Osmotoxicity refers to the toxic effect which is related to the osmolality of a contrast media.

All biological membranes have the property known as semi-permeability, which is the ability to allow water and other small molecules to pass freely through them, but not to allow the passage of large molecules in solution in the water through them. The process of osmosis will inevitably be taking place at blood cell and contrast loaded blood plasma interfaces when the osmolality of the contrast media exceeds that of the blood cells. With high particle concentrations of contrast in the plasma, water will gradually be drawn from cells across their semi-permeable membranes.

High osmolar contrast media have a strong osmotoxicity, while low osmolar contrast media have only very low osmotoxicity, and isotonic solutions have no osmotoxicity at all.

Clinical effects that can be attributed to osmotoxicity are feelings of warmth during injection, reduced peripheral resistance creating hypotension, rigidification of erythrocytes affecting blood pressure and pulmonary function. Other significant effects include damage to the blood–brain barrier, renal damage and disturbance of electrolyte balance in small children.

### Osmolality

The osmolality of a solution is basically dependent on the number of particles dissolved in it. The osmotic pressure exerted by the same solution will depend therefore on the concentration of dissolved particles. The osmolality is therefore expressed in terms of its concentration of particles (osmoles) per unit weight (kilograms) of solvent. In clinical medicine this is expressed in milliosmoles per kilogram of water (mosm/kg$H_2O$).

Ionic contrast will dissolve as an anion and a cation, while the non-ionic contrast media will go into a non-dissociated molecular solution (Table 2.2). This means that an ionic monomer contrast media will have an iodine to particle ratio of 3:2, with a non-ionic monomer which does not ionise in solution having an iodine to particle ratio of 3:1. An ionic dimer in solution ionises into two particles and will have an iodine to particle ratio of 6:2.

A non-ionic dimer which does not ionise in solution will have an iodine to particle ratio of 6:1.

As the osmolality depends on the number of particles in solution, it can be seen that an ionic monomer should theoretically have twice the osmolality at a given iodine concentration of the non-ionic monomers and ionic dimers. Similarly, non-ionic monomers and ionic dimers should theoretically have twice the osmolality of that of the non-ionic dimers with the same iodine content. The non-ionic dimers are isomolar with blood and body fluid at all clinical concentrations.

The benefits of such isomolar contrast media are that they have no osmolality-related side-effects.

**Table 2.2 Comparative chart of contrast media showing iodine concentration, osmolality and viscosity (Courtesy of Schering Health Care Ltd)**

| *Type* | *Composition* (w/v %) | | *Iodine* (mg/ml) | *Osmolality* (mosmol/kg) | *Viscosity* (cps at 37°C) |
|---|---|---|---|---|---|
| High osmolar ionic monomer | Sodium iothalamate | 54% | 325 | 1843 | 2.75 |
| | Meglumine diatrizoate | 65% | 306 | 1530 | 5.0 |
| Low osmolar ionic dimer | Meglumine ioxaglate | 39.3% | 320 | 580 | 7.5 |
| | Sodium ioxaglate | 19.65% | | | |
| Non-ionic monomer | Iopamidol | 61.2% | 300 | 616 | 4.7 |
| | Iohexol | 64.6% | 300 | 640 | 6.3 |
| | Ioversol | 63.6% | 300 | 645 | 5.5 |
| | Iopromide | 62.3% | 300 | 610 | 4.6 |
| Non-ionic dimer | Iotrolan | 64.1% | 300 | 320 | 8.1 |
| | Iodixanol | 65.2% | 320 | 290 | 11.4 |

# 2 Physical Principles of Radiographic Contrast Media

## Pharmacology

### Ionic and non-ionic contrast media

The development in the 1950s of the tri-iodinated benzene ring gave rise to the formulation for the modern iodinated intravascular agents used today. It is important, however, to distinguish between two quite distinct groups of these compounds: ionic, possessing electrical charge, and non-ionic, which have no electrical charge.

**Ionic media**

The ionic media, sometimes referred to as conventional agents, are based on the tri-iodinated benzene ring possessing radicals. Typically they consist of one molecule (monomer) which dissociates in solution into two particles, a large negatively charged ion (anion) containing three iodine atoms and a positively charged ion (cation) which is either sodium or meglumine or a combination of both.

As described earlier, ionic contrast media will have a high osmolality and therefore to reduce the osmolality and the degree of side-effects associated with this phenomenon another type of ionic agent was formulated consisting of two molecules (dimer) joined together. The dimer anion, consisting of six atoms of iodine compared with a monomer anion with three iodine atoms with the same iodine concentration, will have half the osmolality. This is because only half the number of dimer anions are required to produce the same iodine concentration as monomer ions, hence halving the number of particles in solution.

**Non-ionic**

The non-ionic media differ from the ionic group in that they do not ionise in solution. The development of such agents in the 1970s was accomplished by replacing the cation radical portion of the benzene ring with a non-dissociating organic chain. Typically such agents have one molecule and because they remain as one particle when dissolved in solution they possess half the osmolality. Such agents have considerably less toxic effects because of the reduction in osmolality and the elimination of acid groups ($COO^-$) and the emplacement of a large number of hydroxyl groups (—OH) which make them more hydrophilic.

At the time of writing a new non-ionic agent formulated with two non-ionic molecules linked together (dimer) with side chains attached has been produced which reduces even further the degree of osmolality to that of plasma.

The disadvantages of these agents are their cost and their viscosity because of the relatively large size of the molecule. To reduce the viscosity the media should be warmed to body temperature.

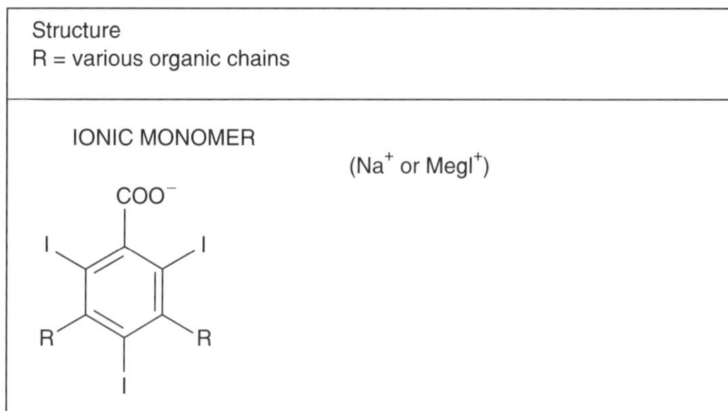


**Figure 2.5a**

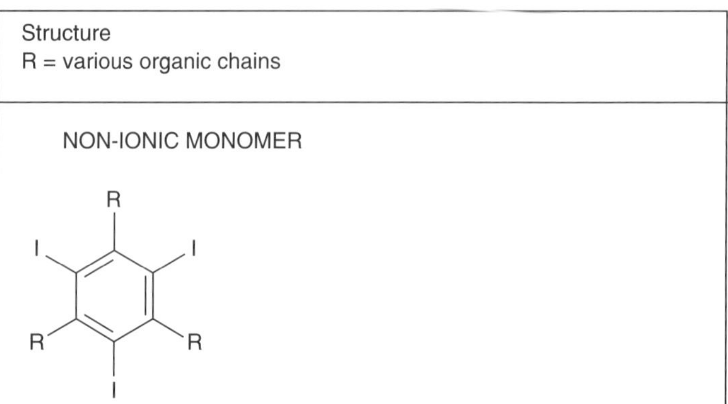


**Figure 2.5b**

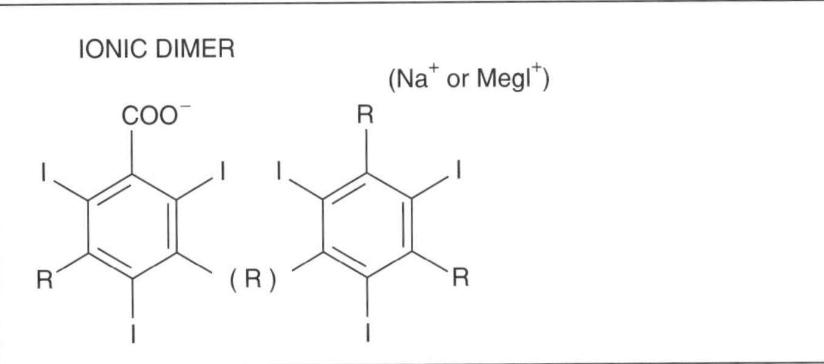


Figure 2.6a

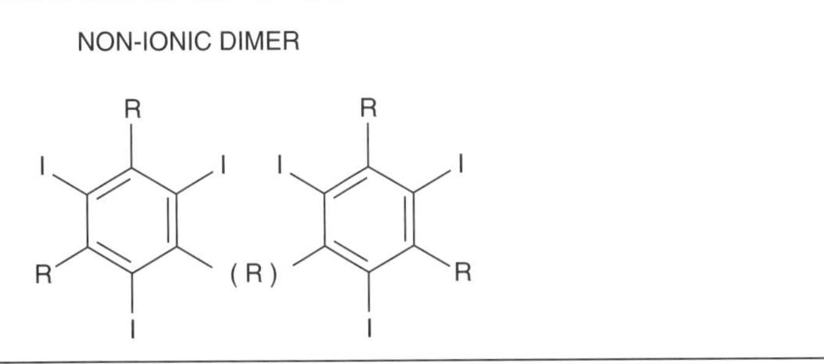


Figure 2.6b

# Physical Principles of Radiographic Contrast Media 2

## Applications of Iodinated Contrast Media

### Vascular

Intravascular contrast media are used to examine both vascular anatomy and the delineation of organs and associated pathology. Their use may be considered under two headings:

- Intravenous, e.g. IVU, CT enhancement, etc.
- Intra-arterial, e.g. angiography, digital subtraction angiography (DSA), etc.

In selecting an agent it is important that in the ideal situation there should be no toxic effect as a result of a pharmacological action, as the sole purpose of the drug is to act as a diagnostic aid. In this instance the radiological efficacy of the examination is achieved without any direct activity on the body, apart from the requisite blood flow for the transportation of the contrast media within the vascular system.

The concentration of the contrast media selected is based on the anatomical region of interest, the prevailing pathology and the sensitivity of the imaging system.

Contrast media concentrations range from 140 to 370 mgIodine/ml (mgI/ml). It is important to select the optimal concentration and volume in order that the vessel, organ or pathology is adequately opacified, but at the same time any toxic risk is minimised. The quantity administered will depend on the above concentration considerations in conjunction with the manufacturer's recommendations in relation to body weight. This information will be found on the data sheet and package insert which are provided by the manufacturer as required by law.

The vascular use of contrast agents should be undertaken with due regard for their potential to affect the normal physiology of the subject and careful attention should be paid to contraindications, precautions and warnings issued.

The route of administration, intravenous or intra-arterial, may determine the choice of medium, as it should be remembered that on intravenous injection the contrast will pass directly into the pulmonary circulation with minimal dilution and therefore potential exists for activation of mast cells and the subsequent release of histamine, one of the major precursors of anaphylactoid-type reactions.

This is predominantly seen when ionic compounds, whether of high or low osmolality, are used; therefore, non-ionic compounds should ideally be used.

In arterial use the direct effect on selected organs should be borne in mind and the relevant nephrotoxicity/neurotoxicity profiles of the contrast media are of major consideration, particularly where manifest vascular disease is present.

# 2 Physical Principles of Radiographic Contrast Media

## Applications of Iodinated Contrast Media

### Renal

The excretion of iodinated contrast media by the kidneys allows renal studies to be made by the intravenous route.

Visualisation of the renal tract occurs with no specific changes occurring to the contrast media, a fact that may be demonstrated by the total excretion of these compounds unchanged and with no metabolites detectable.

The absence of any change to the contrast media is mainly due to the lack of protein binding and a low molecular weight which enhances total excretion by the kidneys, which is by means of glomerular filtration and proximal tubule excretion. Any exchange of water taking place in the proximal tubules does so within the confines of natural physiological need. No contrast is reabsorbed in the distal tubules.

The interest in the nephrotoxocity of the contrast media has led to many studies to try to determine the safest dose levels and also to establish that non-ionic media have an advantage over the older ionic media.

It has proved very difficult to show specific advantages of non-ionic media by the study of conventional parameters, but more recent studies using measurements of the sensitive brush border enzymes have shown that these appear less affected by the non-ionic contrast media than the ionic media.

In terms of the comfort of the patient and in order to minimise the possibility of anaphylactic reaction, non-ionic contrast media should be used in renal studies. However, in cystography ionic contrast media is still used and acceptable where there is little risk of contrast agent absorption.

### Body cavities

The development of non-ionic compounds has led to the demise of the iodised oil contrast media. Examinations of body cavities are now performed using water-soluble non-ionic compounds. The improved endothelial tolerance makes them particularly suitable for examinations of ducts e.g. ERCP, and in areas of tissue sensitivity such as fistulae. Isomolar non-ionic dimers are particularly suitable for bronchography.

### Gastrointestinal

If, as a result of pathological disturbance to the GI tract, i.e. perforation or acute obstruction, barium is an unsuitable contrast medium, it is necessary to use a water-soluble contrast which may be absorbed and will not further complicate the existing condition.

It should be borne in mind when dealing with small infants for GI studies that the hyperosmolality of an ionic compound may be extremely dangerous, as the fluid balance of the child may be compromised. It is therefore becoming recommended practice that non-ionic contrast agents should be used in these cases.

Compounds which do exist for GI studies include those such as sodium diatrixoate, with a flavouring and wetting agent added, but in view of its hyperosmolality this should not be used if perforation or a fistula between the oesophagus and the trachea is believed to be present, as the effect of this material on the pulmonary tissues can be injurious.

The presence of barium sulphate may complicate the surgical management of these patients and therefore a water-soluble low osmolar compound is preferable, e.g. iopamidol with a flavouring agent added.

### Cholecystography and cholangiography

The oral cholecystographic agents are also tri-iodinated benzene ring derivatives with only two side chains, hence a vacancy in the molecular structure for protein binding. Such compounds are excreted by the liver and concentrated in the gallbladder after 12–14 h.

Intravenous cholangiographic contrast agents are meglumine dimer derivatives of a tri-iodinated benzene ring and are dibasic salts excreted by the liver. After injection these show in the bile ducts after a ½–1½ h and after 2–3 h accumulate in the gallbladder. The protein binding effect of these agents gives rise to the concern over their high toxicity and care should be exercised in the selection of patients. They should be injected slowly to judge for any reaction and to allow for maximum protein binding to take place which is necessary to ensure that they are totally excreted by the liver. The use of ultrasound has largely replaced this technique.

### Safety of vascular contrast media

The administration of any contrast medium should only be made after due consideration is given to the risk–benefit ratio. It is the responsibility of the personnel involved in the examination to acquaint themselves with the pharmacological contraindications, precautions and warnings given in the data sheet and package insert provided by the manufacturer.

Familiarisation with emergency procedures and the provision and location of emergency drugs is mandatory. Any serious reaction which may occur should be reported to the manufacturer and to the relevant authorities.

A full and careful explanation of the procedure to the patient, in conjunction with a full history taken of any possible risk factors, will do much to minimise the incidence of adverse events.

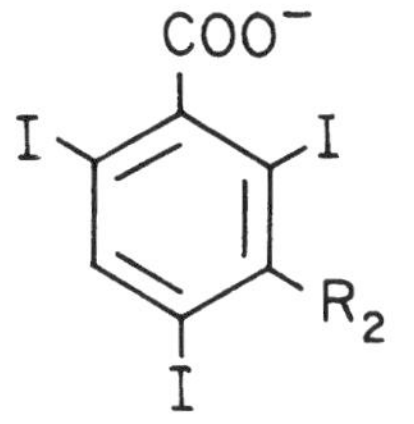

**Figure 2.7a** Oral cholecystographic contrast agent – tri-iodinated benzene ring derivative with two side-chains

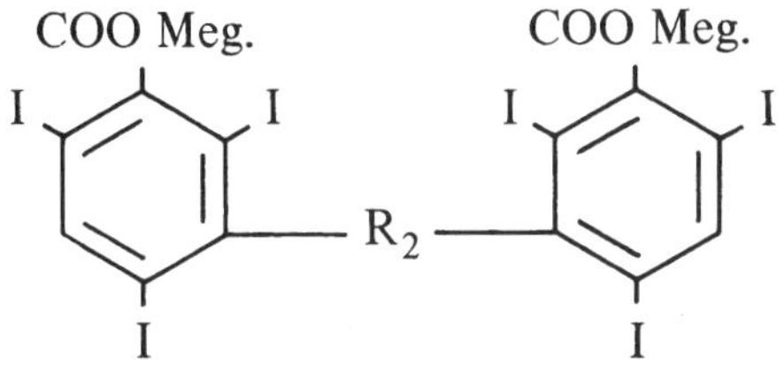

**Figure 2.7b** Intravenous cholangiographic contrast agent – megulamine (Meg.) dimer derivatives tri-iodinated benzene rings

## Applications of Iodinated Contrast Media

### Myelography

Myelography as a procedure is slowly being replaced by MRI. Nevertheless myelography and cisternography will continue to be practised for some years. It is therefore important to consider the nature of a contrast suitable for myelography.

These compounds should be non-ionic in nature, rapidly absorbed by the central nervous system and possess minimal neurotoxicity. The new non-ionic dimers may well have a role in myelographic examinations. They have the ability to reach higher iodine concentration levels while remaining isotonic in nature. This, together with their low neurotoxicity, makes these compounds particularly suitable for examinations of the central nervous system.

### Safety of intrathecal contrast media

The practice of myelography has been associated with particular risk factors both in the physical administration of the contrast and also in relation to the potential side-effects. Scrupulous observation of aseptic techniques is mandatory. The most common side-effect of myelography is post-myelographic headache which can be very severe and prolonged.

Hydration of the patient should be ensured prior to the commencement of the procedure and, very importantly, maintained afterwards.

The ward staff must be constantly reminded of this, as all too often a visit to the X-ray department is associated with the restriction of fluids.

The practice of outpatient myelography carries with it the responsibility of ensuring that the patient understands the importance of maintaining full hydration on return home.

Severe post-myelographic headache is often associated with vomiting which leads to further dehydration, and therefore fluid replacement intravenously may have to be undertaken.

The manufacturer's recommendations as to dosage should be followed, and information as to the side-effects and contra-indications carefully studied.

# 2 Contrast Enhancement Agents

## Barium Preparations

Barium preparations are available either as colloidal barium sulphate, which comprises a suspension of fine barium particles which stay evenly distributed, or more commonly as high-density barium sulphate, which comprises microscopically fine particles of varying size. This preparation results in a higher density and is more resistance to flocculation.

Barium sulphate is supplied either as a powder or in liquid form. The powder may come in large containers for multiple examinations or in a packet for each individual examination, which is subsequently made up to 100–130% weight/volume (w/v) suspensions or to 170% w/v for high-density (HD) preparations.

Liquid barium preparations are colloidal suspensions made up in 100% w/v concentrations. There are also aerated liquid suspensions in tins for double contrast barium meal examinations and individually packed plastic bags for barium enemas.

Barium examinations are performed either as a single or double contrast technique. The method used to obtain double contrast varies throughout the different regions of the GI tract. Swallowed air is used in the oesophagus, gas tablets for the stomach, methylcellulose water solution for the small bowel and air insufflation for the colon. The internal surfaces of these organs are shown by a thin layer of barium while being distended by gas. This produces a detailed view of the surface patterns.

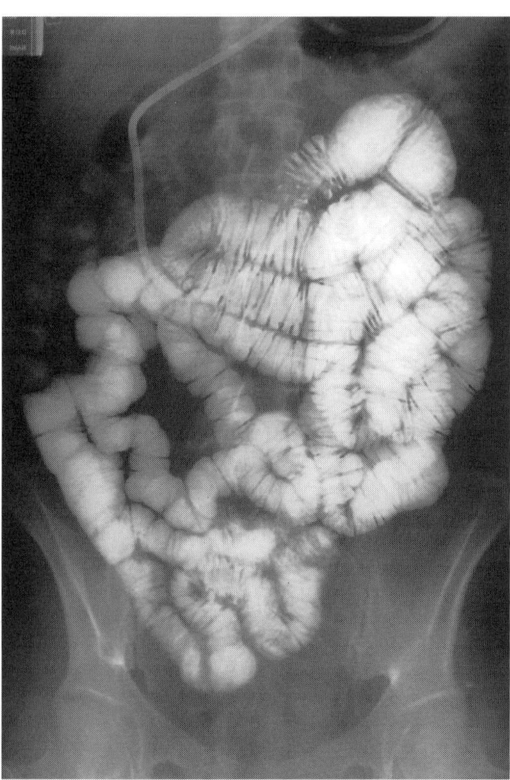

Figure 2.8a Small bowel barium enema

## Applications of Barium Preparations

Barium suspensions vary, dependent on the area of the GI tract under examination.

For single contrast barium examinations, 200–300 ml of 50% w/v barium sulphate is used. For the double contrast examination, either a special liquid barium incorporating a gaseous agent is used or powder is mixed as a 120–130% w/v suspension. Some high-density bariums are given as 170% w/v suspensions, lesser volumes being given, e.g. 120–200 ml. Gas granules, powder or tablets are swallowed just before the barium to produce the double contrast effect. These preparations contain citric acid and sodium bicarbonate which give off carbon dioxide in the stomach as they absorb water.

The small bowel enema technique introduces barium directly into the small intestine via a nasogastric tube. A barium suspension of specific gravity 1.27 is introduced and may be followed by either air or methylcellulose to produce a double contrast effect.

For single contrast barium enema examinations, a dilute barium preparation of approximately 50% w/v is used, 500–600 ml being required to fill the colon to the caecum. In double contrast studies, 100–120% w/v barium is used initially to fill the colon as far as the hepatic flexure. The barium is then drained and air is introduced in order to distend the colon and drive residual barium into the caecum.

The use of barium in the role of a bowel labelling agent (in CT) has led to the development of commercial preparations specifically formulated in order to achieve optimum density without artefacts. The use of water-soluble contrast agents is preferred by many workers as they allow for better control of concentration and are easier to administer.

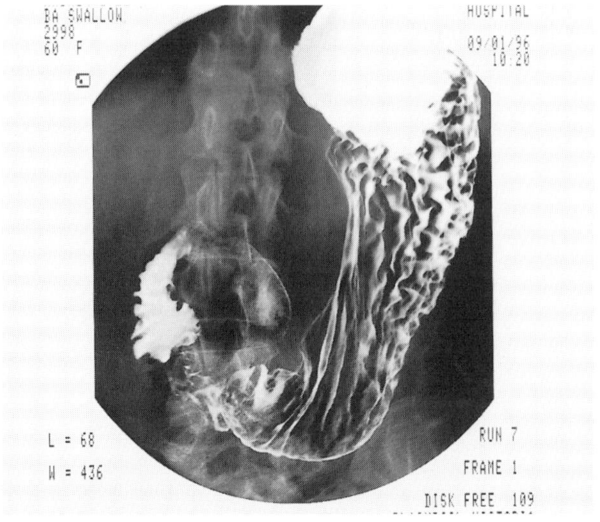


Figure 2.8b Double contrast barium meal

# Enhancement Agents for Magnetic Resonance Imaging

## Introduction

Magnetic resonance imaging has increased the diagnostic potential available to medicine and with the continuing development in both hardware and software this potential is seen to be even greater than first thought.

There remain, however, areas of diagnostic uncertainty and it is in these areas, as in conventional imaging, that the use of contrast media is of benefit.

Contrast media are pharmaceutical agents employed to alter image contrast. Image contrast relates to the signal intensity differences between two tissues, with contrast enhancement accentuating this difference.

MR contrast agents work by altering the magnetic environment (magnetic susceptibility of the local tissue) and are not directly visualised. This is unlike X-ray CT contrast agents which function by their ability to directly alter the image being additive to the normal tissue attenuation.

Although the need for i.v. MR contrast agents was debated in the early years of MRI, as this would make a non-invasive technique into an invasive study, it was soon realised that the use of such agents could increase the sensitivity, specificity and accuracy of the technique. This was particularly evident in the assessment of certain pathological processes, e.g. small meningiomas, intraspinal metastases, etc., which would be missed on non-enhanced studies.

The importance of the i.v. MR contrast agents (of which there are now a number produced) is shown by the current usage in assessment of the brain, spine and musculoskeletal pathology.

The development of suitable contrast media for MRI has posed a completely new set of problems for researchers, as the principle has to be based on the ability of the compound to influence the response of tissues when subjected to a magnetic field.

Many substances exist that possess inherent magnetic characteristics and the choice has to be based on the ability to produce these compounds in a physiologically acceptable form.

The criteria for such compounds is that they affect the following parameters:

- Proton density.
- Spin lattice relaxation time, $T_1$.
- Spin spin relaxation time, $T_2$.
- Flow.

The agents may also be classified in terms of visualisation:

- Directly visualised, e.g. water, lipids, and others which possess inherent contrast.
- Indirectly visualised, e.g. magnetic susceptibility compounds (including paramagnetic/superparamagnetic/ferromagnetic).

Of the directly visualised group it is the water and lipids occurring in tissue which comprise much of the natural contrast effects seen in MRI.

The introduction of water and lipids provides additional contrast to the image, although this has been restricted to use in body cavities.

Possible contrast agents are pharmaceuticals that change the water content of the body, e.g. diuretics. However, in view of the potential side-effects of these compounds and the limited contrast afforded, these are not practical to use. It is therefore the indirectly visualised group of compounds which are considered to be the most useful in MRI.

## Magnetic susceptibility

Magnetic susceptibility of a substance relates to the extent to which the substance is susceptible to magnetisation by an applied magnetic field. Paramagnetic, superparamagnetic and ferromagnetic substances have a magnetic effect (susceptibility) due to the presence of unpaired electrons within their structures. Superparamagnetic and ferromagnetic substances have a much greater magnetic susceptibility effect compared with paramagnetic agents. The difference between superparamagnetic and ferromagnetic substances is that the former, on removal from the external applied magnetic field (i.e. the magnet) do not retain their magnetic memory, unlike ferromagnetic substances.

It is perhaps of value at this stage to consider the difference between paramagnetic and ferromagnetic compounds.

Paramagnetic may be defined as pertaining to the property of any substance (excluding iron and other materials which attract a magnetic field very strongly) which displays a tendency to move to the strongest part of a non-uniform magnetic field. Ferromagnetic (superparamagnetic) substances are those which may be magnetised to a high degree, ultimately reaching saturation value and which possess a high magnetic permeability. Paramagnetic agents such as gadolinium may be considered for use as magnetic resonance imaging contrast.

Gadolinium is a rare earth metal possessing high relaxivity, i.e. an ability to alter relaxation times on adjacent protons in tissue. Paramagnetic media may be considered as 'positive' enhancement, increasing image intensity on $T_1$ weighted images. As the aforementioned metals are potentially toxic, it is necessary to bind them in a stable complex in the form of a chelate, in order that they are delivered in a physiological manner to the body.

## Enhancement Agents for Magnetic Resonance Imaging

These complexes remain intact until such time as the contrast is excreted from the body. Such complexes are DTPA (diethylenetriamine penta-acetic acid) and more recently a chelate of DTPA which is non-ionic. This is achieved by the addition of calcium sodium DTPA BMA. By using these calcium sodium ligands it is possible to reduce the overall osmolality and potential toxicity of the compound. It should be noted, however, that the change in osmolality is likely to have little effect, due to the small volume of contrast injected (typically 14 ml for a 70 kg person, giving a concentration of 0.1 mmol/kg body weight – equivalent to 0.2 ml/kg body weight).

The effect of these compounds is to shorten the $T_1$ of tissues and they are administered as an intravenous injection. They have been extensively used for the central nervous system and in the assessment of musculoskeletal pathology. Subsequent compounds are being developed to study other vascular areas, particularly the liver, biliary system, kidneys and the cardiovascular system.

Superparamagnetic contrast agents form another group of contrast agents. They influence the tissue $T_2$ signal, shortening this, thus producing a low signal intensity. It is appropriate, therefore, to consider such compounds as negative contrast agents. Superparamagnetic agents differ from ferromagnetic agents in their size and configuration; as was stated previously, ferromagnetic agents possess permanent magnetism. If, however, their size is substantially reduced the permanent magnetism is lost and they become superparamagnetic agents.

One such agent is magnetite. When the magnetite is presented in monodispersible spheres it may be used as an oral contrast agent for delineation of the GI tract. It should be remembered, however, that the objective of the exercise is not actually to outline the tract necessarily, but to act as a labelling agent in order that structures within the abdomen may be differentiated, e.g. duodenum from pancreas. These particles have very low absorption and therefore zero toxicity.

## Applications of MR Enhancement Agents

### Central nervous system (including spine)

Enhancement of the central nervous system constitutes the major usage of paramagnetic agents. The ability to differentiate between pathological and non-pathological areas has been demonstrated to increase the confidence level of diagnosis.

In tumours, the differentiation between oedema and active tumour is of particular value in diagnosis, as is the separation of abnormalities such as enhancing epidural fibrosis and non-enhancing disc.

### Musculoskeletal

Intravenous contrast media can be given in cases of suspected tumour or abscess collection. Injection of very dilute gadolinium chelate into joints may have a value in the early evaluation of the synovial surface in the early assessment of joint disease.

### Abdomen and pelvis

As regards MRI of the abdomen, the major problems are found to be with the artefacts which are produced by motion due to respiration, peristalsis and fat layers. A further problem exists in the abdomen in the homogenicity of appearance of the relative tissues. It is in this field that magnetite particles are of considerable value in the form of an oral compound which has the effect that has been previously stated for shortening $T_2$, therefore the image appearing to be black. These oral contrasts may also be extremely valuable in the pelvis for the assessment of lymph nodes and other structures lying within the pelvic cavity which may be difficult to differentiate from bowel.

The use of paramagnetic agents, in conjunction with mannitol, as abdominal agents has also undergone investigation.

New developments continue; among these are blood pool agents and liver specific agents with lipophilic complexes which can be take up by Kupffer cells. Both magnetite particles and derivatives of metals within the ferromagnetic and superparamagnetic groups are being studied for these purposes.

Other areas under consideration are monoclonal antibody bound paramagnetic complexes along with liposomes. Many substances exist which are known to have magnetic effects but their use is restricted by the requirement of safety and specificity.

### Cardiovascular

In terms of MRI in the heart, it is perhaps too early to make definitive assessment of the capabilities of contrast agents, although specific contrast agents are under research for this purpose. It has, however, been seen already that in severely damaged myocardial tissue the $T_1$ signal is shortened following i.v. gadolinium DTPA and therefore it may aid in the distinction between the infarcted and active myocardium.

Examination of the vascular system continues to be investigated and the role of contrast media in conjunction with ultra-fast sequences is proving to be very successful and provides a great challenge for the future.

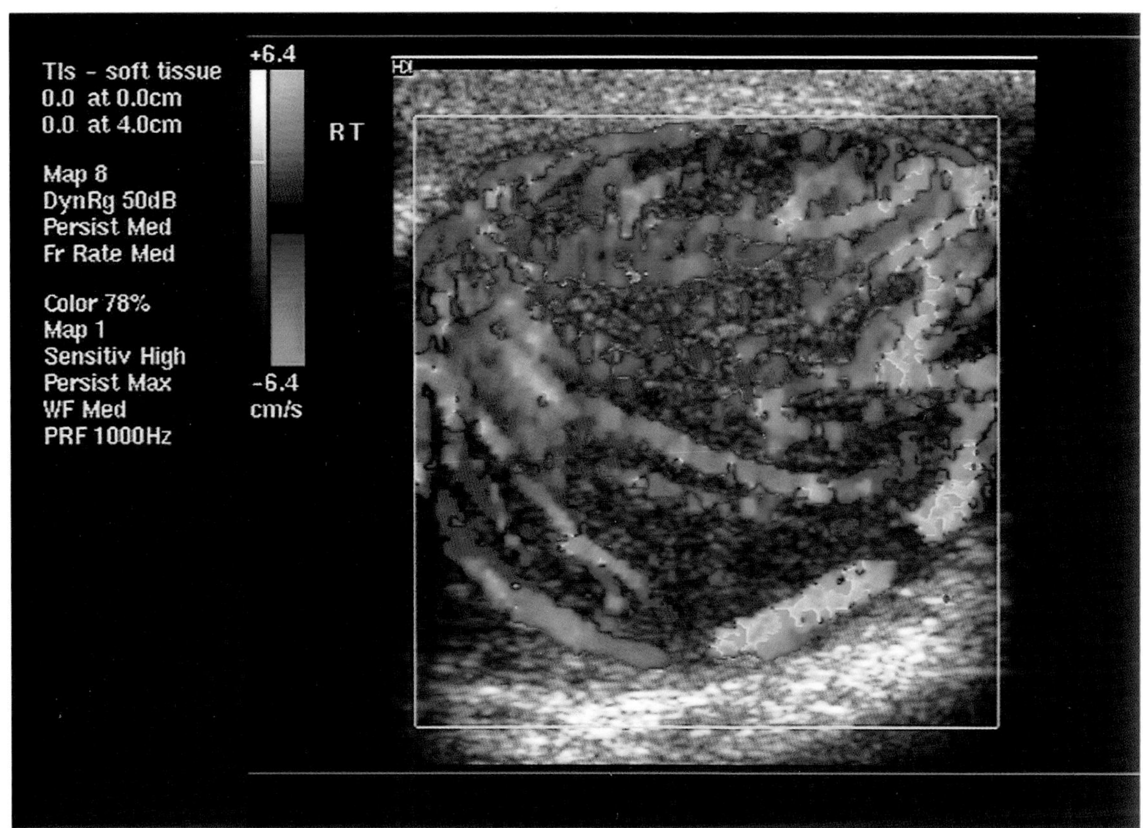


**Plate 3** Colour flow image showing increased blood circulation consistent with orchitis (see text, page 262)

## Enhancement Agents for Ultrasound

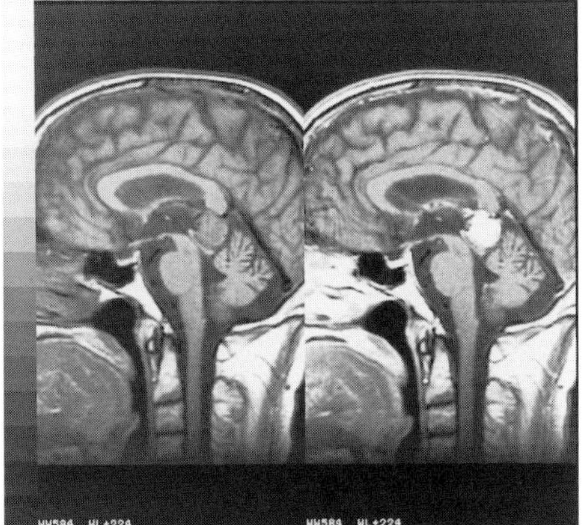


**Figure 2.9a** $T_1$ weighted sagittal images showing effect of contrast enhancement: (i) pre-contrast; (ii) post-contrast

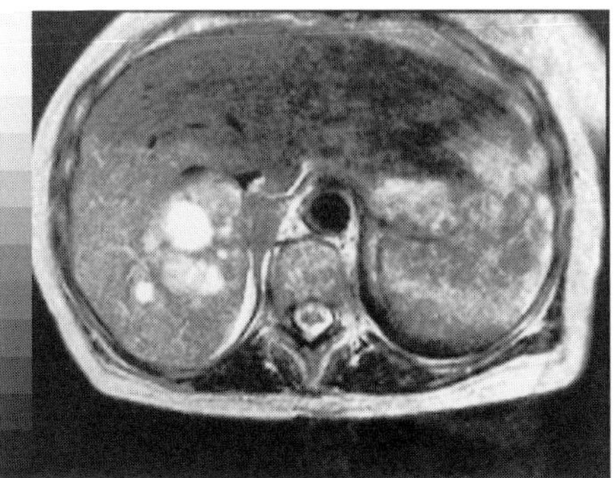

**Figure 2.9b** Pre-contrast $T_2$ weighted MR transaxial image of the liver

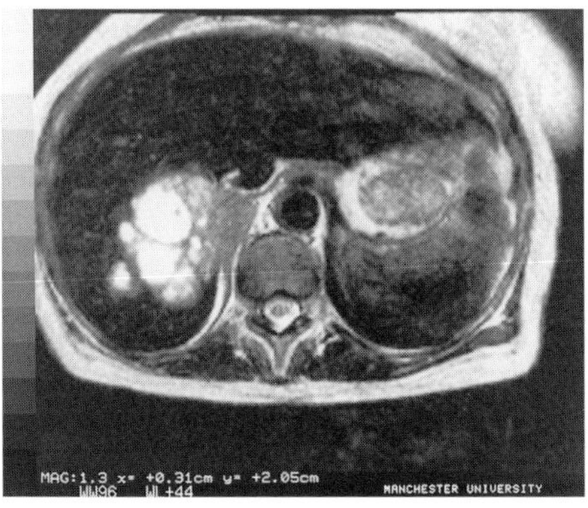


**Figure 2.9c** Post-contrast $T_2$ weighted MR transaxial image of the liver showing drop in signal intensity

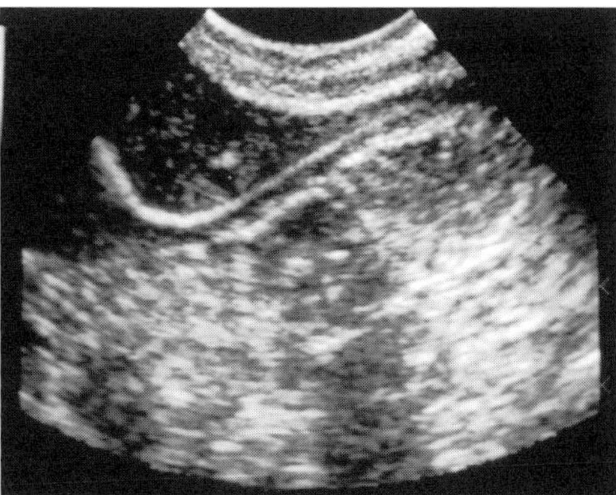

**Figure 2.9d** Ultrasound image of uterus showing effect of ultrasound contrast agent

With the growth of ultrasound has come the need for an image enhancement agent to increase further the information available from this modality. In order to enhance the ultrasound signal it is necessary to increase the relative echogenicity between two adjacent reflective surfaces under examination. The criteria for a contrast media for ultrasound are, first, that it must be echogenic, secondly it must be of low toxicity, thirdly the particles/bubble size must be of a uniform nature, fourthly it must have the ability to traverse the pulmonary capillary bed in order to enter the systematic circulation, and finally it must be stable in solution.

Many attempts to achieve an ultrasound contrast have taken the form of hand-agitated solutions; early work was done using iodinated contrast media which was shaken and then injected. While this in certain instances gave rise to increased echogenicity, there were many problems associated with such a compound. The majority of the bubbles formed would not pass through the pulmonary capillary bed and therefore it was impossible to visualise the left side of the heart.

Feinstein and colleagues, in 1982, described sonication of human serum albumen (HSA) by the use of ultrasound. The resultant bubbles produced by cavitation were of uniform size and small enough to traverse the pulmonary capillary bed. A further advantage of using HSA for this technique was that the base material was of low toxicity and stable in nature.

Other elements for the use as contrast media in ultrasound have been published on the use of gas-free particles, high-density solutions and emulsions.

The most successful of this group has been in the use of soluble galactose microparticles. These microparticles have microbubbles adherent to the surface and on injection into the circulation due to the dissolution of the particles the microbubbles freely circulate.

Early attempts with these compounds were disappointing, in that the microbubbles were absorbed by the capillaries and therefore did not traverse the capillary bed intact and therefore did not have the capability to visualise the left side of the heart and enter into the arterial circulation.

In gynaecology, the examination of the patency of the fallopian tubes and of the inner surface of the uterus by ultrasound contrast offers considerable advantage over the current method of laparoscopic chromopertubation and hysterosalpingography by offering visualisation of these structures without the need for ionising radiation.

Another important area of interest to ultrasonographers is the liver. In view of the fact that neoplastic liver lesions have variable echogenicity which is often subtle in nature, a reliable hepatic contrast agent would be extremely desirable. In conjunction with colour-flow imaging, ultrasound contrast media may give valuable information in renal and hepatic perfusion studies and in vascular studies.

# 2 Contrast Enhancement Agents

## Radiopharmaceuticals

### Introduction

A radiopharmaceutical is a chemical compound containing a radionuclide and formulated in such a way that it can be administered to a patient in order to diagnose, quantify or treat a condition.

## Properties of the Ideal Radionuclide

The ideal radionuclide for imaging should have the following properties:

- The radiation emitted must be detected efficiently by the gamma camera.
- The radiation dose to the patient must be as low as possible.

Optimal performance of gamma camera imaging equipment is achieved by using radionuclides which emit electromagnetic radiation with a monochromatic spectrum of energy 60–200 keV.

The radiation dose to a patient is determined by the type of radiation emitted (and thus absorbed) in the organ or area of the patient; the fraction of the administered activity which localises in the organ or area of interest and the rate which the activity is cleared.

Nuclides which emit $\alpha$ and $\beta$ radiation, both of which are locally absorbed within tissue, give higher radiation doses to the patient and are not ideal for imaging. Therefore, nuclides which decay by electron capture and isomeric transition in which $\beta$ emissions are absent are preferred for imaging applications.

The rate at which a radionuclide is cleared from an organ depends on two factors, the physical half-life of the radionuclide ($1/T_{1/2}P$) and the rate of biological clearance ($1/T_{1/2}B$). The radiation dose will be determined by the effective half-life ($1/T_{1/2}E$) which is given by the equation

$$\frac{1}{T_{1/2}E} = \frac{1}{T_{1/2}P} + \frac{1}{T_{1/2}B}$$

The half-life of the selected radionuclide must, however, allow for the processes of production, administration and subsequent imaging of the patient.

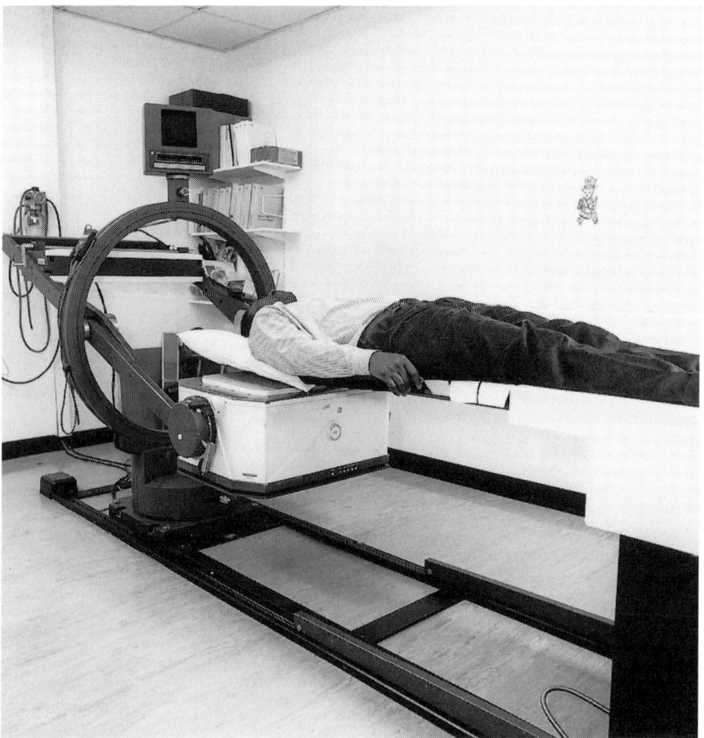

**Figure 2.10a** Gamma camera positioned over patient for image acquisition

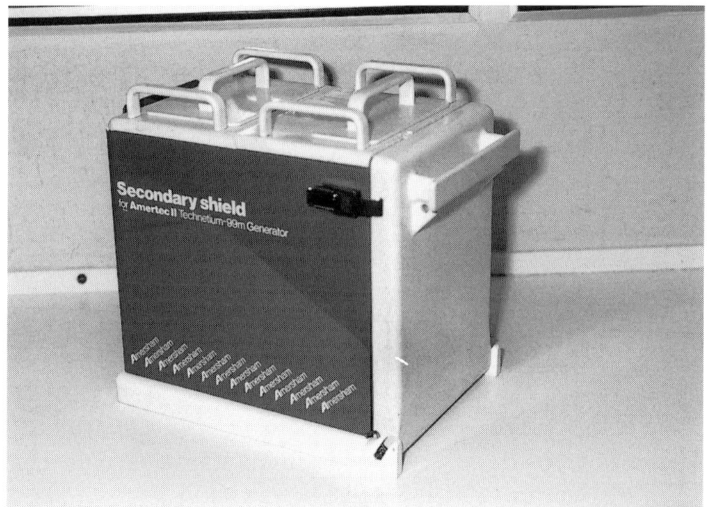


**Figure 2.10b:** Molybdenum generator

**Table 2.3 Some radionuclides and their properties**

| *Radionuclide* | *Type of emission* | *Energy* (keV) | *Half-life* |
|---|---|---|---|
| Chromium-51 | $\gamma$ | 323 | 27.8 d |
| Iodine-123 | $\gamma$ | 159 | 13.3 h |
| Indium-111 | $\gamma$ | 173 | 67.2 h |
| Krypton-81 m | $\gamma$ | 191 | 13 s |
| Thallium-201 | X | 69–83 | 73.1 h |

## Properties of the Ideal Radionuclide

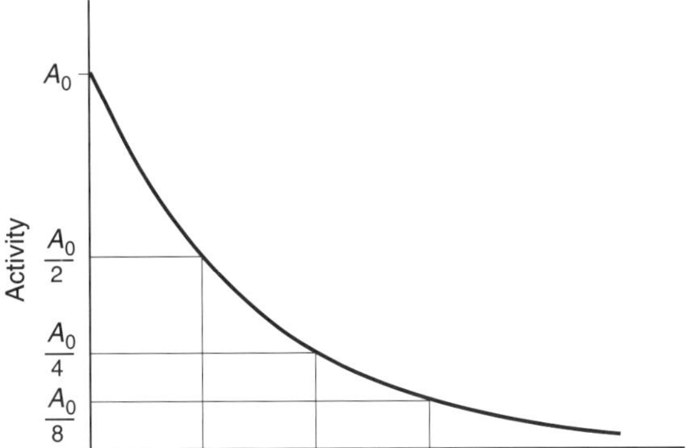


**Figure 2.11a** Half-life decay curve (activity – time)

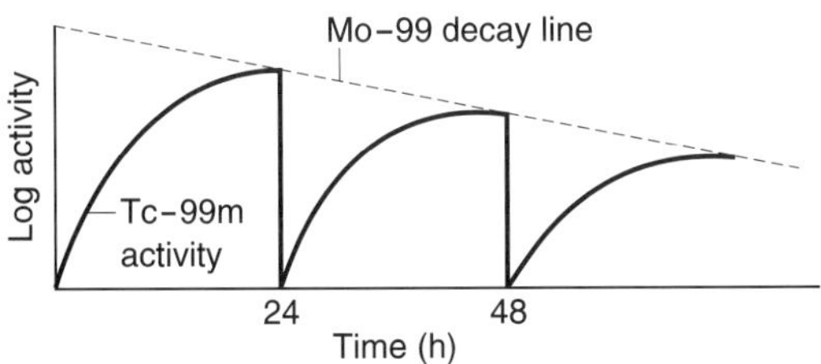


**Figure 2.11b** Curve showing $^{99m}$Tc activity in generator against time (24-hourly elution)

As a result, the physical half-life of a radionuclide used for imaging should ideally be a few hours. There must also be a readily available and inexpensive source of the radionuclide.

The isomer technetium-99m ($^{99m}$Tc) most closely fulfils these requirements. It has the following properties:

- it is a gamma emitter, energy 140 keV
- it has a half-life of 6 h
- it can be obtained from the decay of molybdenum-99, supplied in the form of a generator.

Some other radionuclides and their properties are outlined in Table 2.3.

## Localisation of Radiopharmaceuticals

For a radionuclide to be diagnostically useful it must be coupled to a chemical which will concentrate preferentially in the region of interest or follow a particular physiological process. The bio-distribution will depend on a number of factors. Outlined below are various mechanisms by which organ or pathology specificity is achieved.

### Aerosol

An aerosol is a suspension of minute solid or liquid particles in a gas. In radionuclide imaging, aerosols are principally used in lung ventilation studies, where they are most commonly produced by a jet nebuliser. The droplets produced are deposited on the lining of the airways during inhalation by the patient.

The major factor influencing the site and extent of deposition is the droplet size; the optimum diameter of droplets is in the region of 0.5 μm. Larger droplets may be deposited in the upper respiratory tract, whereas smaller droplets may be exhaled. Other properties affecting deposition include the electrical charge on the particles, their ability to absorb moisture, the nature of the patient's respiration and the state of the respiratory tract.

### Antibodies

Radioimmunoscintigraphy (RIS) is the term given to the process of obtaining images following the administration of radiolabelled antibodies or antibody fragments.

# 2 Radiopharmaceuticals

## Localisation of Radiopharmaceuticals

Labelled antibodies have the ability to bind to particular antigens or receptor sites on the surface of cells. In doing so they deliver the radionuclide to those cells. By using monoclonal rather than polyclonal antibodies a higher degree of target specificity can be achieved. Ideally the antigens should be unique to the pathological tissue; however, this rarely occurs as the surface antigens may be common to many types of cell. Current research is aimed at developing antibodies with greater specificity to receptor sites on certain cell types. One of the apparently truly tissue-specific antibodies is anti-$CD_{20}$ which is directed solely against the $CD_{20}$ antigen on B cells (lymphocytes). This antigen also will not shed into the blood or internalise after antibody binding, thus retaining the antibody–radioisotope conjugate on the B-cell surface.

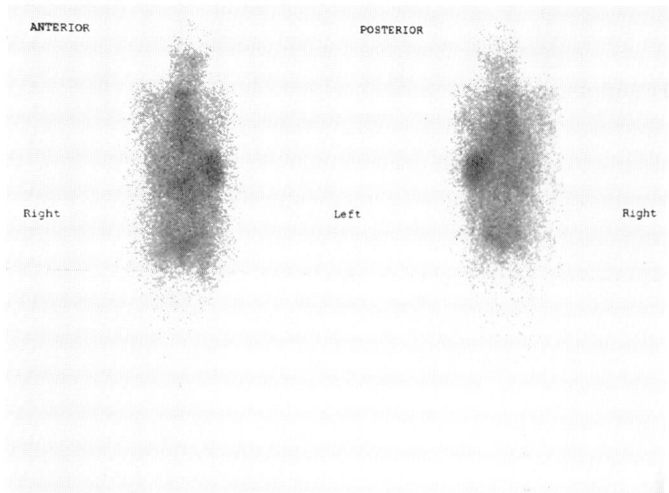


**Figure 2.12a** Antibody scan using anti-$B_1$ labelled with $^{131}I$ in a patient with low-grade non-Hodgkin's lymphoma (Image courtesy of Christie Hospital, Manchester and Coulter Pharmaceutical, Inc., USA)

### Autologous material

Autologous materials are products (such as blood cells) removed from the patient and then introduced back into the same patient. For example, whole blood can be taken from the subject, centrifuged and the required fraction, such as platelets, removed. This fraction is treated with an inhibiting agent to reduce the activity of the cells during processing. The cells are then radiolabelled with an $^{111}In$ complex. The labelled cells behave the same way *in vivo* as normal untreated cells, provided that they have not been damaged. Platelets will, therefore, accumulate at a deep venous thrombosis and white blood cells at a site of infection. In splenic imaging, red blood cells can be deliberately damaged so that they are taken up by the spleen during the normal sequestration process.

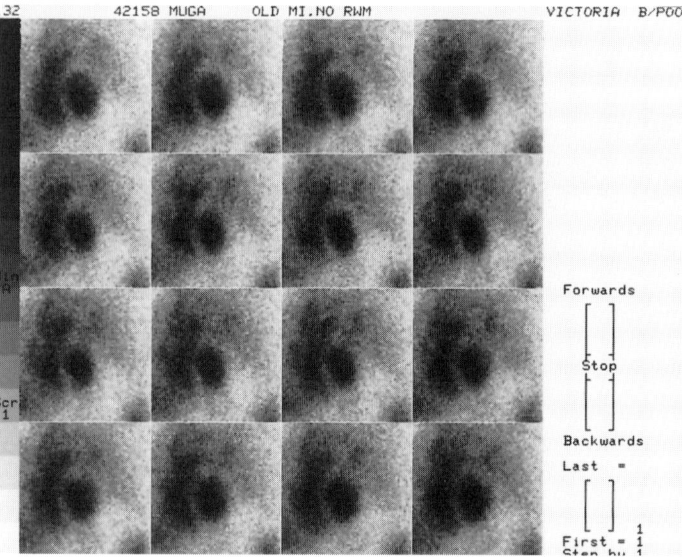


**Figure 2.12b** A dynamic gated blood pool image using a red blood cell agent with *in vivo* labelling

### Capillary trapping

In order to image blood flow in the capillaries, the radiopharmaceutical is designed in such a way that it becomes trapped in the capillaries or precapillary arterioles. Trapping is achieved by injection of a suspension containing radiolabelled particles which have a larger diameter than the blood vessels of interest. Intravenous injection of a particulate suspension results in the radiopharmaceutical being lodged in the pulmonary capillary bed. If the particles are administered intra-arterially, trapping occurs in the coronary circulation. For pulmonary perfusion studies, macroaggregated human serum albumin (HSA) particles are used which have diameters of 10–100 μm. Alternatively, a preparation of HSA microspheres has a narrower size distribution of 20–50 μm.

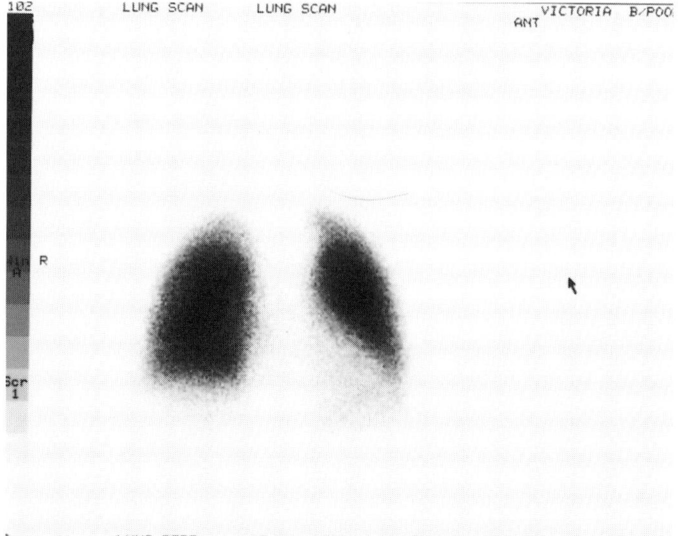


**Figure 2.12c** Image of a lung perfusion scan demonstrating radiolabelled particle trapping in the pulmonary capillary bed

### Gas inhalation

The inhalation of a radioactive gas is an alternative to the aerosol method of administering a radiopharmaceutical during lung ventilation.

## Localisation of Radiopharmaceuticals

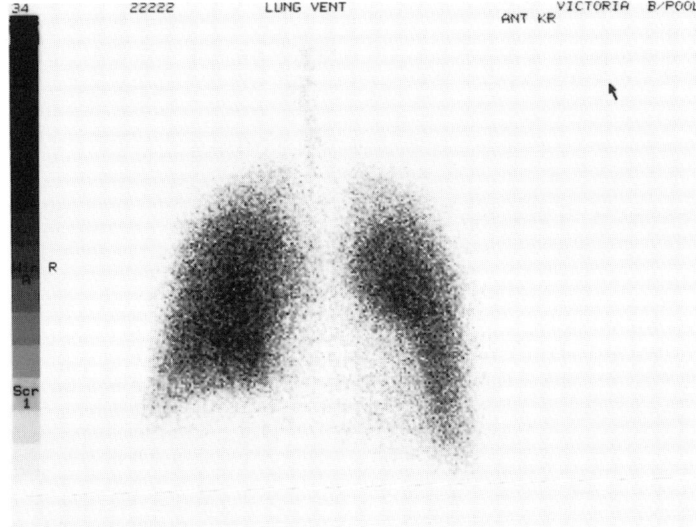


**Figure 2.13a** Image of a lung ventilation scan demonstrating inhalation of radioactive gas

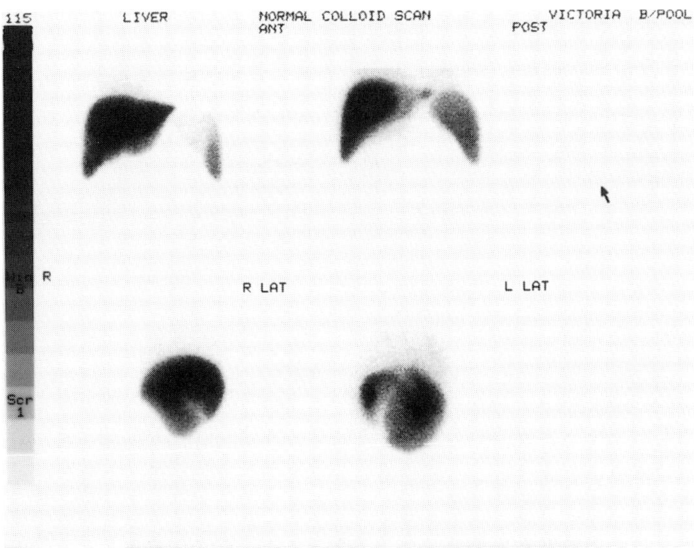


**Figure 2.13b** Images from a liver scan demonstrating phagocytosis of colloid particles as a result of Kupffer cells lining the liver sinusoids

The radioactive gas, mixed with air, is delivered to the patient via a mouthpiece or face mask. The radioactive gas behaves in the same manner as air. Therefore, the distribution of activity will reflect the ventilation of the lungs.

### Ion exchange

Ion exchange occurs when an insoluble material is placed in a solution. Some of the ions on the surface of the insoluble material are replaced by ions of the same charge from the solution.

Radioactivity can be introduced onto the surface of certain structures, for the purposes of imaging, by injecting a solution containing ions of a radioisotope.

### Metabolic localisation

Certain organs may be imaged by introducing into the patient radiopharmaceuticals designed to follow a metabolic pathway specific to that organ. A number of mechanisms are used:

- A metabolite which is chemically identical to those normally found in the body but where one of the elements has been substituted by a radioactive isotope, e.g. $^{123}I$ instead of $^{127}I$.
- A metabolite with an additional 'foreign' radioisotope added to its structure, e.g. fatty acid with an extra $^{123}I$ group added to the end of the carbon chain.
- A radioactive compound which is similar (but not identical) in structure to the naturally occurring metabolite and behaves metabolically in the same manner (a metabolic analogue), e.g. a labelled long-chain diphosphonate binding on the hydroxy-apatate layer of bone.

### Phagocytosis

Phagocytic cells are capable of recognising microscopic particles when they come into contact with receptors on the external cell membrane. After recognition, the cytoplasm of the cell streams outwards and engulfs the particle.

Colloids consist of particles suspended in a fluid medium. They are in an intermediate state between solution and emulsion, the size of the suspended particles being larger than the molecules of the solution in which they are dispersed.

# 2 Radiopharmaceuticals

## Localisation of Radiopharmaceuticals

Preparations consisting of a radiolabelled colloid can be used in the imaging of structures containing reticuloendothelial cells (although it need not necessarily be the reticuloendothelial function that is being investigated).

These structures include the liver, bone marrow, the spleen and lymphatic system.

The major factor affecting the localisation of the colloid is the size of its particles. Particles of most sizes will be trapped by the Kupffer cells lining the liver sinusoids. Particles of 200 nm or more will lodge in the spleen, and those of approximately 80 nm in the bone marrow.

To demonstrate the lymphatic system a very narrow range of particle sizes must be used (5–12 nm), as large particles will remain at the subcutaneous injection site and small particles will not lodge in the lymph nodes

As the phagocytosis of colloid particles occurs in a matter of minutes after their introduction, radionuclides of a short half-life can be employed.

### Transport via permeability barriers

The cell membrane represents a barrier to the passage of materials into the cell.

Movement of radiopharmaceuticals may occur passively by diffusion down an electrochemical gradient, e.g. in lipid-soluble transport. This is a slow process and some structures are impermeable to all but the most essential materials. The blood–brain barrier is a classic example of this. However, if it is disrupted by a pathological process, radiopharmaceuticals such as pertechnetate become free to pass into the area of damage. More rapid mechanisms of transport are mediated by specialised structural components in the cell membrane. Facilitated diffusion results in the rapid transfer of substances along the electrochemical gradient; active transport results in movement against a concentration gradient involving the use of ATP as a source of energy.

Table 2.4 shows a selection of examinations, the radiopharmaceutical utilised and its formulation.

**Table 2.4 Some examinations, with radionuclides and their formulations**

| *Examination* | *Radionuclide* | *Administration* | *Route* |
|---|---|---|---|
| Lung ventilation | $^{99m}Tc$ | Diethylenetriamine penta-acetic acid complex aerosol | Inhalation |
| Lung ventilation | $^{133}Xe$ | Gas and air mixture | Inhalation |
| DVT localisation | $^{111}In$ | Autologous platelets labelled with $^{111}In$ oxine complex | i.v. |
| Lung perfusion | $^{99m}Tc$ | $^{99m}Tc$-labelled macroaggregated HSA | i.v. |
| Ectopic thyroid | $^{123}I$ | Sodium iodide | Oral |
| Liver blood flow | $^{99m}Tc$ | $^{99m}Tc$-labelled albumin colloid | i.v. |
| White cell localisation | $^{99m}Tc$ | Autologous leucocytes labelled with $^{99m}Tc$ hexamethylpropyleneamine oxime complex | i.v. |
| Blood–brain barrier | $^{99m}Tc$ | Pertechnetate | i.v. |
| Myocardial blood flow | $^{99m}Tc$ | $^{99m}Tc$-labelled methoxyisobutyl isonitrile | i.v. |
| Thrombus localisation | $^{131}I$ | Labelled fibrinogen | i.v. |
| Renal scan (static) | $^{99m}Tc$ | $^{99m}Tc$-labelled dimercaptosuccinic acid | i.v. |
| Renal scan (dynamic) | $^{99m}Tc$ | Diethylenetriamine penta-acetic acid complex | i.v. |
| GI haemorrhage | $^{99m}Tc$ | Labelled autologous red blood cells | i.v. |
| Lymph nodes | $^{99m}Tc$ | HSA colloid | i.v. |

# Radiopharmaceuticals 2

## Radiation Protection

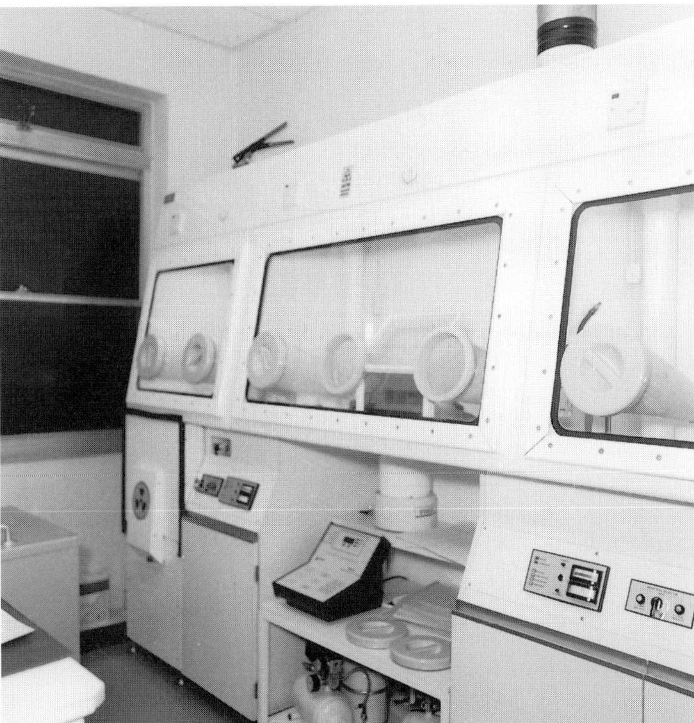

Figure 2.14a Example of a radiopharmaceutical preparation suite

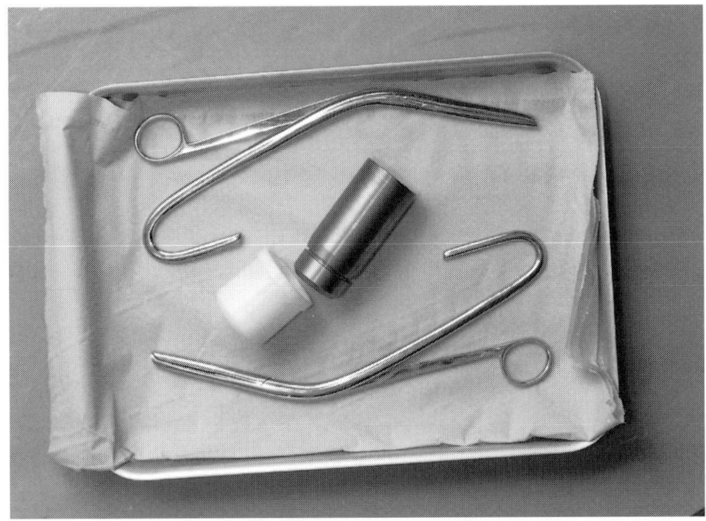

Figure 2.14b Remote handling instruments

Radiopharmaceuticals are products intended for internal use, frequently by parenteral administration. They are therefore subject to the same stringent preparation standards as other drugs. These standards are laid down in official manuals known as pharmacopoeias and may also be under governmental control.

The radioactive nature of these pharmaceuticals does mean, however, that conventional methods of preparation, administration and disposal cannot always be employed. Specific radiation protection principles must also be applied to radiopharmaceuticals, as they may constitute unsealed sources of radiation. These principles are laid down by bodies such as the International Commission on Radiological Protection.

At any stage of handling the operator will be at risk from ionising radiation from the radiopharmaceuticals; however, the fundamentals of radiation protection can still be applied.

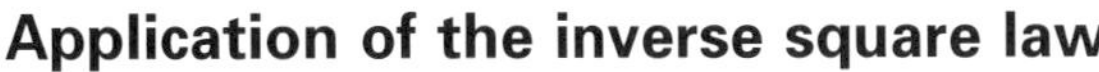

### Application of the inverse square law

The radiation dose rate which the operator receives will decrease with the square of the distance from the source. Safe practice therefore maintains as large a distance as possible between the radiopharmaceutical and the operator. This may be achieved by:

- handling unshielded containers with tongs
- only partially filling unshielded syringes
- using syringes of larger capacity than the amount required.

### Use of protective barriers

Wherever possible a barrier of material appropriate to the energy of the radiation should be interposed between the operator and the source. Examples of this include:

- tungsten syringe shields
- lead pots for vials
- lead glass screens
- lead bricks or castles for larger pieces of equipment.

### Limitation of exposure time

Wherever possible the amount of time spent in the potentially radioactive environment should be kept to a minimum. This can be achieved by:

- careful analysis of systems of work to ensure the quickest techniques are employed
- allowing time to practise techniques before radiopharmaceuticals are introduced
- prompt removal of contaminated equipment.

*continued on next page*

## Radiation Protection

- as much patient liaison as possible before the administration of the radiopharmaceutical, in order to ensure minimum examination time
- introducing policies preventing unnecessary activity in risk areas, e.g. making telephone calls and completion of paper work.

### Contamination

To avoid contamination, stringent precautions must be taken to protect both staff and public. These include:

- Safe and well-designed work areas.
- Use of protective equipment such as overalls and gloves.
- Frequent washing of hands.
- Introduction of a no smoking, eating, drinking or applying of cosmetics policy, to prevent ingestion.
- Provision of an emergency decontamination kit for personnel and equipment in the event of spillage occurring.
- Safe disposal of waste. Waste such as used syringes and dressings may be kept in closed lead lined containers in a secure area until its activity has reduced to a safe level (for $^{99m}$Tc this is about 24 h). After this time it may be disposed of in a conventional manner such as incineration.

  Liquid waste, including unused radiopharmaceuticals and body fluids, can be disposed of down designated drains as long as this is accompanied by large quantities of water to ensure adequate dilution and flushing away of the waste.

### Protection of the public

The patient who has received a dose of radioisotope represents a potential radiation hazard. To reduce this the following considerations should be taken into account:

- The department should have its own waiting and WC facilities for patients.
- Extreme caution should be exercised when considering the use of radionuclides during pregnancy, in order to protect the fetus.
- Nursing mothers should have minimum contact with the infant during the 24 h following injection of radionuclide and should not breast-feed.
- The safety of patients' visitors should be borne in mind, although most imaging radioisotopes do not represent a significant risk.

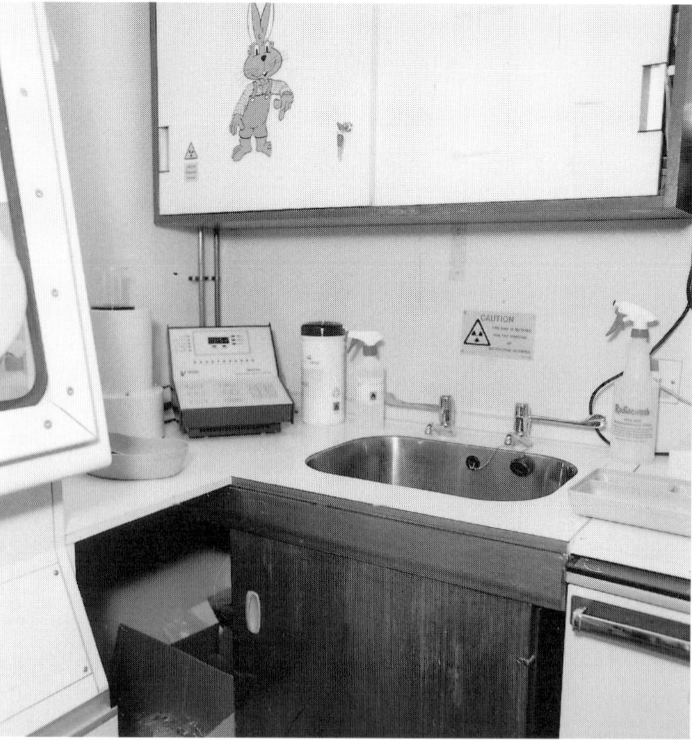


**Figure 2.15a** Work area showing warning signs

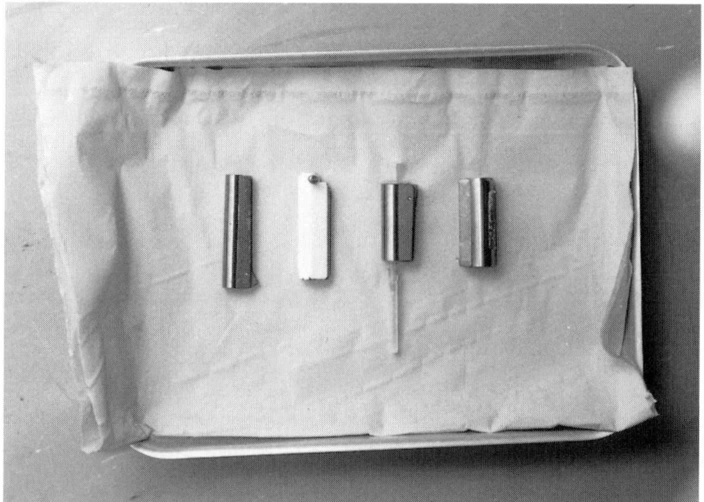

**Figure 2.15b** Selection of tungsten syringe shields

# 3

# Locomotor System

## CONTENTS

# 3 Locomotor System

## Introduction

The locomotor system comprises bone, cartilage and other connective tissue which together form the appendicular and axial skeletons.

The function of the skeleton is to provide a supporting framework for the body, to form boundaries for body cavities and to protect delicate organs. It also gives attachment to muscles and provides levers essential for movement. Bone forms the main store for calcium salts and red bone marrow is responsible for erythropoiesis.

There are five types of bone: long, short, irregular, flat and sesamoid.

Long bones are characterised as possessing a shaft and two extremities. The shaft forms a cylinder of compact bone enclosing a medullary canal which in adult life is filled with yellow bone marrow (adipose tissue).

The outer aspect of the shaft is covered by a fibrous vascular membrane known as the periosteum. In addition to providing an outer protective covering, the periosteum provides attachment to muscle tendons and allows the passage of blood vessels for bone nutrition. The deep (osteogenic) layers contain osteoblasts which are responsible for circular bone growth.

The extremities of long bones comprise a thin layer of compact cortical bone enclosing inner cancellous trabecullar bone.

Short bones are roughly cuboidal in shape, with a thin layer of compact bone surrounding inner cancellous bone. They are found only in the wrist and ankle joints.

Irregular bones have a similar structure to short bones; examples include the bones of the vertebral column and the pelvis.

Flat bones comprise two layers of compact bone with an inner cancellous layer. Their function is normally protective, e.g. the bones of the vault of the skull, ribs and the scapula.

Sesamoid bones comprise outer compact and inner dense cancellous bone tissue. They are situated in tendons to provide additional strength, e.g. the patella.

Joints are formed by the junction of two or more bones or cartilages. There are three major classifications of joints: fibrous (synarthrodial), cartilaginous (amphiarthrodial), and synovial (diarthrodial).

Fibrous joints are fixed joints which allow little or no movement. The bone ends are held together by fibrous tissue, e.g. the sutures of the skull and the inferior tibiofibular joint. There are three subgroups of fibrous joint: suture, gomphosis and syndesmosis.

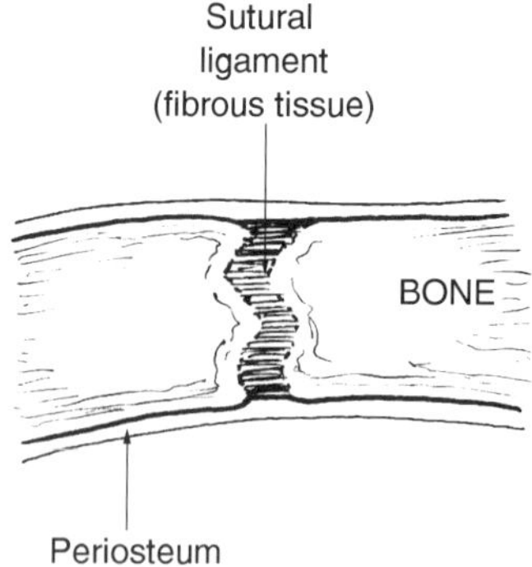


**Figure 3.1a** Fibrous joint

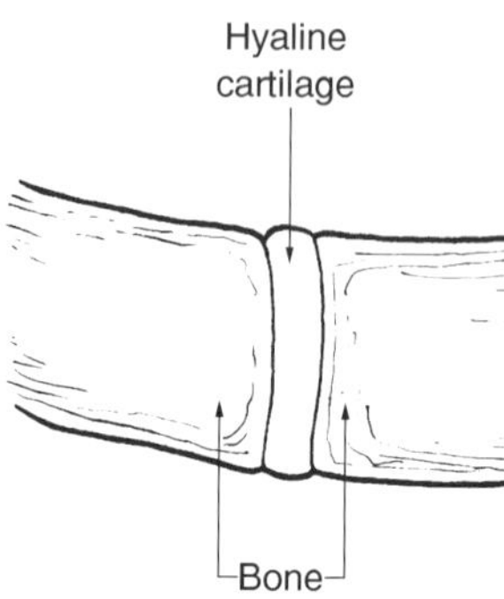


**Figure 3.1b** Cartilaginous joint

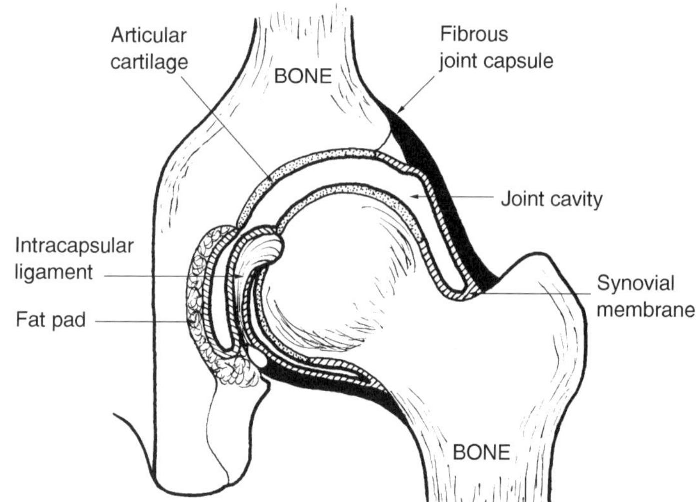


**Figure 3.1c** Synovial joint

# Locomotor System 3

## Introduction

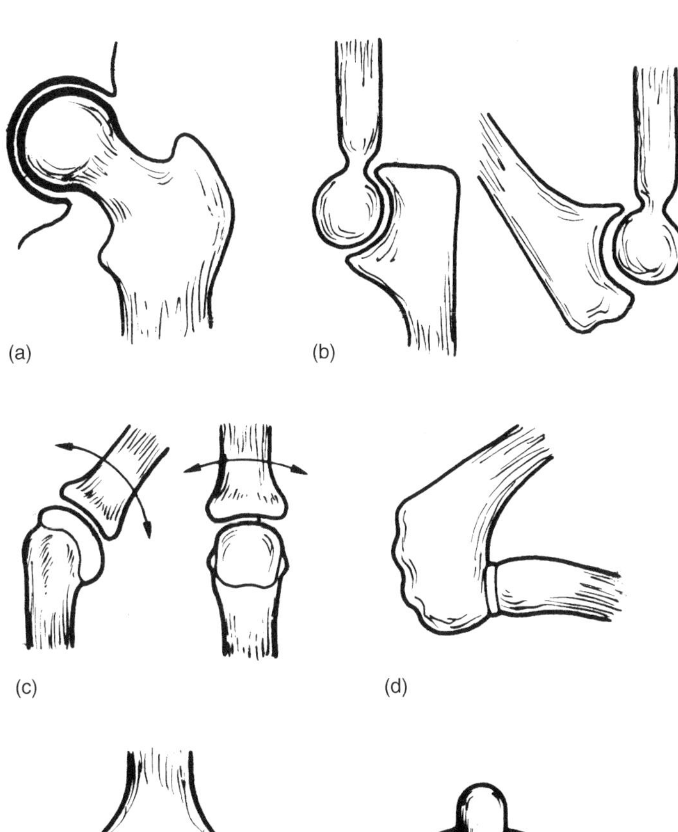


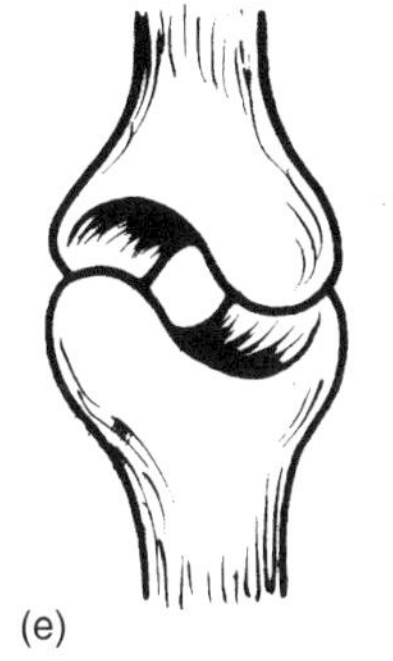


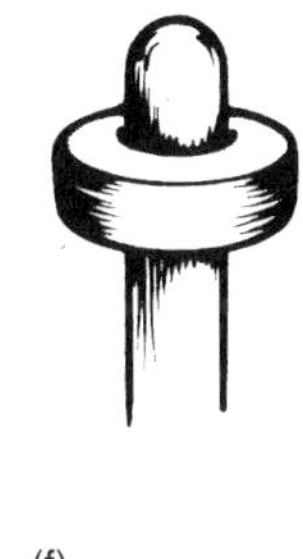


**Figure 3.2** (a) Ball-and-socket joint; (b) Hinge joint; (c) Condyloid joint; (d) Plane joint; (e) Saddle joint; (f) Pivot joint

In a cartilaginous joint the bone ends are lined with hyaline cartilage and a pad of fibrocartilage is situated between the bones. The joint is held together by a fibrous capsule. The cartilage pad may permit a limited degree of movement and can act as a 'shock absorber'. Examples include the joints between the intervertebral bodies and the symphysis pubis. There are two subgroups of cartilaginous joint, primary and secondary.

Synovial joints form the largest group in the body and are generally freely movable, the degree of movement being limited only by the shape of the bone ends. There are seven subdivisions of synovial joints:

- Ball-and-socket joint which consists of a spherical-shaped head which fits into a concave depression and permits all angular and rotational movements, e.g. the hip joint and shoulder joint.
- Hinge joint which consists of a convex surface fitting into a concave surface, e.g. the elbow joint and ankle joint, and permits flexion and extension only.
- Condyloid joint which comprises two rounded condyles, which may be together or separate, fitting into concave depressions, e.g. the knee and the temporomandibular joint, and permits flexion and extension with limited rotation.
- Gliding (plane) joint which consists of two flat surfaces, e.g. the acromioclavicular joint and the intercarpal/tarsal joints, and permits sliding movements only.
- Saddle joint which comprises a concavo-convex surface which fits into a convexo-concave surface, e.g. the first carpometacarpal joint, and permits all angular movements but no rotation.
- Pivot joint which consists of a peg which fits into an articular cylinder, e.g. the atlanto-occipital joint, which permits rotational movements only.
- Ellipsoid joint which consists of an oval convex surface which fits into an oval concave surface, and permits angular movements but not rotational movements e.g. the radiocarpal joint.

# 3 Locomotor System

## Introduction

Most synovial joints share a number of common features, including a white fibrocartilaginous capsule which completely encloses the joint, providing strength and protection, and a synovial membrane which lines all internal parts (except articular surfaces) and secretes synovial fluid for nutrition and lubrication. All synovial joints have articular surfaces lined with hyaline cartilage to reduce friction and protect the bone ends.

Other intracapsular features may include inter-articular cartilages for additional stability, inter-articular ligaments for extra strength, bursae to reduce friction and sesamoid bones.

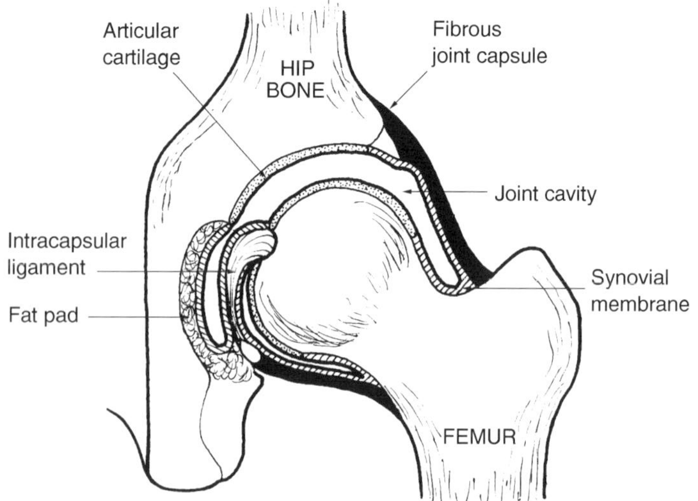


**Figure 3.3a** Typical synovial joint (hip joint)

## Recommended Imaging Procedures

Plain radiography is routinely performed in the examination of the locomotor system.

Single contrast or double contrast arthrography is used to demonstrate the internal anatomy of the joint where internal derangement is suspected, particularly in the shoulder and elbow. The procedure is performed with the aid of fluoroscopy and images recorded either digitally or using a conventional film/screen combination.

Computed tomography may be undertaken to supplement plain film radiographs. Non-contrast enhanced CT sections can be used to demonstrate fractures and some bony anomalies. Contrast enhanced CT may be necessary to define musculoskeletal tumours adequately. It can, however, prove difficult for some patients to maintain the required position and it may involve the risk of increased radiation dose to adjacent structures.

The non-invasive nature of MRI and its superior ability to visualise both internal structures and soft tissues are resulting in the gradual replacement of arthrography in the investigation of tendon abnormalities, loose bodies, meniscal tears, avascular necrosis, rotator cuff injuries, rheumatoid arthritis and osteoarthritis.

The imaging procedure and protocol for MR examinations is common to most sections of the locomotor system. A separate section covering MR techniques is included on pages 98–101.

Ultrasound is also a useful non-invasive technique used to supplement plain radiography, especially in the investigation of the hip joint in children.

Radionuclide imaging and plain radiography are the principal techniques for screening in metastatic disease and in the investigation of bone infection. These may be complemented by CT and MRI for bone marrow assessment.

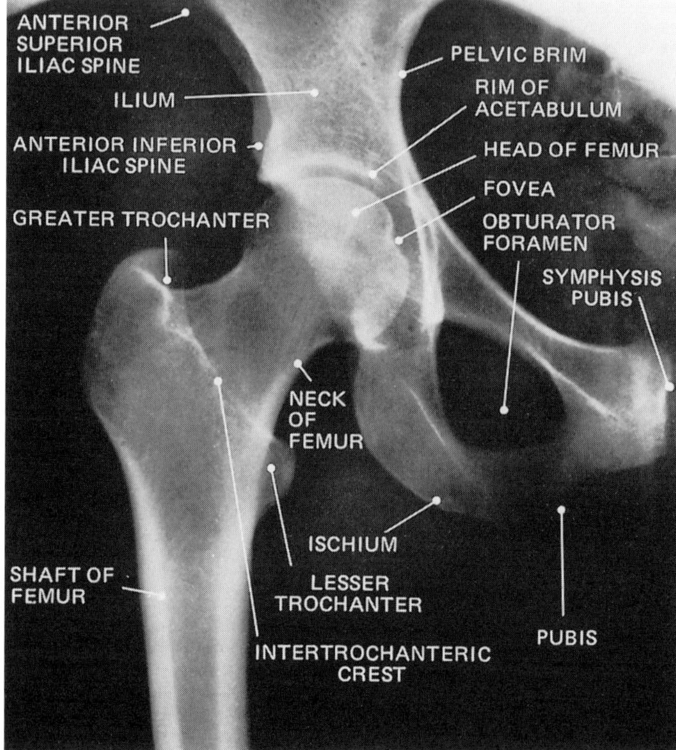


**Figure 3.3b** Radiograph of hip joint

## Wrist Joint

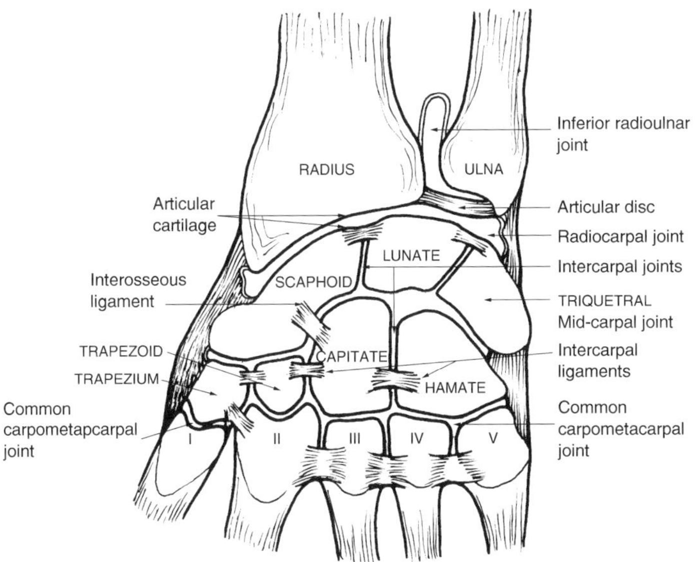


**Figure 3.4a** Schematic diagram of the wrist in the coronal plane

The wrist joint has four major compartments: the radiocarpal joint, the distal radioulnar joint, the mid-carpal space and the carpometacarpal joints.

The radiocarpal joint is a synovial ellipsoid joint formed between the lower end of the radius and an articular disc together with the scaphoid lunate and triquetral.

The joint capsule which is separate from the distal radioulnar joint, encloses the joint and is reinforced by palmar radiocarpal, palmar ulnar-carpal, dorsal radiocarpal, ulna and radial collateral ligaments.

It receives its blood supply from the anterior and posterior branches of the radial and ulnar arteries and the nerve supply is through the anterior and posterior interosseous branches derived from the brachial plexus.

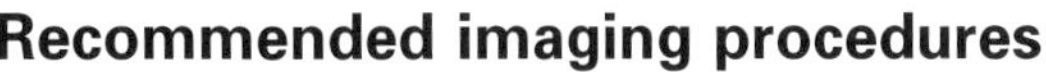

### Recommended imaging procedures

Initially most lesions are investigated with plain radiography including macroradiography. Magnetic resonance imaging is the modality of choice to complement plain films particularly in the investigation of carpal tunnel syndrome, avascular necrosis and tendon disease.

When magnetic resonance imaging is not available computed tomography can play a useful role, particularly in the investigation of bone disease.

Arthrography is occasionally used to demonstrate cartilage tears, ligament damage following trauma and to demonstrate early changes associated with inflammatory arthritis. It is not, however, frequently performed.

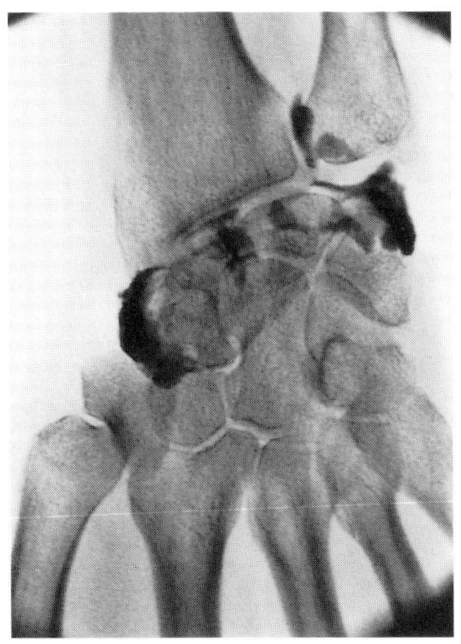

**Figure 3.4b** Wrist arthrogram

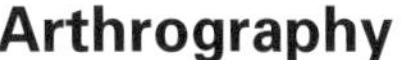

### Arthrography

Wrist arthrography is the radiographic demonstration of the wrist joint following the introduction of a contrast agent. It is a relatively uncommon examination but it can be used to demonstrate the radiocarpal joint following the introduction of a suitable contrast agent into the joint capsule.

Radiographs are taken in the anteroposterior, lateral and oblique positions. Tomography may be employed if an ununited fracture of the scaphoid is suspected.

*Contrast medium and injection data*

| *Volume* | *Concentration* | *Flow rate* |
|---|---|---|
| 6–8 ml | 240–300 mgI/ml | Hand injection |

# 3 Locomotor System

## Wrist Joint

### Computed tomography

Computed tomography of the wrist joint is not an easy procedure to undertake, as it may prove difficult for patients to maintain the required position for the duration of the examination.

It may also involve unnecessary irradiation to the adjacent areas.

It is the normal procedure for both wrists/forearms to be scanned for comparison.

**Indications**

Computed tomography provides good anatomical detail of the joint and may be used to assess the extent of bone and soft tissue tumours, trauma and bony anomalies.

**Position of patient and imaging modality**

The patient lies prone on the scanner table. The arms are extended above the head and supported on a radiolucent pad. The wrists are placed as near as possible to the centre of the scan field with the hands pronated.

The patient is moved into the scanner so that the scan reference point is at the level of the ulnar styloid process.

**Imaging procedure**

An anteroposterior scan projection radiograph is performed, ensuring that all the area of suspected abnormality is imaged.

Usually 3 or 5 mm sections are prescribed from the scan projection radiograph. To improve spatial resolution, the images may be reconstructed either prospectively or retrospectively, using a small display field of view.

A bone reconstruction algorithm is normally selected. This enhances bony structures while still enabling soft tissues to be demonstrated adequately. Further reformatted images in either the coronal or sagittal plane may be useful.

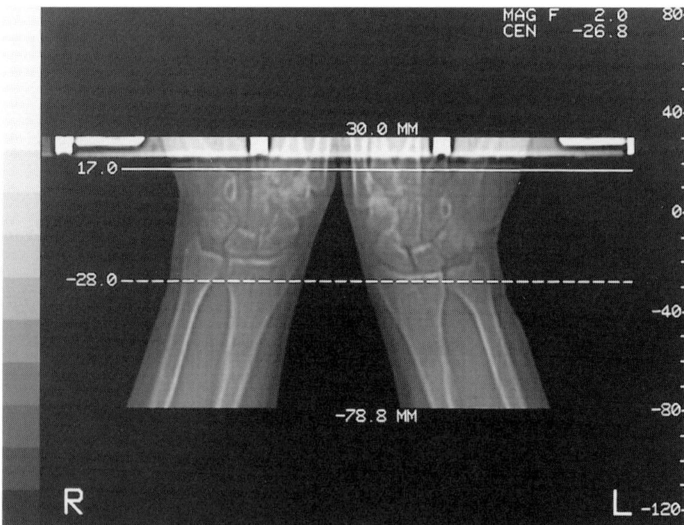


**Figure 3.5a** Scan projection radiograph showing start and end locations

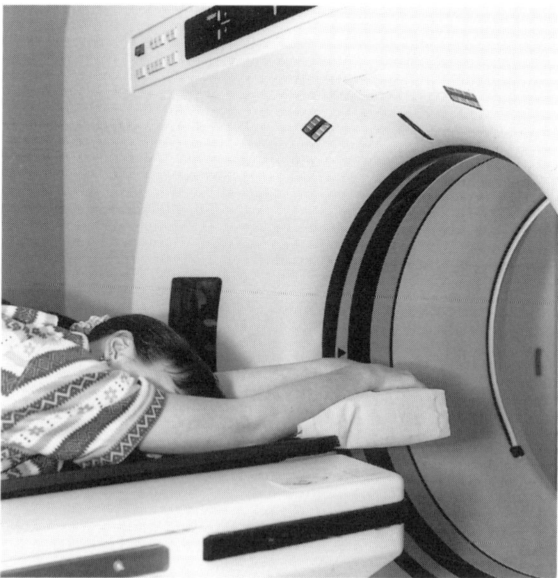

**Figure 3.5b** Patient on a CT scanner

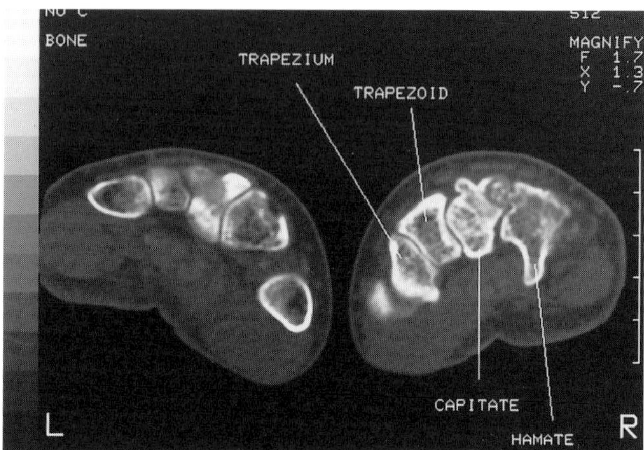


**Figure 3.5c** Transaxial image through the wrist joint

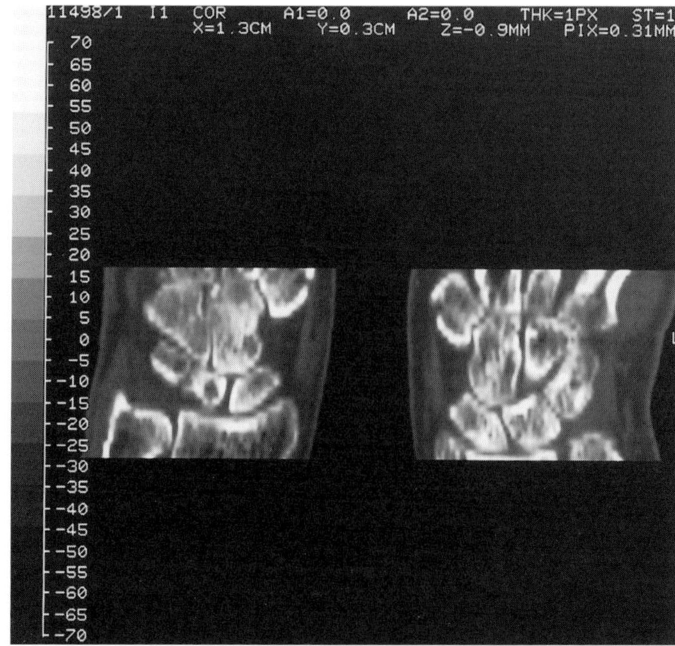


**Figure 3.5d** Reformatted image in the coronal plane

## Elbow Joint

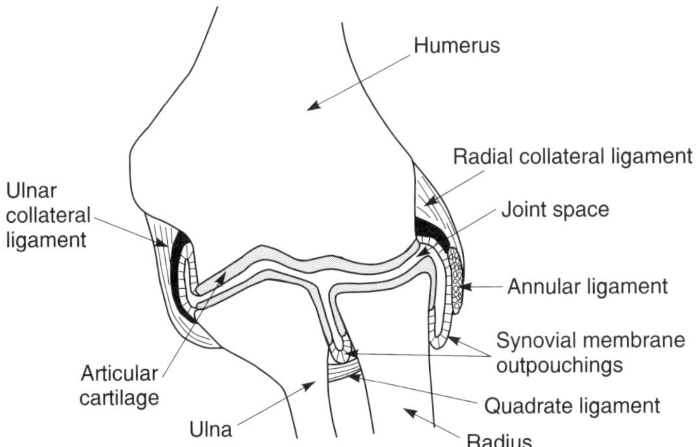


**Figure 3.6a** Coronal section through left elbow joint

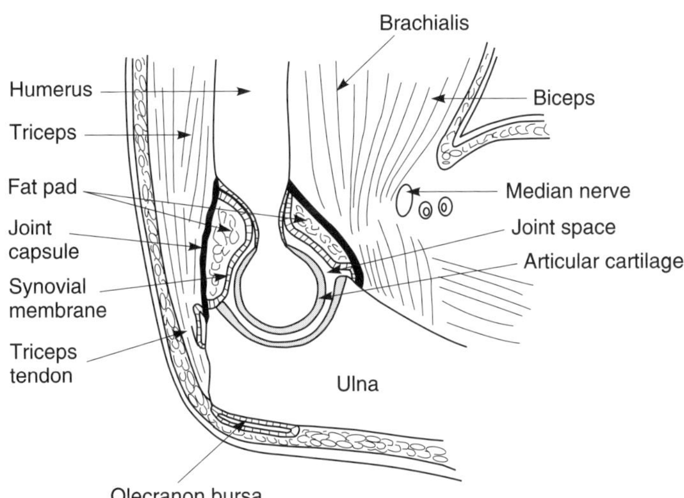


**Figure 3.6b** Sagittal section through elbow joint

The elbow is a synovial hinge joint formed between the lower end of the humerus and the upper ends of the radius and ulna, specifically, the capitellum of the humerus articulates with the head of the radius and the trochlea of the humerus articulates with the trochlear notch of the ulna. The joint space is continuous with that of the proximal radioulnar joint and is collectively known as the cubital articulation.

The joint capsule completely encloses the joint and is continuous laterally with the collateral ligaments. It sometimes forms three compartments: the anterior, posterior and annular recesses. It is attached inferiorly below the head of the radius, enclosing the annular ligament. Projecting into the joint cavity between the radius and ulna from behind is a triangular fold of synovial membrane.

Intrinsic features of the joint include three fat pads situated between the joint capsule and the synovial membrane. They are closely related to the three fossae on the lower end of the humerus, being situated over the olecranon, coronoid and radial fossae.

Extrinsic features include medial and lateral collateral ligaments and a bursa situated between the radius and ulna.

When the elbow joint is extended, the radius and ulna form an angle of approximately 165° (155° in females) to the humerus. This is known as the 'carrying angle'.

Blood supply is derived from the radial and ulnar arteries and the nerve supply is the radial nerve from the brachial plexus.

## Recommended imaging procedures

Subsequent to plain radiography, arthrography is the procedure of choice for investigation of the elbow joint. It may be performed in conjunction with tomography or CT to confirm the presence of loose bodies, and to demonstrate the articular surfaces.

At the time of writing, MRI has yet to make a significant contribution to imaging the elbow joint.

## Elbow Joint

### Arthrography

Elbow arthrography is the radiographic demonstration of the elbow joint following the administration of a water-soluble non-ionic contrast agent into the joint space. A single contrast technique may be used or air may be introduced for double contrast.

The examination is normally performed under fluoroscopic control, and images may be recorded using digital fluoroscopic equipment or using conventional radiographic equipment together with high-definition intensifying screens.

**Indications**

Single contrast arthrography may be performed to assess the synovial membrane and to demonstrate the presence of synovial cysts. A double contrast technique is used to demonstrate loose bodies and the articular surfaces.

**Patient preparation**

Control films are taken in the anteroposterior, lateral and oblique projections.

The patient sits alongside the fluoroscopy table with the arm extended across the table top. The elbow is flexed to 90° and supported on a non-opaque foam pad so that the humerus and forearm are parallel to the table top.

The articulation between the radial head and the capitellum is identified under fluoroscopic control and marked on the skin surface.

The skin is prepared using a suitable antiseptic solution and the surrounding area is covered with sterile towels. A local anaesthetic is introduced into the area adjacent to the skin marker.

**Imaging procedure**

A 22-gauge needle is inserted vertically into the joint space between the capitellum and the head of radius under fluoroscopic control. When the needle enters the joint capsule, a length of sterile tubing is attached to a 2 ml syringe and synovial fluid may be aspirated.

Once the position of the needle is confirmed in the joint capsule, either by aspiration of synovial fluid or a test injection of a small amount of contrast agent, up to 5 ml of contrast medium is introduced. If the double contrast technique is to be employed, up to 10 ml of air are injected. Once this is complete, the needle is removed.

The patient is encouraged to exercise the joint gently to disseminate the contrast agent throughout the joint space.

A series of radiographs are taken immediately after exercise. Further views may be required with varying degrees of extension of the elbow joint, and it is common to include either lateral tomography or CT.

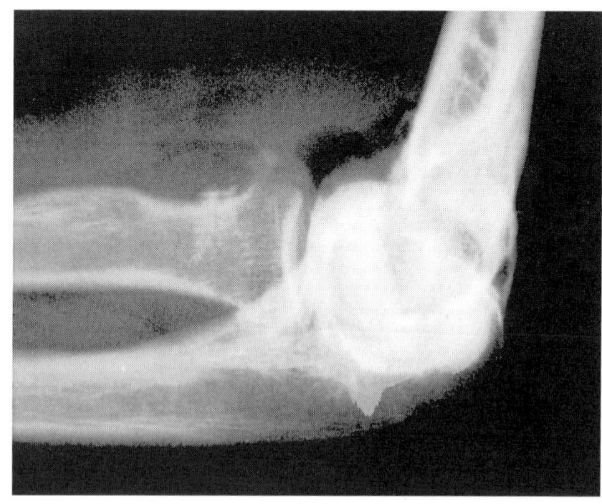

(a)

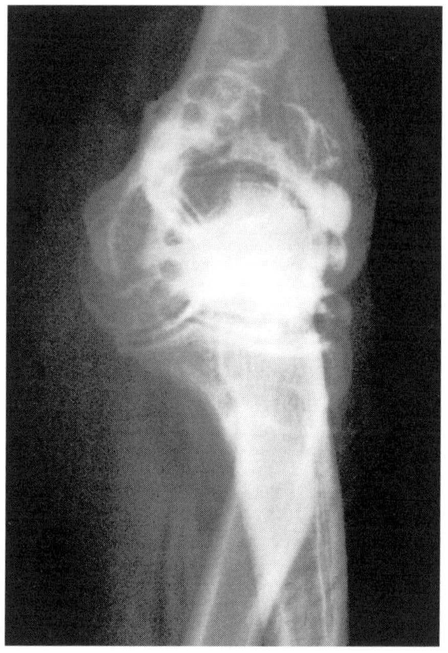

(b)

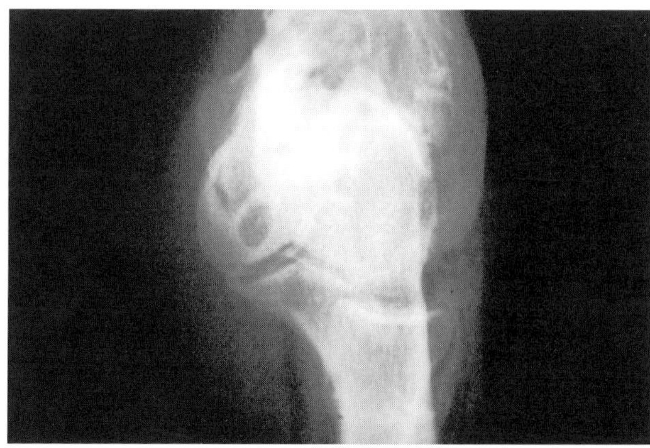

(c)

**Figure 3.7a–c** Series of radiographs demonstrating contrast within the left elbow joint: (a) lateral projection; (b,c) AP oblique projections

## Elbow Joint

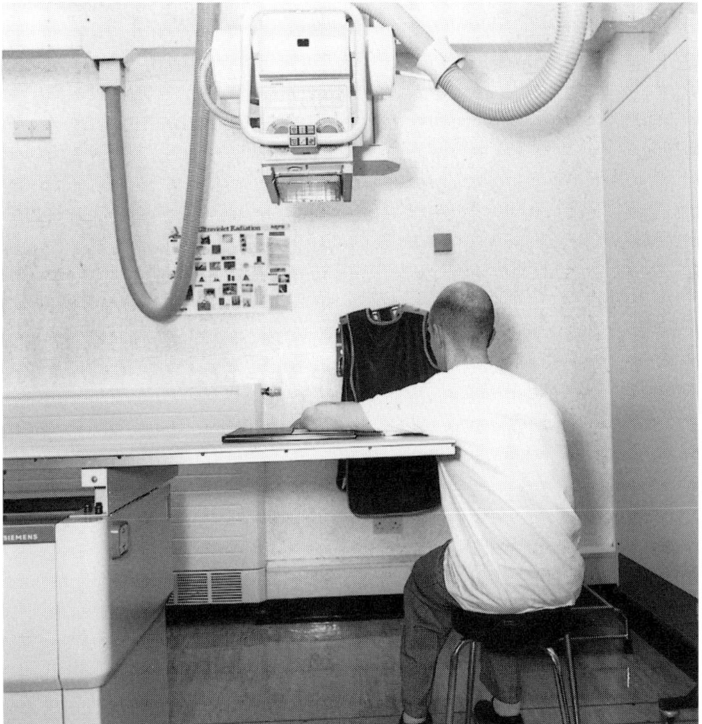

**Figure 3.8a** Patient in lateral position

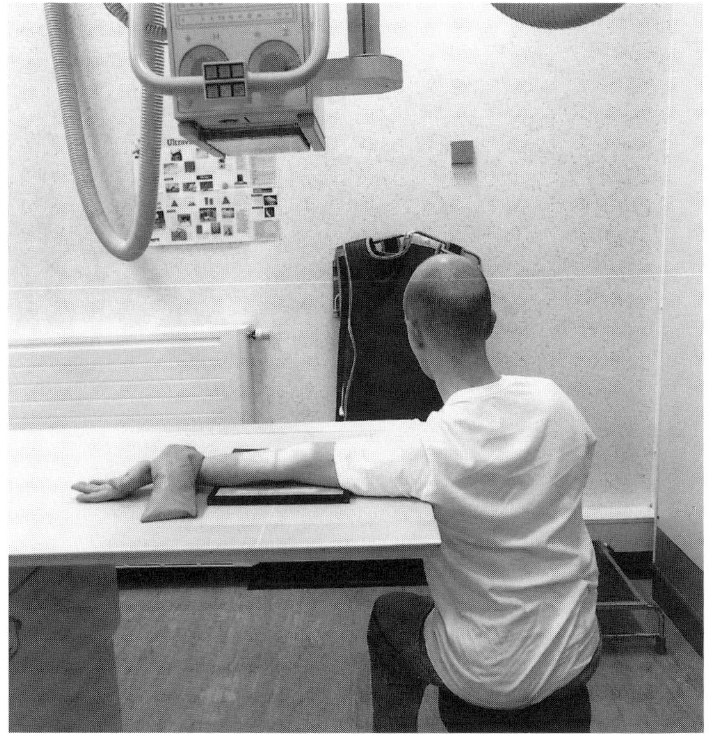

**Figure 3.8b** Patient in AP position

*Contrast medium and injection data*

| *Volume* | *Concentration* | *Flow rate* |
|---|---|---|
| 5–12 ml | 240–300 mgI/ml | Hand injection |
| 10 cm$^3$ | Air | Hand injection |

### Lateral projection

*Position of patient and imaging modality*
The patient's arm is adjusted to ensure that the humerus and forearm are parallel to the table top and the elbow is flexed to 90°. The hand is rotated into the vertical position.

An 18 × 24 cm cassette fitted with high-definition intensifying screens is placed under the elbow joint.

*Direction and centring of the X-ray beam*
The vertical central ray is centred over the lateral epicondyle of the humerus.

### Anteroposterior projection

*Position of patient and imaging modality*
The patient's arm is extended across the table top with the hand supinated. The forearm is rotated slightly externally so that the medial and lateral epicondyles of the humerus are equidistant from the table top.

An 18 × 24 cm cassette fitted with high-definition intensifying screens is placed under the arm and centred to the elbow joint.

*Direction and centring of the X-ray beam*
The vertical central ray is centred between the epicondyles of the humerus and 2.5 cm distally.

### Oblique projections

*Position of patient and imaging modality*
From the anteroposterior position, the arm is rotated 45° medially and then 45° laterally, respectively.

*Direction and centring of the X-ray beam*
The vertical central ray is centred between the epicondyles of the humerus and 2.5 cm distally.

# 3 Locomotor System

## Elbow Joint

### Computed tomography – method 1

Computed tomography of the elbow joint is not an easy procedure to undertake, as it may prove difficult for patients to maintain the required position for the duration of the examination. It may also involve unnecessary irradiation to adjacent areas.

#### Indications

The procedure provides good anatomical detail of the joint and may be used as a supplementary procedure in cases of suspected intra-articular tumours and fractures.

#### Position of patient and imaging modality

The patient lies prone on the scanner table. The affected arm is placed above the head and the elbow joint is extended as far as possible. The arm is supported on a radiolucent pad. The elbow is placed as near as possible to the centre of the scan field with the hand pronated.

The patient is moved into the centre of the scanner so that the scan reference point is at the level of the lateral epicondyle.

#### Imaging procedure

A scan projection radiograph is performed with the tube in either the anteroposterior or postero-anterior position. From this image, 3 or 5 mm sections are prescribed through the area of abnormality.

If spiral scanning options are available these images may be acquired with a volume acquisition, using a 3 mm slice thickness and 3 mm table increments, but with a 2 mm reconstruction index to give overlapping sections.

To improve spatial resolution, the images may be reconstructed either prospectively or retrospectively using a small display field of view.

A bone reconstruction algorithm is normally selected, as this enhances bony structures while still allowing soft tissues to be demonstrated adequately.

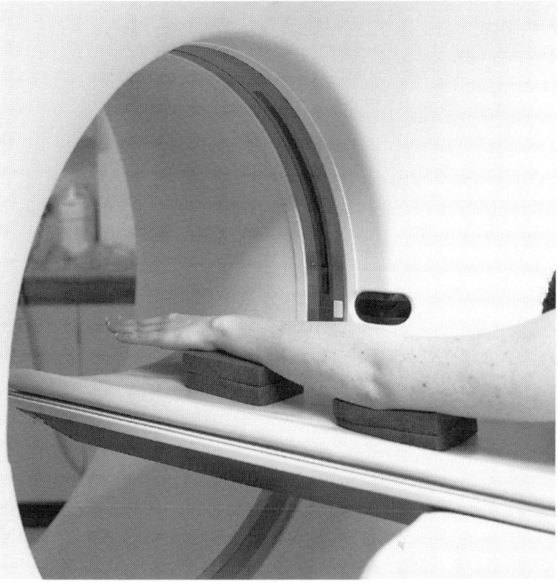

**Figure 3.9a** Photograph of patient position – method 1

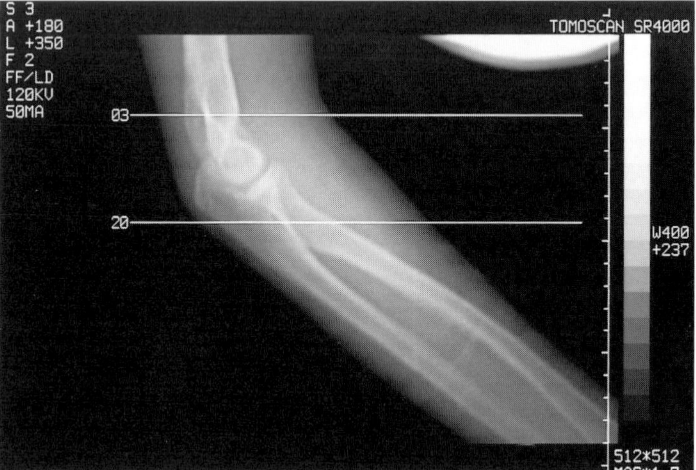


**Figure 3.9b** Scan projection radiograph showing start and end locations

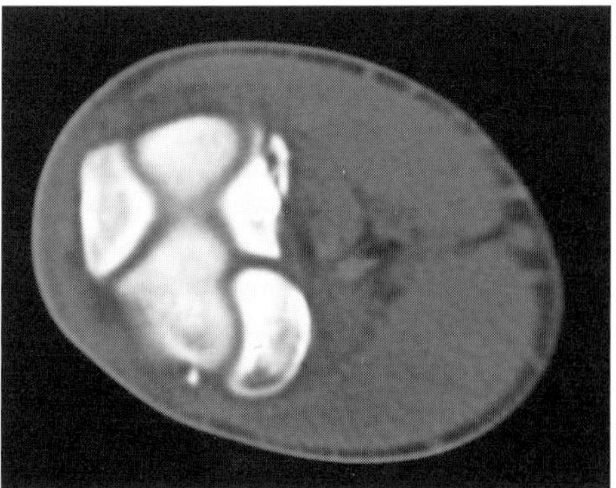

**Figure 3.9c** Transaxial image showing fracture through the coronoid process

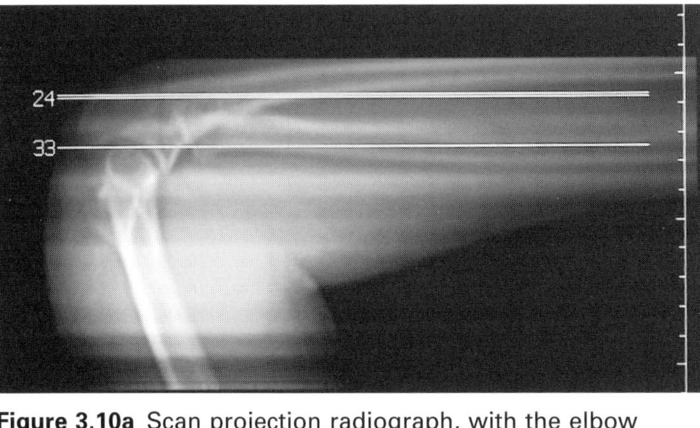


Figure 3.10a Scan projection radiograph, with the elbow flexed, showing start and end locations

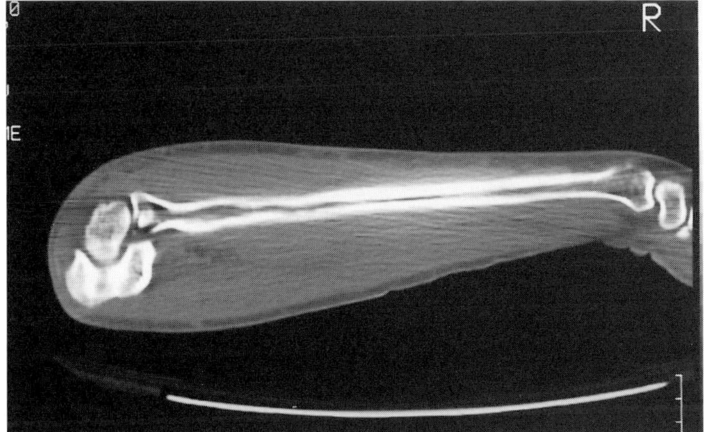


Figure 3.10b Transaxial image showing fracture of the radial head

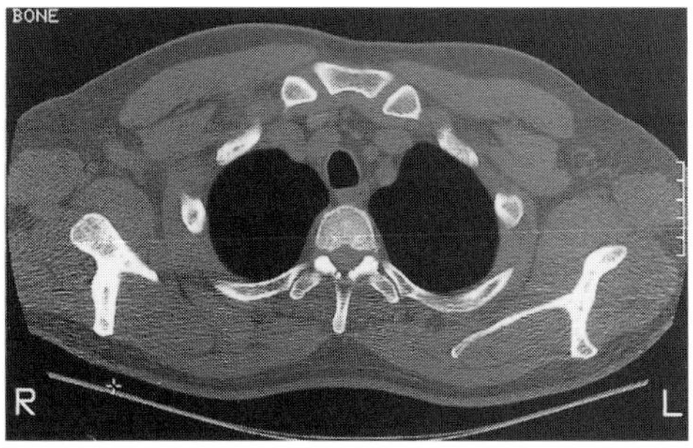

Figure 3.10c Transaxial image showing bilateral sternoclavicular hyperostosis

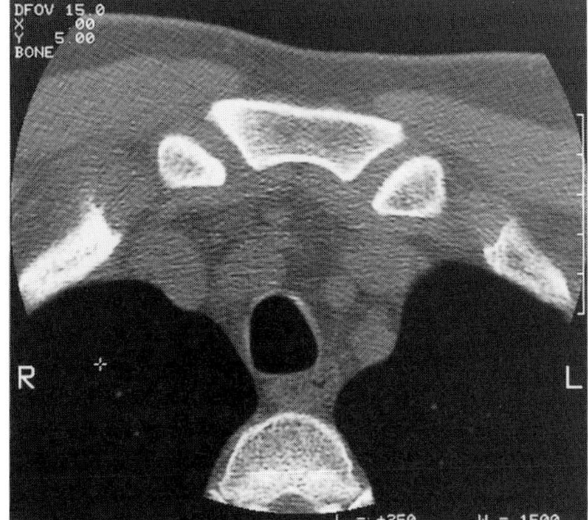


Figure 3.10d Reconstructed image using a small field of view to improve spatial resolution

## Computed tomography – method 2

**Position of patient and imaging modality**

To view the elbow joint and radius the patient is again positioned prone, arm extended above the head. The elbow joint is flexed to 90° and supported on radiolucent pads. Again the wrist is pronated.

The patient is moved into the centre of the scanner so that the scan reference point is at the level of the lateral epicondyle.

**Imaging procedure**

A scan projection radiograph is performed with the tube in either the anteroposterior or postero-anterior position. Usually 3 mm or 5 mm sections are prescribed.

If spiral scanning options are available these images may be acquired with a volume acquisition, using a 3 mm slice thickness and 3 mm table increments, but with a 2 mm reconstruction index to give overlapping sections.

To improve spatial resolution the images may be reconstructed either prospectively or retrospectively using a small display field of view. A bone reconstruction algorithm is normally selected. This enhances bony structures while still allowing soft tissues to be adequately demonstrated.

# Sternoclavicular Joints

Computed tomography is used to demonstrate anomalies of the sternoclavicular joints.

## Position of patient and imaging modality

The patient lies supine head first on the scanner table with the arms resting by the side of the body. Positioning is aided by transaxial, coronal and sagittal alignment lights.

The median sagittal plane is perpendicular and the coronal plane is parallel to the table. The patient is moved until the scan reference point is at the level of the sternal notch and the height adjusted to bring the coronal alignment light to the level of the mid-axillary line

## Imaging procedure

A lateral scan projection is performed on full inspiration. From this image 3 or 5 mm section are prescribed with the gantry angled to align the scan plane with the long axis of the clavicle.

# 3 Locomotor System

## Shoulder Joint

The shoulder joint is a synovial ball-and-socket joint formed between the head of the humerus and the glenoid cavity of the scapula. The glenoid cavity is shallow which makes the joint unstable. It has a wide range of movements and relies on muscle support for stability.

The joint capsule is lax to permit the wide range of movements available at the joint. It attaches close to the margin of the head of humerus, except inferiorly where it attaches 2–3 cm distally.

The capsule is strengthened by four muscles, subscapularis, supraspinatus, infraspinatus and teres minor, which are known collectively as the rotator cuff. Subscapularis originates on the anterior aspect of the scapula and inserts into the lesser tuberosity of the humerus. Supraspinatus originates from the supraspinous fossa of the scapula and inserts into the superior aspect of the greater tuberosity of the humerus. Infraspinatus originates from the infraspinous fossa on the scapula and inserts into the middle portion of the greater tuberosity. Teres minor originates from the upper two-thirds of the axillary border of the scapula (posterior surface) and inserts into the inferior aspect of the greater tuberosity.

Intrinsic features include the glenoid labrum which is a ring of fibrocartilage attached to the periphery of the glenoid fossa to deepen the articular surface.

The long head of biceps arises from the supraglenoid tubercle within the capsule and runs superiorly and laterally to the joint, exiting down the bicipital groove.

Extrinsic ligaments include the coraco-acromial, coracohumeral and glenohumeral. The deltoid muscle covers the joint anteriorly, posteriorly and laterally.

The subdeltoid bursa is situated between the deltoid and the rotator cuff to reduce frictional forces on the rotator cuff tendon. Blood supply is derived from the axillary artery and nerve supply from the axillary, subscapular and lateral pectoral nerves.

### Recommended imaging procedures

Subsequent to plain radiography, MRI with dedicated surface coils is the modality of choice in the evaluation of rotator cuff injury, labrum tear, frozen shoulder or recurrent dislocation.

In the absence of MRI, arthrography can provide a comprehensive investigation of the shoulder joint, particularly when used in conjunction with CT.

Ultrasound, which is non-invasive and less expensive than any of the above techniques, can also prove useful in the investigation of rotator cuff injuries, effusions and cysts.

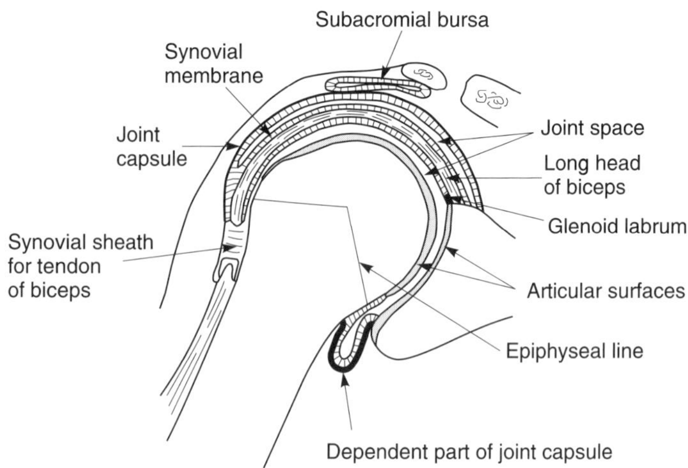


**Figure 3.11** Coronal section through right shoulder joint

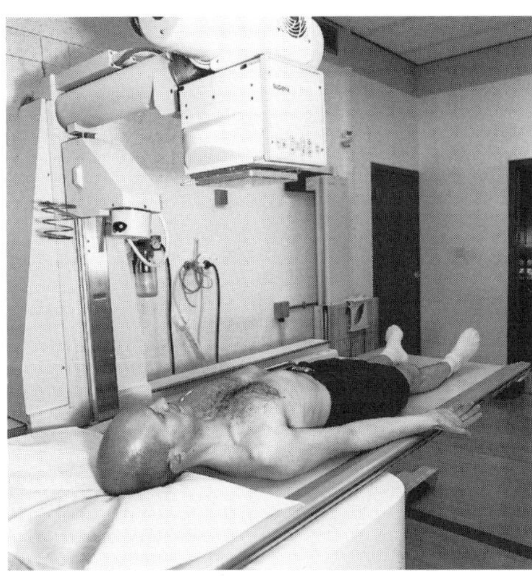

**Figure 3.12a**
Patient positioned for AP shoulder

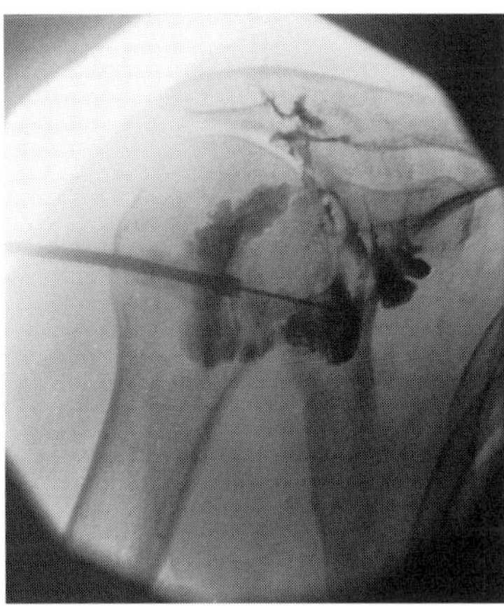

**Figure 3.12b**
Anteroposterior image with needle *in situ*

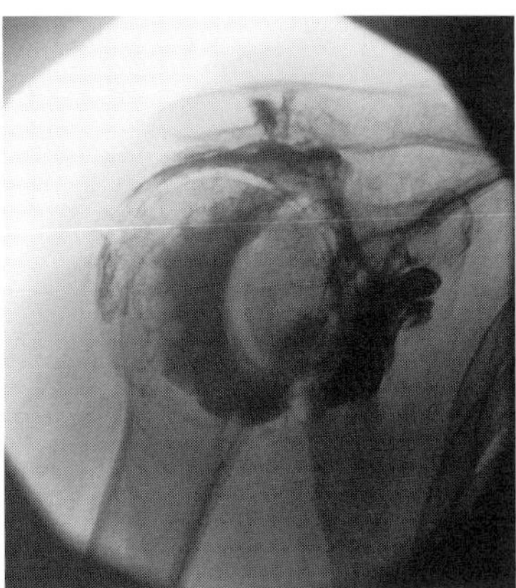

**Figure 3.12c**
Antero-anterior image with internal rotation (showing tear)

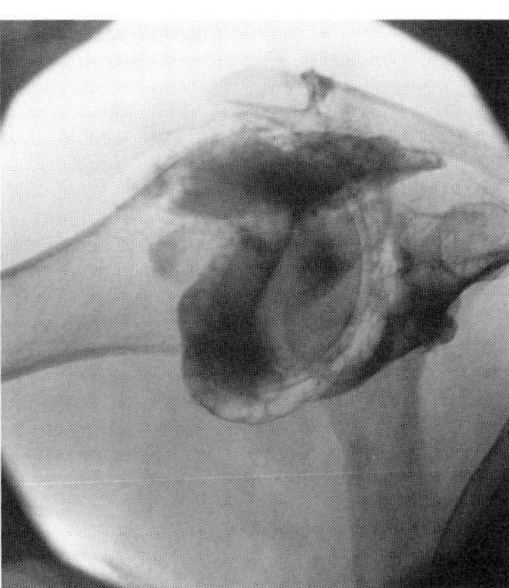

**Figure 3.12d**
Anteroposterior image with abduction

## Arthrography

Shoulder arthrography is the radiographic demonstration of the shoulder joint following the administration of a water-soluble non-ionic contrast agent. A single contrast technique may be used or air may be introduced for double contrast effect. The examination is performed under fluoroscopic control.

### Indications

Arthrography is most commonly performed to demonstrate injury to the rotator cuff. It is also used for recurrent dislocation, capsulitis, loose bodies and to assess the articular surfaces.

### Patient preparation

Control films may be taken in the anteroposterior position with internal and external rotation of the humerus, and a supero-inferior (axial) projection. These radiographs are inspected for the presence of tendon calcification and opaque loose bodies prior to the introduction of a contrast agent.

The patient lies supine on the fluoroscopy table, with the affected arm abducted and externally rotated. The patient's head is supported on a pillow.

The injection site, the junction of the upper two-thirds and lower one-third of the glenohumeral joint, is identified under fluoroscopic control and marked on the skin surface.

The skin is prepared using a suitable antiseptic solution and the surrounding area is covered with sterile towels. A local anaesthetic is introduced into the area adjacent to the skin marker.

### Imaging procedure

A 22-gauge needle is inserted vertically into the glenohumeral joint under fluoroscopic control. The position of the tip of the needle within the capsule can be confirmed by a test injection of 1 ml of contrast agent which should be seen to disperse freely.

Once the position is confirmed, a 20 ml syringe connected to a length of sterile tubing is connected to the needle and the contrast is introduced slowly. If a single contrast technique is employed, 10–12 ml of 240–300 mgI/ml strength contrast is injected. If a double contrast technique is to be employed, a smaller quantity of contrast agent (3–5 ml) is injected, followed by 10 ml of air.

A series of anteroposterior radiographs of the joint, with various degrees of rotation and abduction of the humerus, are taken immediately after injection. If no abnormality is detected the patient is encouraged to exercise gently and the series is repeated. A supero-inferior projection may be taken for rotator cuff injury.

## Computed tomography – method 1

Computed tomography of the shoulder joint may be undertaken either as part of a double contrast arthrogram examination or as a supporting examination in cases of soft tissue or bony tumours adjacent to the shoulder joint.

When a double contrast technique is employed, contrast is injected under fluoroscopic control in a similar way to that described on page 75.

Magnetic resonance imaging is, however, replacing these techniques.

### Indications

The procedure provides useful additional information about the general structure of the shoulder joint and is used to evaluate the extent of any damage to the glenoid labrum.

### Position of patient and imaging modality

The patient lies supine head first on the scanner table with the affected arm resting by the side and the unaffected arm raised above the head. Positioning is aided by transaxial, coronal and sagittal alignment lights.

The patient is offset to the affected side to ensure that the entire shoulder joint is within the scan field of view.

The median sagittal plane is perpendicular and the coronal plane is parallel to the scan table. The table height is adjusted to bring the coronal plane alignment light to the level of the mid-axillary line. The patient is moved into the scanner until the scan reference point is at the level of the sternal notch.

### Imaging procedure

An anteroposterior scan projection radiograph is performed commencing 12 cm above and ending 12 cm below the reference point. From this image, 3 or 5 mm sections are prescribed through the area of suspected abnormality.

If spiral scanning options are available these images may be acquired with a volume acquisition, using a 5 mm slice thickness and 5 mm table increments, but with a 3 mm reconstruction index to give overlapping sections.

To improve spatial resolution the images may be reconstructed either prospectively or retrospectively using a small display field of view.

A bone reconstruction algorithm is normally selected to enhance bony structures while still allowing soft tissues to be demonstrated adequately.

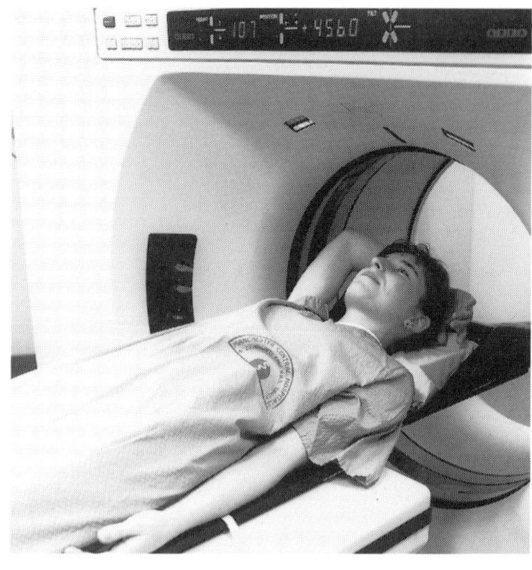

**Figure 3.13a** Method 1 position

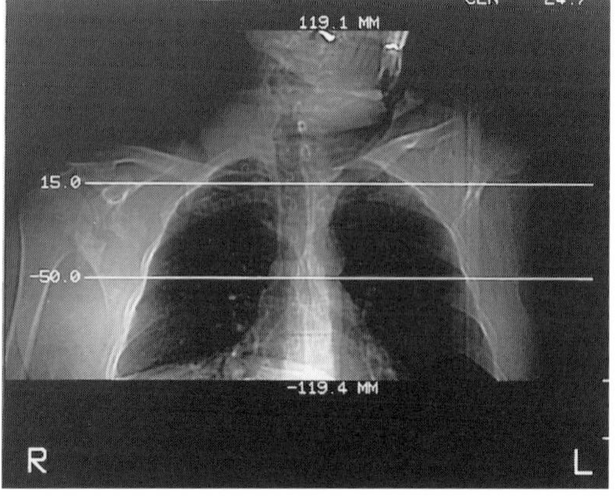


**Figure 3.13b** Scan projection radiograph showing start and end locations

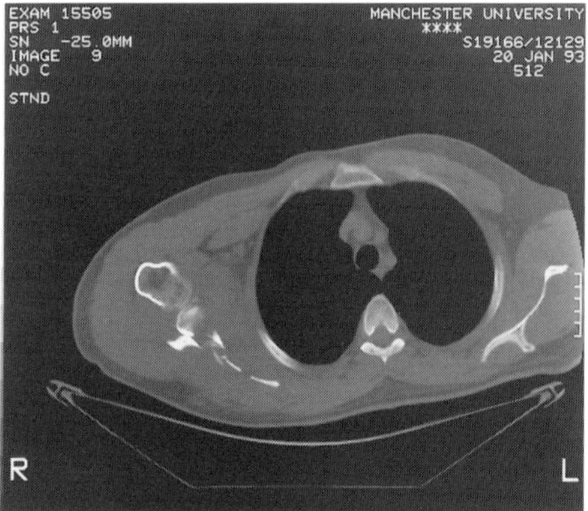


**Figure 3.13c** Transaxial image

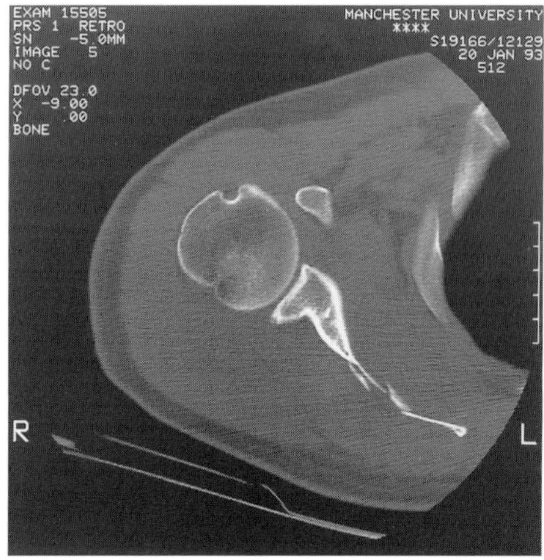


**Figure 3.13d** Reconstructed image on a small field of view demonstrating a fractured scapula

## Computed tomography – method 2

**Position of patient and imaging modality**

This procedure may be used as an alternative to the supine technique in double contrast arthrography of the shoulder. It has the advantage of bringing the glenoid articular surface parallel to the scanner table.

The patient lies head first on the scanner table, on the affected side, arm by the side, and the opposite arm held straight above the head. From this position the patient is rotated forward approximately 30° until the glenoid articular surface is parallel to the table top. A pad is placed under the chest to help maintain this position, preventing the patient from rolling forward.

The patient is moved into the scanner until the scan reference point is over the shoulder joint.

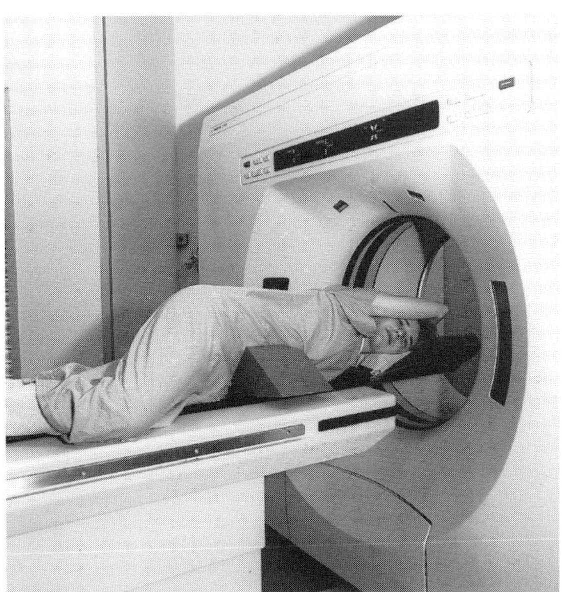

**Figure 3.14a** Method 2 position

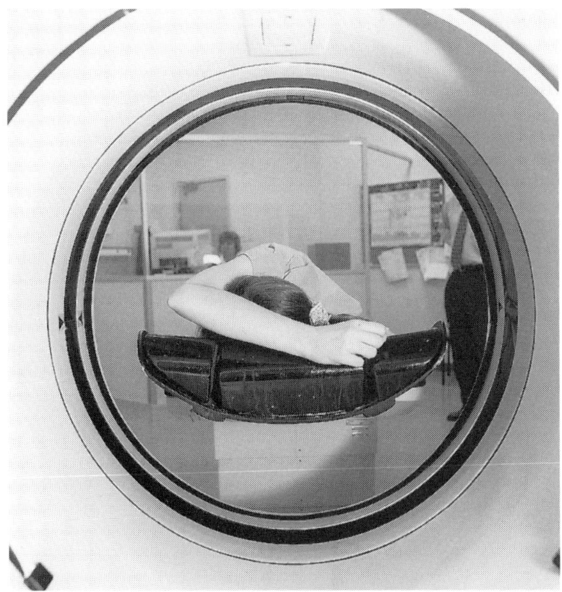

**Figure 3.14b** Method 2 from a different angle

**Imaging procedure**

An anteroposterior scan projection radiograph is performed to include the shoulder joint and upper humerus. From this image 3 or 5 mm sections are prescribed through the area of suspected abnormality.

If spiral scanning options are available these images may be acquired with a volume acquisition, using a 5 mm slice thickness and 5 mm table increments, but with a 3 mm reconstruction index to give overlapping sections.

To improve spatial resolution the images may be reconstructed either prospectively or retrospectively using a small display field of view.

A standard algorithm is normally selected to demonstrate soft tissue adequately.

*Contrast medium and injection data*

| *Volume* | *Concentration* | *Flow rate* |
|---|---|---|
| 3 ml | 320 mgI/ml | Hand injection |
| 15 $cm^3$ | Air | Hand injection |

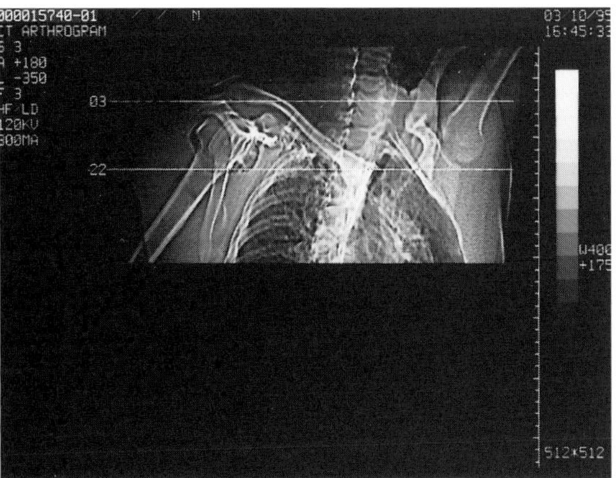


**Figure 3.14c** Scan projection radiograph showing start and end locations

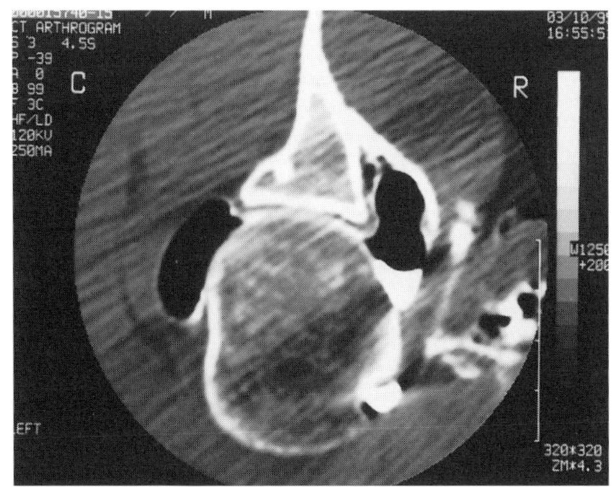


**Figure 3.14d** Transaxial image showing air and contrast medium in the joint space

## Shoulder Joint

### Ultrasound

Ultrasound provides a non-invasive, painless method of imaging the muscle and tendon attachments of the shoulder joint. It can provide useful additional information to supplement plain radiography and can be used to examine both shoulders for comparison.

**Indications**

To confirm the presence and extent of rotator cuff tears, effusions and cysts.

**Position of patient and imaging modality**

The patient is seated on a low stool alongside the ultrasound couch. The arm is abducted, with the elbow flexed to 90°, and supported on the couch.

**Imaging procedure**

The examination is performed using a 7.5 or 5 MHz linear array transducer.

A range of parasagittal and coronal scans are performed to demonstrate the biceps tendon, subscapularis, supraspinatus, infraspinatus and teres minor muscles/tendons, and the subdeltoid bursa.

Dynamic imaging can be performed by rotating, adducting or abducting the arm. This is necessary to demonstrate the tendons in their entirety.

Both shoulders should be examined for comparison.

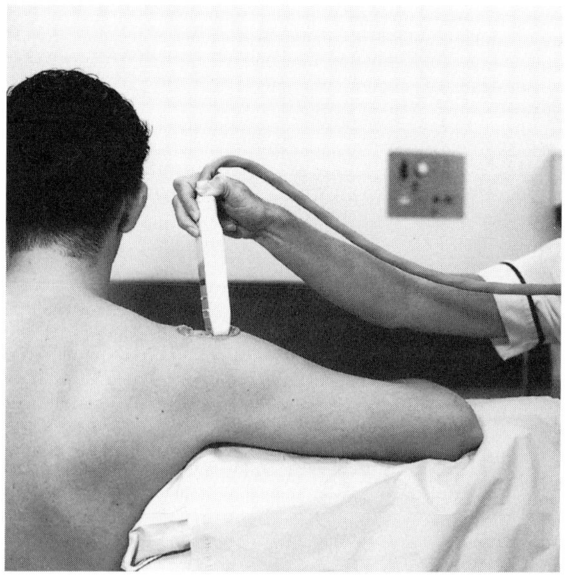

**Figure 3.15a** Transducer positioned for a parasagittal scan

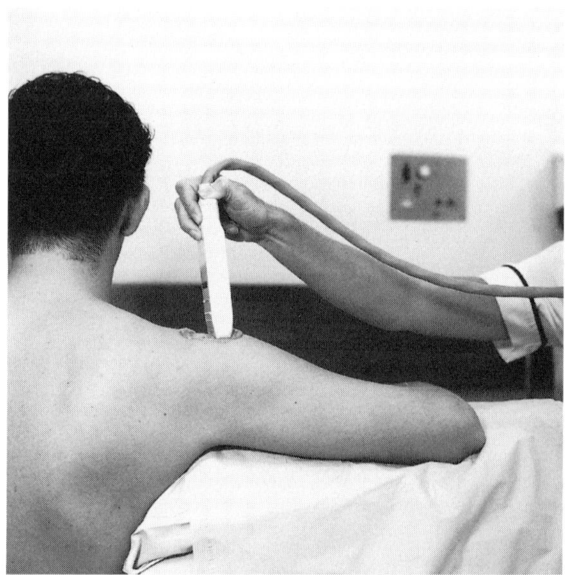

**Figure 3.15b** Transducer positioned for a coronal scan

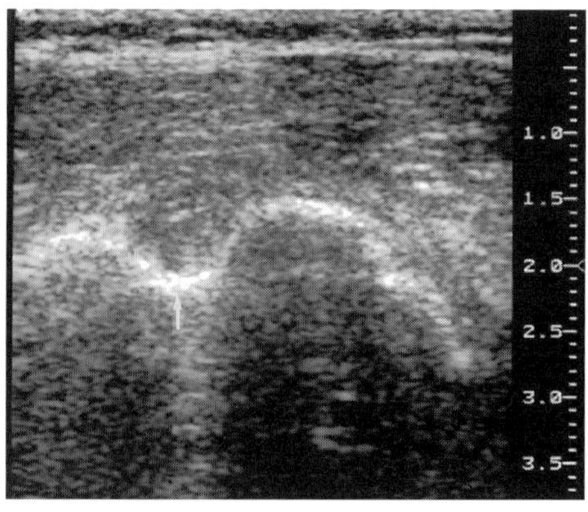


**Figure 3.15c** Coronal image showing the bicipital grove and biceps tendon

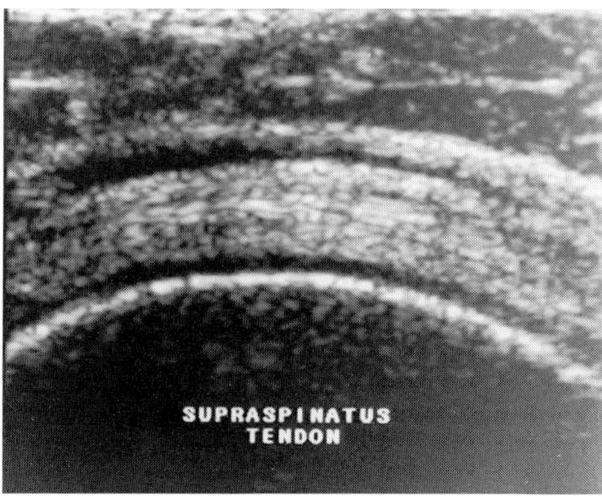


**Figure 3.15d** Parasagittal image showing a normal supraspinatus tendon

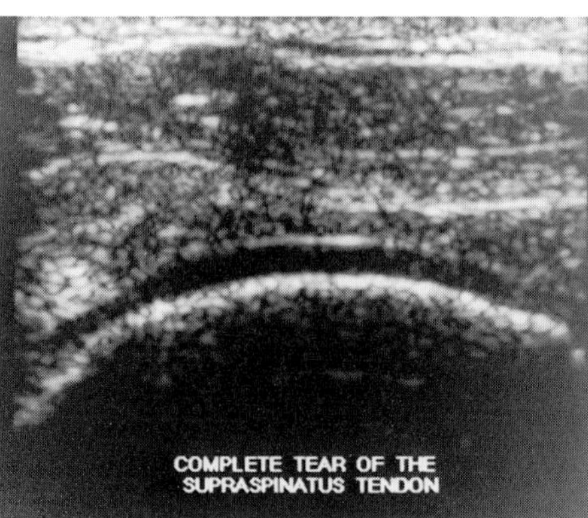


**Figure 3.15e** Parasagittal image showing a complete tear of the supraspinatus tendon

## Ankle Joint

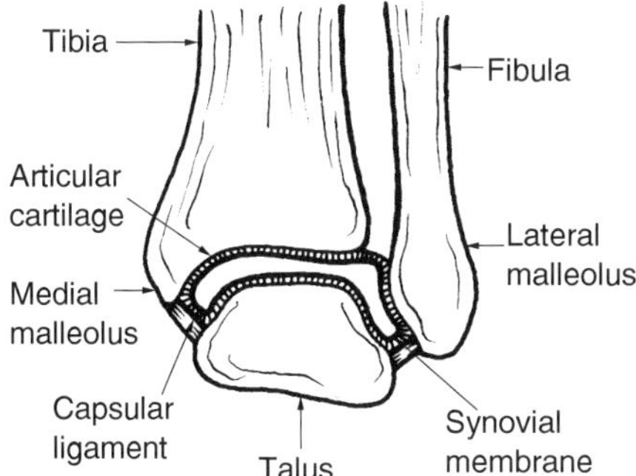


**Figure 3.16a** Schematic diagram of the ankle joint in the coronal plane

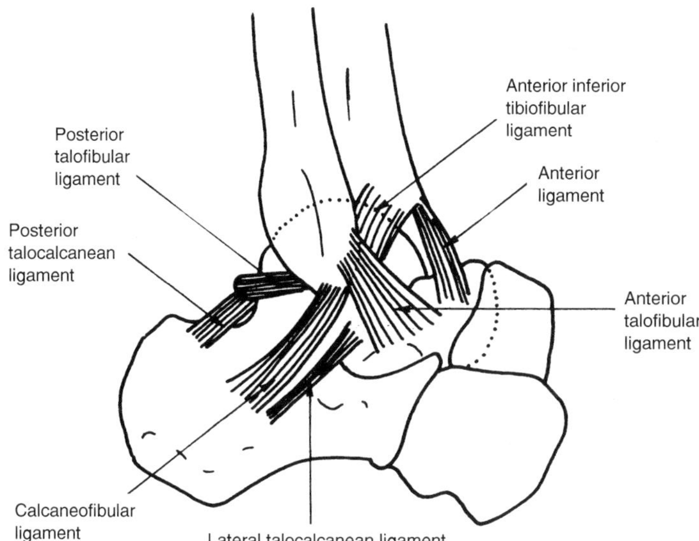


**Figure 3.16b** Schematic diagram showing medial aspect of ankle joint

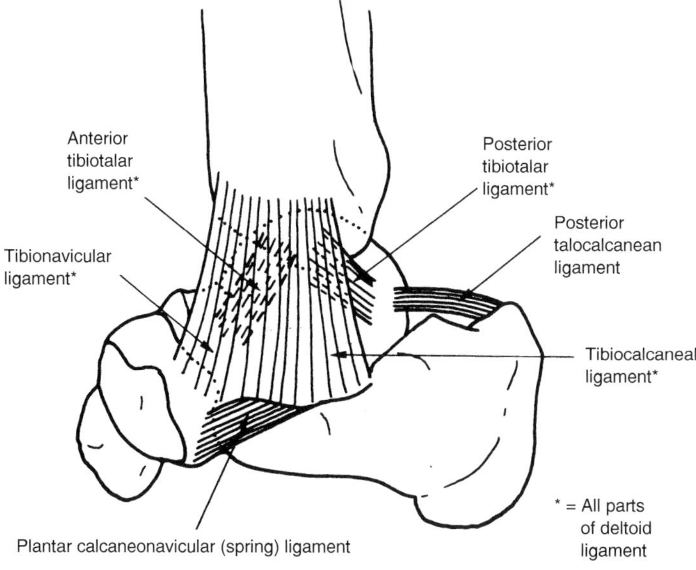


**Figure 3.16c** Schematic diagram showing lateral aspect of ankle joint

The ankle joint is a synovial hinge joint formed between the distal end of the tibia and fibula in articulation with the upper surface of the talus. The tibia and fibula together form a mortice which is narrower posteriorly, thereby reducing the incidence of posterior dislocation of the ankle joint.

The joint capsule is white fibrocartilage and completely surrounds the joint, attaching superiorly and inferiorly to the edge of the articular surfaces, and anteriorly to the neck of the talus. It is relatively thin on its anterior and posterior aspects, with strong lateral and medial collateral ligaments. The extrinsic ligaments are the deltoid on the medial aspect, and the tripartate laterally.

The deltoid ligament is triangular, attaching superiorly to the medial malleolus and inferiorly to the tubercle of the navicular, the sustentaculum tali and the medial surface of the talus.

The lateral or tripartite ligament has three components: anterior talofibular, posterior talofibular, and the calcaneofibular.

Blood supply is derived from the anterior and posterior tibial arteries and the nerve supply is from the peroneal branches of the anterior and posterior tibial nerves.

### Recommended imaging procedures

Plain radiography, which may include stress views, is always undertaken as a primary investigation in cases of chronic instability, although the value of stress views in acute injury is debatable.

Arthrography is a straightforward and relatively simple technique which is ideal for the assessment of joint integrity, to assess the condition of the articular cartilage and to visualise loose bodies.

Computed tomography is ideal where bony abnormalities are suspected.

Magnetic resonance imaging is superior in the visualisation of ligament and tendon abnormalities and in the examination of soft tissues.

# 3 Locomotor System

## Ankle Joint

### Computed tomography – method 1

**Indications**
Computed tomography can be used to assess the extent of tumours and soft tissue infiltration, the degree of bony injury in trauma cases, congenital abnormalities and assessment of the tarsal bones of the feet.

**Position of patient and imaging modality**
The patient lies supine, feet first in the middle of the scanner table with the legs extended. Both joints may be scanned for comparison or the unaffected limb may be positioned out of the scan field by flexion of the knee joint. The legs are internally rotated to ensure that the malleoli, of both ankles, are equidistant from the scanner table. Sandbags should be placed against the knees and positioning straps around the feet to minimise the risk of patient movement.

Positioning is aided by transaxial, coronal and sagittal alignment lights, ensuring that the median sagittal plane is perpendicular and the coronal plane parallel to the scanner table. The scan plane is now perpendicular to the long axis of the body.

The patient is moved into the scanner until the scan reference point is at the level of the malleoli and the table height adjusted until the coronal light is at the level of the lateral malleolus.

**Imaging procedure**
A lateral scan projection radiograph is taken approximately 12 cm above to 6 cm below the scan reference point. From this image either 3 or 5 mm contiguous slices are prescribed through the suspected area of abnormality.

If spiral scanning options are available, these images may be acquired with a volume acquisition, using a 5 mm slice thickness and 5 mm table increments, but with a 3 mm reconstruction index to give overlapping sections.

To improve spatial resolution the images may be reconstructed either prospectively or retrospectively using a small display field of view.

A bone reconstruction algorithm is normally selected to enhance bony structures while still allowing soft tissues to be demonstrated adequately. Further reformatted images in either the coronal or sagittal plane may be useful.

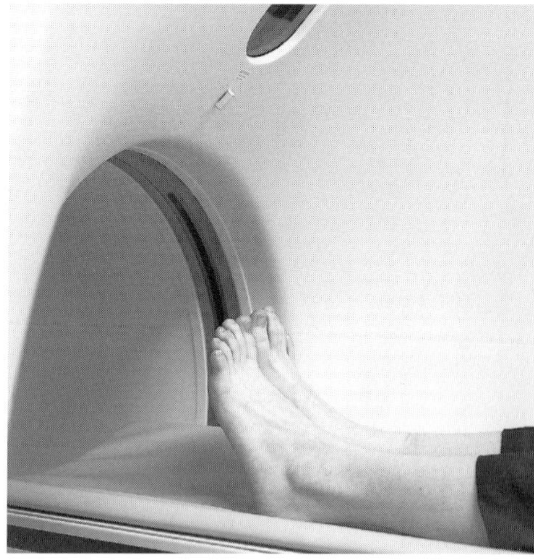

**Figure 3.17a** Method 1 position

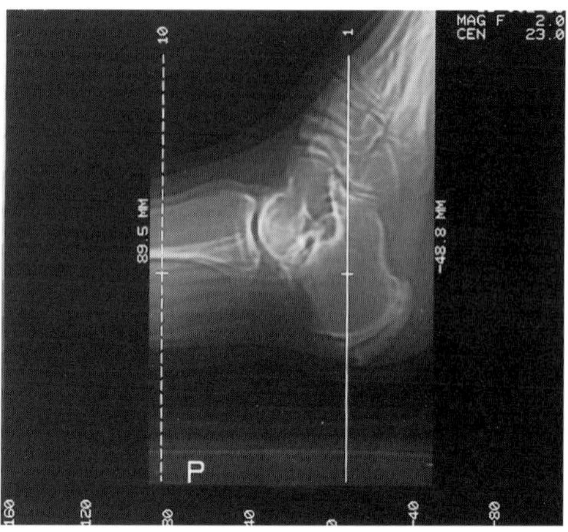


**Figure 3.17b** Scan projection radiograph showing start and end locations

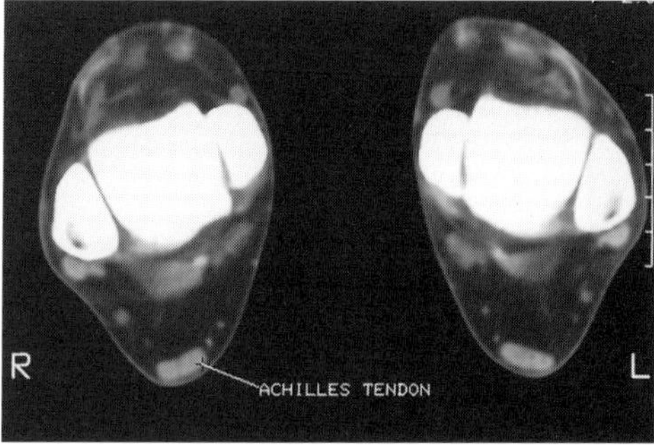


**Figure 3.17c** Transaxial image showing Achilles tendon (soft tissue window width/level)

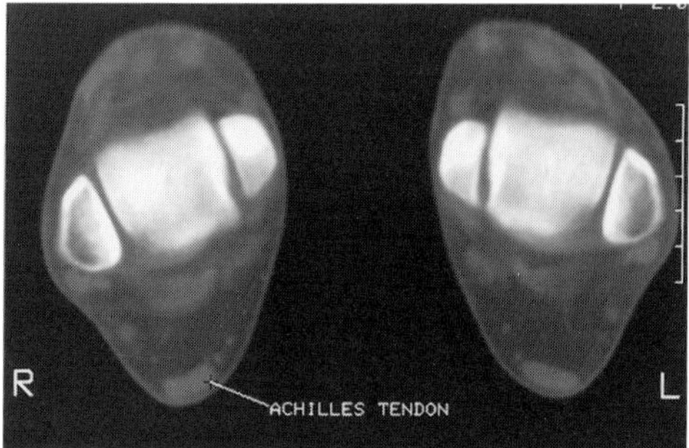


**Figure 3.17d** Transaxial image as above (bone window width/level)

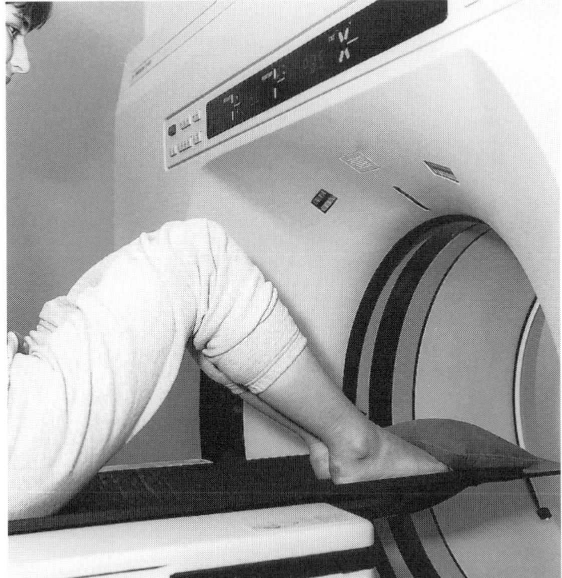

Figure 3.18a Method 2 position

## Computed tomography – method 2

**Position of patient and imaging modality**

The patient sits on scanner table with both knees flexed and the plantar aspect of the feet resting on the table top. Both joints may be imaged for comparison. The feet are immobilised using sandbags or straps positioned over the toes.

The patient is moved into the scanner until the scan reference point is at the level of the malleoli and the table height adjusted until the coronal alignment light is at the level of the lateral malleolus.

**Imaging procedure**

A lateral scan projection radiograph is performed from 5 cm above to 7 cm below the scan reference point. From this image either 3 or 5 mm sections are prescribed through the area of suspected abnormality.

If spiral scanning options are available, these images may be acquired with a volume acquisition, using a 5 mm slice thickness and 5 mm table increments, but with a 3 mm reconstruction index to give overlapping sections.

To improve spatial resolution the images may be reconstructed either prospectively or retrospectively using a small display field of view.

A bone reconstruction algorithm is normally selected to enhance bony structures while still allowing soft tissues to be demonstrated adequately.

Further reformatted images in either the coronal or sagittal plane may be useful.

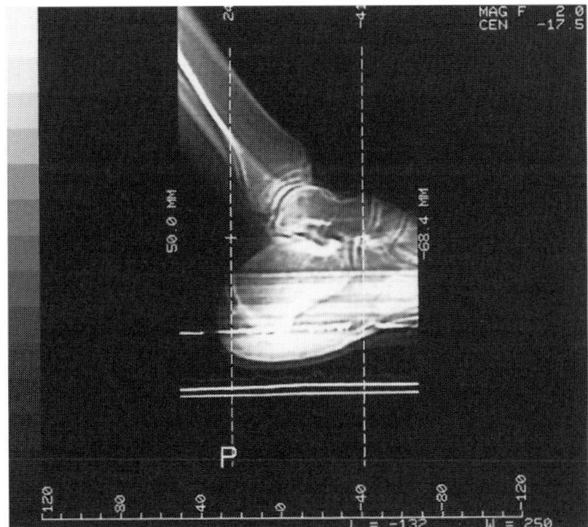


Figure 3.18b Scan projection radiograph showing start and end locations

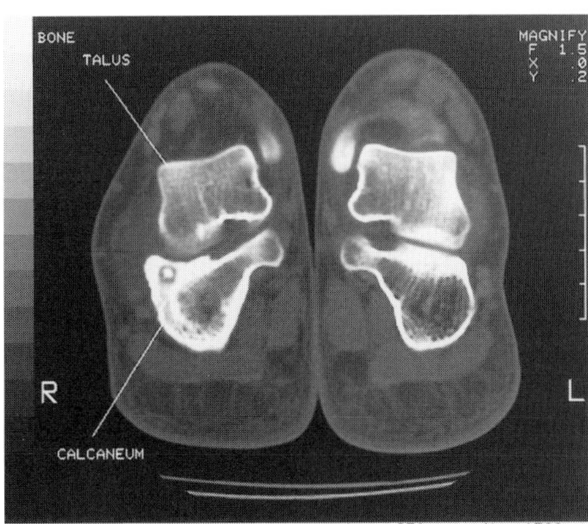


Figure 3.18c Transaxial image through the tarsal bones showing talus and calcaneum

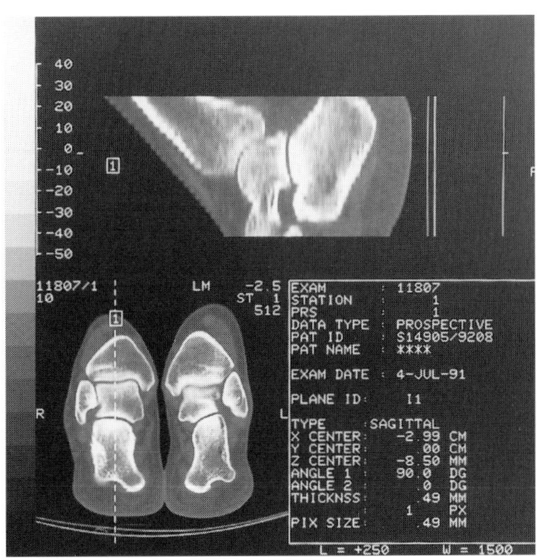


Figure 3.18d Reformatted image showing talocalcaneal joint

## Ankle Joint

### Arthrography

Ankle arthrography is the radiographic demonstration of the ankle joint following the administration of a water-soluble contrast agent.

A single contrast technique may be employed using either a radio-opaque contrast agent or air, or a double contrast technique may be undertaken.

The examination is performed under fluoroscopic control and images may be recorded using digital fluoroscopy equipment or conventional radiography using high-definition intensifying screens.

#### Indications

A single contrast technique using a radio-opaque contrast agent is used in the assessment of ligamental injury, air alone may be used in the investigation of loose bodies, and the double contrast technique is superior in the investigation of the articular cartilage.

#### Patient preparation

Control films are taken in the anteroposterior, lateral and oblique positions. Stress views may also be taken in cases of chronic joint instability.

The patient lies supine on the fluoroscopy table, with head resting on a pillow. The path of the dorsalis pedis artery is identified and marked on the skin surface.

The anterior aspect of the joint is identified under palpation and fluoroscopic control. A point is marked on the skin surface approximately in the midline over the joint space.

The skin is prepared using a suitable antiseptic solution and the surrounding area is covered with sterile towels.

Local anaesthetic is introduced into the area around the skin marker.

#### Imaging procedure

A 22-gauge needle is inserted into the joint space under fluoroscopic control, with the ankle rotated into the lateral position. The needle is inserted slightly upwards to avoid the anterior margin of the tibia.

Once the position of the needle is confirmed in the joint capsule, either by aspiration of synovial fluid or by a test injection of a small amount of contrast agent, the syringe containing the contrast agent is attached to the needle and approximately 6–8 ml of 240–300 mgI/ml strength contrast is injected. If a double contrast technique is to be undertaken, a smaller quantity of radio-opaque contrast is introduced followed by 6–8 ml of air.

Following gentle exercise of the joint a series of anteroposterior, anteroposterior oblique and lateral images are acquired.

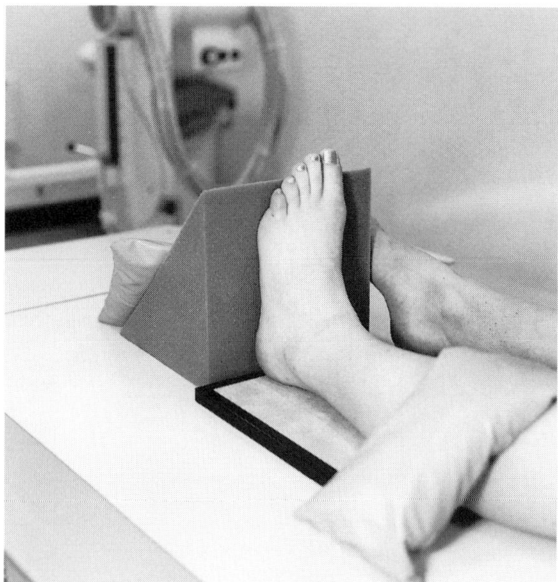

**Figure 3.19a** Position for anteroposterior projection

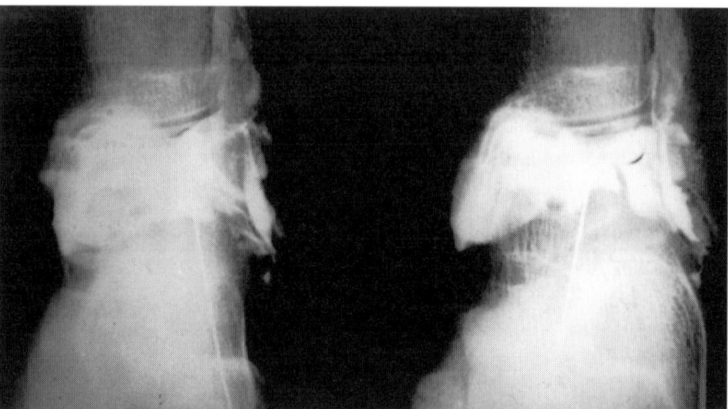

**Figure 3.19b** Anteroposterior radiographs of both ankle joints

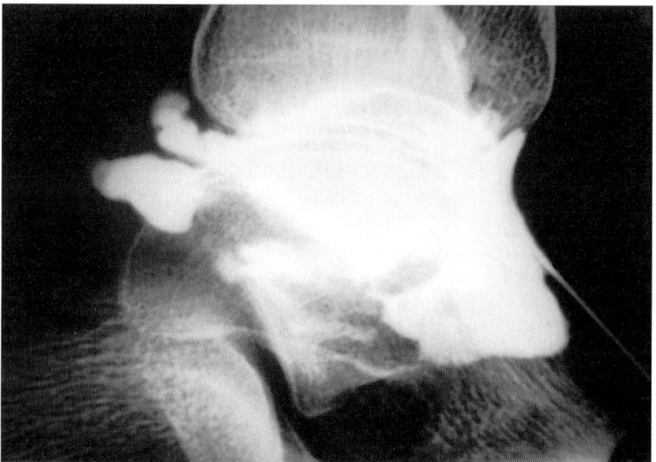

**Figure 3.19c** Lateral radiograph of ankle joint

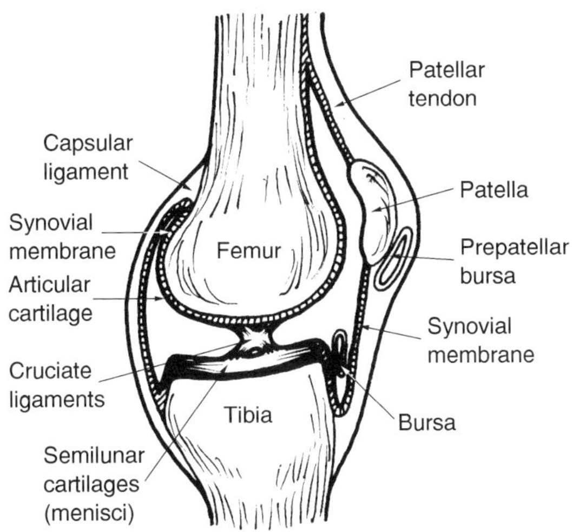


**Figure 3.20a** Sagittal section through knee joint

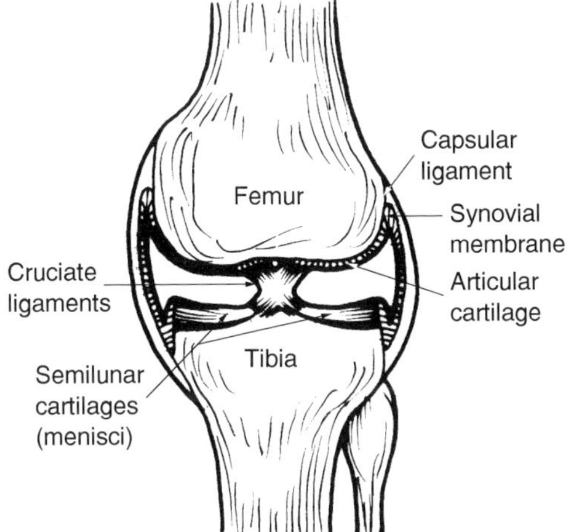


**Figure 3.20b** Coronal section through knee joint

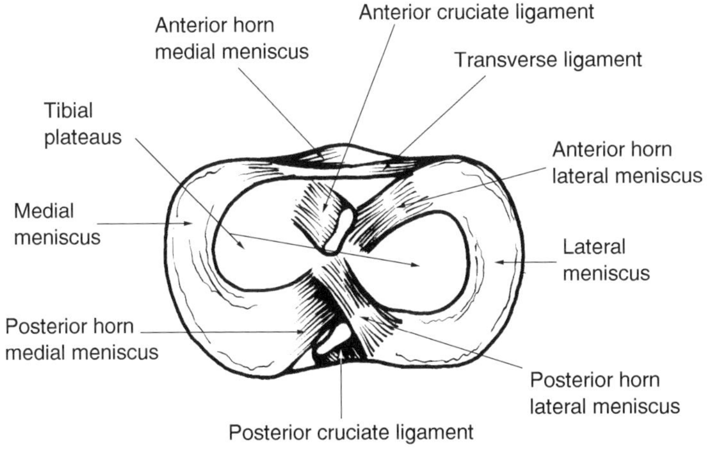


**Figure 3.20c** Superior aspect of tibia

The knee joint is a compound joint. The joint formed between the condyles of the femur and the tibia is a synovial double condyloid joint and the joint between the patella and the femur is a synovial plane joint.

It is the largest joint in the body and the joint capsule is complex and very strong. It is not a separate structure, being absent in some places, notably over and above the patella, and in other places it is replaced by tendons of muscles surrounding the joint.

There are a number of intrinsic features, including the prepatella, suprapatella and infrapatella bursae. There are two cruciate ligaments. The anterior arises from the posterior aspect of the medial surface of the lateral condyle of the femur and passes inferiorly and medially, attaching to the anterior part of the intercondylar area of the upper surface of the tibia. The posterior cruciate ligament arises from the lateral surface of the medial condyle of the femur and passes inferiorly and laterally, attaching to the posterior part of the intercondylar area of the tibia.

The menisci are crescent-shaped cartilages which are wedge shaped in cross-section and are situated on the articular surfaces of the tibia. The transverse ligament joins the anterior ends of the two menisci.

The patella is a sesamoid bone and is situated in the ligamentum patellae, the central part of the quadriceps tendon.

The joint is surrounded by the ligamentum patellae, quadriceps femoris, oblique popliteal ligament, arcuate popliteal ligament, and tibial and fibular collateral ligaments.

The movements of the joint between the femur and the tibia are complex. Flexion involves slight medial rotation of the tibia on the femur, and extension involves slight lateral rotation of the tibia on the femur.

The blood supply is derived from the popliteal and anterior tibial arteries and the nerve supply from the femoral, obturator and tibial nerves.

## Recommended imaging procedures

Plain radiography is the initial imaging technique in the investigation of the knee joint.

Magnetic resonance imaging has to a large extent replaced CT and arthrography of the knee joint. Arthroscopy is now routinely used in the investigation of the menisci without the need for imaging.

Ultrasound is restricted to the investigation of fluid-filled cysts such as Baker's cyst and associated aneurysms, although arthrography may be used to support the findings.

## Computed tomography

**Indications**

Transaxial CT can be used to assess the extent of tumours and soft tissue infiltration, the degree of bony injury in trauma cases, and congenital abnormalities, and provides a useful assessment of joints prior to prosthetic surgery.

**Position of patient and imaging modality**

The patient lies supine, feet first, in the middle of the scanner table, arms folded across the chest.

Ideally the femoral condyles of each limb should be equidistant from the table as both limbs are scanned for comparison. If it is impossible for both knees to be straightened, they should have the same degree of flexion.

Sandbags should be placed against the ankles and positioning straps around the feet to reduce the risk of patient movement. Positioning is aided by transaxial, coronal and sagittal alignment lights to ensure that the median sagittal plane is perpendicular and the coronal plane parallel to the scanner table. The scan plane is now perpendicular to the long axis of the body.

The patient is moved into the scanner until the scan reference point is at the level of the femoral condyles and the table height adjusted until the coronal light is at the level of the lateral femoral condyle.

Trauma patients must be made as comfortable as possible on the scanner table to avoid movement and further injury to the affected area.

**Imaging procedure**

An anteroposterior scan projection radiograph is taken from approximately 5 cm above to 24 cm below the scan reference point. From this image, 3 or 5 mm sections are prescribed through the suspected area of abnormality.

If spiral scanning options are available, these images may be acquired with a volume acquisition, using a 5 mm slice thickness and 5 mm table increments, but with a 3 mm reconstruction index to give overlapping sections.

To improve spatial resolution the images may be reconstructed either prospectively or retrospectively using a small display field of view.

The digital data may be reformatted to produce images in either the coronal or sagittal plane.

A bone reconstruction algorithm is normally selected. This enhances bony structures while still allowing soft tissues to be adequately demonstrated.

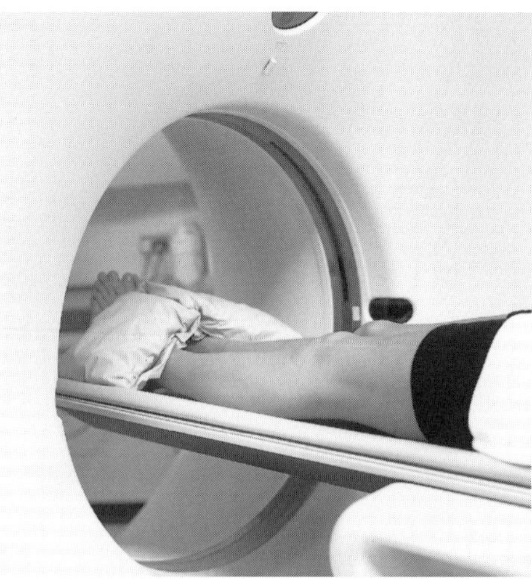

**Figure 3.21a** Patient in CT scanner

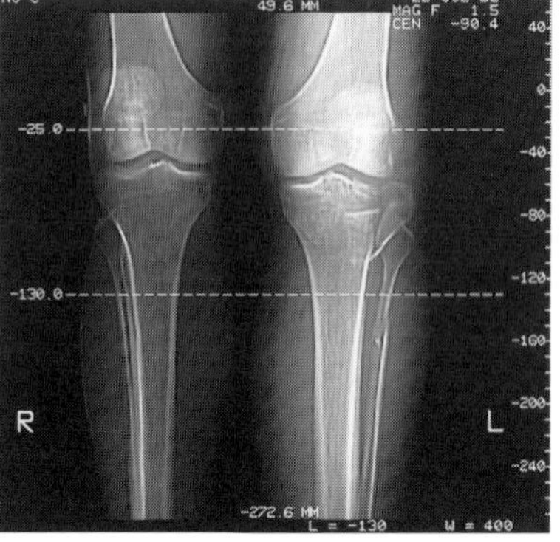


**Figure 3.21b** Scan projection radiograph showing start and end locations

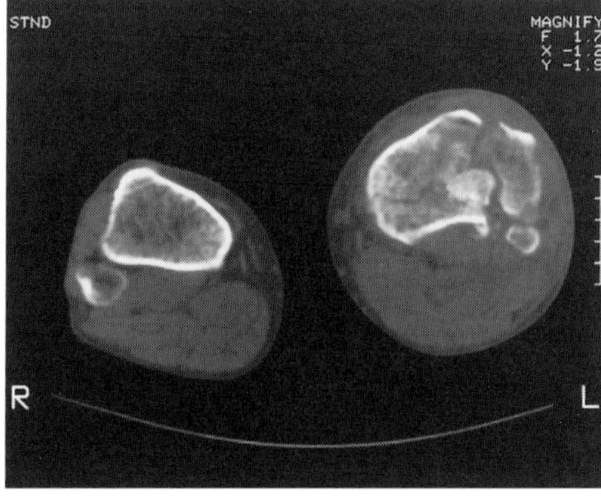


**Figure 3.21c** Transaxial image through the tibial plateau showing a fracture

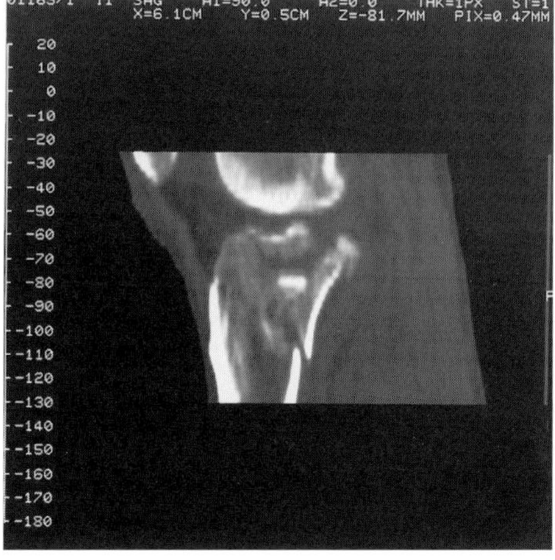


**Figure 3.21d** Sagittal re-formation

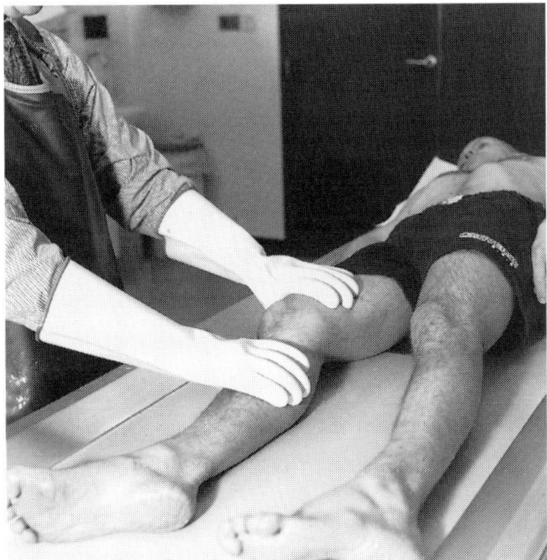
**Figure 3.22a** Patient positioned for oblique stress views of the knee

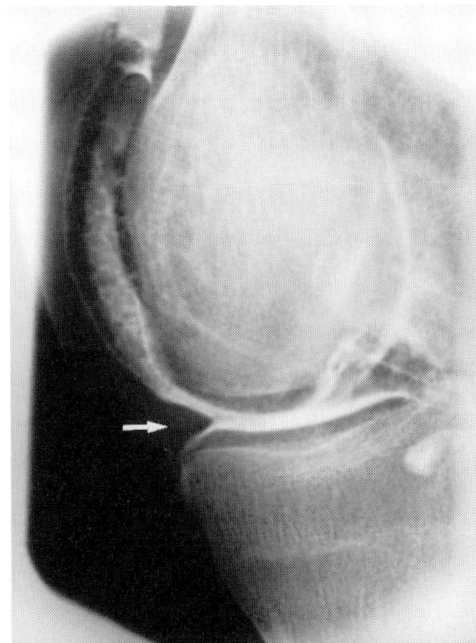
**Figure 3.22b** Oblique view of knee showing normal meniscus cartilage

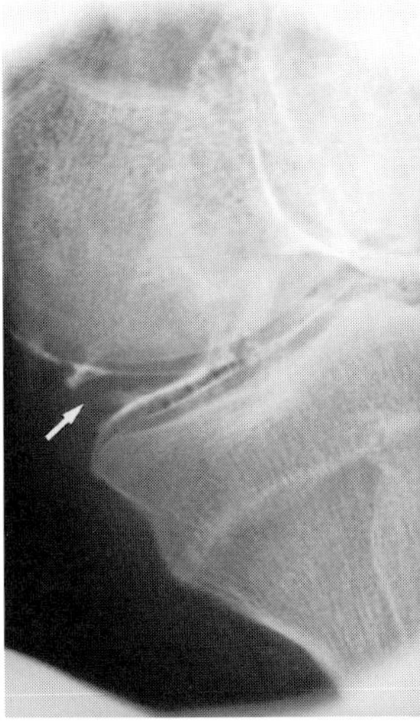
**Figure 3.22c** Oblique view of knee showing meniscal tear

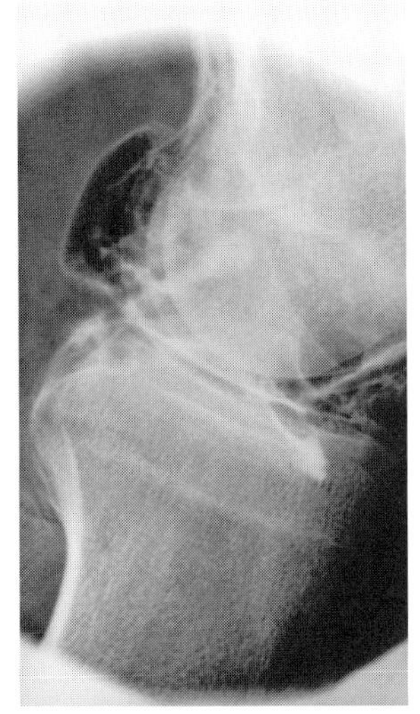
**Figure 3.22d** Lateral image of knee showing posterior capsular structures and cruciate ligaments

## Arthrography

Knee arthrography is the radiographic demonstration of the knee joint following the administration of a non-ionic water-soluble contrast agent. A double contrast technique is normally employed, but a single contrast technique may be employed for suspected loose bodies or a Baker's cyst.

The examination is performed under fluoroscopic control and images may be recorded using digital fluoroscopy equipment or a combination of fluoroscopic spot films and conventional radiography. A fine focal spot, together with regular speed intensifying screens, is required.

### Indications

Double contrast arthrography is used in cases of suspected ligamental, cartilaginous or capsular damage.

### Patient preparation

Control films may be taken with the patient in the prone position. The patient is then turned supine and the knee is supported on a non-opaque triangular foam pad.

The skin is prepared using a suitable antiseptic solution and the area around the knee is draped with sterile towels. Local anaesthetic may be introduced into the surrounding tissues.

### Imaging procedure

The needle is introduced using either a medial or lateral approach. The medial approach offers the advantage of access to a larger area of the joint space, whereas the lateral approach traverses less soft tissue.

A 21-gauge needle is inserted into the joint space at a point between the mid-point of the patella and the femoral condyle. Any effusion is aspirated and 3–5 ml of water-soluble contrast agent (240–300 mgI/ml) is introduced under fluoroscopic control, followed by approximately 40 ml of air to produce the double contrast effect.

The needle is removed and the knee is exercised to distribute the contrast within the joint capsule.

The patient is turned prone and the knee is placed under stress, either by the use of a stress immobilising device or by hand traction applied to the lower leg. Suitable additional radiation protection is required for the operator.

Each meniscus is examined in turn by applying rotation, flexion, extension and stress. Internal rotation is used to demonstrate the anterior horn of the medial meniscus and for the posterior horn of the lateral meniscus; lateral rotation is used to demonstrate the posterior horn of the medial meniscus and the anterior horn of the lateral meniscus.

The cruciate ligaments may be examined with the patient rotated into the lateral position for lateral and oblique views under stress. Spot films are taken as required.

## Knee Joint

### Ultrasound

Ultrasound provides a useful, inexpensive and non-invasive method of determining the presence of cysts and vascular abnormalities. However, due to the shape of the knee joint, ultrasound examination is limited to the articular surfaces, and para-articular and superficial structures.

The procedure is rarely generally specific and sensitive and is often performed in conjunction with another imaging modality for accurate diagnosis.

**Indications**

Superficial structures such as a Baker's cyst are easily demonstrated and it is an excellent alternative to plain film radiography, arthrography and arthroscopy for examination of lateral joint margin masses and effusions. It may also be useful in determining meniscal cysts, large meniscal tears, rupture of the anterior cruciate ligament in the presence of haemarthrosis and in the assessment of patellar tendonitis.

Doppler ultrasound, especially colour flow imaging, may be useful in the differentiation of abnormalities such as popliteal aneurysms, deep vein thrombosis and suspected benign or malignant tumours.

**Position of patient and imaging modality**

The patient lies prone or supine on the table, depending on the structures to be examined. The knee is slightly flexed and the transducer held over the joint.

**Imaging procedure**

The examination is performed using a high-resolution 5 or 7.5 MHz linear array probe.

Scanning in multiple planes needs to be undertaken and comparison with the normal side is essential.

Most of the cartilage on the femoral condyle may be studied by flexing and extending the limb, but large areas on the retropatellar surface and tibial plateau are hidden from examination.

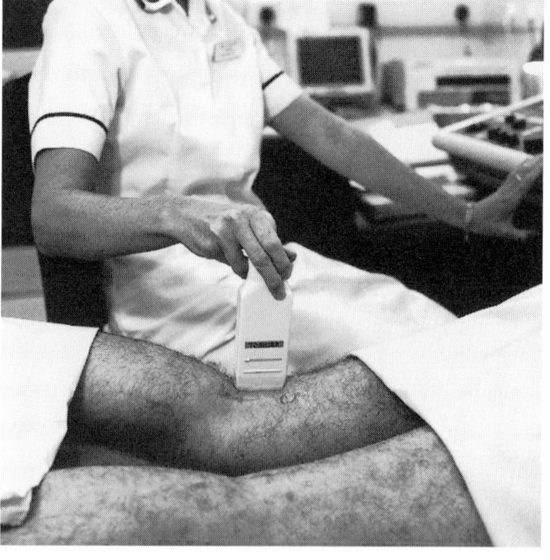

**Figure 3.23a** Transducer positioned for a longitudinal scan

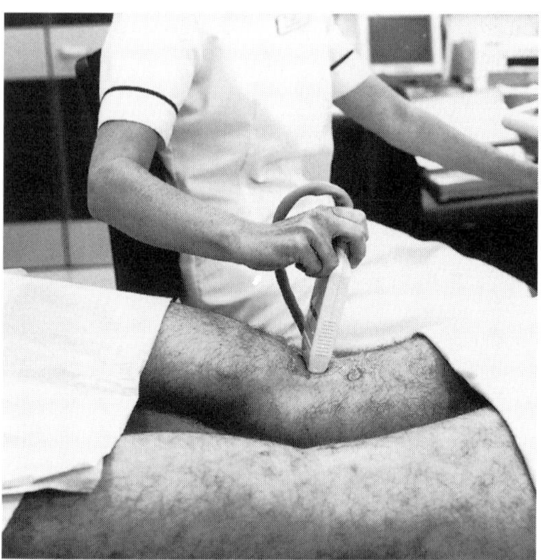

**Figure 3.23b** Transducer positioned for a transverse scan

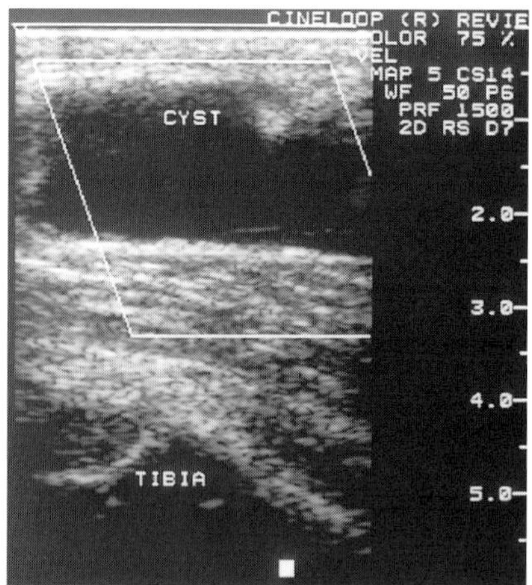


**Figure 3.23c** Image showing a Baker's cyst

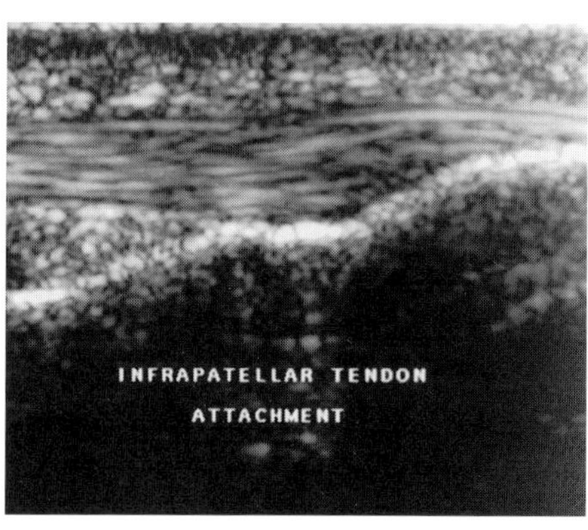


**Figure 3.23d** Image showing the infrapatellar tendon attachment

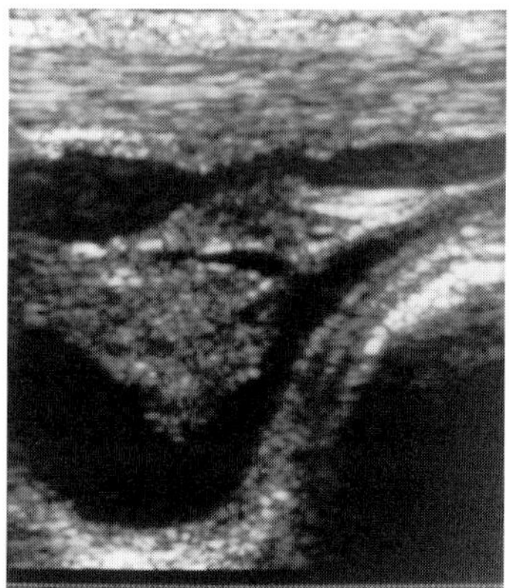

**Figure 3.23e** Image showing Osgood–Schlatter disease

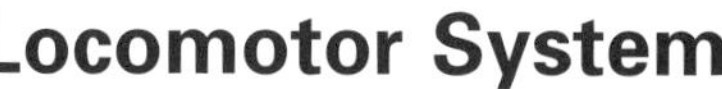



# Hip Joint

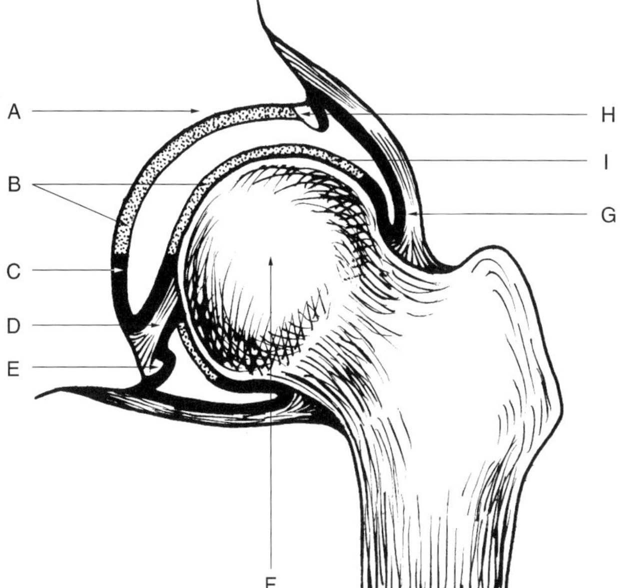


**Figure 3.24** Left hip joint, anterior aspect (A, acetabulum; B, hyaline cartilage; C, synovial membrane; D, ligamentum teres; E, transverse acetabular ligament; F, head of femur; G, fibrous capsule; H, acetabular labrum

The hip joint is a synovial ball-and-socket joint formed between the head of the femur and the acetabulum of the innominate bone. The head of the femur comprises two-thirds of a sphere and the articular surface of the acetabulum is formed by a horseshoe-shaped ring of fibrocartilage. The femoral neck forms an angle of approximately 125° to the shaft and is directed anteriorly and superiorly to it. This requires the limb to be internally rotated if the neck is to be imaged without foreshortening.

The joint capsule is a strong tense cylindrical sleeve which encloses the joint and the majority of the neck. It attaches to trochanteric line on the femur anteriorly and 1 cm above the trochanteric crest posteriorly. It attaches to the rim of the acetabulum beyond the acetabular labrum where it merges with the tranverse ligament.

Intrinsic features of the joint include the acetabular labrum which is a horseshoe-shaped ring of fibrocartilage. It is shaped in profile and deepens the articular surface of the acetabulum significantly. The transverse acetabular ligament which is partly intrinsic and partly extrinsic completes the horseshoe inferiorly. The ligamentum teres, which is triangular in shape, attaches by its apex to a depression in the head of the femur, the fovea capitis, and by its base to the acetabular notch and blends with the transverse ligament.

Extrinsic ligaments which strengthen the joint capsule include the iliofemoral (anterolaterally), the ischiofemoral (posterolaterally) and the pubofemoral (inferiorly).

Blood supply is derived from the medial circumflex, internal iliac and femoral arteries, and the nerve supply is via the sacral plexus.

## Recommended imaging procedures

Plain radiography is usually undertaken as the primary method of investigation of the hip joint.

Arthrography is a straightforward technique and is used primarily in the adult to assess joint integrity including suspected prosthetic loosening. It may also be used in children to assess the condition of the articular cartilages.

Computed tomography is particularly useful in the investigation of suspected bony abnormalities.

Magnetic resonance imaging provides additional information of ligamentous and soft tissue structures.

Ultrasound is the modality of choice for the investigation of hip dysplasia in infants.

Radionuclide imaging can provide useful additional information in cases of suspected infection and loosening of prostheses.

## Computed tomography – method 1

**Indications**

Transaxial CT can be used to assess the extent of tumours and soft tissue infiltration, the degree of bony injury in trauma cases, and congenital abnormalities, and provides a useful assessment of joints prior to prosthetic surgery.

**Position of patient and imaging modality**

The patient lies supine, feet first, on the scanner table, with arms extended and supported above the head. The anterior superior iliac spines are equidistant from the table top, and the lower limbs are and internally rotated and supported by sandbags and positioning straps. Positioning is aided by transaxial, coronal and sagittal lights, ensuring that the median sagittal plane is perpendicular and the coronal plane parallel to the table top. The scan plane is now perpendicular to the long axis of the body.

The scanner table height is raised until the mid-axillary line is at the centre of the scan field. The patient is moved into the scanner until the scan reference point is at the level of the iliac crest.

Trauma patients must be made as comfortable as possible on the scanner table, with as little movement as possible to avoid further injury to the affected area.

**Imaging procedure**

An anteroposterior scan projection radiograph is performed from 2 cm above to 25 cm below the scan reference point. From this image, 5 mm contiguous sections are prescribed either through the whole pelvis or the hip joints.

The large scan field of view must be selected to ensure that all the bony areas are included in the transaxial images.

If spiral scanning options are available, these images may be acquired with a volume acquisition, using a 5 mm slice thickness and 5 mm table increments, but with a 3 mm reconstruction index to give overlapping sections.

To improve spatial resolution the images may be reconstructed either prospectively or retrospectively using a small display field of view.

A bone reconstruction algorithm is normally selected to enhance bony structures while still allowing soft tissues to be demonstrated adequately.

Further reformatted images may be useful.

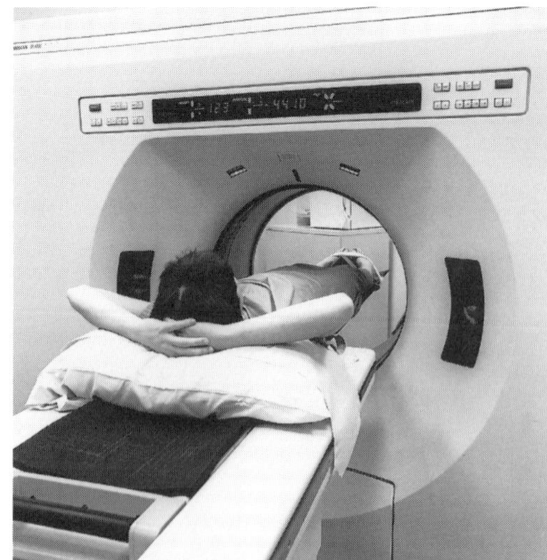

**Figure 3.25a** Method 1 position

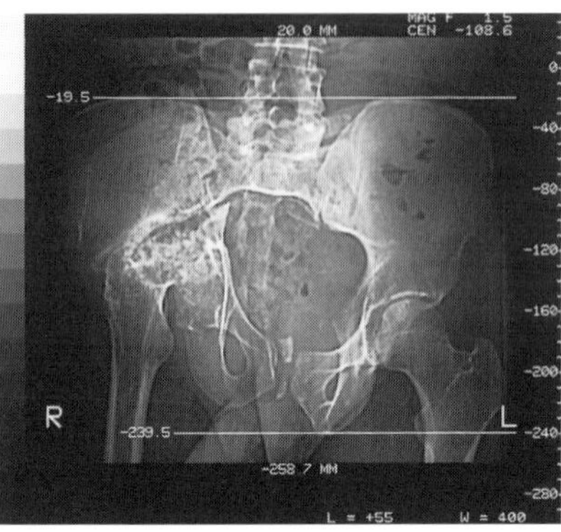


**Figure 3.25b** Scan projection radiograph showing start and end locations

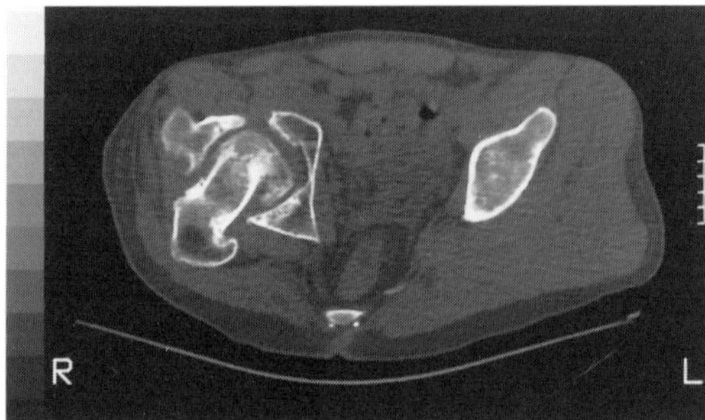


**Figure 3.25c** Transaxial image

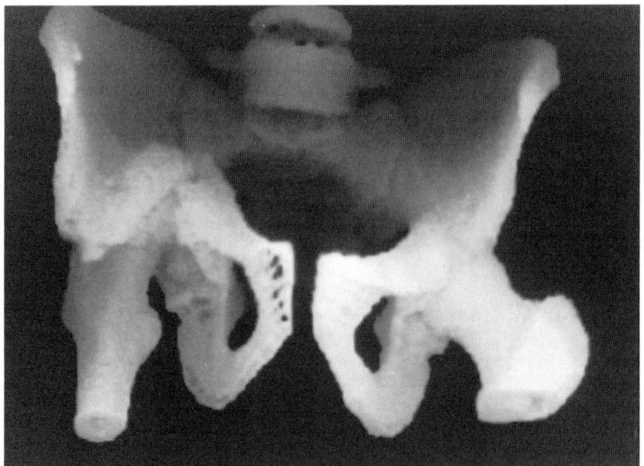

**Figure 3.25d** Reformatted 3D image of pelvis

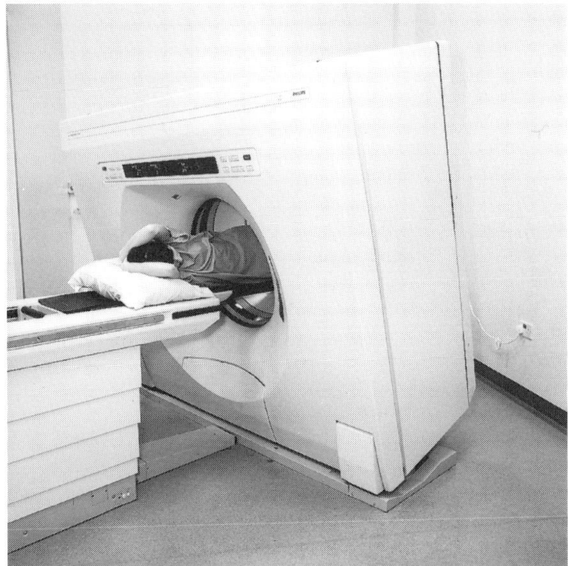

Figure 3.26a Method 2 position

## Computed tomography – method 2

**Position of patient and imaging modality**

This technique may be used to assess the opposite hip in patients who have already undergone a total hip replacement.

The patient is turned onto the side to be examined, with the knees slightly flexed and arms raised onto the pillow.

The table is raised until the coronal alignment light is at the level of the median sagittal plane. The patient is moved into the scanner until the scan reference point is at the level of the iliac crest.

**Imaging procedure**

A scan projection radiograph is taken with the tube in the lateral position, starting 5 cm above and ending 25 cm below the scan reference point.

To prevent image degradation from streak artefacts the gantry is angled cranially until the hip prosthesis is clear of the scan plane and 5 mm sections are prescribed through the joint.

If spiral scanning options are available, these images may be acquired with a volume acquisition, using a 5 mm slice thickness and 5 mm table increments, but with a 3 mm reconstruction index to give overlapping sections.

To improve spatial resolution the images may be reconstructed either prospectively or retrospectively using a small display field of view.

A bone reconstruction algorithm is normally selected to enhance bony structures while still allowing soft tissues to be demonstrated adequately.

Further reformatted images may be useful.

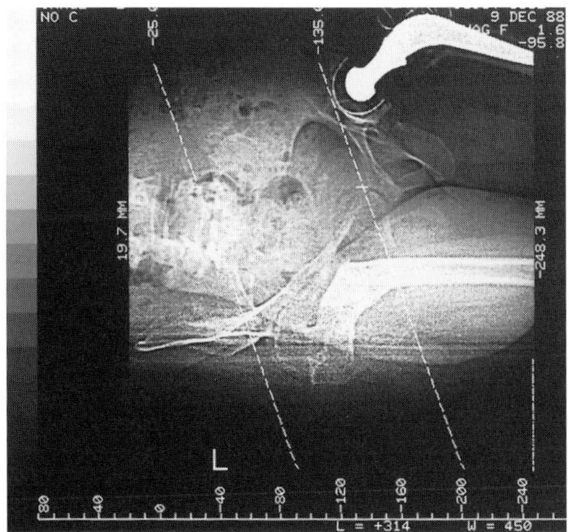


Figure 3.26b Scan projection radiograph showing start and end locations and gantry angulations

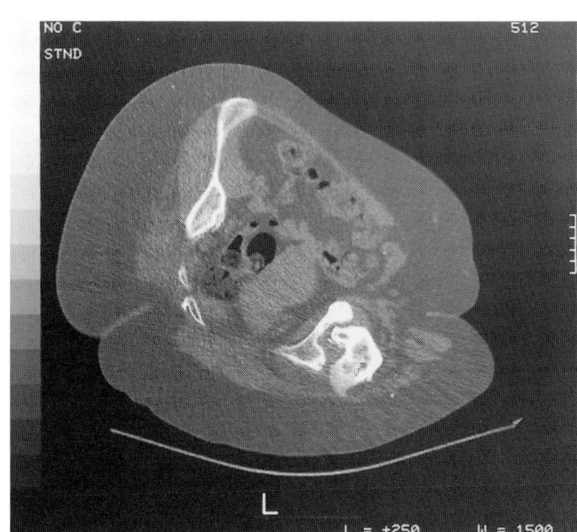


Figure 3.26c Transaxial image through the affected hip joint showing deformity of the joint

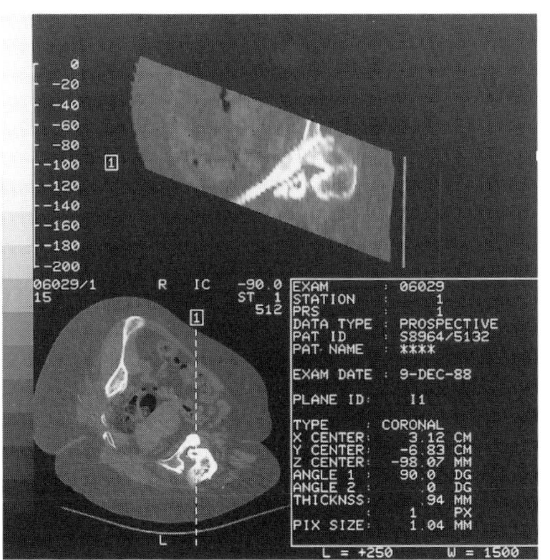


Figure 3.26d Reformatted oblique image through the area of deformity

## Hip Joint

### Arthrography

Hip arthrography is the radiographic demonstration of the hip joint following the administration of a non-ionic water-soluble contrast agent. A single contrast technique is normally employed.

The examination is performed under fluoroscopic control and images are recorded digitally or on conventional radiographs.

**Indications**

The most common indication for arthrography of the hip is pain following prosthetic replacement of thc head of the femur. Additionally it can also be used for suspected loose bodies or 'clicking hip syndrome' and is usefully employed in conjunction with steroid injection of the joint to ensure correct location of the needle within the joint space. It is also used to investigate congenital hip dislocation.

**Patient preparation**

The patient lies supine on the fluoroscopy table, with head resting on a pillow. Control films are taken with the affected hip in the relaxed or neutral position.

A support may be positioned under the patient's knee to provide a small degree of flexion of the hip joint which relaxes the capsule. With the leg in a relaxed position, the head of the femur is identified under fluoroscopic control. A marker is placed on the skin surface over the middle of the femoral neck.

For safety purposes the path of the femoral artery is identified by palpation and delineated on the surface of the skin. This normally lies medial to the above marker.

The skin is prepared using a suitable antiseptic solution and the surrounding area is covered with sterile towels.

Local anaesthetic is introduced into the area around the skin marker.

The procedure may also be performed under general anaesthetic when used to investigate congenital hip dislocation in infants.

**Imaging procedure**

A 22-gauge needle is inserted vertically through the capsule at the point marked on the skin surface. The progress of the needle is checked periodically under fluoroscopic control until the tip of the needle strikes the neck of the femur.

The position of the needle is confirmed either by aspiration of synovial fluid or, if this is not possible, by the introduction of a small quantity of contrast agent under fluoroscopic control. Once the position of the needle has been confirmed, up to 15 ml of 240–300 mgI/ml strength contrast is introduced. Anteroposterior images of the joint are acquired immediately following the introduction of contrast, with the leg in the neutral position and with internal and external rotation. The patient is instructed to exercise and the film series is repeated.

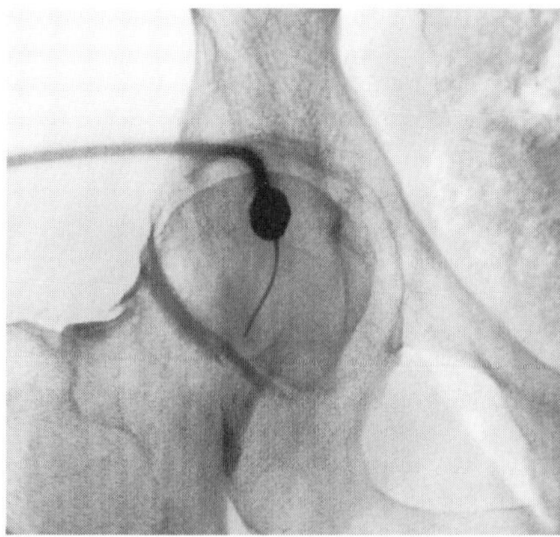

**Figure 3.27a** Anteroposterior image of right hip joint (neutral position) to ensure correct position of needle in joint space prior to steroid injection

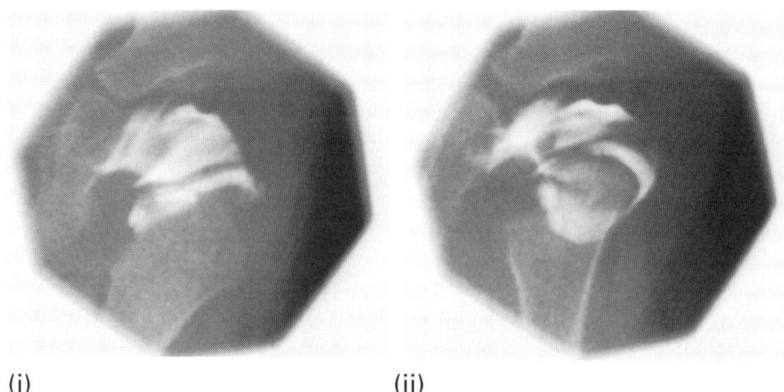

(i) (ii)

**Figure 3.27b** (i) AP with internal rotation; (ii) AP with external rotation

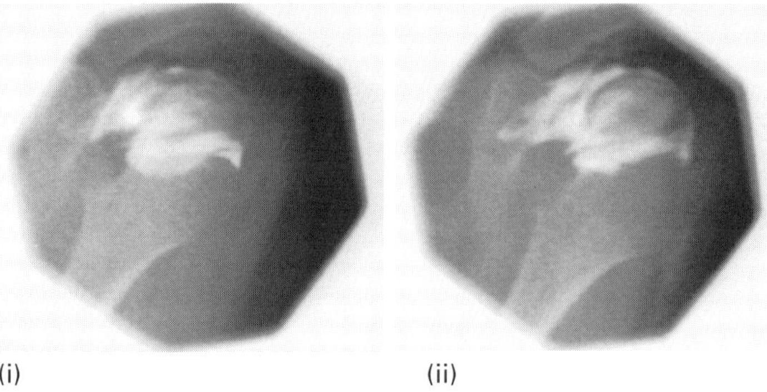

(i) (ii)

**Figure 3.27c** (i) AP with adduction; (ii) AP with adduction and internal rotation

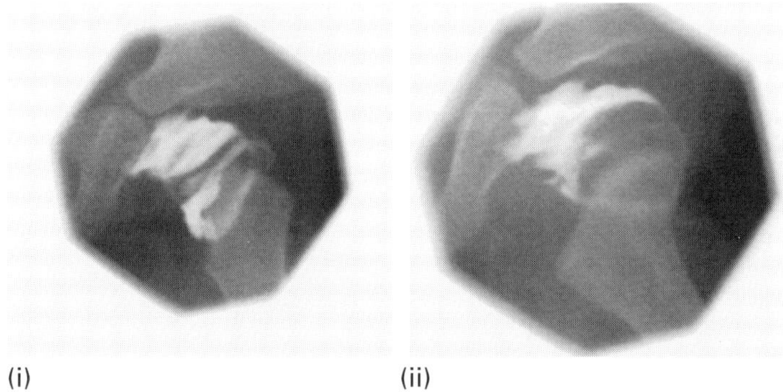

(i) (ii)

**Figure 3.27d** (i) AP with abduction and internal rotation; (ii) AP with abduction and external rotation

**Figure 3.27(b–d) Series of images of an infant's left hip, acquired with a mobile image intensifier in theatre, with various degrees of movement and rotation**

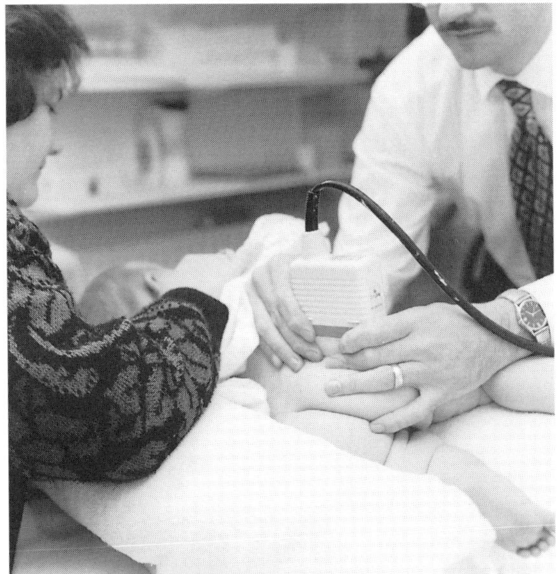

**Figure 3.28a** Imaging procedure

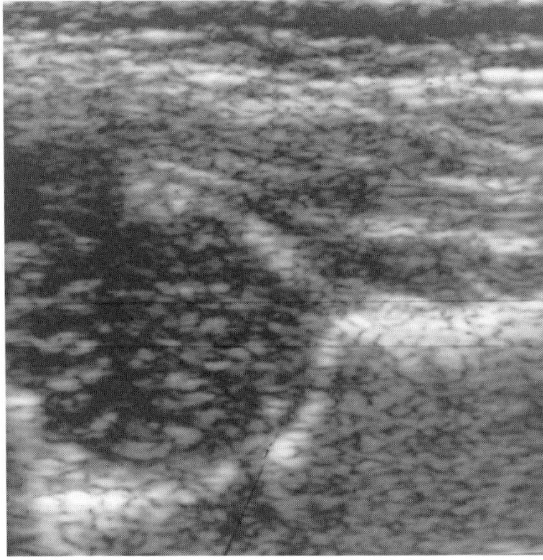

**Figure 3.28b** Coronal image of normal hip using a linear transducer. The cartiliginous labrum and soft tissues of the hip are demonstrated

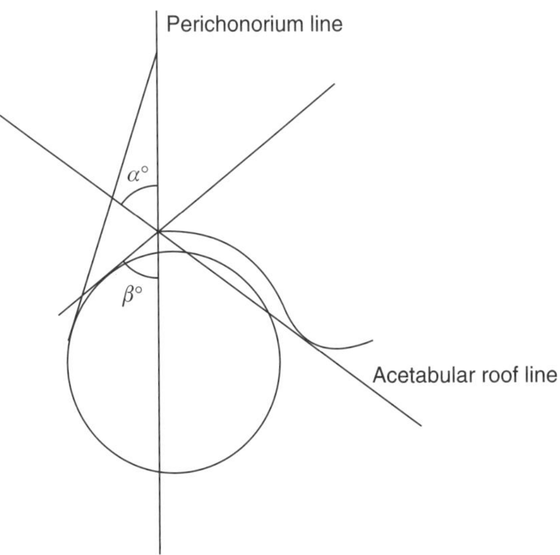


**Figure 3.28c** Graf method of drawing lines to measure alpha and beta angles

## Ultrasound

Ultrasound is a non-invasive and widely used modality in the investigation of hip conditions in the neonate. It offers the advantage over conventional radiography of imaging cartilage which enables more accurate assessment of hip dysplasia. It may be used in the way advocated by H. Prof. Reinhart Graf so that the hip is imaged in the coronal plane, giving the equivalent of an anteroposterior radiograph.

Using the ultrasound equipment software or alternatively drawing directly on a hard copy, image lines are drawn between specific landmarks and angles measured to assess acetabular shape and depth. Alternatively, dynamic studies in the coronal and transverse planes may be performed to demonstrate any hip instability.

Adult investigation using ultrasound is limited due to the bony anatomy which obscures most of the joint space.

### Indications

Ultrasound is used to confirm the clinical suspicion of congenital dislocation of the hip (CDH) and to determine the degree of severity. It is also used as a follow-up during and after treatment. It may be used as a screening tool, especially when there is a family history of CDH or following breech delivery.

In the older child and adult it is used mainly to detect effusion of the joint.

### Position of patient and imaging modality

Ideally the baby either lies supine in a special harness or is held secure in the lateral position in a trough device made up of paper rolls or foam pads covered with blankets. The affected side is uppermost and the femur slightly flexed.

### Imaging procedure

The examination is performed using a 5–7.5 MHz linear array probe. Both hips are scanned for comparison. Coronal scans are obtained through the midline of the hip. The transducer is placed over the lateral trochanter, parallel to the line of the baby's spine, and held in position using both hands. The probe is moved back along the baby's thigh to bring the femoral head into view. The probe is then moved across the femoral head to locate the midline of the joint, and normally two images are recorded of each joint.

### Image analysis

Lines are drawn on the image. The baseline is the line of the lateral border of the ilium and the roof line is drawn along from the lower limb of the ilium to the acetabular margin. A third line is drawn from the tip of the cartilaginous labrum to the bony acetabular margin. From the intersection of these lines an alpha and beta angle are measured (Figure 3.28c), allowing classification of the degree of dysplasia.

# 3 Locomotor System

## Temporomandibular Joints (TMJs)

The TMJ is a synovial condyloid joint formed between the head (condyle) of the mandible and the mandibular fossa of the temporal bone. The anterior part of the mandibular fossa, with which the head of the mandible articulates when the mouth is opened, is termed the articular tubercle.

The joint capsule is attached superiorly to the rim of the articular surface and inferiorly to the neck of the mandible. The capsule is strengthened laterally to form the lateral or temporomandibular ligament.

Intrinsically there is an interarticular disc (meniscus) which divides the joint into the superior and inferior cavities. It is attached to the periphery of the capsule and is situated over the head of the mandible, projecting anteriorly towards the tubercle.

A number of small muscles combine to produce depression, elevation, protrusion, retraction and lateral movements of the mandible. These movements are complex, and the action of opening the mouth results in the head of the mandible moving downwards and forwards. Excessive movement can result in anterior dislocation of the head of the mandible on the articular tubercle.

The joint derives its blood supply from the temporal and maxillary branches of the external carotid artery.

### Indications

Pain and dysfunction of the joint caused by either misalignment, dislocations, bony abnormalities or damage of the meniscus.

### Recommended imaging procedures

The bony structure of the joints may be demonstrated by plain film radiography using lateral 25° caudal projections of both joints with the teeth clenched, mouth closed and with the jaws relaxed and the mouth open as far as possible. These projections may be supplemented with either postero-anterior 10° cephalad or fronto-occipital 35° caudal projections, with the mouth open and closed.

Tomography may also be employed using an exposure angle of 5–10° (zonography), with either a linear or multidirectional X-ray tube movement. Alternatively, an orthopantomogram (OPG) of the jaw may be taken.

Computed tomography may be used, but arthrography is used in preference as this will also demonstrate, when used with fluoroscopy, motion of the joint as well as any pathology present.

Magnetic resonance imaging will demonstrate with more clarity the soft tissue structures of the joint.

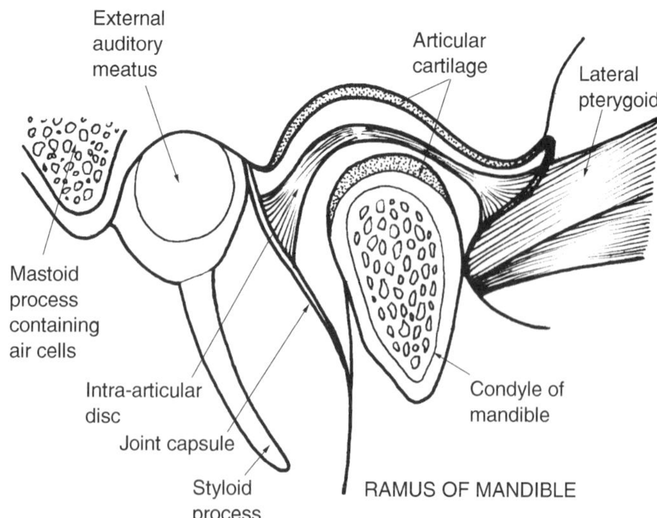


**Figure 3.29a** Temporomandibular joint, sagittal section

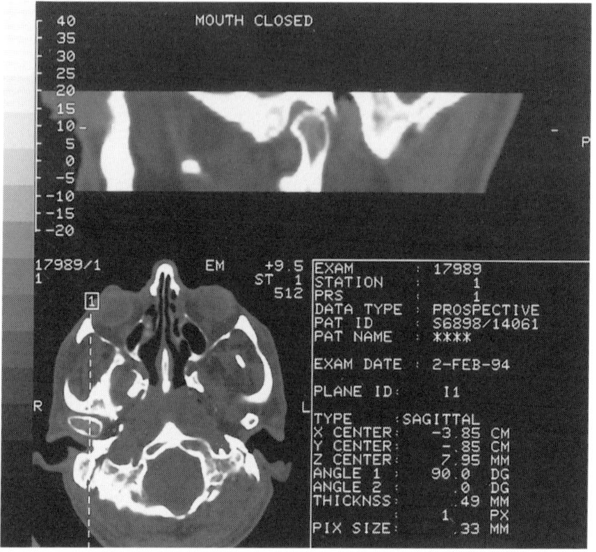


**Figure 3.29b** CT sagittal re-formation image through the right TMJ – mouth closed

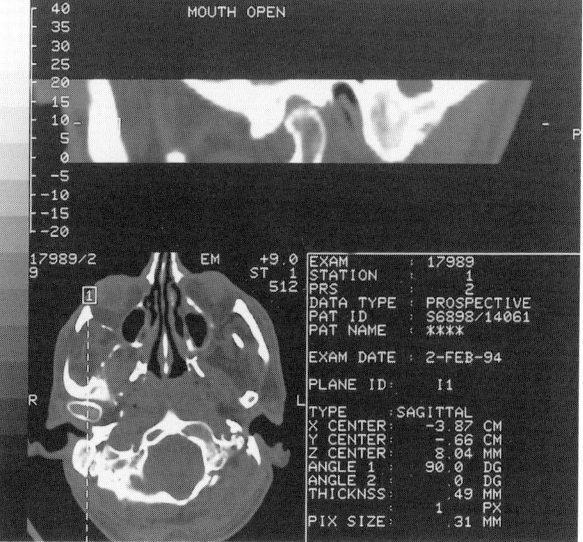


**Figure 3.29c** CT sagittal re-formation image through the right TMJ – mouth open

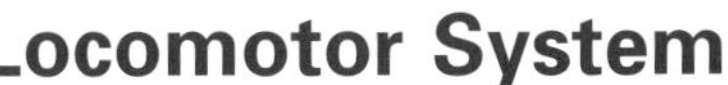


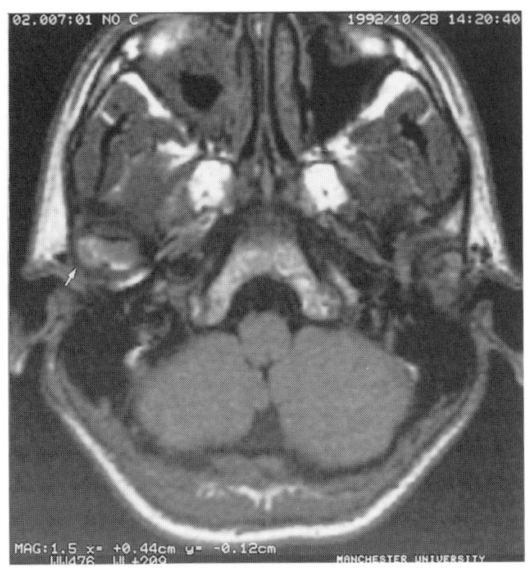


**Figure 3.30a** MR $T_1$ weighted transaxial image of TMJs

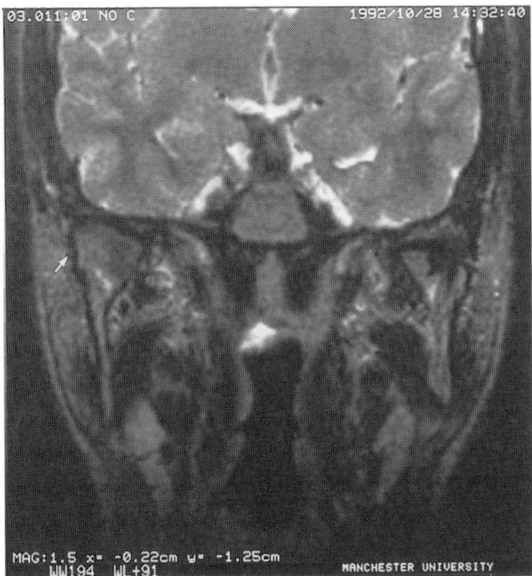


**Figure 3.30b** MR $T_1$ weighted coronal image of TMJs

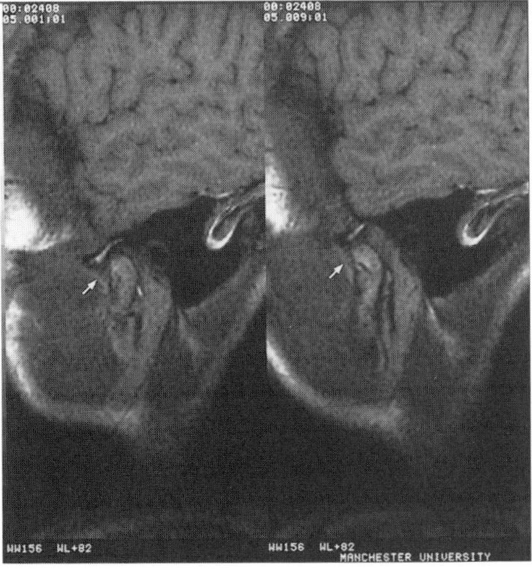


**Figure 3.30c** MR multi-displayed sagittal images; (left) mouth closed; (right) mouth open

## Computed tomography

Computed tomography may be used to evaluate the internal and bony structures of the joint. Routinely, high-resolution images are acquired in the transaxial plane. Two series are taken, one with the mouth closed and the other with the mouth open. The digital data are reformatted to produce images of each side in the sagittal plane.

### Imaging procedure

Positioning of the patient is similar to that described for the standard brain protocol on page 342.

Initially a lateral scan projection radiograph is obtained, starting 10 cm above and ending 10 cm below the external auditory meatus. From this image a series of 1.5–2 mm contiguous transaxial scans are prescribed through the joints, with the patient's mouth closed.

This series is then repeated with a mouth-opening device in position.

The digital data acquired from the high-resolution transaxial sections can be reformatted in the sagittal plane to show the relationship of the meniscus and the bony structures. Three-dimensional reformations may be useful in demonstrating bony abnormality of the condyle and mandibular head.

## Magnetic resonance imaging

The availability of small dedicated surface coils, enabling bilateral imaging of each joint, has increased the use of MRI in TMJ imaging.

### Imaging procedure

With the patient supine and central on the scanning table, the coils are placed adjacent to each joint. Using the external alignment lights, the table is moved until the external reference point is at the centre of the coils. From this position the patient is driven the fixed distance to the isocentre of the magnet.

Initially a transaxial localiser image is obtained. From this image, sagittal oblique $T_1$ weighted spin-echo sections (TR 500 ms/TE 25 ms) are prescribed through each joint, perpendicular to the condyles of the mandible. This series is acquired with mouth closed and then repeated several times if necessary, using a device which gradually opens the mouth at graded intervals.

Further $T_1$ weighted images may be acquired in the coronal plane with the mouth in the closed position.

Routinely, 3 mm sections with no spatial gap are used, with a field of view of 12 cm for the sagittal oblique images and 16 cm for the coronal series. A matrix of 256 × 256 is used with 1 NEX.

# Temporomandibular Joints

## Arthrography

Temporomandibular joint arthrography is the radiographic demonstration of the TMJs following administration of a water-soluble contrast agent. A single contrast technique is normally employed, with the contrast injected into the inferior joint space. This enables the relationship of the condylar head and the under-surface of the meniscus to be studied both in motion and in static imaging.

The examination is performed under fluoroscopic control, using magnification and a fine focus, with static images recorded either using digital imaging equipment or conventional film. Dynamic imaging of the joint as it opens and closes may be recorded on video tape.

The following description assumes the use of remote control equipment, but the procedure can be performed on conventional fluorography equipment.

### Indications

To differentiate between dysfunction and pain caused by misalignment and dislocation of the bony structures and that associated with damage or dislocation of the meniscus.

### Patient preparation

A set of radiographs of both joints may be required with the mouth open and closed, using lateral 25° caudal projections. Alternatively, OPG or tomography may be requested. The patient lies semi-prone on the fluoroscopy table, with the head turned in a lateral position and the joint under investigation uppermost. The patient is made comfortable, with the raised shoulder and knee supported by pads and the patient's hand at the level of the chin but out of the primary beam. The opposite arm is extended alongside the trunk.

The skin around the pre-auricular region is prepared using a suitable antiseptic solution and the surrounding area is covered with sterile towels. Local anaesthetic is introduced into the skin and subcutaneous tissues over the lateral pole of the condyle and over the lateral tip of glenoid fossa.

### Imaging procedure

The inferior joint space is cannulated using a 23-gauge needle attached to an extension tube. With the head in the lateral position and the mouth closed, the needle is first directed towards the condyle in the 11 o'clock position. After downward and forward movement of the condyle, the needle should slip into the joint space and adopt a more vertical position. Confirmation that the needle is in the joint is made by asking the patient to open and close the mouth and observing that the needle moves forward and backward in step with these movements. Once the needle is confirmed in the joint, 0.3–0.7 ml of 280–320 mgI/ml strength contrast medium is injected under fluoroscopic control, with the patient's head in the lateral oblique position.

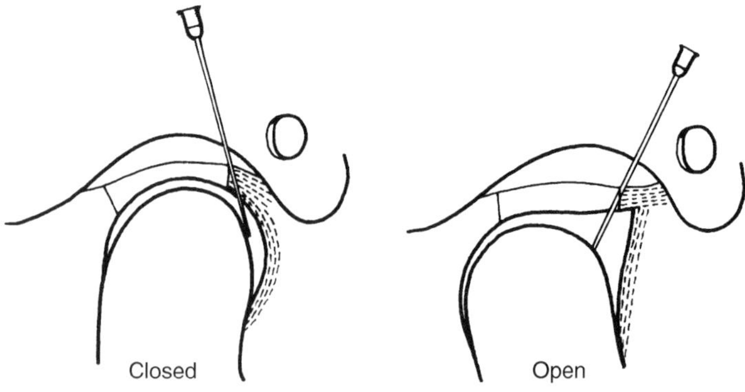


**Figure 3.31a** Cannulation of the temporomandibular joint space, with mouth closed and open, showing forward movement of the needle within the joint space

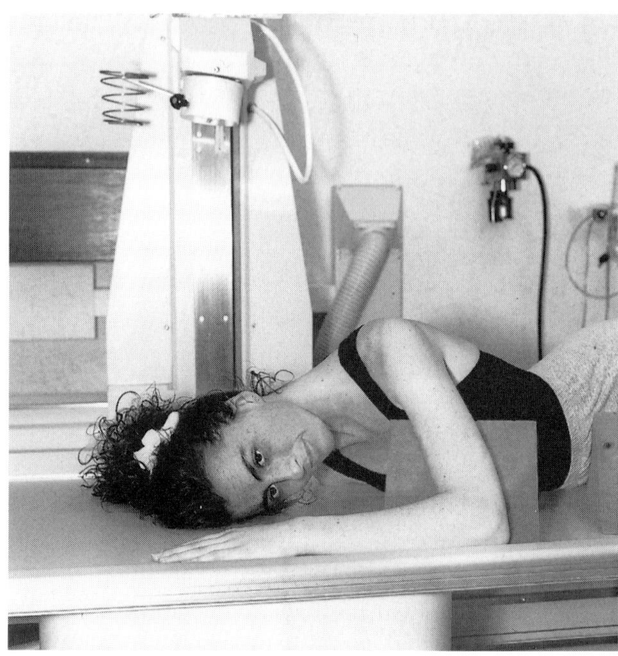

**Figure 3.31b** Modified lateral projection with the joint under investigation nearest the X-ray tube

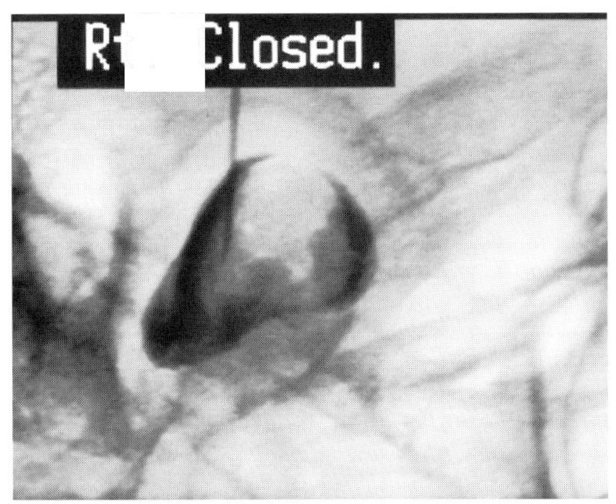


Figure 3.32a Image of joint with mouth closed

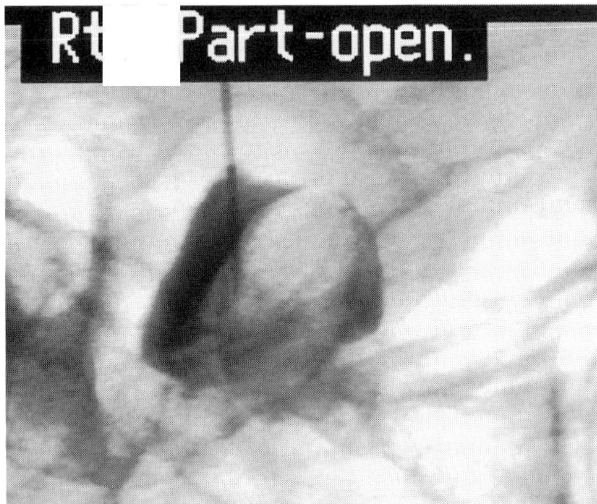


Figure 3.32b Image of joint with mouth partly open

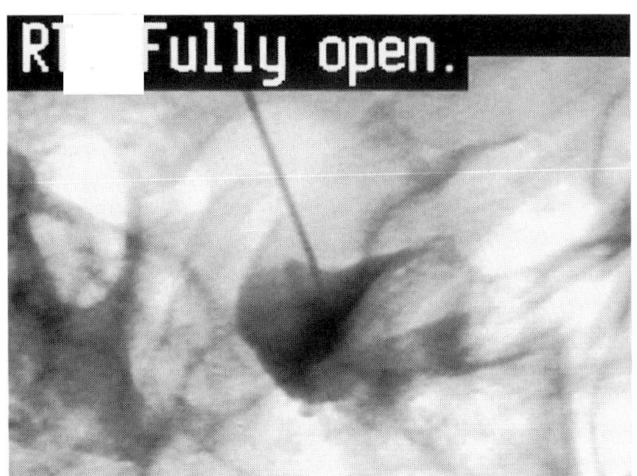


Figure 3.32c Image of joint with mouth fully open

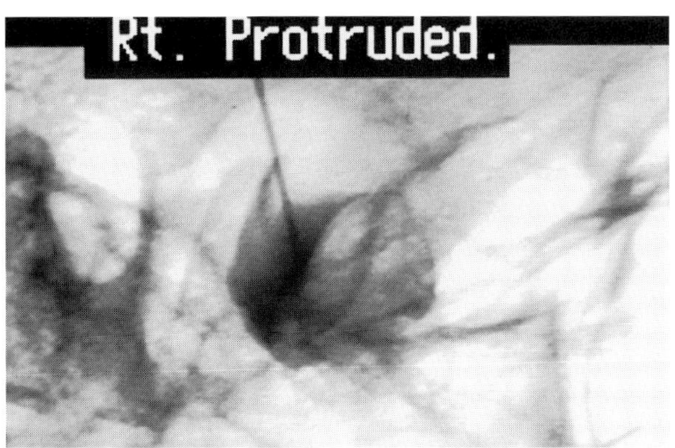


Figure 3.32d Image of joint with jaw protruded

The contrast medium should be seen to flow freely from anterior to posterior recesses as the mouth opens and closes. With the aid of fluoroscopy, a series of images of the joint are acquired, with the mouth in different stages of opening. Visualisation of the actual joint and meniscal motion, recorded digitally or on video, is the major advantage of arthrography.

## Lateral oblique projection (modified)

The projection used is an unconventional approach, as the joint under investigation is nearest the X-ray tube. To demonstrate the joint space optimally, the relationship of the skull planes to the film is determined under fluoroscopic control. Rotation of the neck may be restricted in some patients, in which case angulation of the X-ray tube may be necessary. Images are routinely taken with the mouth open and closed.

*Position of patient and imaging modality*

The patient lies semi-prone on the fluoroscopy table, with the head turned in a lateral position and with the joint under investigation uppermost. Ideally the glabella and external occipital protuberance are equidistant from the table top. From this position the head is tilted, with the chin raised, to separate the joints until the joint is superimposed over the opposite temporal area nearest the image intensifier. The interpupillary line is at an angle of approximately 20° to the table top.

*Direction and centring of the X-ray beam*

The vertical central ray is directed to a point 1 cm anterior to the external auditory meatus.

*Image analysis*

In the normal arthogram the contrast medium is seen to fill the recesses of the inferior joint space 360° around the junction of the condylar head and neck, as well as outlining the inferior surface of the meniscus. During opening and closing of the joint the meniscus should be seen to move smoothly and freely.

With the mouth in the tightly closed position the posterior recess is collapsed and the anterior recess is distended and filled with contrast. As the mouth opens, a shift of fluid is observed with the anterior recess closing as the posterior recess starts to distend. At the halfway stage the thinnest part of the meniscus is seen interposed between condylar head and the temporal eminence. With the mouth fully open, the condylar head translates beyond the anterior tubercle with the anterior recess fully collapsed and the posterior recess fully open and filled with contrast. In this position the meniscus is seen as a sigmoid curve.

# 3 Locomotor System

## Contrast Enhanced Computed Tomography

Contrast enhanced CT can be used to delineate tumours of the musculoskeletal system, particularly if MRI is unavailable. This technique may also complement MRI in cases where there is gross bone destruction.

If the tumour is malignant, CT scanning of the chest is routinely performed to identify secondary metastatic deposits.

### Indications

Contrast enhanced images give information on the vascularity of the lesion and its relationship to normal anatomical structures.

### Positioning of patient and imaging modality

Positioning of the patient is as described previously for the various anatomical areas.

As some of the positions are difficult to maintain, the patient must be supported and made as comfortable as possible. It is important that there is no movement between the non-enhanced and enhanced image series, in order to make direct comparisons between the scan series.

### Imaging procedure

The appropriate anteroposterior or lateral scan projection radiograph is performed. The length of the scan projection radiograph must include the nearest joint space to enable accurate anatomical location of the abnormality.

From this image a series of non-enhanced transaxial sections are prescribed. The slice width and table increment depend on the size of the lesion; 3 or 5 mm contiguous sections are chosen for small lesions. Either 10 mm contiguous scans or 10 mm sections with a table increment of 15–20 mm are necessary for large lesions.

The scan field of view is selected to ensure that all the soft tissue component of the area of interest is imaged.

After review, the appropriate sections are rescanned during the infusion of a non-ionic contrast medium. Scanning commences 60 s after the start of the injection.

To improve the spatial resolution of these contrast enhanced images a narrower slice width and table increment may be selected.

### Image analysis

For the scans, a soft tissue algorithm is normally selected. However, it may be necessary to reconstruct the non-enhanced images retrospectively using a bone algorithm which will highlight any calcification within the lesion. Regions of interest applied to both series of images will give information on the uptake of contrast medium within the lesion.



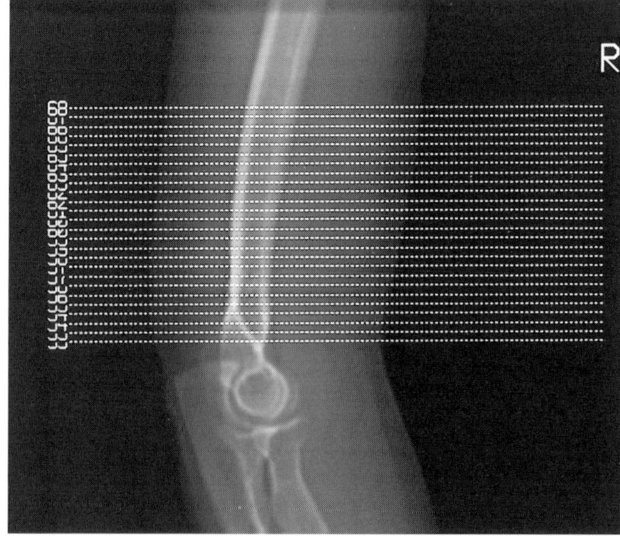


**Figure 3.33a** Scan projection radiograph of lower humerus showing prescribed scanning levels

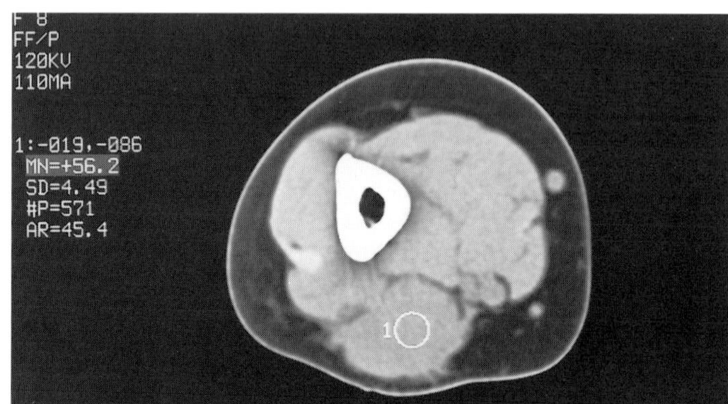


**Figure 3.33b** Pre-contrast enhanced scan through a suspected abnormal mass in the lower humerus (ROI – CT number recorded as 56.2)

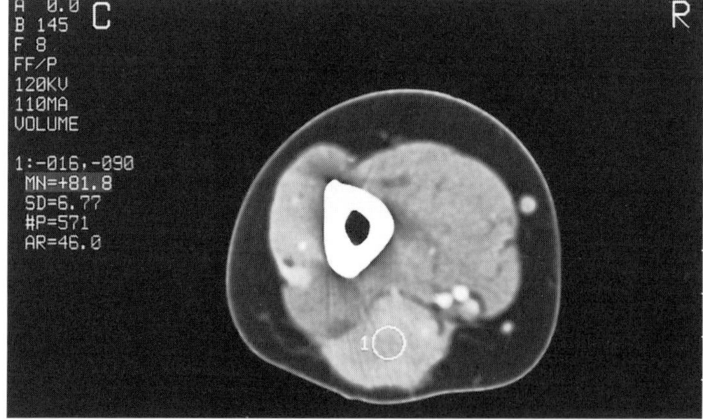


**Figure 3.33c** Contrast enhanced scan of same section as above (ROI – CT number increased to 81.8)

*Contrast medium and injection data*

| *Volume* | *Concentration* | *Flow rate* |
|---|---|---|
| 100 ml | 300 mgI/ml | 2 ml/s |

Scanning commences 60 s after the start of the injection.

## Contrast Enhanced Computed Tomography

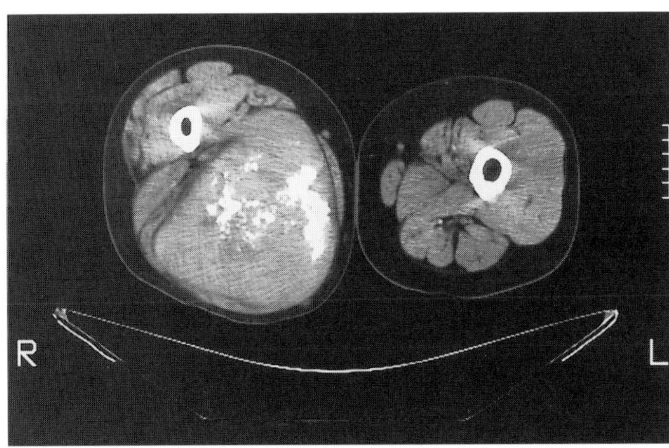


**Figure 3.34a** Pre-contrast enhanced scan showing a large identified mass in the right mid-femur

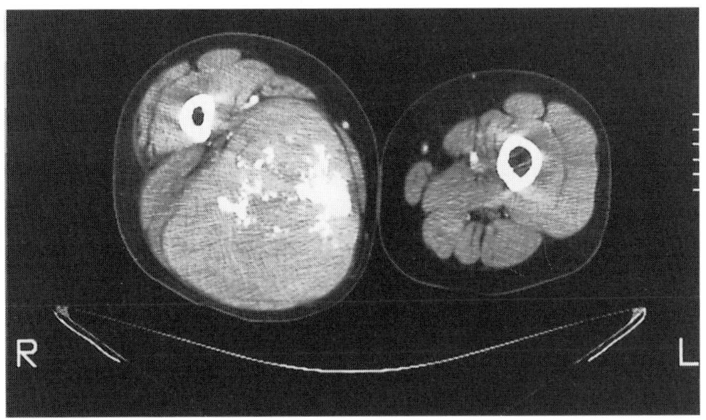


**Figure 3.34d** Post-contrast enhanced scan showing no contrast enhancement in the mass identified in the image opposite

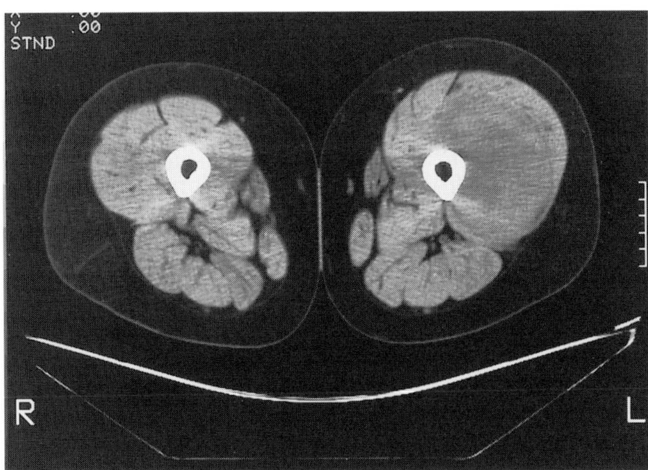


**Figure 3.34b** Pre-contrast enhanced scan at the level of the mid-femur

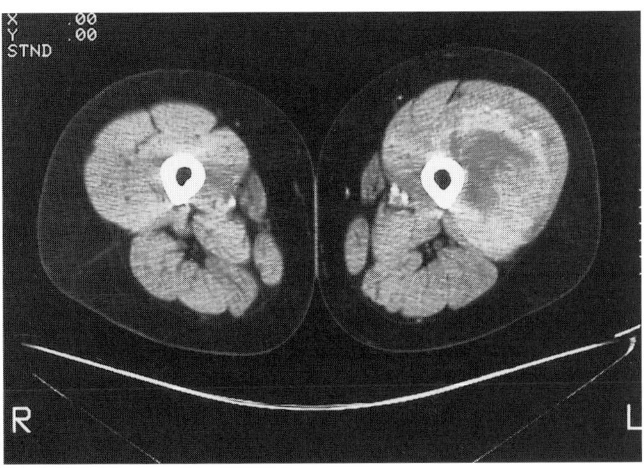


**Figure 3.34e** Post-contrast enhanced scan at the same level as the image opposite showing a mixed attenuated structure (osteosarcoma)

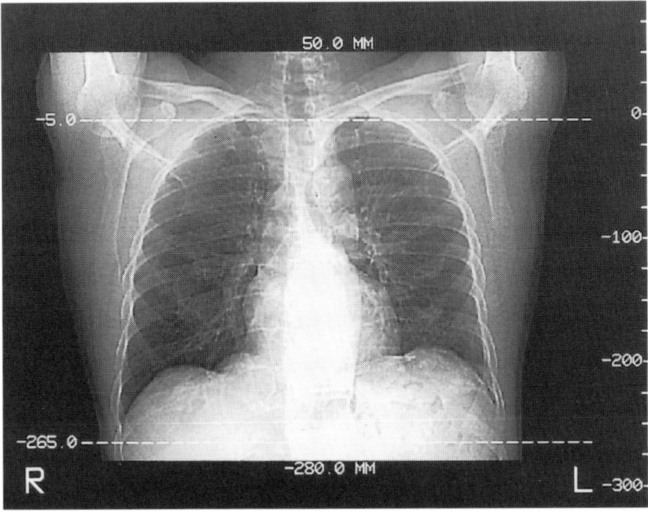


**Figure 3.34c** Scan projection radiograph of the thorax

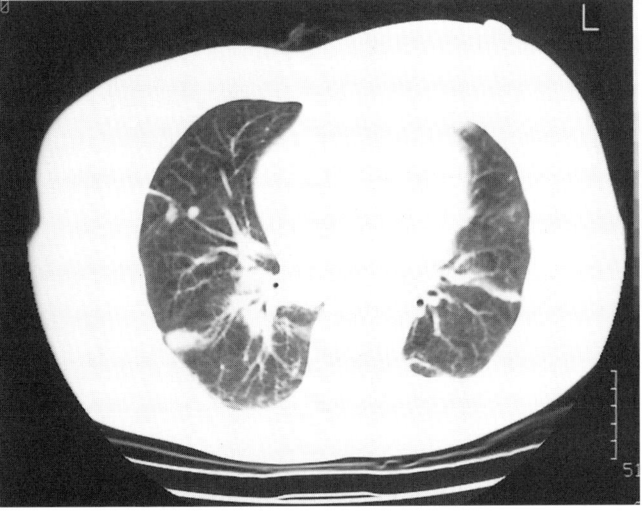


**Figure 3.34f** CT section of thorax showing metastatic deposits

# 3 Locomotor System

## Magnetic Resonance Imaging

Magnetic resonance imaging is now playing an important role in the investigation of abnormalities of the locomotor system. Its superior ability to demonstrate both internal structures and soft tissue surrounding the joints, together with its non-invasive nature, has in many instances made it the imaging modality of choice.

The technique and protocols throughout the locomotor system are very similar. Surface coils are preferred as they give an improved signal-to-noise ratio, thereby increasing resolution. A variety of coils exist (see Chapter 1), and generally the closer the coil is to the region of interest, the better the quality of the images produced. The disadvantage of smaller coils however, is the loss of signal as you move away from the coil, limiting the examination to more superficial structures. When surface coils are used, the examination is normally confined to one point only. If a simultaneous bilateral examination of the lower extremities is required, larger surface coils must be used.

The field of view (FOV) must be selected to cover the appropriate area. For example, an examination of the wrist, using the appropriate surface coil, requires a FOV of between 8 and 15 cm, whereas an examination of both hips uses the conventional body coil with a FOV between 35 and 40 cm.

A combination of $T_1$ and $T_2$ weighted sequences in a minimum of two anatomical planes is normally used to assess a joint and surrounding structures. Three-dimensional volume acquisition, with subsequent post-processing to give images in any anatomical plane, is now being used more extensively.

Additional $T_1$ weighted images following intravenous contrast enhancement may be required to further define a lesion. If available a $T_1$ weighted sequence using a fat suppression technique may be selected pre- and post-contrast enhancement, again to highlight any abnormality. These images are repeated in the plane which best demonstrates the abnormality.

### Indications

Where MRI is available it is replacing conventional arthrography as a diagnostic technique, and should ideally be done prior to any invasive procedure which could result in a localised area of high signal intensity leading to difficulty in true interpretation of the MR images. It is the modality of choice in the investigation of tendon and ligament abnormalities, meniscal tears, loose bodies, avascular necrosis, and in inflammatory conditions. It is also used to diagnose and monitor treatment of soft tissue and bony tumours.

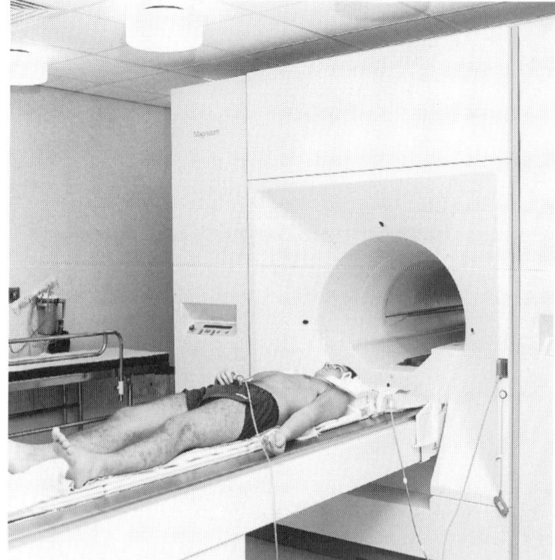

**Figure 3.35a** Positioning of coil and shoulder

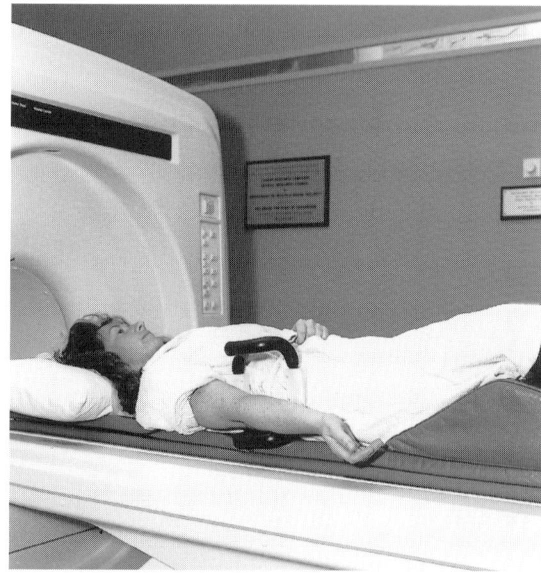

**Figure 3.35b** Positioning of coil and elbow

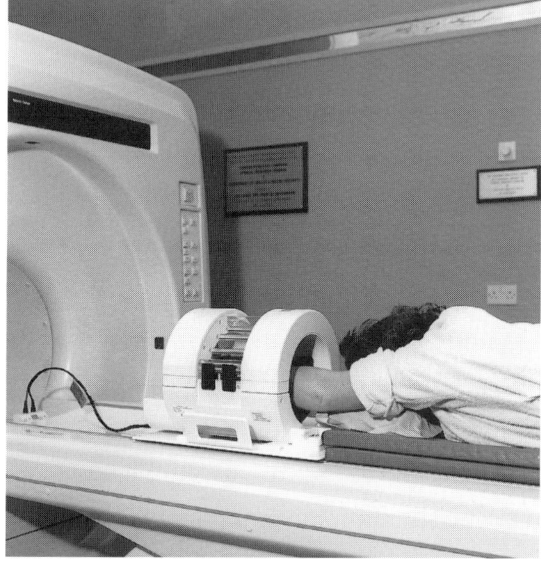

**Figure 3.35c** Positioning of coil and wrist

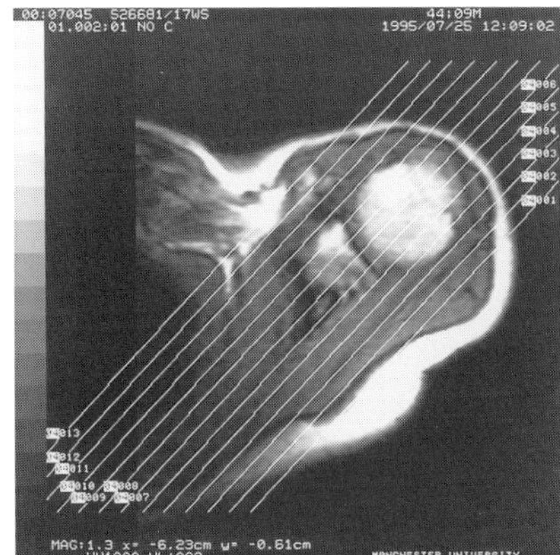


**Figure 3.36a** MR localiser image of shoulder

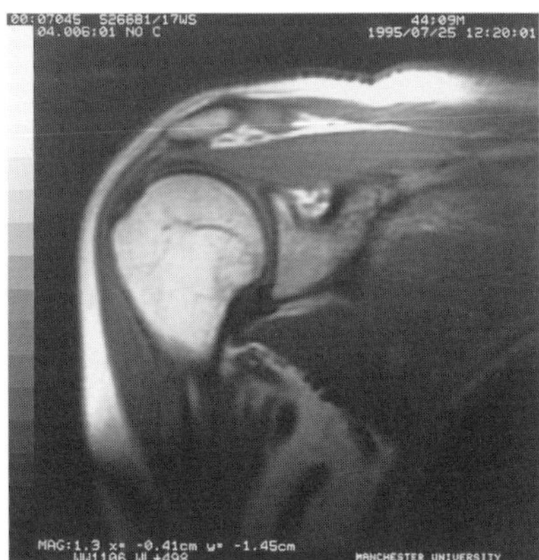


**Figure 3.36b** Spin-echo $T_1$ weighted oblique image through the shoulder joint

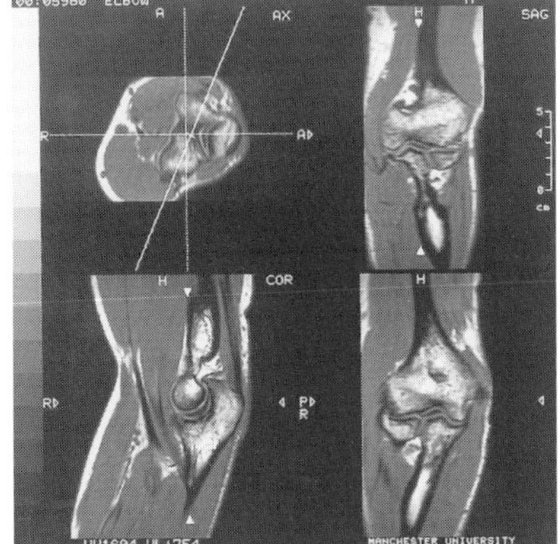


**Figure 3.36c** 3D SPGR image set of the elbow joint

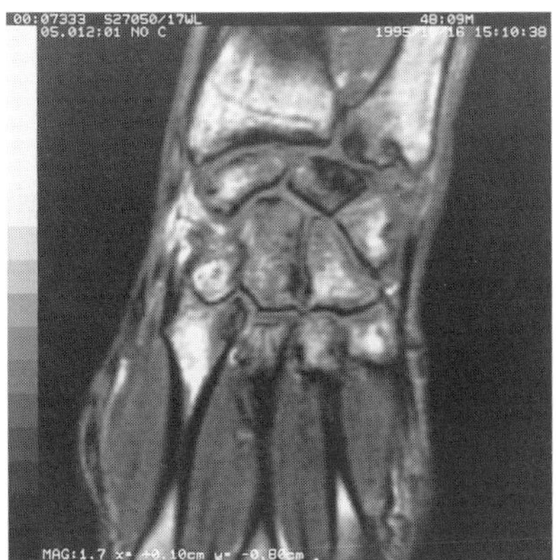


**Figure 3.36d** 3D SPGR $T_1$ weighted coronal image of the wrist joint

## Upper limb

### Position of patient and imaging modality

*Shoulder and elbow*

The patient lies supine, head first on the scanner table. The affected arm is placed by the side and is externally rotated to bring the palm of the hand uppermost. The appropriate coil is then placed in close proximity to the joint.

*Wrist*

For the wrist the patient lies prone, head first on the scanner table. The affected arm is extended, palm downwards and the wrist placed over the surface coil.

For each joint using the halogen alignment lights, the external reference point is obtained at the centre of the surface coil. From this position the patient is moved to the isocentre of the magnet, which is also the centre of the radiofrequency transmitter coil.

### Imaging procedure

Initially, localiser scans are obtained in the transverse, coronal and sagittal planes. From these images a series of $T_1$ weighted and $T_2$ weighted images are acquired in the appropriate anatomical planes. The slice width and field of view are determined by the size of the area to be imaged.

Additional $T_1$ weighted sequences combined with the option of fat suppression may be used pre- and post-contrast enhancement to highlight any abnormality.

In complex situations a 3D volume acquisition uses $T_1$ or $T_2$ weighting, and a slice width of 1 mm may be considered. With post-processing of the data, images may be displayed in any anatomical plane.

**Table 3.1 Optimum plane**

| *Joint* | *Coronal* | *Sagittal* | *Transaxial* | *Other* |
|---|---|---|---|---|
| Shoulder | | | ✓ | Coronal oblique parallel to supraspinatous tendon |
| Elbow | ✓ | ✓ | ✓ | |
| Wrist | ✓ | | ✓ | |

# 3 Locomotor System

## Magnetic Resonance Imaging

### Lower limb

**Position of patient and imaging modality**

*Hips*

For hips, the conventional body coil is used routinely.

The patient lies supine, feet first on the scanner table, with the arms folded across the chest. If possible the feet are internally rotated through 45° and strapped together to prevent movement.

*Knee joint*

With the patient supine on the scanner table the knee in question is positioned in the quadrature knee coil. The limb is externally rotated 15–20° to bring the lateral femoral condyle parallel to the sagittal plane to demonstrate the cruciate ligaments.

*Ankle/lower tibia and fibula*

Both joints are usually imaged using the conventional head coil.

The patient lies supine on the scanner table. Both ankles are placed in the head coil with the feet, if possible, perpendicular to the scanner table.

Using halogen alignment lights, the following **external scan reference points** are obtained:

- **hips** at the level of the greater trochanters
- **knees and ankles** at the centre of the surface coil.

From the appropriate external scan reference point the patient is moved to the isocentre of the magnet which is also the centre of the radiofrequency coil.

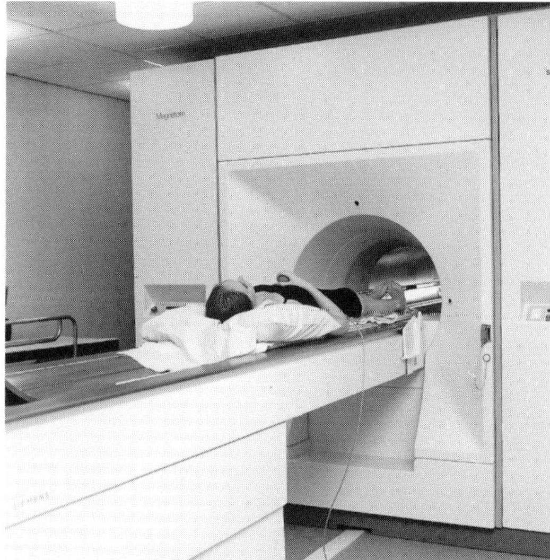

**Figure 3.37a** Patient positioned for hips with the feet internally rotated

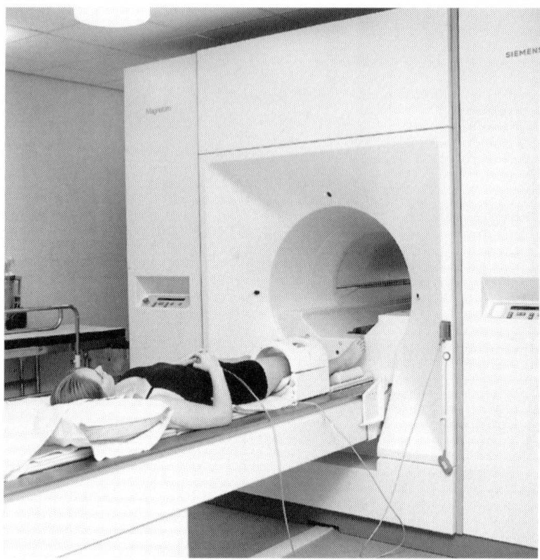

**Figure 3.37b** Knee positioned showing external rotation of the limb

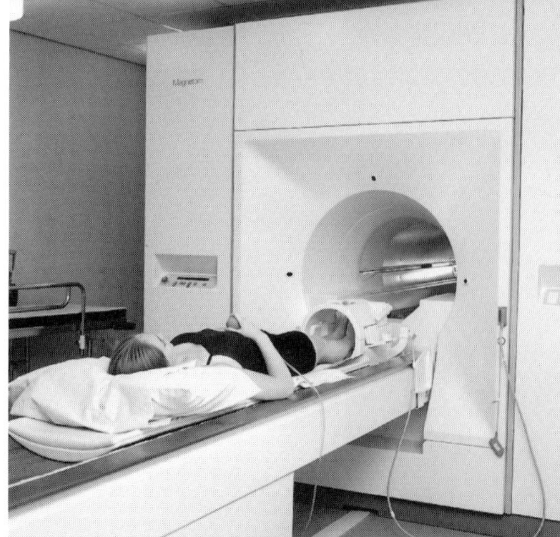

**Figure 3.37c** Ankle joints positioned with the conventional head coil

**Table 3.2 Optimum planes**

| *Joint* | *Coronal* | *Sagittal* | *Transaxial* |
|---|---|---|---|
| Hips | ✓ | | ✓ |
| Knees | ✓ | Parallel to the lateral condyle of femur | |
| Ankles | ✓ | ✓ | ✓ |

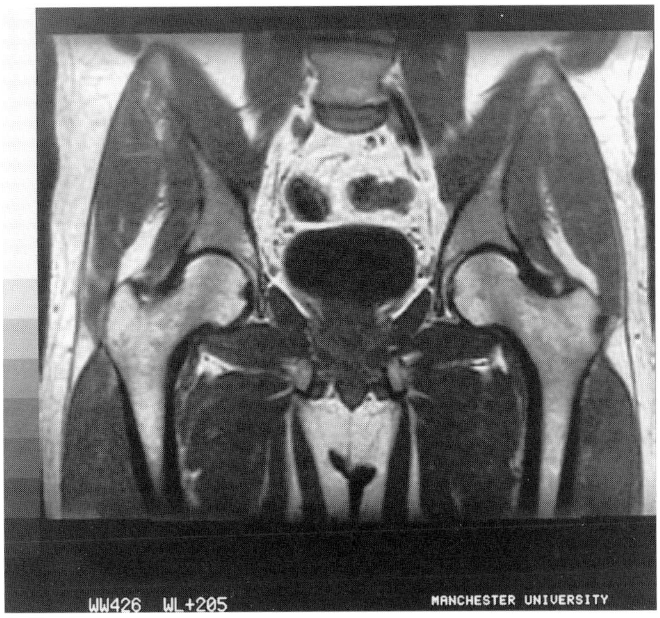

Figure 3.38a Coronal spin-echo $T_1$ weighted image of both hips (large field of view)

**Imaging procedure**
Initially, localiser scans are obtained in the transverse, coronal and sagittal planes. From these images a series of $T_1$ weighted and $T_2$ weighted images are acquired in the appropriate anatomical planes. The slice width, field of view and repetition time are determined by the size of the area to be imaged. For example, for coverage of the knee joint the repetition time of the $T_1$ weighted sequence may be increased from 500 to 820 ms.

Additional sequences may include fat suppression techniques, 3D volume acquisition with subsequent post-data processing into the optimum anatomical plane, and the use of i.v. contrast enhancement agents.

Also in imaging of the knee joint a sagittal $T_2$ gradient echo sequence may be used to demonstrate a meniscal tear.

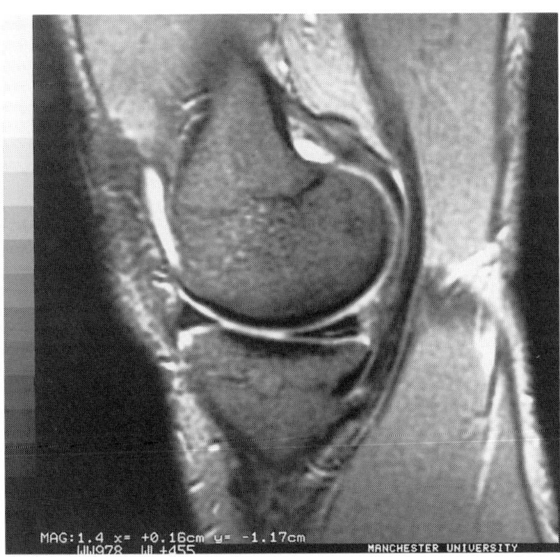


**Figure 3.38b** Sagittal gradient-echo $T_2$ weighted image of the knee joint

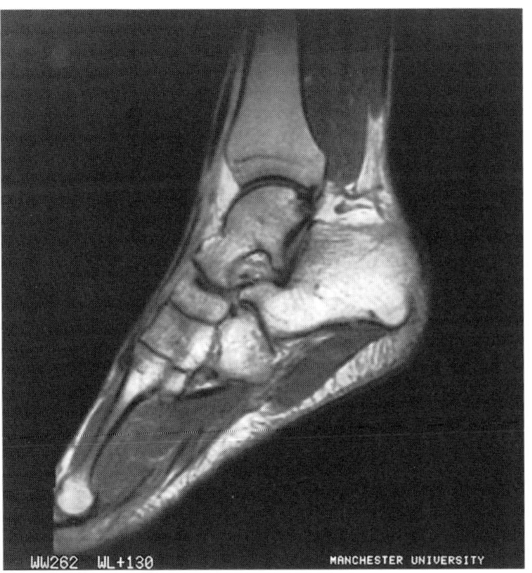


**Figure 3.38c** Sagittal spin-echo $T_1$ weighted image of the ankle joint

**Table 3.3 Imaging parameters**

| *Imaging sequence* | *TR* | *TE* | *Field of view* (cm) | *No. of NEX* | *Slice width/ gap* (mm) | *Matrix* (horizontal–vertical, to cover anatomical area) |
|---|---|---|---|---|---|---|
| Spin-echo $T_1$ weighted | 500 | 20 | 8–40 | 2 | 3–5/1 | 160 × 256<br>256 × 160 |
| Fast spin-echo $T_2$ weighted | 3500<br>echo train length – 12 | 90 | 8–40 | 3 | 3–5/1 | 160 × 256<br>256 × 160 |
| 3D volume SPGR with flip angle 45° | 50 | 12 | 8–30 | 1 | 1–2 | 160 × 256<br>256 × 160 |
| Gradient-echo $T_2$ weighted with flip angle 35° | 920 | 25 | 20 | 2 | 5/1 | 160 × 224<br>(sagittal plane) |

# 3 Locomotor System

## Radionuclide Imaging – Bone Scan

Radionuclide imaging is usefully employed in examining both bone and bone marrow. The bone scan is the most sensitive way of detecting changes in bone physiology and changes in normal blood supply associated with lesions, trauma or infection in adults and children. In the majority of cases, disorders are detected by observing an increase in activity or alternatively an absence or diminished uptake of the radiopharmaceutical.

A radiopharmaceutical such as $^{99m}$Tc-labelled MDP (methylene diphosphonate) or $^{99m}$Tc-labelled HDP (oxidronate), which have a high uptake in bone, is injected intravenously. The procedure usually involves both anterior and posterior whole body scanning 2–4 h after the injection, to demonstrate the total skeleton combined with static views of specific regions of interest.

'Three – phase bone scanning' is employed when investigating infections at a suspected bone region. As the name suggests, this procedure is divided into three phases:

- Phase 1, the vascular phase, involves dynamic imaging immediately following intravenous injection of the radiopharmaceutical, to investigate blood flow to a region. Any increase in activity seen during this phase will confirm hypervascularisation of the region consistent with infection.
- Phase 2, the blood pool phase, after reaching equilibrium at 2–5 min following injection, consists of a static image of the soft tissues to demonstrate any areas of differential areas of uptake of activity. An area of infection will show increased blood pool activity.
- Phase 3, the bone phase, consists of a static image taken 2–4 h following injection. Infection will be shown as increased uptake in the suspected region.

## Indications

Metastases, especially from breast, prostate and lung tumours. Benign bone tumour such as osteoid osteoma. Primary bone tumours to check for metastasis or in case of osteoid sarcoma to detect a nidus of activity. Staging of malignant bone tumours. Trauma and sports injuries, including stress fracture and shin splints, non-accidental injury, and identification of undisplaced fractures from injuries such as those associated with the scaphoid and hip. Metabolic bone disease associated with osteomalacia, osteoporosis and hyperparathyroidism. Paget's disease and mapping of rheumatoid arthritis and osteoarthritis. Inflammatory disease such as osteomyelitis, inflammation of the spine, e.g. discitis and spondylitis, and infected bone associated with a loose prosthesis, e.g. hip or knee. Vascular disorders, including diagnosis of sickle cell disease associated with infarcts, Caisson disease, Perthe's disease and trauma.

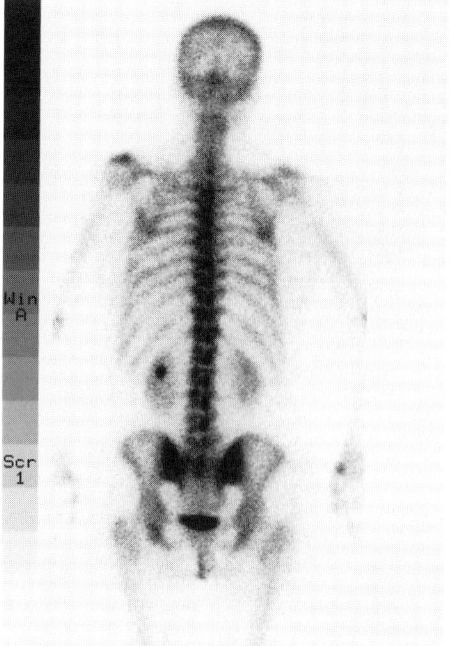


**Figure 3.39a** Normal bone body scan image

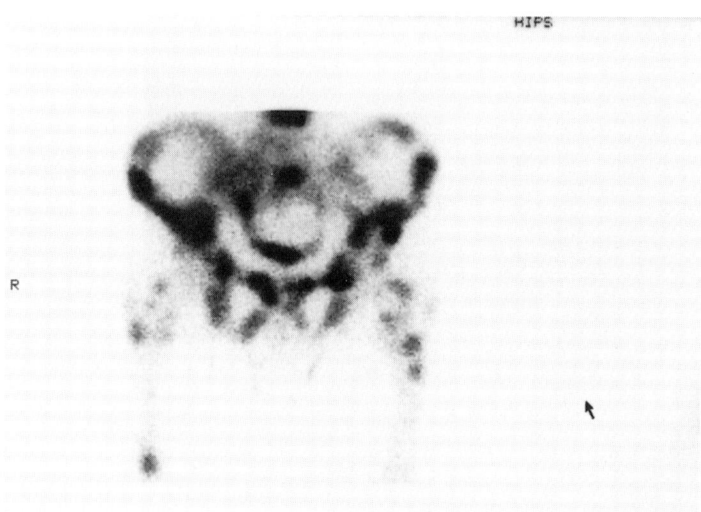


**Figure 3.39b** Image of pelvic region showing bony metastases from Ca prostate

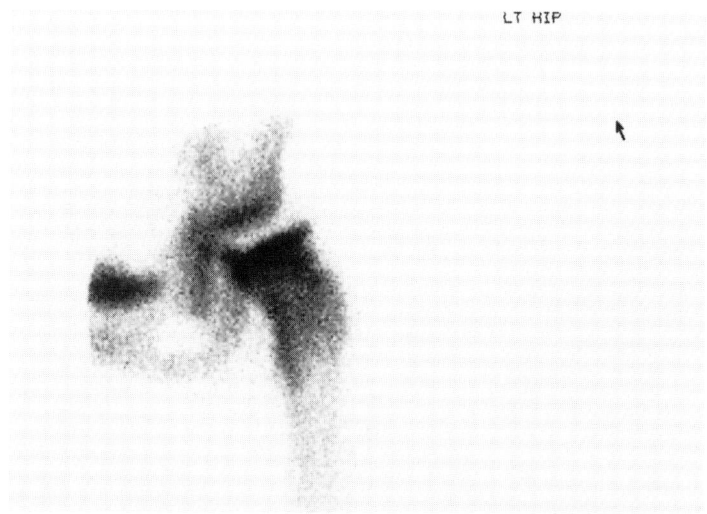


**Figure 3.39c** Image of hip showing Perthe's disease

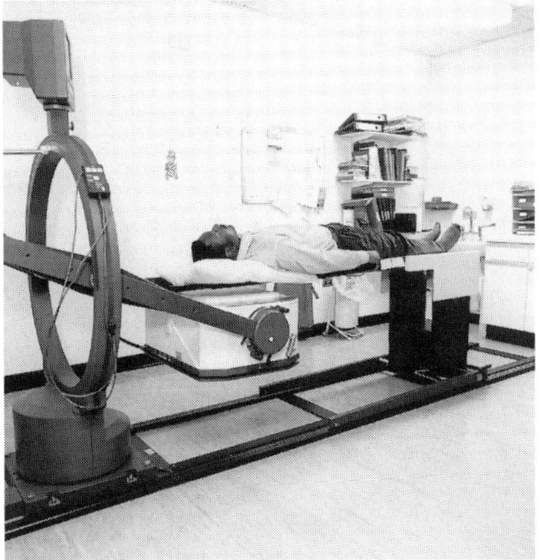

**Figure 3.40a** The gamma camera

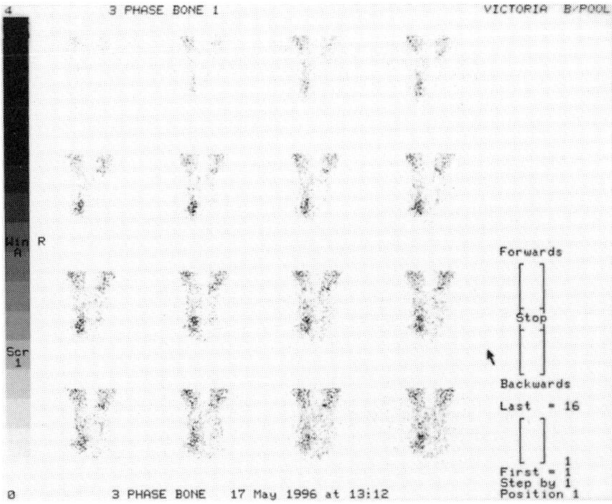


**Figure 3.40b** Arterial phase images of both feet (first phase of a three-phase bone scan)

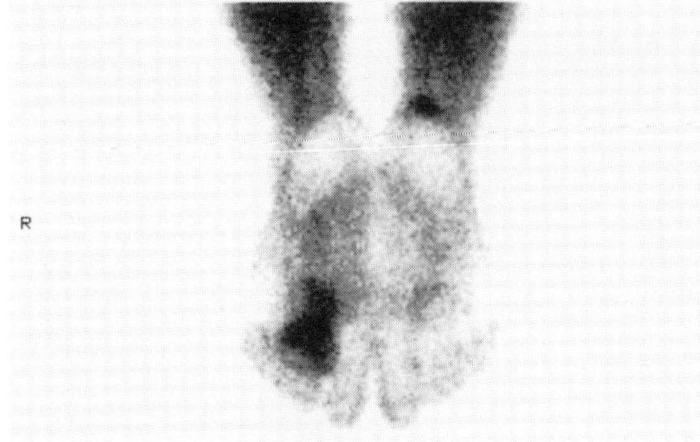


**Figure 3.40c** Equilibrium blood pool image of the feet (second phase of a three-phase bone scan)

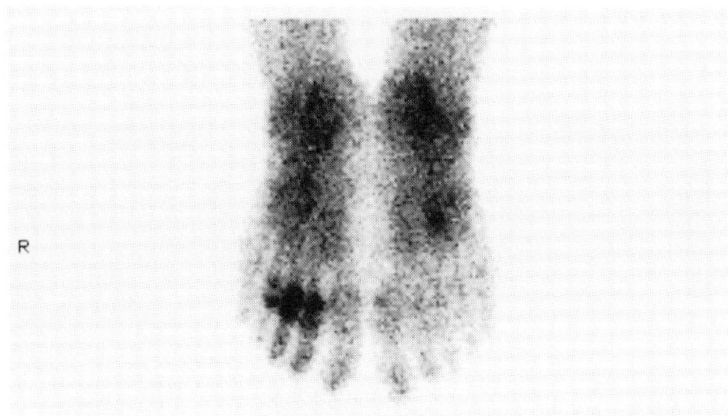


**Figure 3.40d** Bone phase image of the feet (final phase of a three-phase bone scan)

## Position of patient and imaging modality

For whole body scanning the patient is scanned from head to foot. A variety of equipment is available for such procedures. In one example the camera head is moved from head to foot, with the camera positioned in turn above and below the patient for anterior and posterior views.

The patient is supine on the imaging couch, with the centre of the camera positioned initially to commence scanning at the vertex of the skull. In another example the table moves in relation to the camera which is in a fixed position.

For static scanning the camera is positioned above the patient for the anterior and below the imaging couch for the posterior view of the regions concerned. For some images the patient may sit erect directly in front of the camera.

## Imaging procedure

A high-resolution collimator is employed for whole body scanning and static scans, while a general-purpose camera is used for dynamic imaging. A pinhole collimator may be selected for joints or specific areas of interest, e.g. scaphoid.

For whole body imaging the radionuclide is administered intravenously either 2 or 4 h prior to image acquisition. The exact scanning time depends on the bone agent used: with HDP, imaging may commence at 2 h post-injection, while with MDP it may start at 3–4 h post-injection.

The patient is positioned on the imaging couch for head to foot scanning and during image acquisition the camera is moved automatically, using a floor track system, at a predetermined speed towards the feet. Movement can be terminated when images of the feet are acquired.

When whole body scanning facilities are unavailable the patient is placed supine on the couch for static anterior and posterior images of the pelvis and thorax, together with anterior and lateral views of the skull. Additional views are acquired, showing images of the extremities. Normally two views of each extremity are required to cover the full extent of the limbs.

For three-phase bone scanning the patient is positioned comfortably on the imaging couch with the camera directly over the suspected region. Dynamic imaging of blood flow commences as soon as the isotope appears on the display monitor following a bolus injection of the radiopharmaceutical. A total of 16 images are acquired in 32 s, with a 2-second image acquisition time for each frame. The blood pool phase image is acquired at 2–5 min following injection and the bone phase image 2–4 h following injection.

*Imaging and radiopharmaceutical parameters*

| *Type* | *Administered activity* | *Principal energy* |
|---|---|---|
| $^{99m}$Tc-HDP | 500 MBq | 140 keV |
| *Window width* | *Acquisition counts/time* | |
| 20% | 500–750 counts (static image) | |

# 3 Locomotor System

## Bone Densitometry

### Introduction

Bone mineral analysis plays an important role in both the prevention and management of osteoporosis. The adult skeleton consists of two types of bone tissue, namely cortical and trabecular bone. The former is found mainly in the appendicular skeleton and the latter in the axial skeleton. Two types of bone cells, osteoblasts and osteoclasts, are continually forming and reabsorbing bone. These events, known collectively as bone 'turnover', occur at the bony surfaces and are normally linked in an organised fashion. From approximately 40 years of age, however, changes in bone turnover occur, resulting in both sexes losing bone at a slow continuous rate of 0.3–0.5% per annum. At the female menopause this loss is accelerated to 2–3% per annum but can, in some individuals, be as high as 10% per annum, resulting in generalised osteopenia or the clinical syndrome of osteoporosis, where bone mineral density is reduced to such a low level that easy fracture of the skeleton can occur. Certain metabolic diseases (e.g. hyperparathyroidism) and long-term drug therapies (e.g. corticosteroid therapy) also have an adverse effect on the skeleton, with the possibility of easy fracture.

Several techniques are now commercially available to assess the amount of bone mass present and to monitor any subsequent response to prescribed treatment. The prerequisites for any method used to measure bone loss and to monitor longitudinal changes (i.e. with time) in osteoporosis and other metabolic bone disease are that it is accurate and precise, sensitive, simple, inexpensive and the associated radiation dose is as low as reasonably achievable.

Accuracy is the ability of the equipment to obtain results that reflect the 'true' value of the quantity being measured. Precision is the measure of the variation (usually the standard deviation of a series of measurements) in values obtained when measurements are repeated in the same individual or phantom on the same day (short-term precision) or over several months (long-term precision). Sensitivity is the ability of the technique to differentiate normal from abnormal or to detect changes in bone mineral density with time and treatment.

Whichever method is employed, the equipment must be supplied with software incorporating population reference data against which the patient's value can be plotted. Due to differences in measurement sites, calibration, software, algorithms and reference data, results from one manufacturer's equipment cannot be directly compared with those results obtained from another. It has been proved in centres specialising in bone mass measurement that the greatest source of error is related to the ability of the operator to position the patient correctly. To reduce this and thus maintain a high precision, it is desirable that only a limited number of dedicated operators perform these examinations.

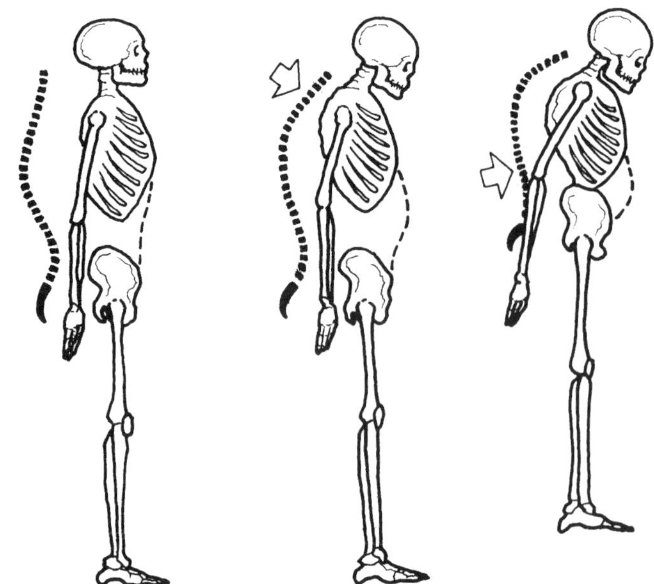

**Figure 3.41a** Diagrams showing spinal deformity with age

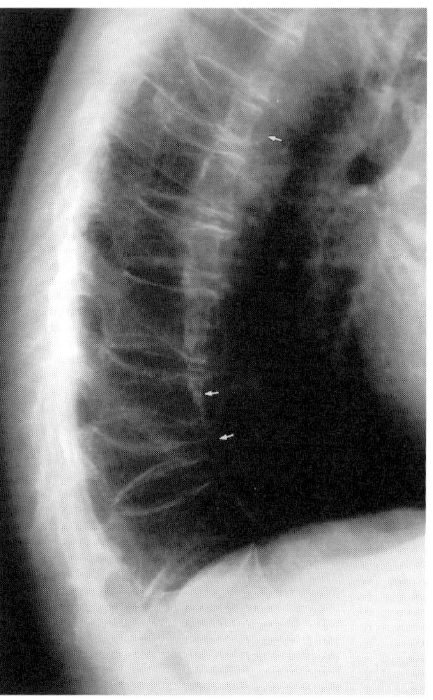

**Figure 3.41b** Radiograph of lateral thoracic spine showing an osteoporotic wedge fracture

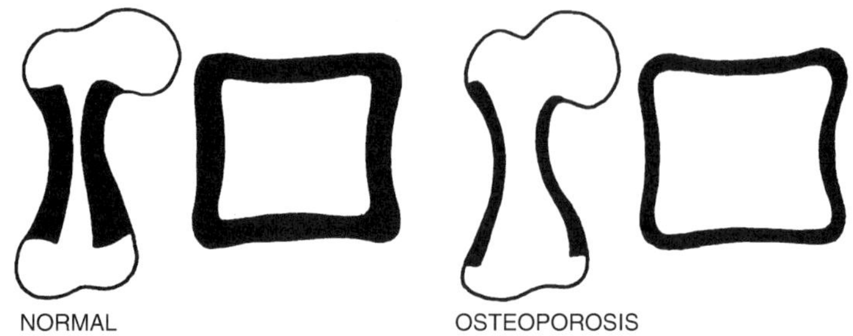


**Figure 3.41c** Diagram showing normal and osteoporotic trabecular bone pattern

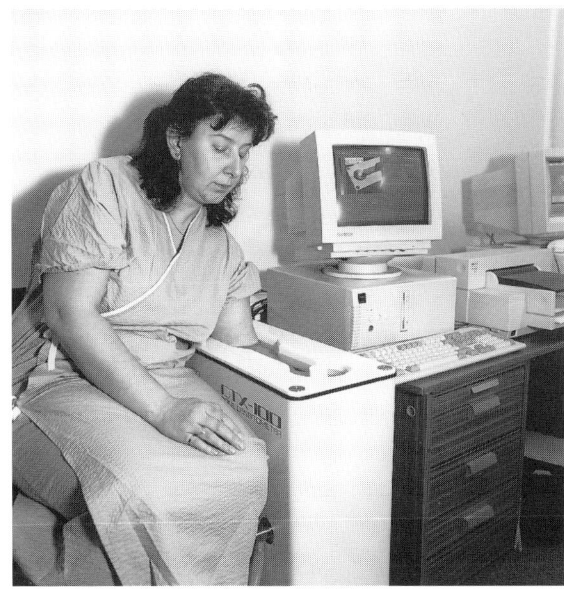

**Figure 3.42a** Single energy X-ray bone densitometry equipment

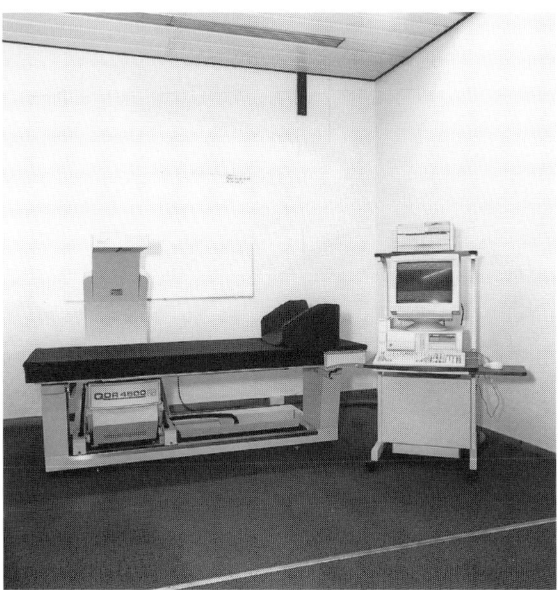

**Figure 3.42b** Dual energy X-ray absorptiometry equipment

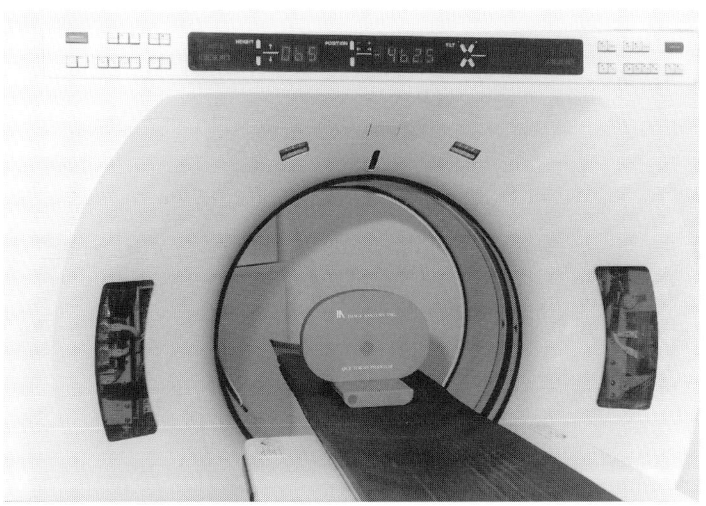

**Figure 3.42c** Quantitative CT equipment

## Recommended modalities

The techniques which will be described are:

- Single energy X-ray bone densitometry (SXA) – applicable to the forearm.
- Dual energy X-ray absorptiometry (DXA) – applicable to the femoral neck, lumbar spine and total body.
- Quantitative computed tomography (QCT) – applicable to the lower thoracic and lumbar vertebrae.

Other methods, such as QCT of the forearm and broad band ultrasound of the calcaneum, are currently used in research establishments and although these may be available clinically in the near future, the techniques are not described here.

## Contraindications

Bone densitometry measurements must not be undertaken if the patient has recently undergone investigations involving the use of either radiopharmaceuticals or radiological contrast agents. The former adds to the photon count recorded at the detector system; the latter, by absorbing radiation, lowers the photon count. Therefore all traces must have left the body before carrying out the examination. In the case of radiopharmaceuticals, a 72-hour delay is recommended. Dense contrast agents such as barium sulphate may require the examination to be postponed for 10 days and bowel purgatives prescribed.

## Preparation of patient

All radio-opaque objects must be removed from the area of interest. The patient's sex, weight, height and date of birth must also be recorded. It is also advisable to obtain a recent medical history, including menopausal age, drug therapies and previous skeletal fractures, and to complete a lifestyle questionnaire highlighting certain 'risk' factors such as excessive alcohol consumption and smoking. These may help validate any abnormal results.

# 3 Locomotor System

## Bone Densitometry

### Single energy X-ray bone densitometry (SXA)

This is a simple technique used to assess the bone mineral content of the distal radius.

The equipment consists of an X-ray source and a sodium iodide/ photomultiplier detector system, mounted opposite each other and surrounding a water bath of a fixed thickness and linked to a computer system. The X-ray beam is filtered with tin to produce an effective energy of 29 keV. The water bath is used to provide a uniform baseline against which the bone is measured. The baseline counts are recorded through water only. Any reduction in photon count below this baseline is due to attenuation of the photons by bone. As skeletal muscle has a similar attenuation coefficient to water, the effects of different amounts of muscle within the forearm can be eliminated. Fat attenuates radiation less than water, resulting in a photon count higher than the baseline value. By assuming that this effect is present across the width of the forearm, a correction to the baseline is made proportional to the amount of adipose tissue present. Therefore the total area measured below the baseline is proportional to the amount of bone present and the results given as a bone mineral content (BMC) expressed in grams of bone per centimetre of bone length.

#### Position of patient and imaging modality

The non-dominant wrist is normally scanned unless there is a previous history of fracture or, in the case of renal dialysis patients, if a shunt is in situ. The patient sits with the side to be measured against the water bath and with the arm submerged in tepid water. The wrist is positioned laterally, with the posterior aspect of the wrist resting firmly against the side of the tank. A hand grip and elbow rest are present to assist immobilisation and to raise the forearm sufficiently to enable baseline measurement to be recorded through water only.

#### Imaging procedure

Once a patient is positioned satisfactorily, the scanning arm is moved into a start position approximately 1 cm proximal to the radial styloid process. At this point the interosseous space between the cortices of the ulna and radius is approximately 8 mm. From this starting point six consecutive rectilinear scans, each 4 mm apart and moving proximally, are obtained. Immediately after this data acquisition the scanner arm moves back to the start position and, moving distally, completes four rectilinear scans each 2 mm apart.

#### Image analysis

A computer printout is obtained showing the area measured for distal and ultra-distal sites, and the BMC measurement and its value plotted against an age/sex matched reference population.

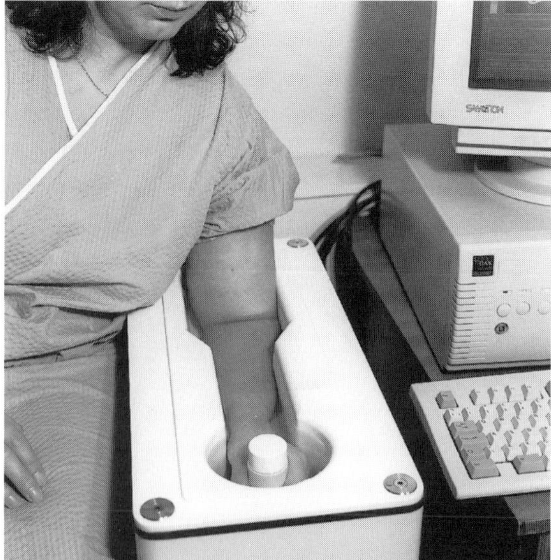

**Figure 3.43a** SXA equipment

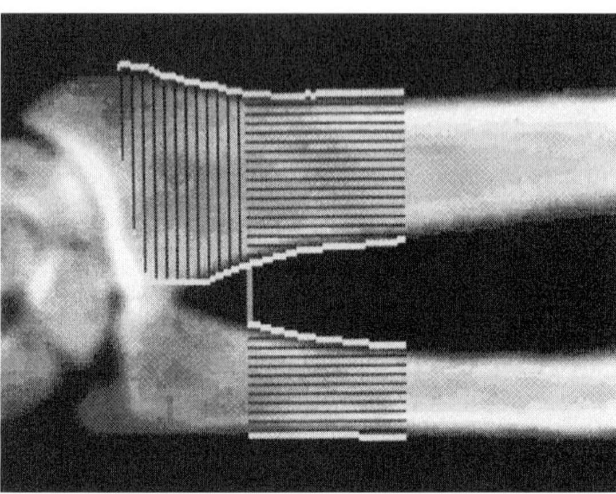

**Figure 3.43b** Image showing scanning pathway and area for image analysis

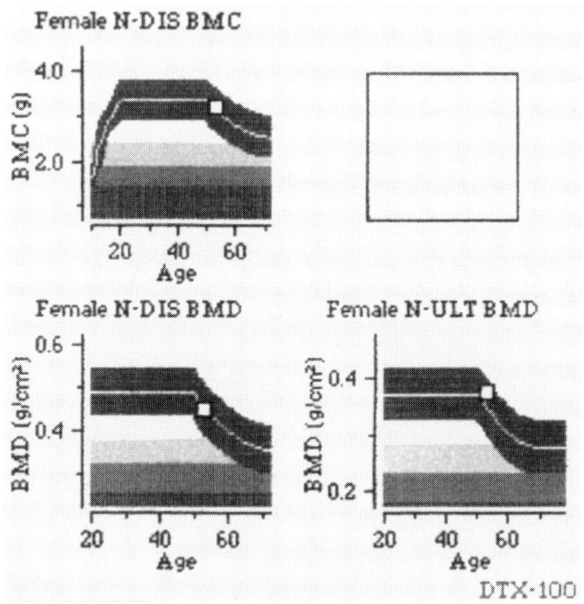


**Figure 3.43c** Result sheet showing patient data plotted against age/sex related reference population

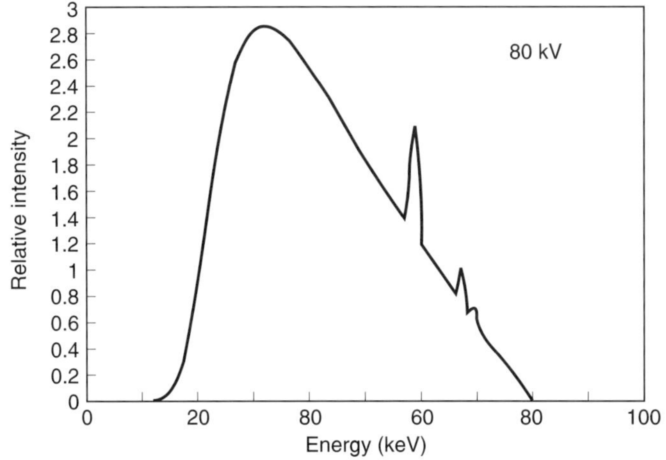


**Figure 3.44a** Relative intensity plotted against energy with peak energies from a pulsed X-ray tube

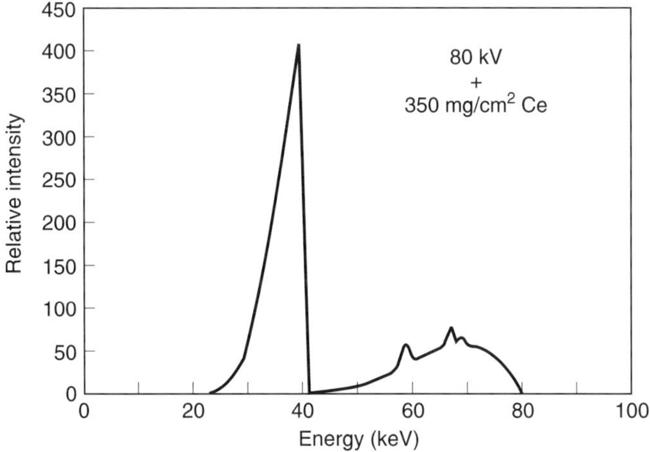


**Figure 3.44b** Relative intensity plotted against energy with the effect of a cerium filter

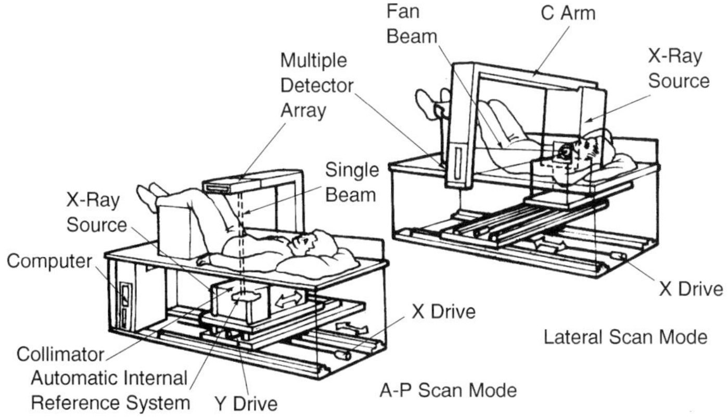


**Figure 3.44c** Schematic diagram of a DXA system (Courtesy of Hologic INC)



## Dual energy X-ray absorptiometry (DXA)

This scanning technique enables bone mineral density measurements to be made in the following areas: lumbar vertebrae, femoral neck, and total body scanning which provides information on body composition as well as bone mineral content.

The technique has superseded dual photon absorptiometry (DPA) and uses a low-output X-ray tube to produce X-ray beams which correct for overlying soft tissue and fat. Equipment manufacturers use different methods to obtain the peak energies. An X-ray tube pulsed on two alternative kVp settings (70 kVp and 140 kVp) can be used or a rare earth 'K' edge filter can shape the broad spectrum from the X-ray tube into two narrow energy bands. A cerium filter, for example, produces two peaks at 38 keV and 70 keV. The detector system coupled to the X-ray tube allows the transmitted photons of each energy to be counted separately. The differential in relative attenuations of these two photon energies corrects for overlying soft tissue and allows the mass of bone mineral in the beam to be estimated. The results obtained are given as a bone mineral content (BMC) expressed in grams (g) or bone mineral density (BMD). The BMD is the BMC divided by the estimated area measured and is expressed in grams per centimetre squared ($g/cm^2$). The X-ray tube is situated beneath the scanning table with the detector system above the patient. All mineral within the track of the X-ray beam adds to the measurement, therefore aortic calcification, degenerative and hyperostotic changes in the spine can cause inaccuracies. To overcome this, lateral DXA scanning has been developed, but overlying rib or iliac crest can often result in only one vertebral body (L3) being assessed. As precision for this measurement is poorer than conventional anteroposterior DXA, its full clinical role has still to be established.

Further advances may extend the role of DXA into orthopaedics and paediatrics and give scan times in the region of 1 min.

### Image analysis

Computer software supplied to manufacturers enables analysis of the scan data with minimal operator intervention. During scanning the detector system records photon counts at each sample point and calculates the density. Bone density is then obtained by subtracting the soft tissue density from the total density.

# 3 Bone Densitometry

## Dual energy X-ray absorptiometry

### Lumbar vertebrae

*Postero-anterior scan*

The patient lies supine in the middle of the scanner table, with the anterior superior iliac spines equidistant from the table top and arms resting by the patient's side. To reduce lumbar lordosis, the knees are flexed over a 90° support pad. A compression band may be applied across the abdomen to reduce patient movement and thickness.

With the aid of a positioning light, the scanner arm is centred in the midline 1.5 cm below the level of the iliac crest. From this start position, scanning continues cranially, covering a maximum distance of 200 mm and including the lumbar region. Scanning time for this is 2–10 min.

*Lateral scan*

Lateral scanning may be undertaken either by rotating the patient into the left lateral position or by rotating the scanner gantry through 90°. Scanning commences 10 mm below iliac crest, covering a distance of 150 mm cranially.

*Image analysis*

*Postero-anterior* lumbar spine analysis gives bone mineral densities for individual vertebrae L1–L4 plus a summation of all the individual results.

Lateral lumbar spine analysis involves defining the region of interest over the trabecular bone within the vertebral body, taking care to exclude vertebral end-plates. Overlying ribs may exclude a particular vertebra, usually L1 or L2, from the final analysis.

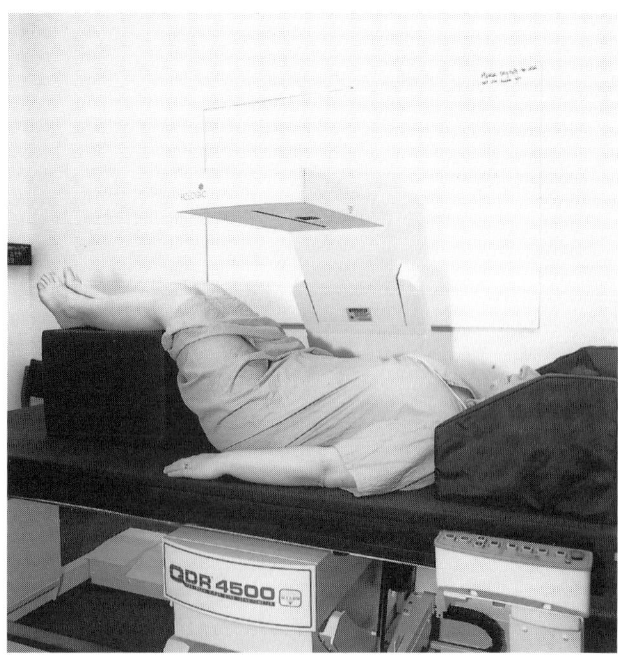


**Figure 3.45a** Patient in PA position

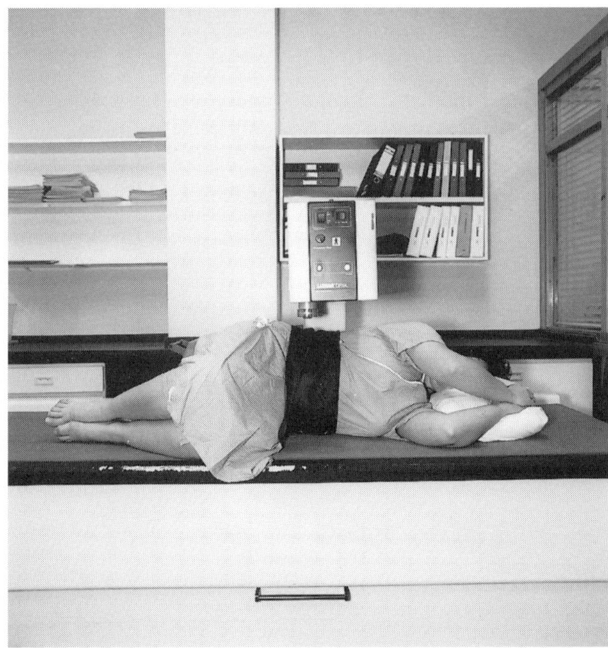

**Figure 3.45b** Patient in lateral 1 position

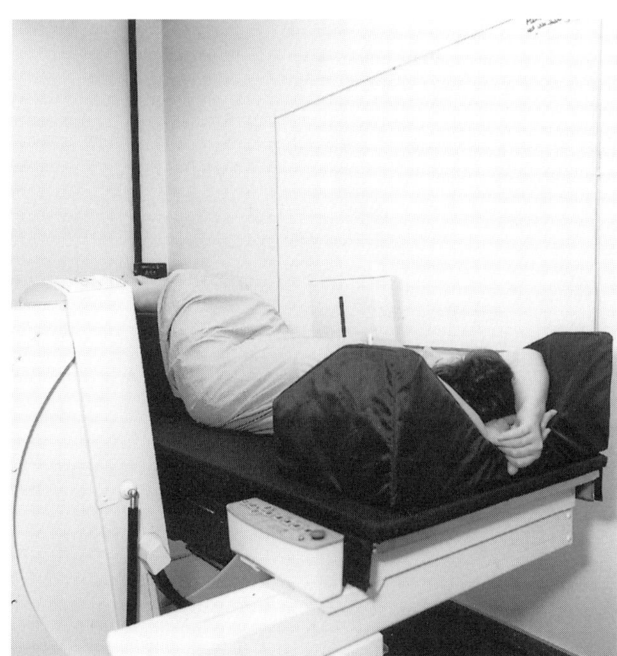

**Figure 3.45c** Patient in lateral 2 position

## Lumbar vertebrae continued

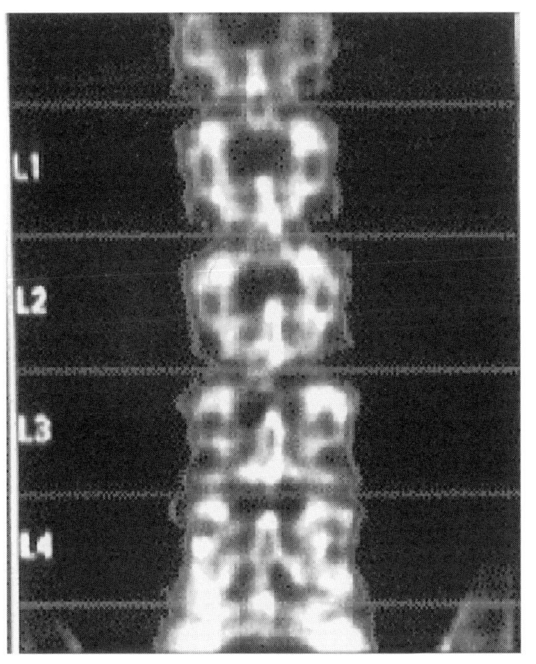

(a)

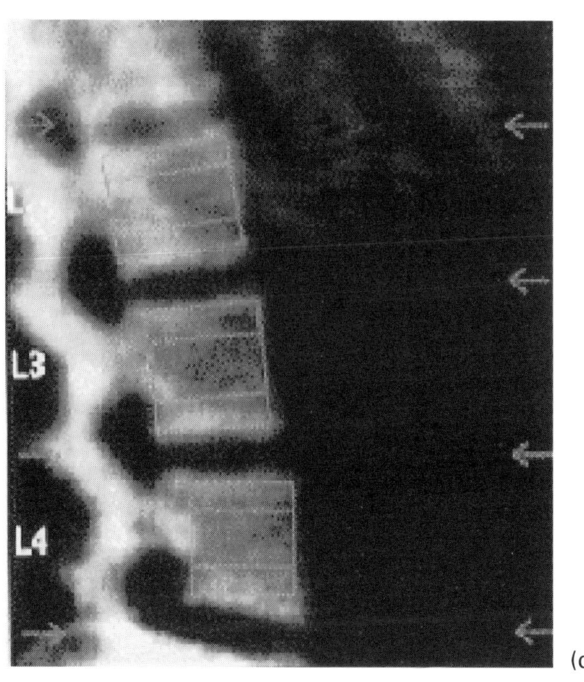

(d)

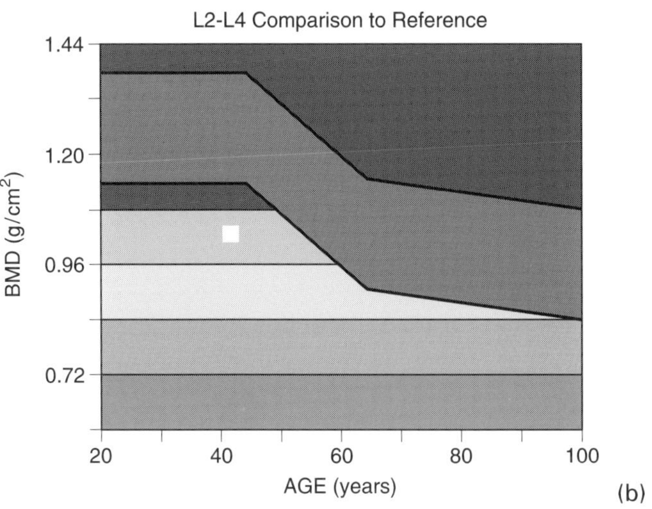

(b)

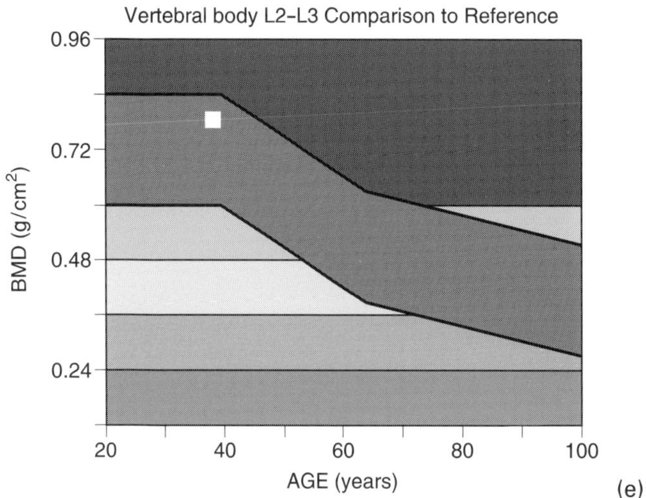

(e)

**Bone Results**

| Region | BMD $g/cm^2$ | Young Adult % | Young Adult T | Age Matched % | Age Matched Z |
|---|---|---|---|---|---|
| L1 | 0.862 | 76 | −2.24 | 85 | −1.25 |
| L2 | 1.021 | 85 | −1.49 | 94 | −0.51 |
| L3 | 1.093 | 91 | −0.98 | 101 | 0.09 |
| L4 | 1.102 | 92 | −0.81 | 102 | 0.17 |
| L2-L4 | 1.075 | 90 | −1.04 | 99 | −0.06 |

(c)

**Bone Results**

| | |
|---|---|
| B2-B3 BMD $(g/cm^2)^1$ | $0.791 \pm 0.01$ |
| B2-B3 % Young Adult[2] | $110 \pm 3$ |
| B2-B3 % Age Matched[3] | $111 \pm 3$ |

B = Vetebral body L2/L3

(f)

**Figure 3.46** DXA analyses of lumbar vertebrae

## Dual energy X-ray absorptiometry

### Femoral neck

The patient lies supine in the middle of the scanner table, ensuring that the anterior superior iliac spines are equidistant from the table top and the arms are placed across the chest. The selected limb is abducted to move the lesser trochanter away from the ischium of the pelvis and medially rotated through 25°, bringing the femoral neck parallel to the scanner table. By doing so the greater trochanter is rotated forward and the lesser trochanter backwards, bringing the femoral neck parallel to the table, thus avoiding foreshortening of the neck due to normal femoral anteversion, and giving adequate bone for analysis. The foot is secured to a dedicated support to maintain the required position.

With the aid of a positioning light, the scanner arm is centred over the femur 2 cm below the lower border of the symphysis pubis. From this start point, scanning continues cranially covering a maximum distance of 200 mm.

Although the procedure may be stopped by the operator at any time, scanning must commence at least 20 mm below the lesser trochanter and end no less than 30 mm above the greater trochanter to give adequate coverage for accurate measurements. Scan time varies depending on the equipment and the supporting software used. A typical scan time is approximately 2 min.

*Image analysis*

For the femoral neck region, measurements are obtained for three areas, namely femoral neck, greater trochanter and Ward's triangle. Information on the femoral neck and trochanteric regions is important as these are two main sites for fracture. Ward's triangle is an area where there is early loss of trabecular bone in osteoporosis, but the measure is less precise than other sites in the hip.

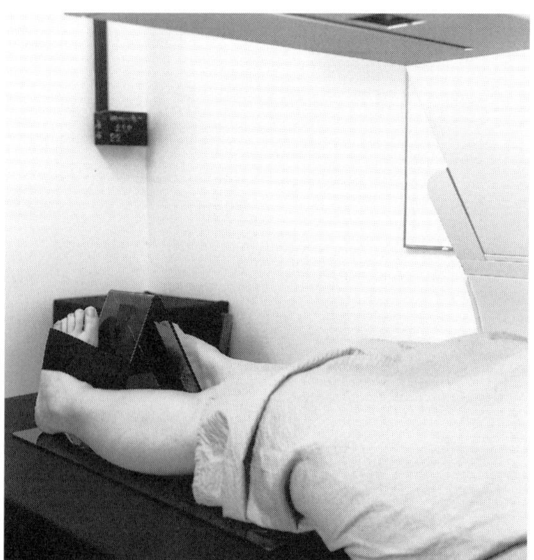

(a)

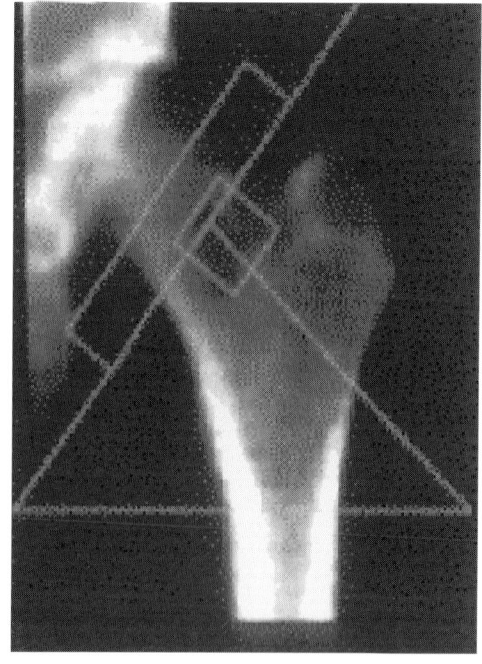

(b)

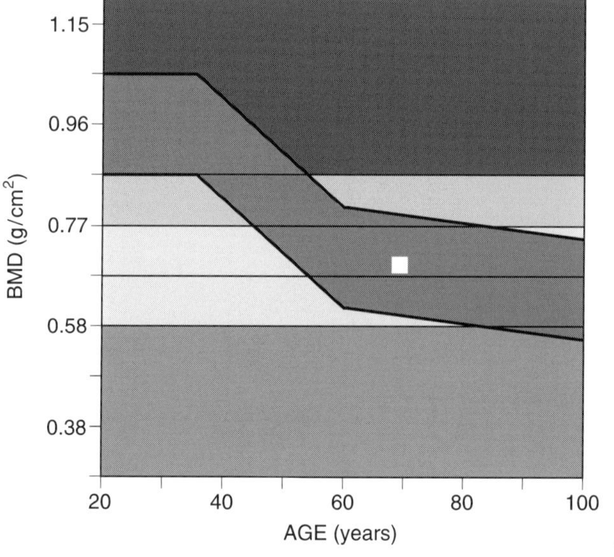


(c)

| Bone Results DEXA Calibration | | | |
|---|---|---|---|
| Region | BMD g/cm$^2$ | % Young Adult | % Age Matched |
| **Neck** | **1.221** | **114** | **107** |
| Wards | 1.031 | 107 | 99 |
| Troch | 1.101 | 118 | 110 |
| Shaft | 1.545 | 122 | 115 |
| **Total** | **1.307** | **120** | **112** |

(d)

**Figure 3.47a,b,c and d** DXA equipment and analyses of femoral neck

## Total body scanning

For total body DXA to be performed successfully, no part of the body should lie outside the boundary lines marked on the scanner table top. If this is not achieved, falsely low measurements will be obtained. The patient lies supine in the middle of the scanner table, with legs together. Positioning straps are applied to the knees and ankles to help immobilisation and maintain position. The patient's arms rest on the table, preferably with palms downwards, ensuring that the fingers are not in contact with the lateral aspect of the pelvis but within the transverse rectilinear travel limits of the scanner gantry. The patient's head should be 2 cm below the top boundary line.

For rectilinear systems, scanning commences at a point 1 cm above the top of the head and is terminated 1 cm below the toes. The patient must remain still throughout the whole examination, and the imaging time is approximately 15–30 min. When using fan beam systems the data are collected in three scanning sweeps, starting from the top of the patient, scanning the right side, returning to the head of the patient over the midline, and ending with the third sweep over the left side. The patient must remain still throughout the whole examination. The imaging time for rectilinear pencil beam systems is approximately 30 minutes, compared to 3 minutes for fan beam systems

*Image analysis*

Total body analysis as well as providing bone mineral density values for the body as a whole subdivides the body into specific regions, namely head, arms, legs, ribs, pelvis, and thoracic and lumbar spine. Three sets of body composition values are also calculated – grams of fat tissue, grams of lean tissue and the percentage of body mass compared with total soft tissue mass. At present, this additional information is used in research only.

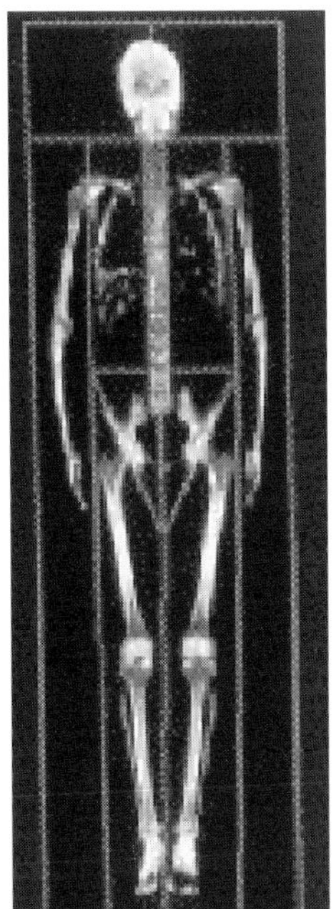

(b)

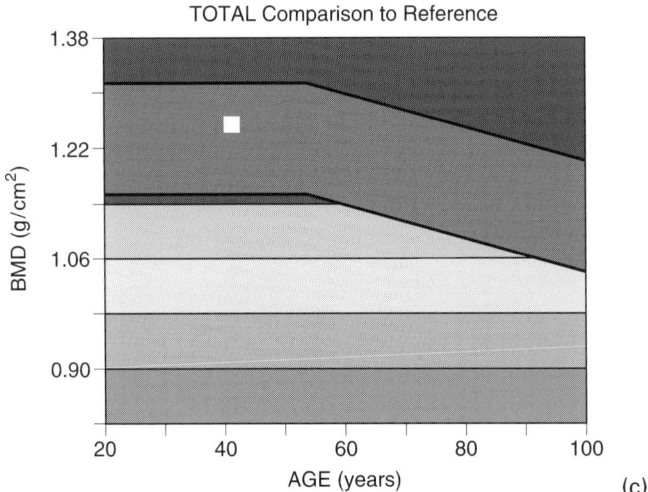


(c)

**Bone Results**

| Region | BMD g/cm$^2$ |
|---|---|
| Head | 2.024 |
| Arms | 0.959 |
| Legs | 1.382 |
| Trunk | 0.983 |
| Ribs | 0.742 |
| Pelvis | 1.051 |
| Spine | 1.019 |
| Thoracic | 0.967 |
| Lumber | 1.137 |
| **Total** | **1.151** |

(d)

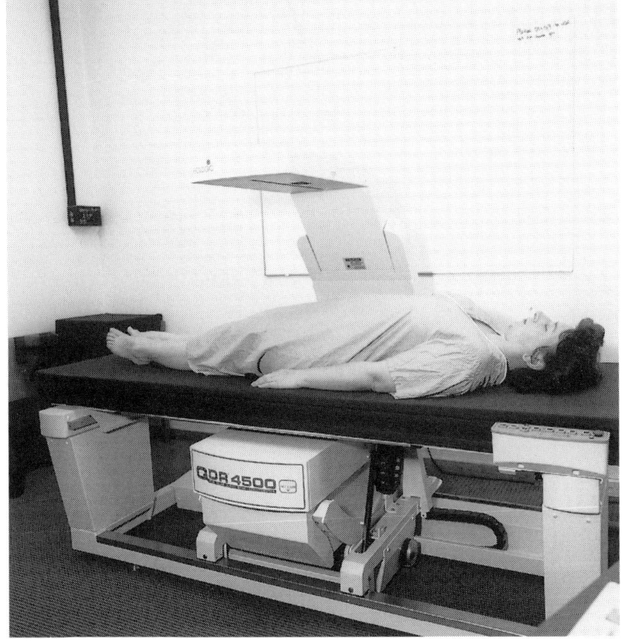


(a)

**Figure 3.48a,b,c and d** DXA equipment and analyses of total body

## Quantitative computed tomography (QCT)

Computed tomography not only demonstrates cross-sectional anatomy, but also gives precise measurements of the linear attenuation coefficient of the various structures of the body. By using this numerical data, bone mineral density measurements can be obtained of the trabecular bone in the lower thoracic and lumbar vertebral bodies. As CT attenuation values are energy dependent and susceptible to errors, a fixed kVp must be selected and a calibration phantom consisting of different densities of bone mineral equivalent material (cither dipotassium hydrogen phosphate or calcium hydroxyapatite) must be used to correct for slight variations in X-ray output. Because CT attenuation values change across the scan field, a consistent table height is required to keep the vertebrae and the phantom in the same position within the scan field. This level must be recorded and selected at subsequent follow-up examinations.

### Position of the patient and imaging modality

The calibration phantom is placed centrally on the scanner table and the patient positioned with the thoracolumbar region adjacent to the phantom, knees are flexed over a 60° support pad to reduce the lumbar curvature and arms are elevated out of the scan field. The patient is moved into the scanner so that the scan reference point is at the level of the xiphisternum. The vertical table height is raised to the predetermined level.

### Imaging procedure

Anteroposterior and lateral scan projection radiographs are taken, starting 5 cm above the reference point and ending 25 cm below. The AP projection is used to assess any scoliosis which may be present. From the lateral projection, one 10 mm section is prescribed at each of the vertebral levels T12–L3. Meticulous care must be taken to ensure that the section is at the mid-point of the vertebral body and parallel to the vertebral end-plates. To minimise radiation dose, the technique factors are reduced. Typical scan values are 80 kVp, 70 mA and 2-second scan time. All scans are taken on suspended expiration. The total examination time is approximately 15 min.

### Image analysis

Computer software enables image analysis to be carried out in approximately 10 min. A region of interest (ROI), in the form of an elliptical cursor, is positioned over the vertebral body to include only trabecular bone and to exclude the cortex and the entry point of the basivertebral vein. The attenuation values of each calibration material are measured and from the regression line the ROI of the trabecular bone is converted into a bone mineral density (BMD), expressed as bone mineral equivalent in $mg/cm^3$. To ensure that the same area is sampled at subsequent visits, the analysis should be recorded on 'hard copy'.

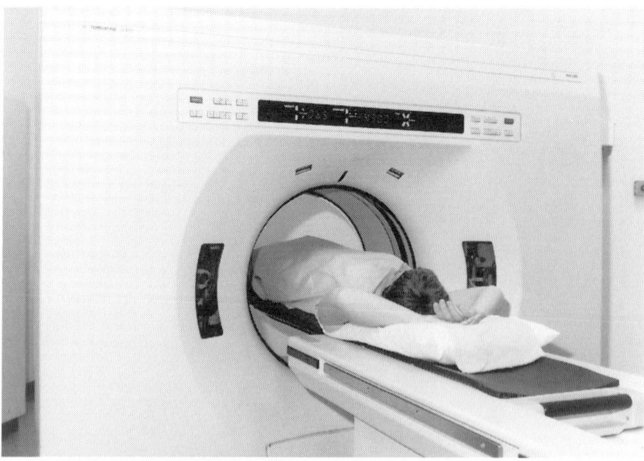

**Figure 3.49a** QCT equipment

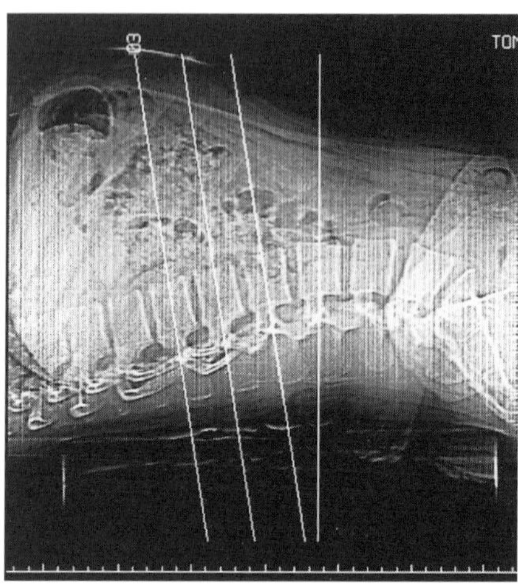

**Figure 3.49b** Scan projection radiograph showing scanning levels

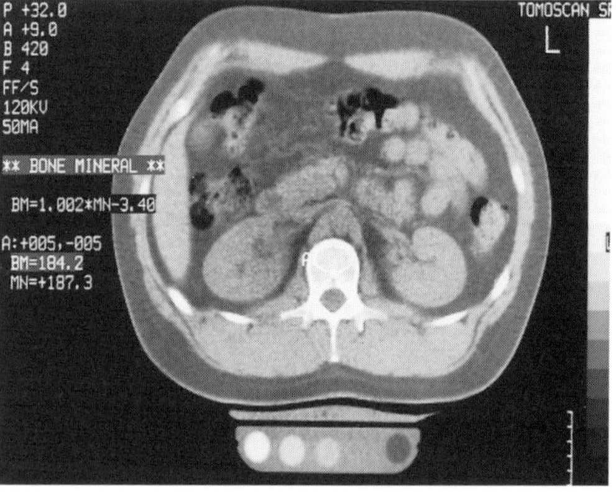


**Figure 3.49c** Transaxial image showing ROI for analysis

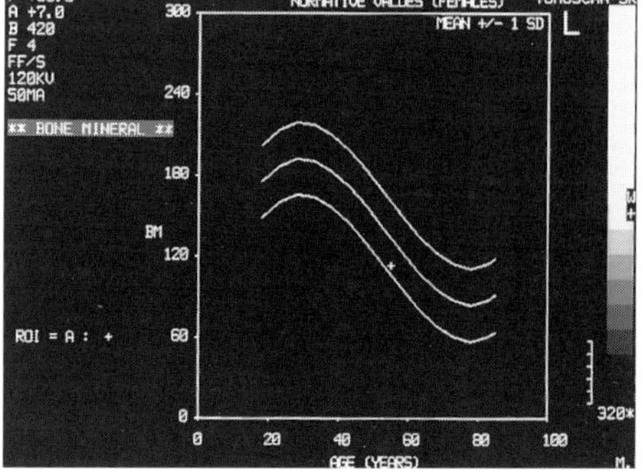


**Figure 3.49d** Bone mineral density measurement plotted against normal population reference age

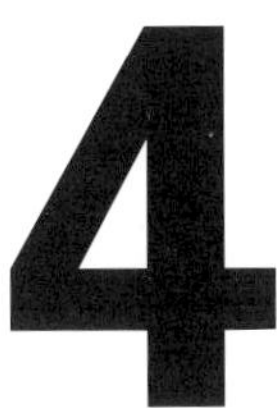

# Respiratory System

## CONTENTS

# 4 Respiratory System

## Pharynx

### Phonation following laryngectomy

The alimentary function of the pharynx is considered in Chapter 5. In this section, consideration is given to its role in phonation following laryngectomy.

In normal circumstances air passes from the lungs through the larynx, where sound is made, into the pharynx. However, following laryngectomy voice restoration is achieved by training the patient first to move air into the oesophagus and then to remove this air past the pharyngo-oesophageal (P-E) segment as opposed to the vocal cords in the larynx.

Oesophageal voice is achieved if the P-E segment is relaxed, allowing air to pass into the oesophagus, following which the P-E segment becomes the vibratory source for sound. However, a number of patients find difficulty with this technique and in order to establish any anatomical or physiological reasons a barium swallow combined with attempted phonation or an 'air insufflation test' is done to assess the tonicity of the P-E sphincter. Failure may be due to hypotonicity of the P-E muscles, hypertonicity, spasm and stricture.

### Barium swallow and air insufflation test

**Indications**

Assessment for surgical voice reconstruction either prior to or following laryngectomy associated with failed speech.

The assessment of the patient is divided into two procedures, first the barium swallow, followed by the air insufflation test.

A single contrast technique is selected and no special patient preparation is required. Fluoroscopic equipment incorporating videotape and sound recording is required to record and play back the dynamic processes under investigation. A specially adapted chair may be necessary during fluoroscopy for those patients unable to stand without assistance during the procedure.

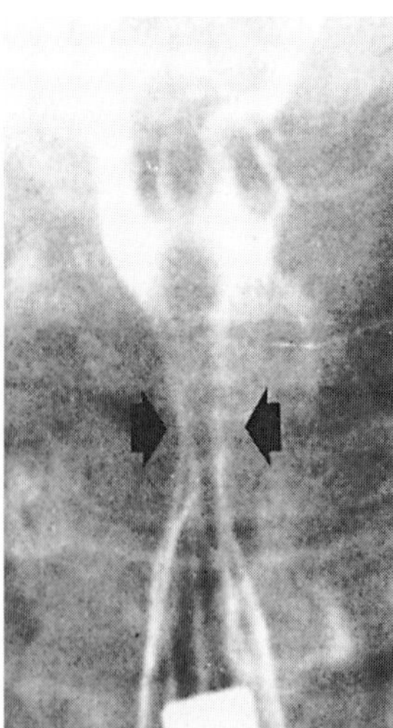

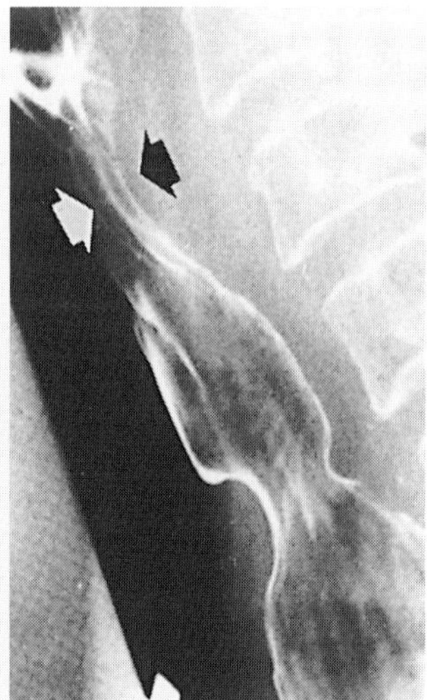

**Figure 4.1a** AP and Lateral images of a good oesophageal speaker during phonation. Vibrating P-E segment is marked with arrows

**Imaging process**

*Barium swallow*

Lateral projection images of the neck are acquired with the fluoroscopic table erect and the patient standing or sitting in the lateral position, so that the median sagittal plane is parallel to the image intensifier input face which is positioned over the neck region. The chin is elevated and the shoulders depressed to permit maximum visualisation of the neck. The patient is asked to swallow a good mouthful of barium, during which dynamic real-time images of this process are recorded on videotape under fluoroscopic control.

The patient is instructed to attempt phonation, during which images of the air-filled oesophagus and P-E segment are recorded. Good oesophageal speakers exhibit an open oesophagus with fast motility of the bolus and a visible P-E segment on phonation, with a good oesophageal air reservoir.

*Air insufflation test*

The patient's P-E segment is then assessed independent of their ability to direct air into the oesophagus using the 'air insufflation test'. Prior to the procedure a radio-opaque marker is secured on the patient's neck near the laryngectomy stoma to act as a landmark.

After the pharynx is coated with barium a flexible rubber tube, with a radio-opaque tip and two opposing side holes, is passed through the nose and P-E segment and the tip positioned at the level of the tracheostomy, with the radiographic marker acting as a guide. Dynamic images of the pharynx are then acquired as the patient attempts to produce oesophageal voice while air flows through the tube at the rate of approximately 0.5 litres/min.

*Contrast medium and injection data*

| *Volume* | *Concentration* | *Flow rate* |
|---|---|---|
| 70–150 ml | Barium, low viscosity high density | Oral |

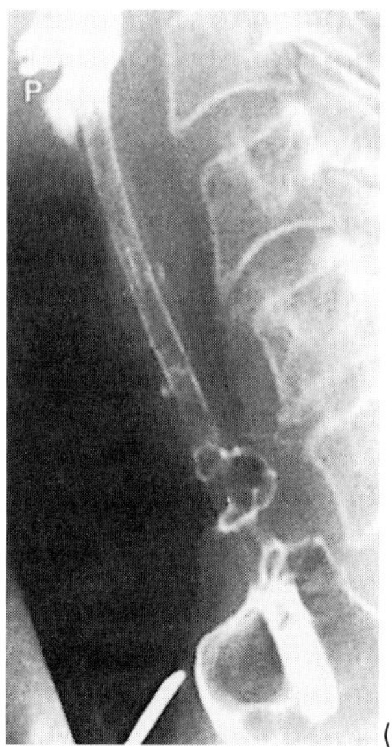


(b)

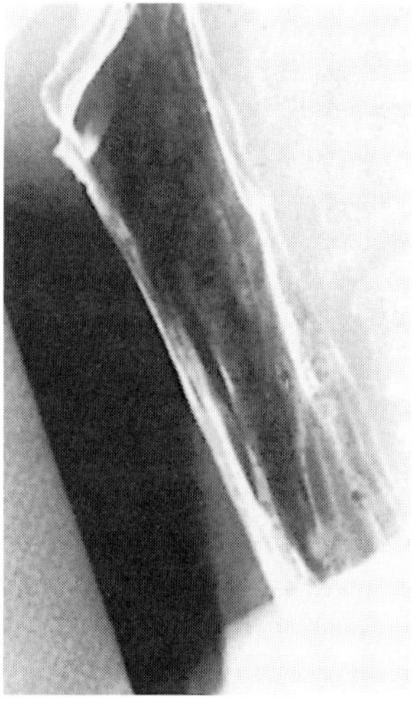

(c)

**Figure 4.1b,c** Examples of: (i) hypotonic patient during phonation with widely separated anterior and posterior walls and no P-E segment and no voice; (ii) spastic patient during attempted phonation with air insufflation showing severe narrowing of the reconstructed pharynx with no vibrating P-E segment and no voice (Images courtesy of J. McIvor, P.F. Evans, A. Perry and A.D. Cheesman, Charing Cross Hospital, London)

## Larynx

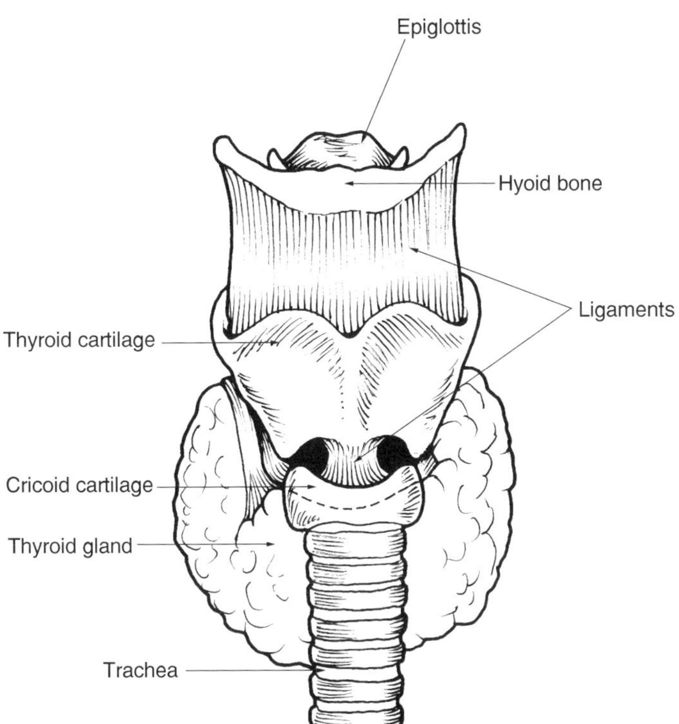


**Figure 4.2a** Larynx – anterior aspect

The larynx, the organ of voice, lies between the base of the tongue and the trachea. It is situated in the upper and anterior aspect of the neck anterior to the oropharynx. In the adult it lies between the fourth and sixth cervical vertebrae.

It consists of nine cartilages, the largest three being the thyroid, cricoid and epiglottis.

The air-filled cavity of the larynx is divided into two parts by the true vocal cords which are separated in the midline by a narrow triangular fissure called the rima glottidis.

Sound is produced when the vocal cords vibrate; this happens when the cords are close together but not touching. When fully open or closed the cords cannot vibrate.

Speech occurs on the commencement of and during breathing out as the cords begin to close and vibrate. Speech stops as the cords start to open and no longer vibrate, with silence continuing during the breathing-in phase.

### Recommended imaging procedures

Plain film radiography is limited to demonstrating the air-filled larynx, which is useful in foreign body localisation or demonstrating the presence of a laryngocele which is filled with air from the larynx.

The larynx may be examined using a number of imaging procedures, including fluorography, CT, MRI, tomography and laryngography.

Of these, CT and tomography are perhaps the most frequently requested examinations. Prior to any of these procedures the larynx will be examined directly by laryngoscopy when surface abnormalities of internal structures can readily be visualised and biopsy made of suspected tissues.

### Indications

Speech difficulties, tumours and congenital abnormalities.

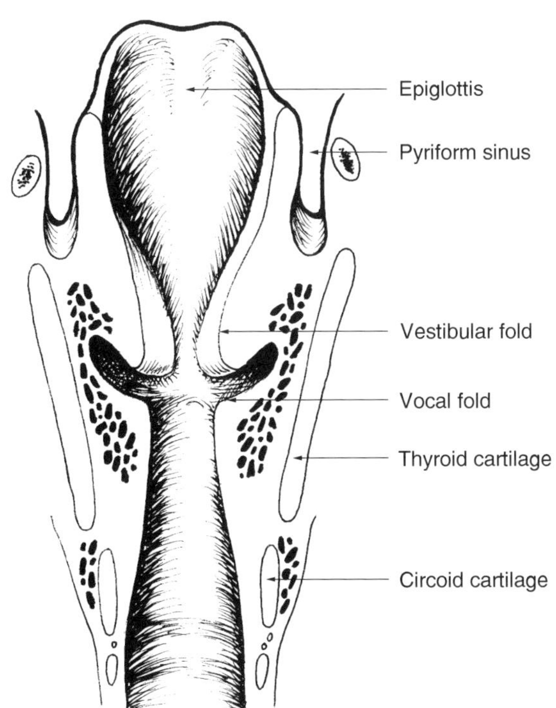


**Figure 4.2b** Diagrammatic coronal section of the larynx (posterior aspect)

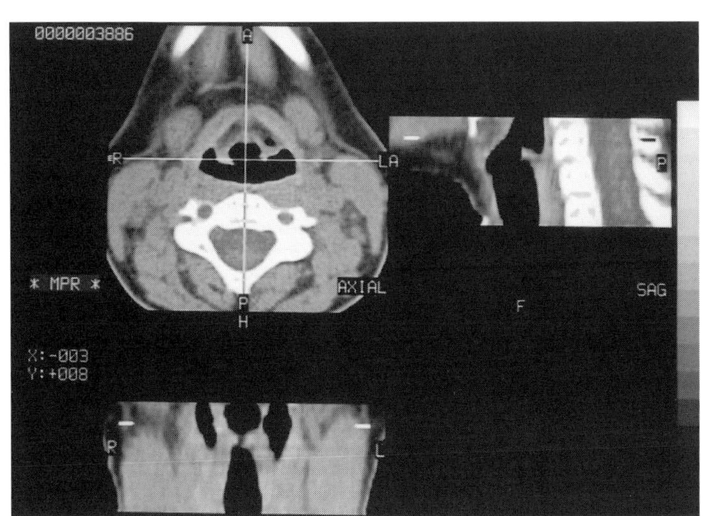


**Figure 4.2c** CT section through the larynx with corresponding sagittal and coronal reformations

# 4 Respiratory System

## Larynx

### Computed tomography

Transaxial images of the larynx are obtained with no specific patient preparation.

Contrast enhanced scans may be prescribed when staging tumours to assist detection of involved cervical nodes.

#### Indications

Tumours of the larynx, including the vocal cords.

#### Position of patient and imaging modality

The patient lies supine, head first on the scanner table. The arms are placed by the side and the neck is extended and supported on a positioning pad. Positioning is aided by transaxial, coronal and sagittal alignment lights. The median sagittal plane is perpendicular and the coronal plane is parallel to the scanner table.

The scanner table height is adjusted to ensure that the coronal plane alignment light is approximately 1 cm posterior to the laryngeal prominence. The patient is moved into the scanner so that the scan reference point is at the level of the sternal notch.

#### Imaging procedure

A lateral scan projection radiograph of the neck is performed, starting 12 cm above and ending 12 cm below the reference point. From this image, 3 mm contiguous sections are prescribed through the larynx, starting from the hyoid bone and ending at the first tracheal cartilage ring, with the gantry angled so that the scan plane is parallel to the hyoid bone.

If spiral scanning options are available, these images may be acquired with a volume acquisition, using a 3 mm slice thickness and 3 mm table increments, but with a 2 mm reconstruction index to give overlapping sections.

Scans are initially taken on arrested inspiration and may be repeated either on arrested expiration or during a Valsalva manoeuvre.

When investigating or staging tumours the same area is rescanned, using the same imaging parameters, during the infusion of a non-ionic contrast agent. It is important that the patient does not move between these scanning sequences.

For cervical node involvement the field of view must include the neck region.

*Contrast medium and injection data*

| *Volume* | *Concentration* | *Flow rate* |
| --- | --- | --- |
| 100 ml | 240 mgI/ml | 2 ml/s |

Scanning commences 20 s after the start of injection.

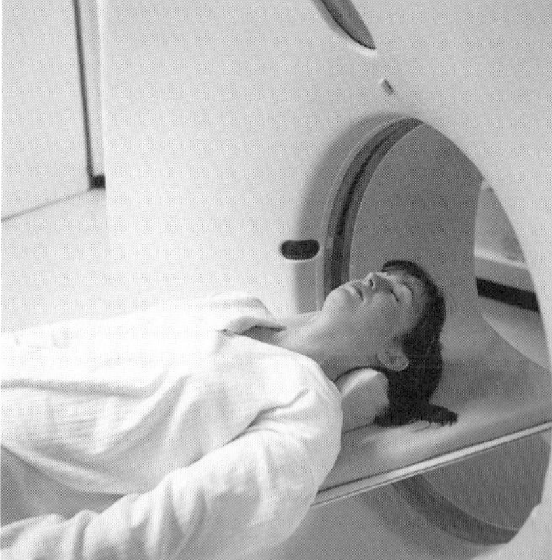

**Figure 4.3a** The CT scanner with patient in position

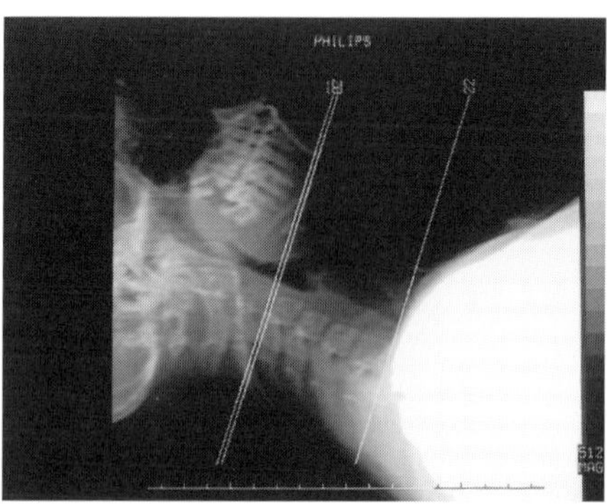


**Figure 4.3b** Lateral scan projection radiograph showing start and end locations

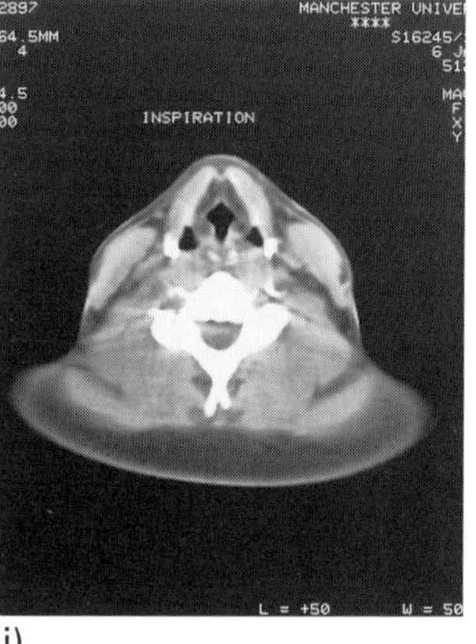


(i)

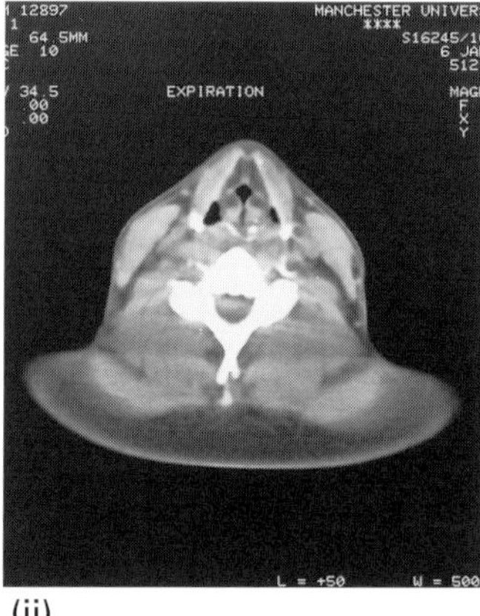


(ii)

**Figure 4.3c** (i,ii) Transaxial images on inspiration and expiration at the level of the aryepiglottic folds

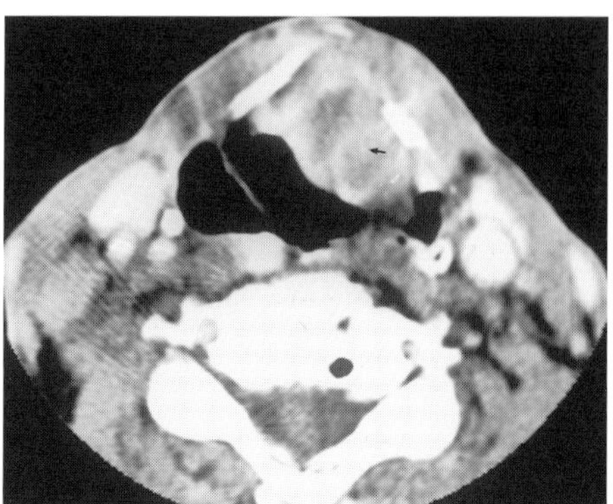

**Figure 4.3d** Post-contrast image through a laryngeal tumour

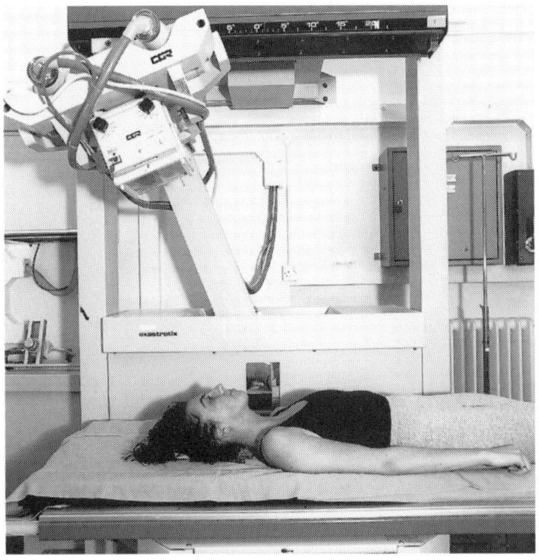

Figure 4.4a Tomography equipment with patient in position for scanning of the larynx

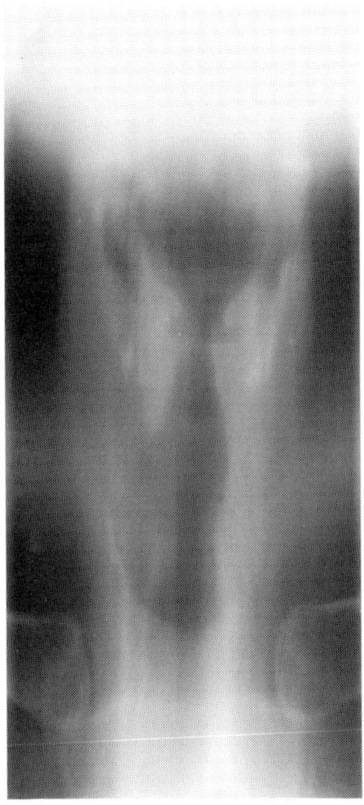

**Figure 4.4b** Linear tomograph through a normal larynx

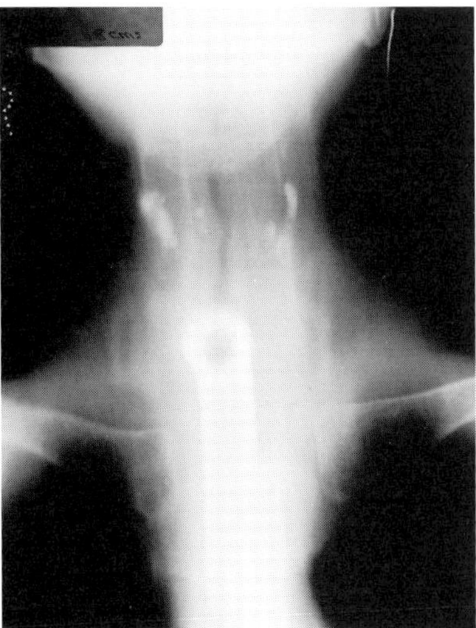

**Figure 4.4c** Linear tomograph showing compression of the larynx (NB tracheotomy)

## Tomography

Tomography is usually performed in the absence of CT. Because of the high inherent contrast of air and soft tissues in the larynx, when combined with higher kilovoltages, excellent thin sections of 1 mm thickness can be used to demonstrate vocal cord tumours. No special patient preparation is required and the patient is positioned to enable a series of anteroposterior projections through the larynx, with lateral projections if required.

### Indications

Tumour of the larynx including the vocal cords.

### Position of patient and imaging modality

The patient lies supine on the imaging table, with the median sagittal plane at right angles to and in the midline of the table.

The patient is located on the table so that a vertical central ray would pass 1 cm inferior to the eminence of the thyroid cartilage.

### Imaging procedure

A longitudinal linear tomographic tube movement employing a 40° angle is selected. The X-ray tube is set up to move in a caudal to cranial direction using only the first half of the 40° movement (20° exposure angle), to avoid superimposing the images of the mandible and facial bones onto those of the larynx. The first tomogram is taken on a 18 × 24 cm cassette placed longitudinally in the cassette tray, with the pivot height set at 0.5 cm deep to the skin surface centring point. A series of further tomograms are taken at 3 mm intervals through the whole of the larynx. All images are acquired on arrested inspiration. A repeat series of tomograms are then made at each level during phonation of the letter 'E'.

The use of high kilovoltages (90 kV plus) will also help to reduce linear streak artefacts on the image.

# 4 Respiratory System

## Larynx

### Magnetic resonance imaging

This procedure, employed with the use of an anterior or volumetric surface coil, enables images of the larynx to be obtained in various anatomical planes. Coils used for the cervical spine rarely produce satisfactory images due to anterior signal loss. $T_1$ and $T_2$ weighted spin-echo sequences are used to obtain excellent anatomical details of the larynx and surrounding structures.

**Indications**

Tumours of the larynx and surrounding structures.

**Position of patient and imaging modality**

The patient lies supine on the imaging couch with the median sagittal plane perpendicular to the imaging couch. The neck is positioned within the volumetric surface coil. The head is secured in position by Velcro straps across the forehead and chin to minimise patient movement. Using the alignment lights the couch is moved to bring the external scan reference point at the centre of the surface coil, after which the patient and coil are driven into the isocentre of the magnet. The patient is instructed to remain as still as possible, with no tongue movements or swallowing, during each scan.

**Imaging procedure**

An initial sagittal localiser scan is performed, from which a coronal $T_1$ weighted series of images are prescribed through the larynx to assess anatomy. From these images further transaxial $T_1$ and $T_2$ weighted series are prescribed. In all instances the section width is 5 mm, with a gap of 1 mm. To further delineate a tumour mass, the $T_1$ weighted images may be repeated after the administration of a paramagnetic contrast agent. Also, MRA may be useful to visualise the tumour in relation to the blood vessels of the neck.

*Contrast medium and injection data*

| *Volume* | *Pharmaceutical* | *Flow rate* |
|---|---|---|
| 0.2 ml/kg body weight | Gadolinium DTPA | Hand injection |

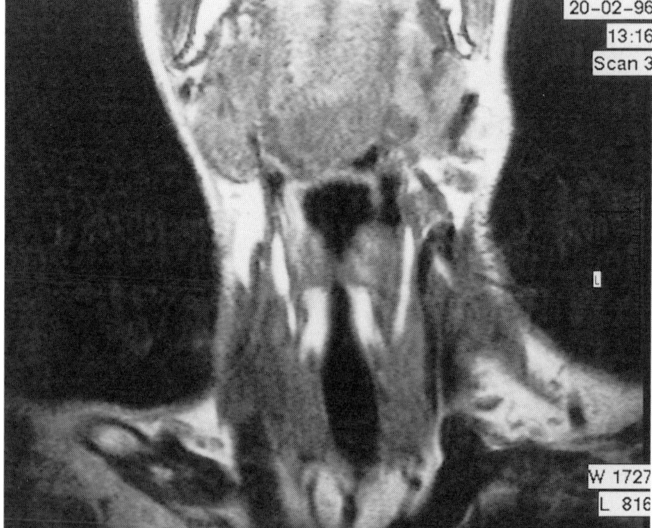


**Figure 4.5a** Coronal $T_1$ weighted image of normal larynx

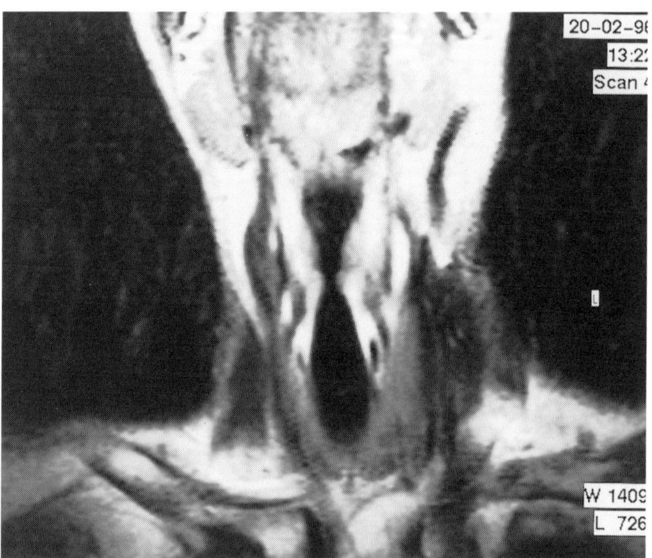


**Figure 4.5b** Coronal $T_2$ weighted image of normal larynx

**Table 4.1 Imaging parameters**

| *Imaging plane* | *Imaging sequence* | *TR* | *TE* | *Field of view* (cm) | *No. of NEX* | *Slice width/gap* (mm) | *Matrix (horizontal–vertical)* |
|---|---|---|---|---|---|---|---|
| Coronal and transaxial | Spin-echo $T_1$ weighted | 500 | 25 | 25 | 4 | 5/1 | 160 × 256 |
| Transaxial | Fast spin-echo $T_2$ weighted echotrain length –6 | 3000 | 100 | 20 | 3 | 5/1 | 160 × 256 |
| Transaxial | 2D time of flight Flip angle 90° | 60 | 10 | 20 | 2 | 2/0 | 128 × 256 (rectangular pixel) |

## Trachea

The trachea is a cartilaginous and musculomembranous tube approximately 10 cm in length and 2 cm in diameter. It is made up of 16–20 incomplete cartilagous rings and descends from the cricoid cartilage of the larynx through the neck and thorax where it divides at its bifurcation, called the carina, into the two main bronchi supplying air to the lungs. It commences at the level of the sixth cervical vertebra and terminates at the level of the fifth thoracic vertebra.

In the neck it is related anteriorly to the isthmus of the thyroid gland and laterally to the lateral lobes of the thyroid gland and the common carotid arteries. In the thorax it lies in the superior mediastinum and is related anteriorly to the anterior mediastinum and posteriorly to the oesophagus.

The right main bronchus approximately, 2.5 cm in length, enters the right lung at the level of the fifth thoracic vertebra and is shorter, wider and more vertical in direction than the left. Due to this vertical orientation, inhaled foreign bodies are more likely to become lodged in the right bronchus than the left.

The left main bronchus, approximately 5 cm in length, enters the left lung at the level of the sixth thoracic vertebra and is narrower and longer than the right.

### Recommended imaging procedures

Plain film radiography using well-penetrated anteroposterior and lateral projections (including lateral thoracic inlet projection of the upper thoracic trachea) will demonstrate the normal air-filled trachea. This will enable any deviation of the trachea due to pathological abnormalities of the thyroid or parathyroid glands to be detected.

Special investigation of the trachea is usually confined to CT or tomography to demonstrate more clearly its relationship with surrounding structures.

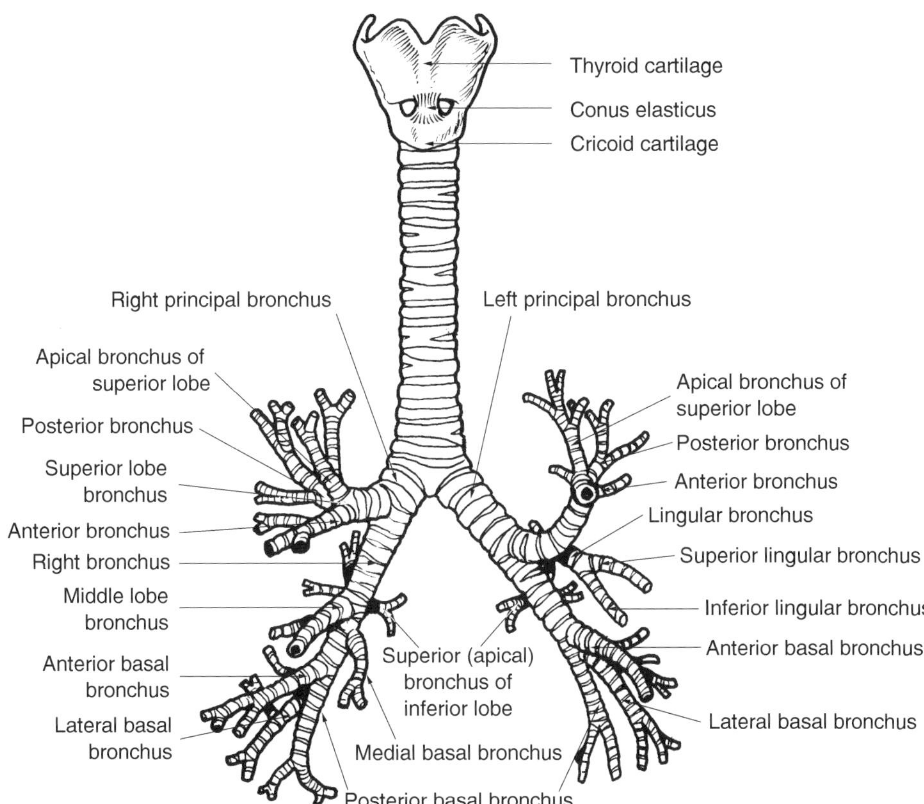


**Figure 4.6** Trachea and bronchial tree – anterior aspect

# 4 Respiratory System

## Trachea

### Computed tomography

Transaxial images of the trachea are obtained with no specific patient preparation. Contrast enhanced scans may be prescribed when staging tumours to show the relationship of the trachea to surrounding anatomy and tumour masses.

**Indications**

Obstructive large airways disease, tracheal compression, tracheomalacia and tumour.

**Position of patient and imaging modality**

The patient lies supine, head first on the scanner table, with the arms raised and placed behind the head, out of the scan plane for the thoracic trachea. For the cervical trachea the arms are placed by the side. Positioning is aided by transaxial, coronal and sagittal alignment lights. The median sagittal plane is perpendicular and the coronal plane is parallel to the scanner table. The scan plane is now perpendicular to the long axis of the body to enable transaxial cross-sectional imaging to be undertaken. The scanner table height is adjusted to ensure that the coronal plane alignment light is at the level of the mid-axillary line. The patient is then moved into the scanner so that the scan reference point is at the level of the sternal notch.

**Imaging procedure**

For the cervical trachea a postero-anterior scan projection radiograph is performed, starting 12 cm above and ending 12 cm below the reference point. For the thoracic trachea a scan projection radiograph may be taken, starting 4 cm above and ending 25 cm below the reference point. A postero-anterior projection is selected to reduce the radiation dose to the thymus and breast tissue.

For a general survey of the trachea, 10 mm contiguous sections through the trachea are acquired on arrested inspiration. After review, a suspected lesion may be rescanned during the infusion of a contrast agent using 10 mm contiguous sections. In order to avoid contrast streak artefacts from the brachiocephalic vein when scanning the upper trachea, it may be necessary to commence scanning at the lower margin of the abnormality and continue scanning in a cranial direction over the entire lesion.

If spiral scanning options are available, all scans may be acquired in one breath hold using a 10 mm slice thickness and 10 mm table increments, but with a 5 mm reconstruction index to give overlapping sections.

When investigating tracheomalacia a series of images are acquired in both arrested inspiration and expiration to compare the integrity of the structure of the trachea in these phases of respiration. Scans using 5 mm sections are prescribed at three different levels, the first immediately below the larynx, the second at the level of the sternal notch and the third just above the bifurcation.

*Contrast medium and injection data*

| *Volume* | *Concentration* | *Flow rate* |
|---|---|---|
| 100 ml | 240 mgI/ml | 2 ml/s |

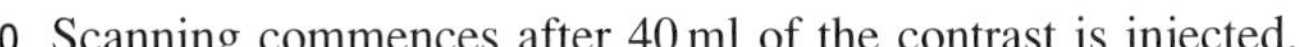

Scanning commences after 40 ml of the contrast is injected.

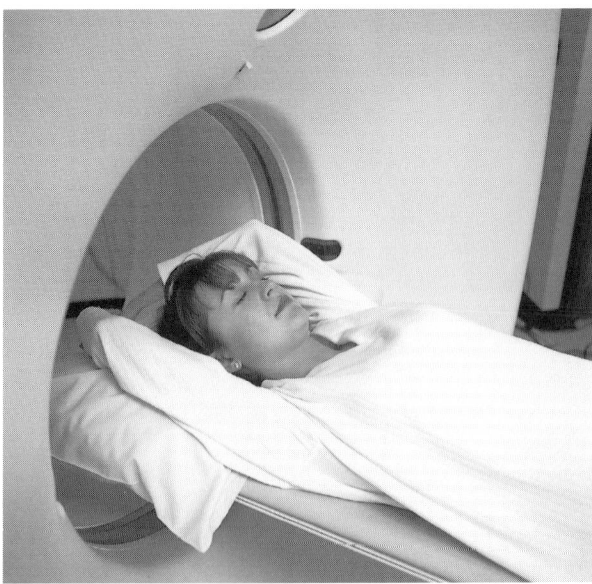

**Figure 4.7a** Patient in position for CT scanning of the trachea

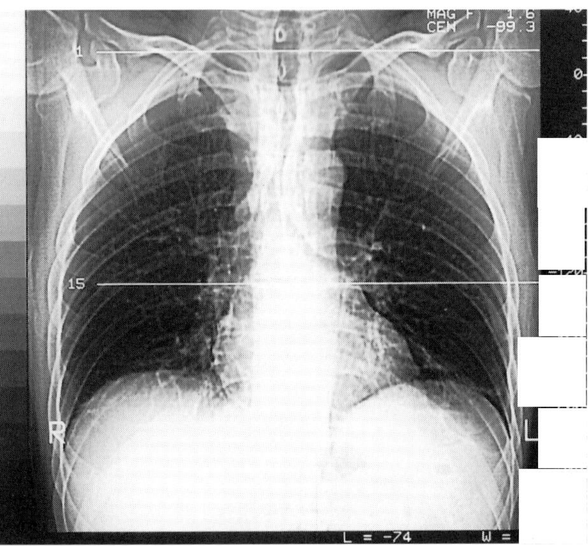


**Figure 4.7b** Scan projection radiograph showing start and end locations

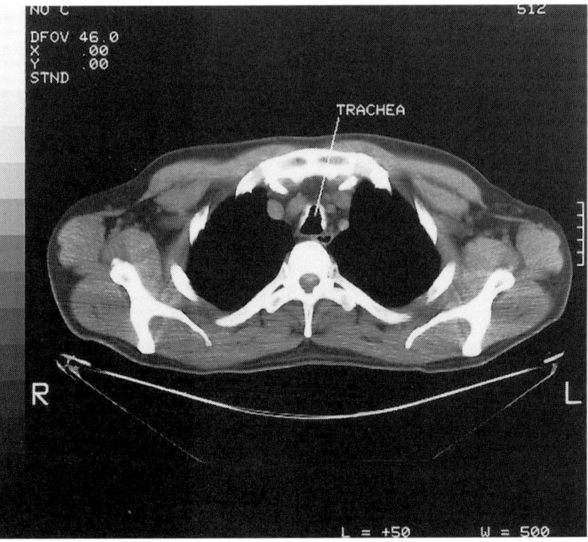


**Figure 4.7c** Transaxial image showing abnormal triangular-shaped trachea with calcifications within the walls

## Tomography

Tomography, using a linear movement, is performed to demonstrate abnormalities associated with the trachea. With this procedure the full extent of the trachea can be demonstrated in a single breathhold technique. No special patient preparation is required and the patient is positioned on an imaging couch adapted for tomography to enable a series of anteroposterior projections to be taken. Reference to a lateral radiograph of the chest will assist in determining the tomographic pivot height, which is measured from the posterior skin surface of the trunk to the centre of the trachea, and determining the amount that the lower trunk has to be raised to bring the trachea parallel to the film by observing by angle of the trachea in the thorax relative to the posterior chest wall.

**Figure 4.8a** Tomography equipment with patient in position for scanning of the trachea

### Indications

To identify the cause of obstruction of the trachea.

### Position of patient and imaging modality

The patient lies supine on the imaging table with the median sagittal plane at right angles to and in the midline of the table. The lower trunk is raised to bring the trachea parallel to the film. The patient is located on the table so that a vertical central ray would pass mid-way between the cricoid cartilage and the sternal angle.

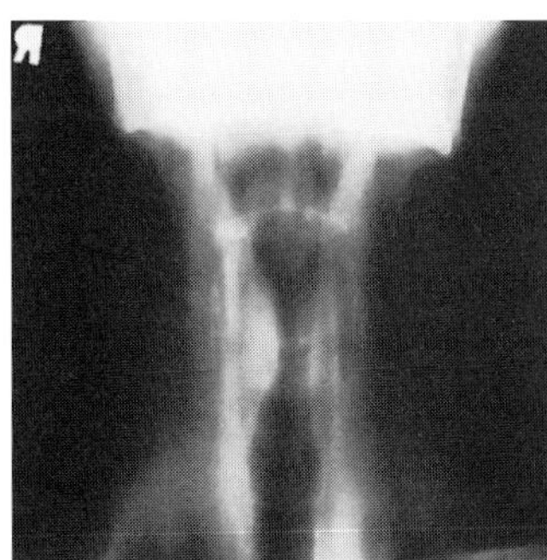

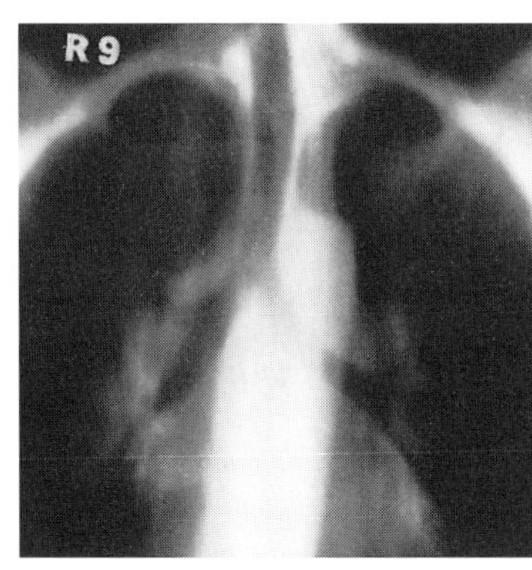


**Figure 4.8b** Lateral CT scan projection radiograph of thorax showing relationship of trachea

### Imaging procedure

A linear transverse movement using a 10 degrees exposure angle, giving a 5.5 mm layer, is preferred to avoid streak artefacts from the spine. If not available, longitudinal movement is used. For the transverse movement, the X-ray tube is moved to its start position either to the left or right of the thorax, where it is set up to move across the patient at right angles to the spine. The first tomogram is taken on a 24 × 30 cm cassette placed longitudinally in the cassette tray, with the pivot height set at 4–5 cm deep to the suprasternal notch. This radiograph is reviewed to assess if further tomograms above or below this level are required. Thinner layers may be followed at different levels using larger angulations or adapting, if available, complex large-angle movements.

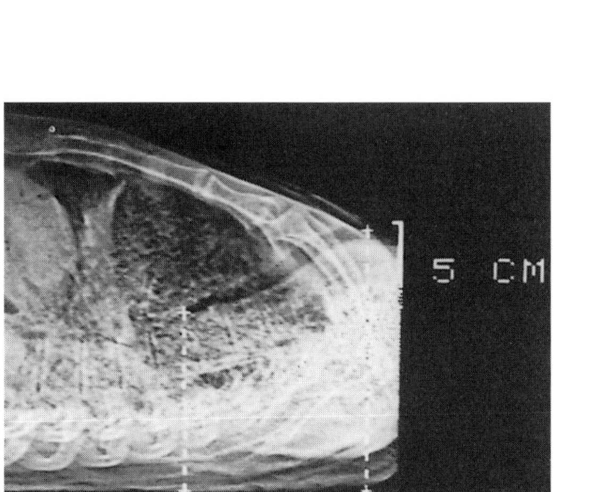


**Figure 4.8c** Tomograph of upper trachea

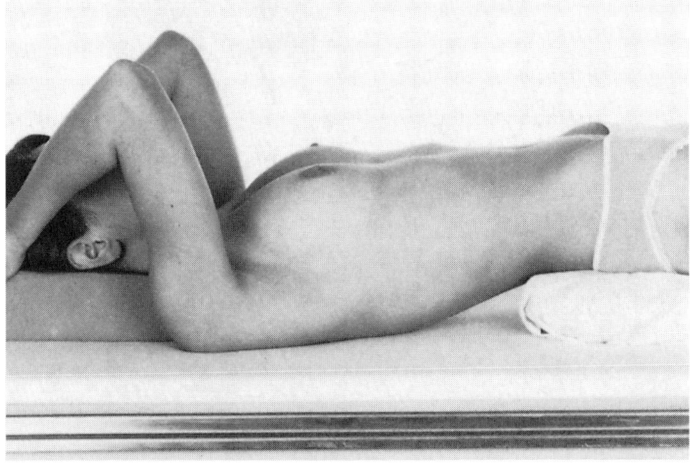

**Figure 4.8d** Tomograph of lower trachea and bifurcation

# 4 Respiratory System

## Lungs

The lungs, the organs of respiration, lie in the thoracic cavity and consist of two distinct structures, the right lung and the left lung. Both lungs are conical in shape and covered by a serous coat called the pleura. Each lie within its pleural cavity, separated from the other lung by the mediastinum containing the heart and great vessels.

The right lung is slightly larger than the left and has three lobes: upper, middle and lower. It is also shorter and wider than the left, due partly to the bulk of the right lobe of the liver pressing the right side of the diaphragm to a higher level than the left side and partly to the heart and pericardium lying a little to the left of the midline.

The left lung has two lobes: upper and lower. In its anterior border is found the cardiac notch which lies in contact with the left ventricle of the heart. Accessory lobes may be present in either lung.

Entering each lung at its root is the main bronchus which divides upon entering the lung at the hilum to form the bronchial tree. The pulmonary artery and pulmonary veins associated with each lung are also found at the root, enclosed by pleura.

The pulmonary artery divides into many branches, accompanying the bronchial tree to convey systemic venous blood to pulmonary capillaries which are associated with the alveoli. Pulmonary veins return oxygenated blood from the alveoli to the left atrium of the heart. Each lung is divided into a number of segments (10 or 8). Each segment is further subdivided into lobules which make up the lung parenchyma. Lobules vary in size and are closely connected together by interlobular areolar tissue. Each lobule is composed of one of the ramifications of a bronchiole and its terminal air sacs, called alveoli, and minute branches of the pulmonary artery, pulmonary capillaries and veins.

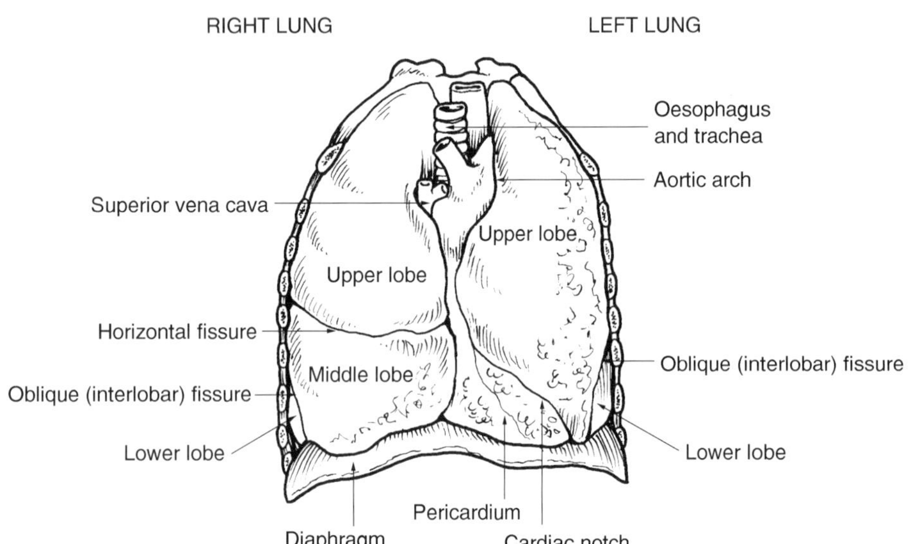


**Figure 4.9a** Schematic diagram of lungs and pericardium – anterior view

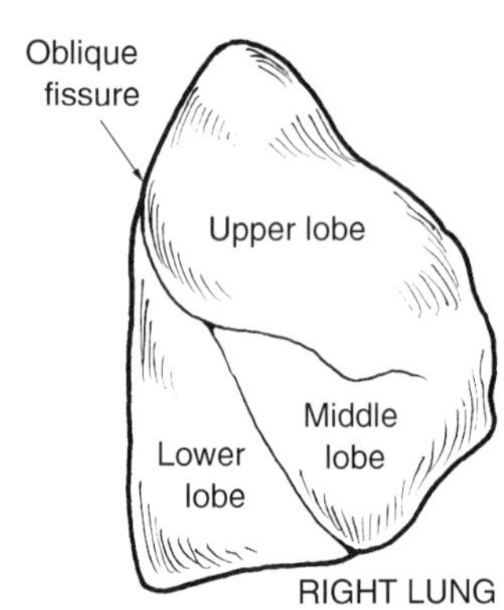


**Figure 4.9b** Lateral plane

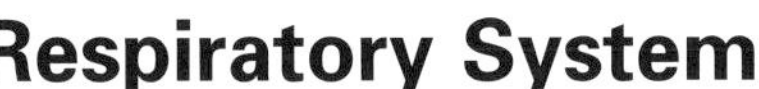

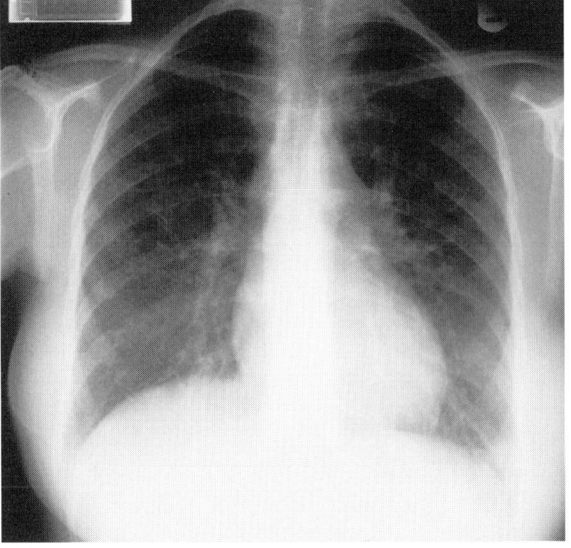

**Figure 4.10a** Conventional radiograph – postero-anterior projection

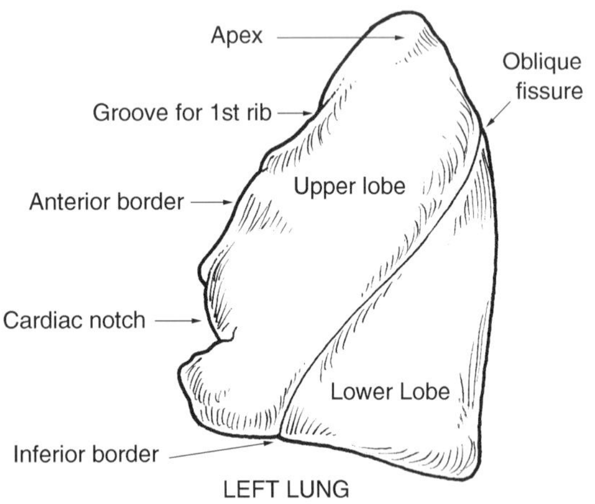


**Figure 4.10b** Left lung: lateral view

## Recommended imaging procedures

Conventional chest radiography is carried out initially when investigating suspected disease or abnormalities of the respiratory system. The type of imaging procedure then selected will depend on the sensitivity of the procedure in detecting the disease process under investigation.

Bronchoscopy with biopsy are used initially to investigate a lung mass seen on a plain film.

Computed tomography has largely replaced bronchography and is used to stage tumours, investigate pleural disease, and is used to delineate interstitial lung disease (with high-resolution CT). CT angiography, made possible with spiral scanning, may be employed to demonstrate the pulmonary arteries for pulmonary embolus and is used as an alternative or to supplement radionuclide imaging.

Bronchography is used only to assess bronchial stenosis and forms part of a bronchoscopy investigation in cases of bronchiectasis in a selected lung area.

Radionuclide imaging is performed using either perfusion lung scanning or ventilation lung scanning, thus enabling functional assessment of the pulmonary vasculature or bronchial tree to be demonstrated in real time. A combination of ventilation and perfusion scanning, commonly known as VQ scintigraphy, is used to diagnose pulmonary embolism.

Angiography is rarely used, but may be employed to detect abnormalities of the pulmonary arteries.

Ultrasound is not used routinely, but does have a place in investigating pleural effusion as it is extremely sensitive in detecting fluid and its application assists in the placement of chest drains when appropriate. It is also used to assess diaphragmatic movement.

Magnetic resonance imaging, at the time of writing, does not offer the same image resolution as that of CT. It is effective, however, at demonstrating soft tissue invasion of a lung tumour affecting the chest wall, spine or brachial plexus and showing mediastinal vessels and blood flow.

Tomography, although allowing imaging in the coronal, sagittal and oblique planes, has limited resolution and has mainly been replaced by CT.

## Indications

Disorders are many and range from those affecting the alveoli, interstitial tissues and rib cage, to those affecting the bronchial tree, mediastinum and lymphatic system.

Abnormalities demonstrated include tumours, bronchiectasis, immunological disorders, the result of infection, complications affecting the vascular supply and those industrial in origin.

# 4 Respiratory System

## Lungs

### Computed tomography – standard chest protocol

Transaxial images of the lungs are routinely obtained with the patient in the supine position. For biopsy of a posterior lesion, however, the patient may be examined prone or lateral with the affected side uppermost.

To reduce radiation dose, the lowest mA and scan time combined with a high kVp technique compatible with acceptable image quality are selected. Images are recorded using an appropriate soft tissue window level and width (50 L, 500 W) and an extended lung tissue window level and width (–700 L, 1000 W).

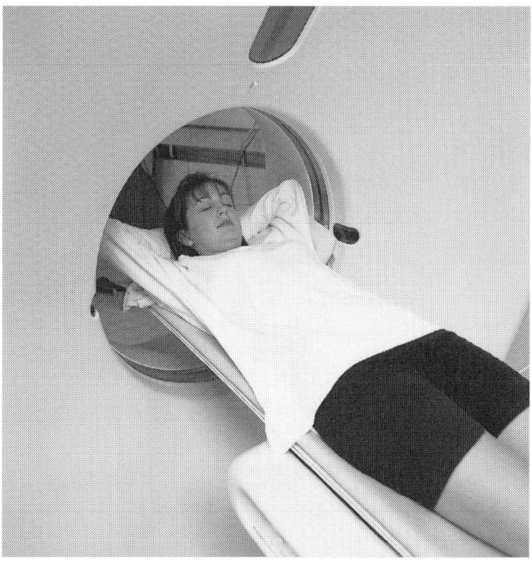

**Figure 4.11a** The CT scanner with patient in position – standard chest protocol

**Indications**

Intrathoracic assessment of benign and malignant tumours of the pleura, lung and mediastinum. Assessment of fluid collections and in interventional procedures as a guide to tissue biopsy and chest drainage.

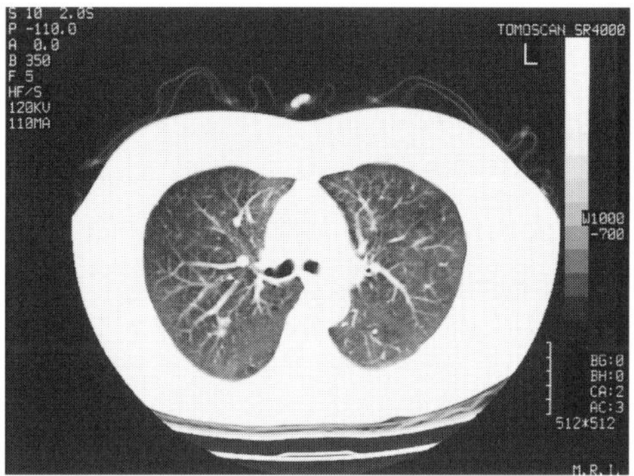


**Figure 4.11b** Transaxial image on soft lung setting

**Position of patient and imaging modality**

The patient lies supine, head first on the scanner table. Arms are raised and placed behind the patient's head, out of the scan plane. Positioning is aided by transaxial, coronal and sagittal alignment lights. The median sagittal plane is perpendicular and the coronal plane is parallel to the scanner table top. The scan plane is perpendicular to the long axis of the body to enable transaxial cross-sectional imaging to be undertaken. The scanner table height is adjusted to ensure that the coronal plane alignment light is at the level of the mid-axillary line. The patient is now moved into the scanner until the scan reference point is at the level of the sternal notch.

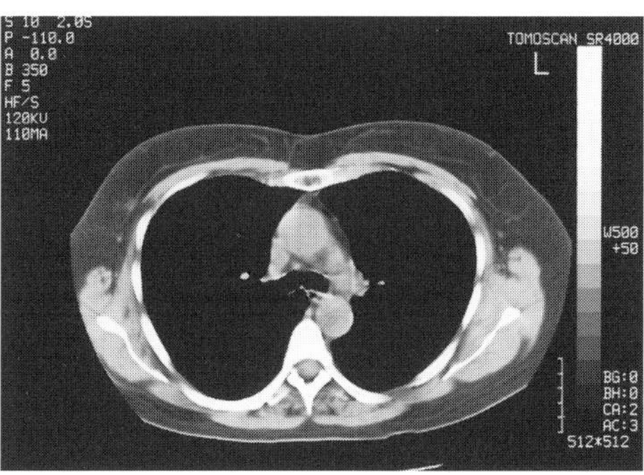


**Figure 4.11c** Transaxial image on soft tissue setting

**Imaging procedure**

A postero-anterior scan projection radiograph is acquired, starting 5 cm above and ending 28 cm below the scan reference point. A postero-anterior projection is selected to reduce the radiation dose to the thymus and breast tissue. From this scan image, 10 mm contiguous sections are prescribed through the lung fields and upper abdomen, starting at the lung apices and ending just below the costophrenic angles. Scans are acquired during arrested inspiration.

In suspected bronchial carcinoma, scanning continues through the adrenal glands to check for metastatic spread.

If volume acquisition is available, scanning of the chest may be performed in two blocks, with each block containing 15 sections, with an acquisition time of approximately 30 s, during which the patient is asked to suspend respiration.

Again a 10 mm slice thickness is selected, with 10 mm table increments, but with a 5 mm reconstruction index to give overlapping sections.

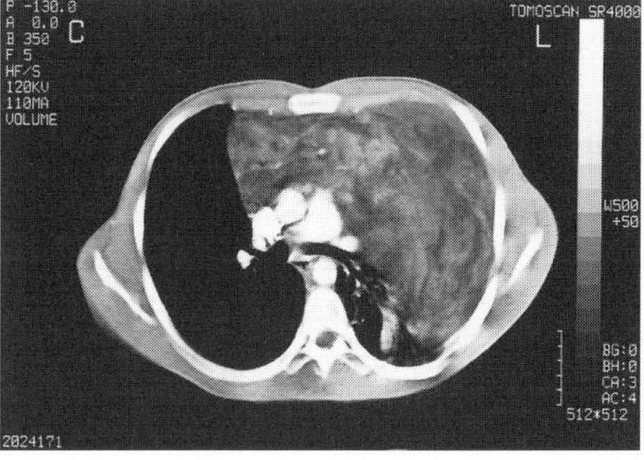


**Figure 4.11d** Image showing tumour on soft tissue setting

## Computed tomography – high-resolution protocol

This technique is used to provide transaxial high-resolution images of the lung parenchyma.

### Indications

Identification and characterisation of diffuse lung disease, assessment and delineation of bronchiectasis and emphysema, pleural disease involving plaques, and characterisation of a focal pulmonary mass.

### Position of patient and imaging modality

Transaxial images of the lungs are obtained with the patient positioned on the scanner table in a similar manner as that for the standard chest protocol.

### Imaging procedure

A postero-anterior scan projection radiograph is performed, starting 5 cm above and terminating 28 cm below the scan reference point. The postero-anterior projection is selected to reduce the radiation dose to the thymus and breast tissue. From the scan image, sections are prescribed through the lung fields using a 1–3 mm slice width and 10–20 mm table increments.

A high spatial resolution algorithm is used and the scan data processed using zoom facilities to define each lung segment further. Scans are routinely taken on suspended inspiration, but in cases of air trapping within the lungs, sections may be repeated on suspended expiration.

Further scans may be necessary in the prone position to redistribute hypostatic changes occurring at the lung bases.

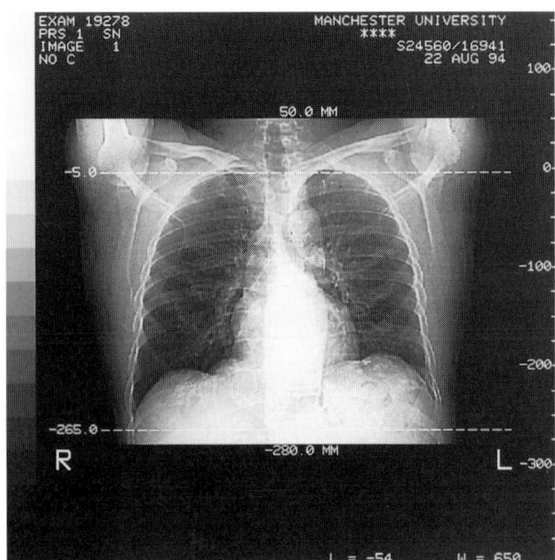


**Figure 4.12a** Scan projection radiograph showing start and end locations

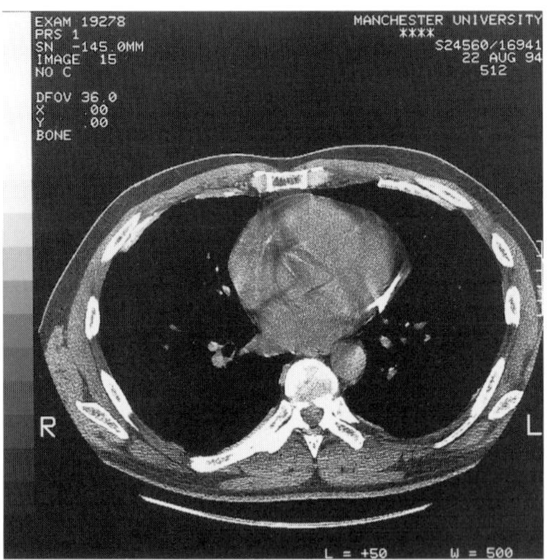


**Figure 4.12b** Transaxial CT section using soft tissue setting

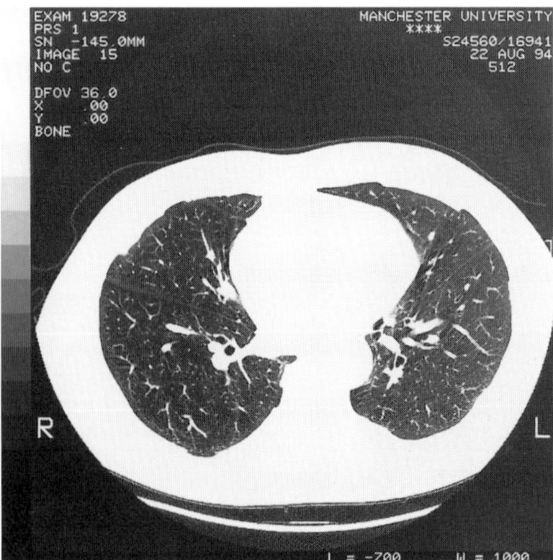


**Figure 4.12c** Transaxial CT section using lung tissue setting (NB patient supine)

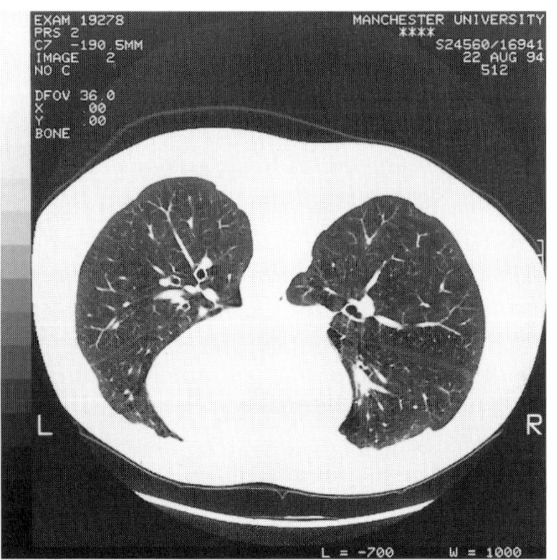


**Figure 4.12d** Transaxial CT section using lung tissue setting (NB patient prone)

# 4 Respiratory System

## Lungs

### Computed tomography – mediastinum

Transaxial images of the mediastinum are routinely obtained in the supine position. Contrast enhanced scans using a non-ionic contrast medium may be necessary to evaluate any lesion and to assess spread of disease.

**Indications**

To assess the extent and position of a mediastinal lesion identified on a chest radiograph. To assess the spread of disease into the mediastinal lymph nodes.

**Position of patient and imaging modality**

The patient lies supine, head first on the scanner table, and is positioned in a similar way to that described for the standard chest protocol on page 124.

**Imaging procedure**

A postero-anterior scan projection radiograph is acquired, starting 5 cm above and ending 25 cm below the scan reference point. A postero-anterior projection is selected to reduce the radiation dose to the thyroid gland and breast tissue. From this scan image, 10 mm contiguous sections are prescribed to cover the full extent of the mediastinum. Scans are acquired during arrested inspiration.

These pre-contrast images are reviewed, following which a selected region may be rescanned during the infusion of a non-ionic contrast medium using the same imaging protocol.

If spiral scanning options are available, these images may be acquired with a volume acquisition, using a 10 mm slice thickness and 10 mm table increments, but with a 5 mm reconstruction index to give overlapping sections.

### Computed tomography angiography

Computed tomography angiography, using CT volume acquisition, is employed to look at the pulmonary arteries for pulmonary embolus when VQ radionuclide imaging is unequivocal.

**Imaging procedure**

The procedure is similar to that described for the standard chest protocol on page 124. Standard pre-contrast images are first acquired to ensure there are no undetected lesions. Contrast enhanced images, using volume acquisition, are now obtained from the mid-atrium to the aortic arch.

A non-ionic contrast agent, 150 ml (180–200 mgI/ml) is injected at the rate of 5 ml/s through a 19–20 gauge venous cannula. Scanning commences 10 s after the start of the injection. By scanning in reverse order (i.e. cranially), streak artefacts from the contrast medium in the inferior vena cava may be minimised.

Images are acquired using a 5 mm slice thickness, with 5 mm table increments and a 3 mm reconstruction index.

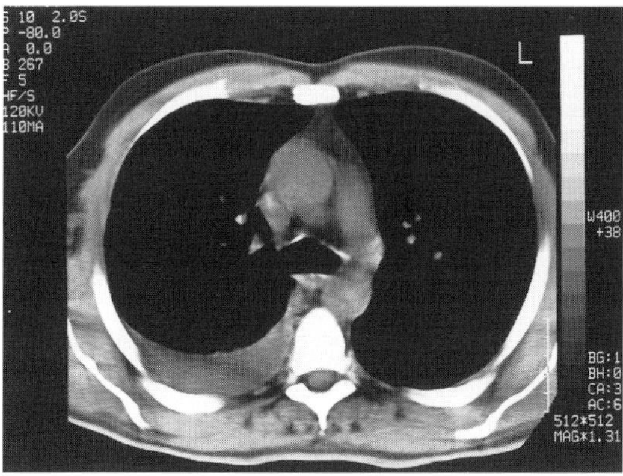


**Figure 4.13a** Pre-contrast section through the mediastinum

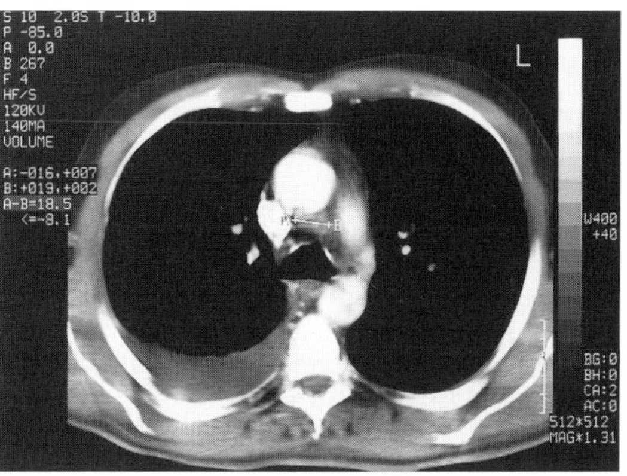


**Figure 4.13b** Post-contrast section through the mediastinum showing contrast enhancement of the ascending and descending aorta and a large non-enhanced mediastinum lymph node (measuring 18.5 mm)

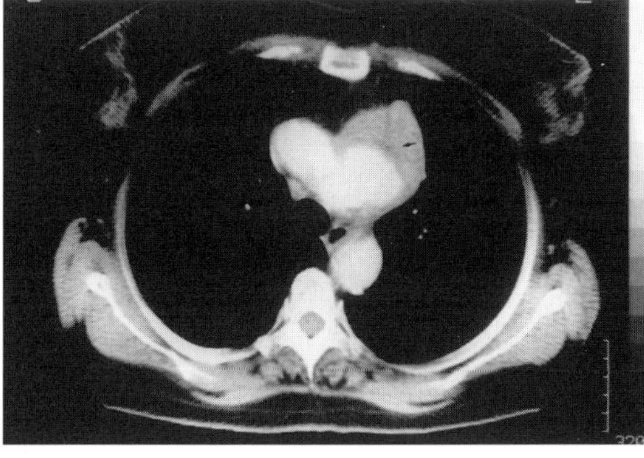

**Figure 4.13c** Contrast enhanced CT section demonstrating a large tumour

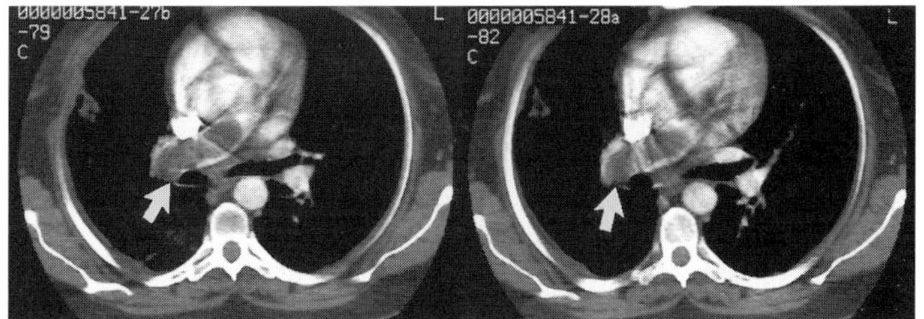

**Figure 4.13d** Post-contrast enhanced transaxial images showing thrombus in the right pulmonary artery

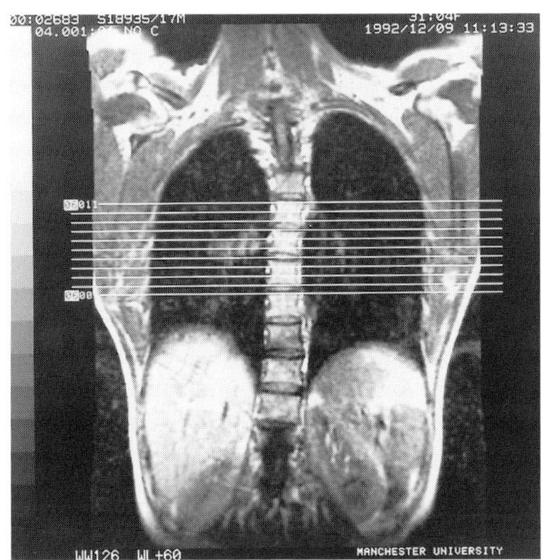


**Figure 4.14a** Coronal localiser image showing the prescribed positions for transaxial images

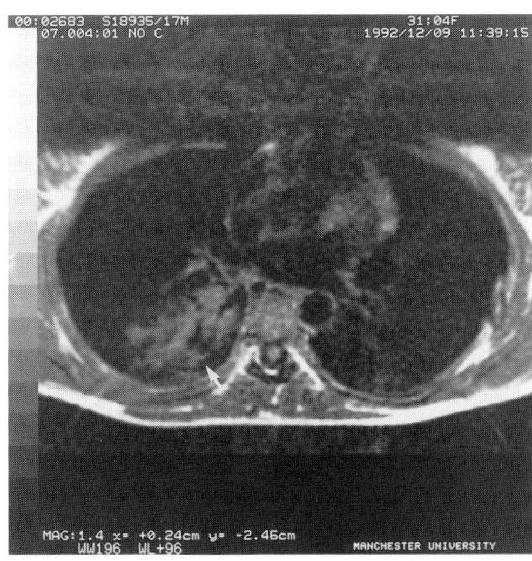


**Figure 4.14b** Transaxial $T_1$ section through a lung lesion

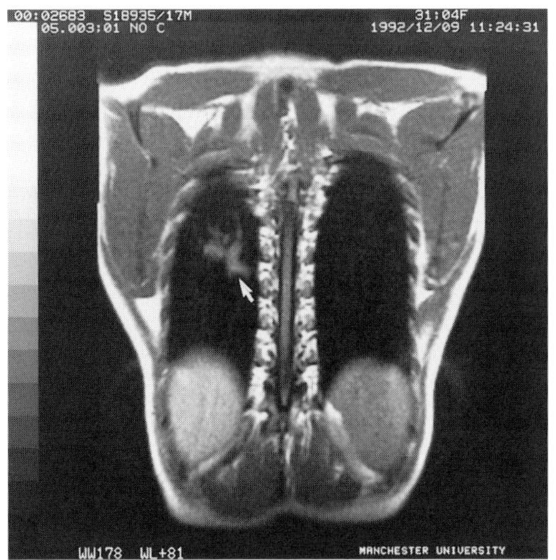


**Figure 4.14c** Further coronal $T_1$ image showing the extent of the lesion shown on the $T_1$ image above

## Magnetic resonance imaging

At the time of writing, MRI has not been fully developed to demonstrate the lung parenchyma in as fine detail as that obtained using CT. It does, however, have a place when lung tumours have been diagnosed in determining if there is any soft tissue invasion of the tumour affecting the chest wall, spine or brachial plexus.

$T_1$ weighted spin-echo pulse sequences with cardiac gating, to improve image quality, are used initially to demonstrate anatomy and pathology. Respiratory artefacts may be overcome by using respiratory ordered phase encoding (ROPE) compensation.

Cine flow-enhanced sequences with gating and breath holding may also be performed to determine any arterial involvement.

### Position of patient and imaging modality

The patient lies supine, head first on the scanner table, and if necessary the cardiac gating facility is applied. The median sagittal plane is perpendicular to the centre of the table and coincident with the sagittal alignment light, and the table is moved until the transaxial alignment light is at the level of the manubrium. From this position the patient is moved the fixed distance to the isocentre of the radiofrequency receiver/transmitter coil.

### Imaging procedure

Initially a series of $T_1$ weighted coronal localiser scans, using thick slices and large gaps, are performed to obtain reference points for image acquisition in the transaxial plane.

$T_1$ weighted spin-echo transaxial sections of the tumour and surrounding tissue are prescribed, employing a slice thickness of 5–10 mm with a gap of 2 mm. Coronal sections may also be obtained to assess craniocaudal extension followed by sagittal sections to obtain anteroposterior extension of a tumour. A STIR sequence which suppresses fat may be employed to reduce the artefact caused by respiratory motion of chest wall fat.

A $T_2$ weighted spin-echo sequence may also be used for mediastinal involvement.

To eliminate arterial involvement, a gated cine acquisition or flow-sensitive breath-hold sequence in the relevant plane is used to show blood flow through a vessel.

# 4 Respiratory System

## Lungs

### Radionuclide imaging

Two distinct types of radionuclide imaging procedures are employed in investigating defects of the pulmonary vascular supply and the lung air passages.

Perfusion lung scanning enables the pulmonary blood flow in the lungs to be investigated. This involves the use of a suspension containing a radionuclide such as $^{99m}$Tc labelled with aggregates of human serum albumin (HSA) ranging from 10 to 100 $\mu$m in size. After an intravenous injection, these minute particles are carried in the venous blood to the right side of the heart where they are pumped via the pulmonary artery and its branches to both lungs and the capillaries. The size, shape and number of these particles are important. The size of each particle should be just slightly larger than the size of a capillary in the lungs, where it will be trapped due to the physical size and shape of the capillary. The adult dose injected should also contain approximately 500 000 particles which will ensure that 1 in 1000 capillaries will be physically blocked. This combination of conditions will result in both lungs being visualised as a function of the blood supply. Any obstruction to the blood supply will be demonstrated as an area of inactivity.

Lung ventilation scanning, however, enables the air-expanded passages and spaces of both lungs to be demonstrated. A suitable radioactive gas, e.g. $^{81m}$Kr, is inhaled by the patient prior to or during the procedure, with the result that images of the lung fields are obtained. The radioactive gas should have a relatively short half-life, as the radiation dose must be low to both the patient and staff. The gas should not be absorbed into the tissues which if it occurs reduces the true ventilated volume. Ideally, the gamma energy of this nuclide should be greater than the gamma energy of the nuclide used for lung perfusion studies. As a perfusion study usually precedes a ventilation study as part of a combined investigation, it is important that ventilation images are free from contamination by scattered radiation from the material used for the perfusion images. This can only be achieved if the gamma energy of the nuclide is higher than $^{99m}$Tc, i.e. $^{81m}$Kr.

These procedures are usually combined when investigating perfusion and ventilation defects. A normal lung is void of any image defects on either set of scans. However, a ventilation (V)/perfusion (Q) mismatch is indicative of an abnormality in the vascular supply or air passages and is characterised by lung image defects on either the perfusion or ventilation scans. Matched defects occur in various conditions and do not indicate pulmonary embolism.

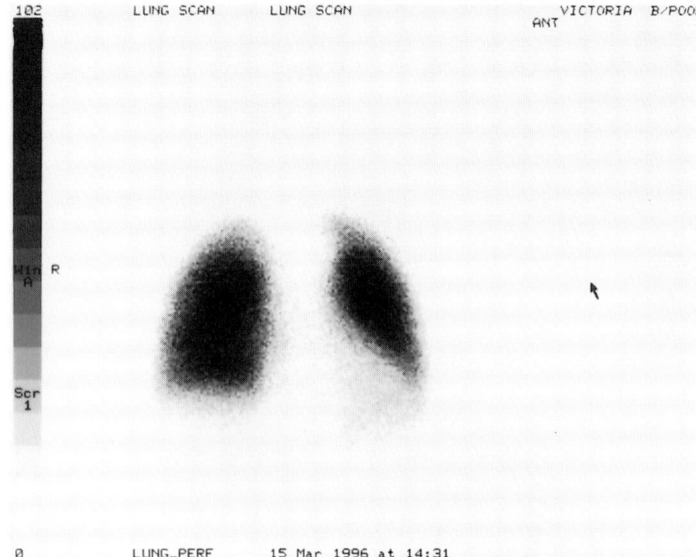


**Figure 4.15a** Image of perfusion lung scan (anterior view)

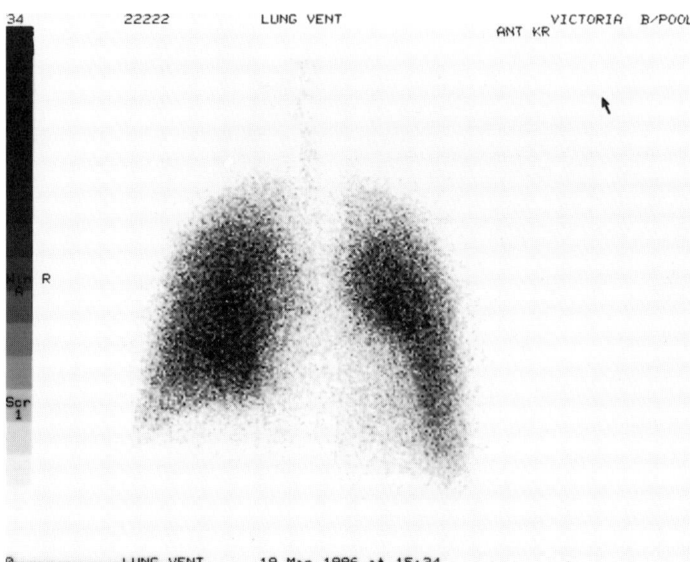


**Figure 4.15b** Image of ventilation lung scan (anterior view)

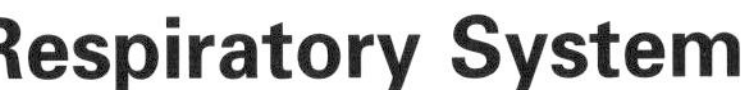



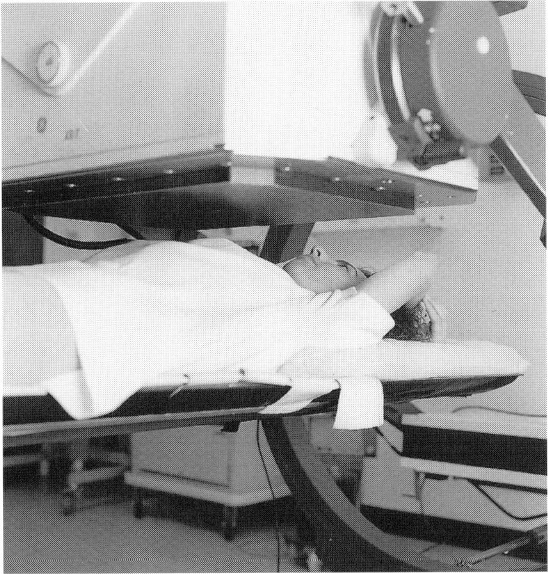

**Figure 4.16a** Patient in position for anterior view

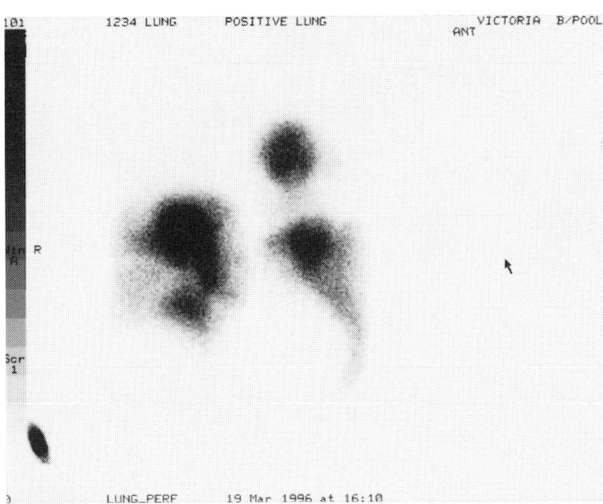



**Figure 4.16b** Anterior view image showing large lung defects

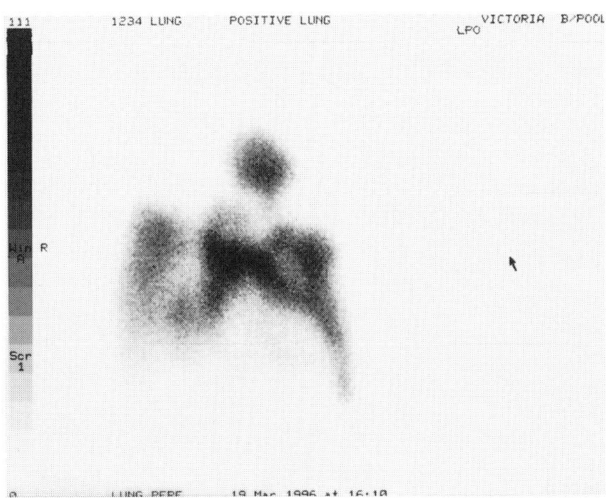



**Figure 4.16c** Left posterior view image showing large lung defects

## Radionuclide imaging – perfusion studies

A low-energy general-purpose collimator is selected. Patient preparation consists of the removal of artefacts from the chest area and a full explanation of the procedure. A radiopharmaceutical such as $^{99m}$Tc pulmonate is prepared for i.v. injection.

**Indications**

Pulmonary embolism (PE) may be confirmed by V/Q mismatch, with an embolic area seen as an area of decreased intensity in the perfusion image. When ventilation scans are not possible, a normal chest radiograph and persistent symptoms will also be strongly suggestive of PE.

**Position of patient and imaging modality**

The patient is less likely to move position if examined supine. This is an important consideration if the procedure is combined with ventilation studies, when an exact match of both sets of images is a requirement. The imaging protocol consists of six static views taken in the following order: posterior, left posterior oblique, left anterior oblique, anterior, right anterior oblique and right posterior oblique.

For the posterior view the camera is positioned below and parallel to the patient and as close to the imaging couch as reasonably possible. From this position the camera is rotated around the patient for each of the other views. For the oblique views the camera is angled 45° relative to the sagittal plane, with the arm of the side being examined raised above or below the chest during the procedure.

**Imaging procedure**

With the patient positioned comfortably and the camera in the operative mode, the radiopharmaceutical is injected into an antecubital vein. It may be helpful to raise the patient's arm after the injection to ensure that the isotope moves quickly to the lungs. Once the operator is satisfied that the isotope has reached the lungs, the imaging sequence is initiated. All six views are acquired in sequence and stored by the system for display at a later time. For the posterior oblique views the imaging couch arm rests should be removed to avoid artefacts.

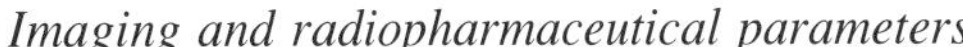

*Imaging and radiopharmaceutical parameters*

| *Type* | *Administered activity* | *Principal energy* |
|---|---|---|
| $^{99m}$Tc pulmonate | 75 MBq | 140 keV |
| *Window width* | *Acquisition counts/time* | |
| 20% | 500 K counts/view | |

## Radionuclide imaging – ventilation studies

Lung ventilation studies are normally combined with lung perfusion studies to distinguish between pathology associated with the pulmonary vascular supply and that involving the lung air passages. The procedure described below assumes the same positioning criteria as that described on the previous page, with the acquisition of the same static images, but in this case the images are acquired in reverse order. The procedure, however, can also be carried out as a separate examination, in which case the patient may be examined erect. A dynamic inhalation study can also be performed as a separate procedure which enables a comparative quantitative analysis of both lungs to be produced in graphical form.

A radioactive gas such as $^{81m}$Kr, with a half-life of 13 s, and therefore demonstrating only the wash-in phase of the respiration process, is used for the procedure. Alternatively, $^{133}$Xe or technegas, an ultra-fine dispersion of technetium-labelled carbon, may be used for the procedure.

A low-energy general-purpose collimator is selected and the patient preparation consists of the removal of artefacts from the chest area, with a full explanation of the procedure.

### Indications

Obstructive lung disease by means of mismatched ventilation defects when combined with perfusion studies. It can also be employed in case of abnormal air cysts to demonstrate the presence of any bronchial communication.

### Position of patient and imaging modality

As this procedure, in the majority of cases, normally follows a perfusion study, the patient will already be in the supine position on the imaging couch. The imaging protocol will consist of the same static views as that prescribed for the perfusion studies described on the preceding page: posterior, LPO, LAO, anterior, RAO and RPO; however, the acquisition will start with the RPO, the final view in the perfusion series, and terminate with posterior view, the first in the perfusion series. This will ensure an almost exact match of the images taken during perfusion and ventilation which will assist in identifying the presence of any mismatch in radioactivity.

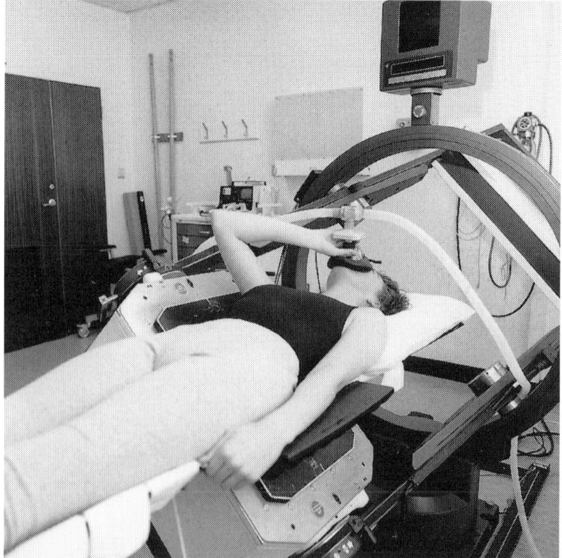

**Figure 4.17a** Patient positioned for right posterior oblique view

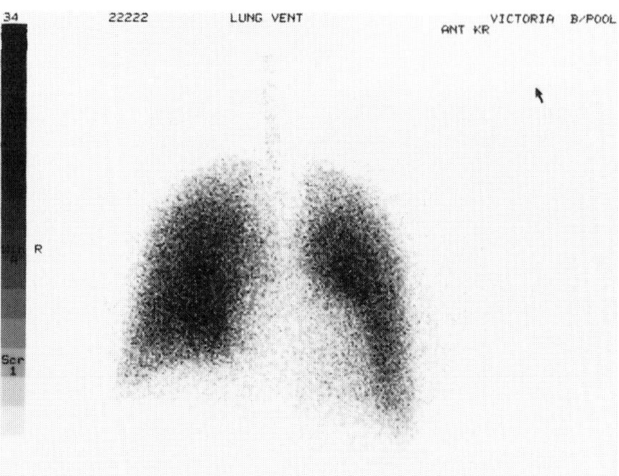


**Figure 4.17b** Normal anterior view image using krypton gas

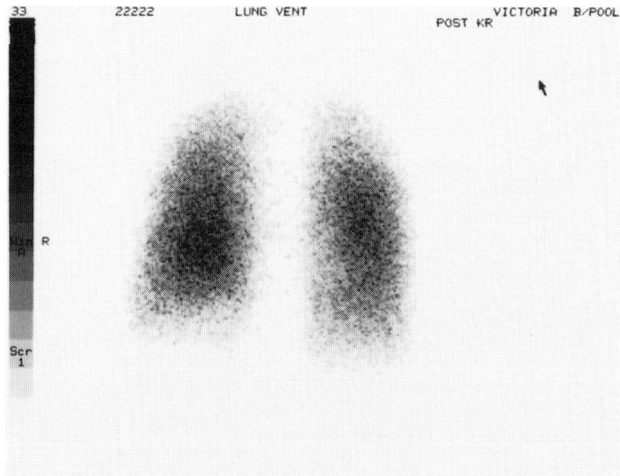


**Figure 4.17c** Normal posterior view image using krypton gas

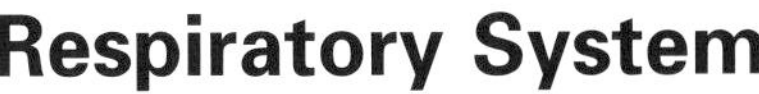


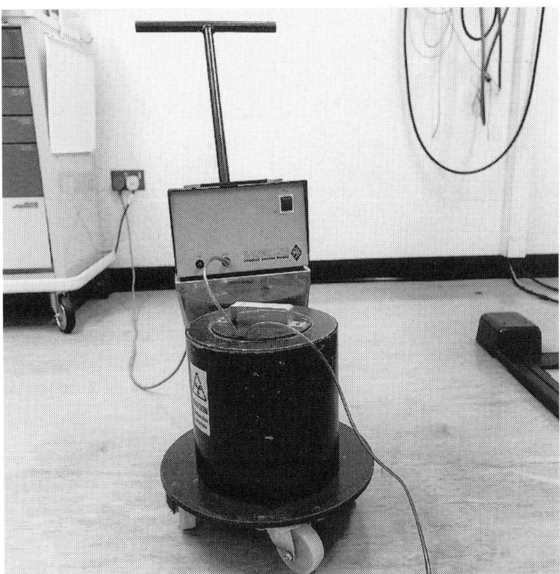
Figure 4.18a Krypton generator

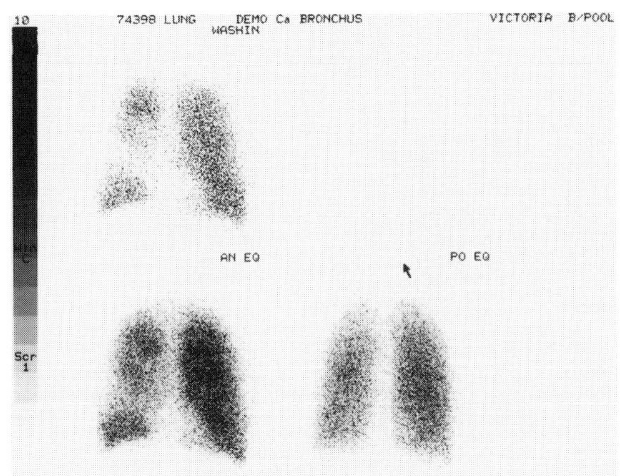

**Figure 4.18b** Selection of wash-in images, using xenon gas, showing a large filling defect from a Ca bronchus

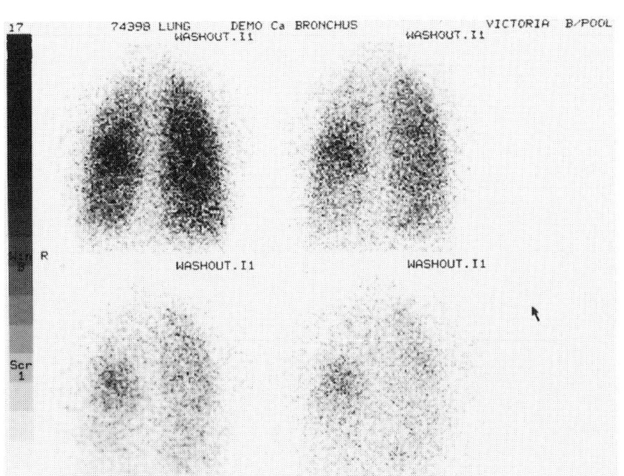

**Figure 4.18c** Selection of wash-out images, using xenon gas, showing trapped gas as a result of a Ca bronchus

The $^{81m}$Kr gas generator is positioned near the imaging couch and its inlet is connected via a thin-bore tube to a compressed air supply using a cylinder, wall supply or pump, a pressure-reducing valve, flowmeter and humidifier. A length of thin tubing is connected to the generator outlet which in turn is connected to a reservoir system consisting of a combination of two 1 m lengths of 'elephant' tubing, fitted either side of an anaesthetic face mask and a low-resistance one-way valve. The tubing from the generator is connected close to the valve inlet by connecting it to a wide-bore needle and pushing this into the elephant tubing near the valve, or alternatively feeding the fine tubing inside the elephant tubing and stopping just prior to the inlet valve.

**Imaging procedure**

Just before imaging commences, the air supply is turned on and the patient is asked to breathe normally through the face mask which must be airtight to the face. The inlet tube is allowed to fill continuously from the generator at 1 litre/min, and as this happens with each inspiration the patient will inhale a mixture of krypton and air, pulling air in from the elephant tube.

Acquisition of the first static image commences immediately and when complete the air supply to the generator is turned off until the gamma camera has been positioned for the next view.

The expired air will still be radioactive, but will be contained in the outlet tube which should be vented away from the operators and the gamma camera. However, with the half-life of krypton being only 13 s, no special disposal arrangements of the gas or tubing are required.

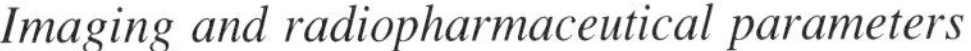

*Imaging and radiopharmaceutical parameters*

| *Type* | *Administered activity* | *Principal energy* |
|---|---|---|
| $^{81m}$Kr gas | 370 MBq/min at 1 litre/min | 191 keV |
| *Window width* | *Acquisition counts/time* | |
| 20% | 200 K counts | |

# 4 Respiratory System

## Lungs

### Radionuclide imaging – pulmonary disease

Static imaging using $^{67}Ga$ is commonly used to determine activity of lung disease. The procedure is particularly useful in distinguishing whether disease scarring visualised in a recent chest radiograph is active or not. For instance, in cases involving sarcoidosis the patient's lungs will remain permanently scarred, but by using this technique the gallium will concentrate in an active lesion and allow this activity to be marked by the gamma camera. The procedure is also used for monitoring other non-infective disease such as fibrosing alveolitis and infective *Pneumocystis carinii*.

A medium-energy high-resolution collimator is selected for maximum resolution.

#### Imaging procedure

Imaging of the lungs is performed at 48 and 72 h after the patient has been injected with the radiopharmaceutical. The patient lies supine on the imaging couch with the camera positioned parallel to the couch first above and then below, to enable anterior and posterior views of the lung fields to be obtained. When investigating for sarcoidosis, the patient is positioned to include the salivary glands in the field of view.

In the case of active disease, areas of increased radioactivity will be acquired by the gamma camera which will be set at three different photopeaks. Permanent images of these lesions will be made onto hard copy film.

*Imaging and radiopharmaceutical parameters*

| *Type* | *Administered activity* | *Principal energies* |
|---|---|---|
| $^{67}Ga$ | 80 MBq | 93 keV, 185 keV, 300 keV |

| *Window widths* | *Acquisition counts/time* |
|---|---|
| 25%, 20%, 20% | 500 K counts |

Images acquired at the three photopeaks simultaneously to achieve 500K total counts.

*Contrast medium and injection data*

| *Volume* | *Concentration* | *Flow rate* |
|---|---|---|
| 40 ml | 350 mgI/ml | 20 ml/s |

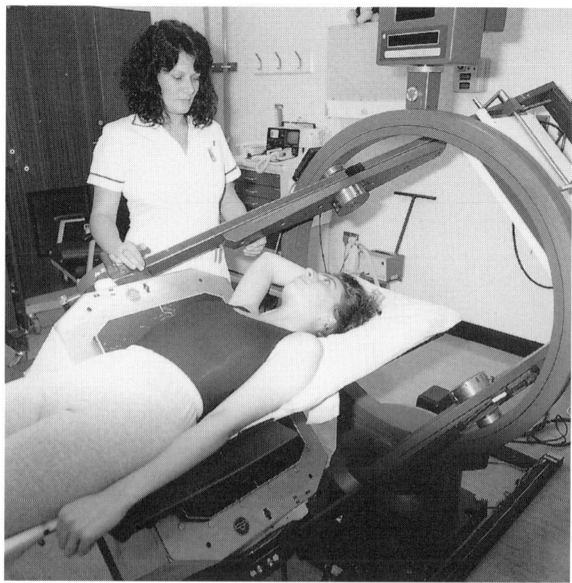

**Figure 4.19a** Patient positioned for right posterior oblique image

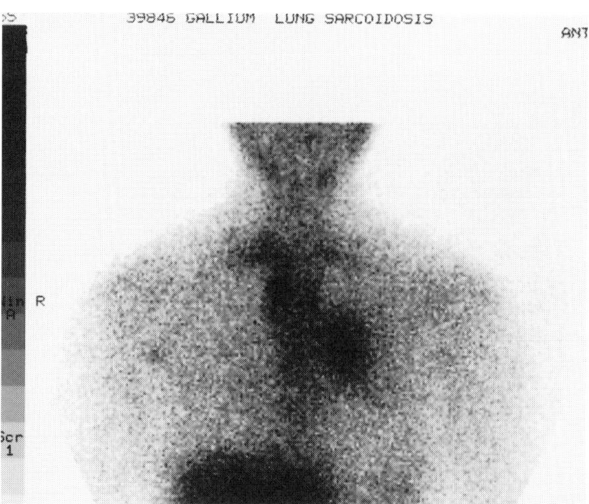


**Figure 4.19b** Anterior gallium scan image taken at 48 h post-injection, demonstrating active sarcoid disease in the left hilar area

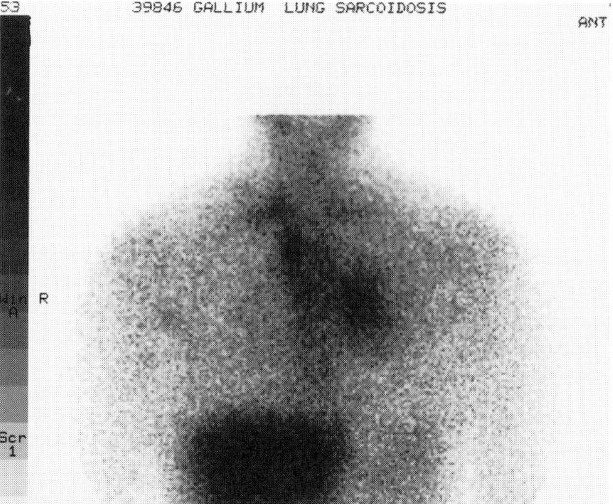


**Figure 4.19c** Anterior gallium scan, of the same patient, taken at 72 h post-injection, confirming lung sarcoidosis

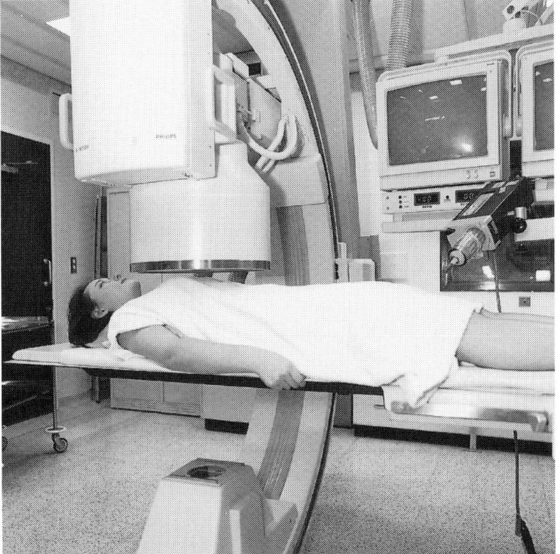

Figure 4.20a Position of equipment and patient for postero-anterior projection

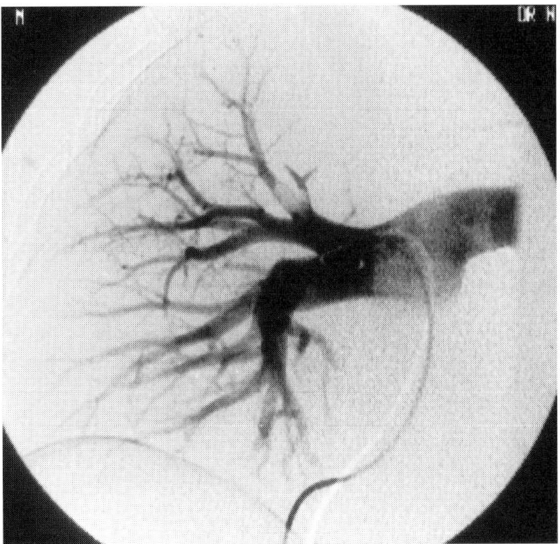

Figure 4.20b Postero-anterior image of the right lung

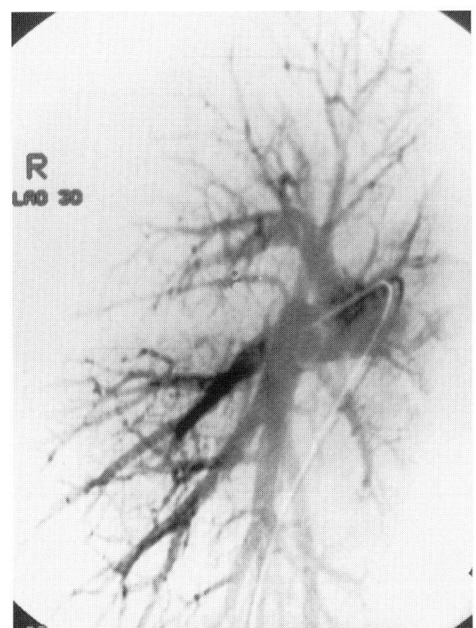


Figure 4.20c 30° left anterior oblique image of the right lung

## Angiography

Pulmonary angiography, the investigation of the vascular supply to the lungs is an established procedure but has been replaced by non-invasive radionuclide perfusion lung scanning. When employed, it requires specialised angiographic equipment similar to that used for cardiovascular procedures, but instead of a small field image intensifier it requires an intensifier large enough to include the thorax. Image acquisition is by means of either digital subtraction angiography, 35 × 35 cm rapid film changer or cine fluorography.

Bi-plane equipment allows simultaneous acquisition of postero-anterior and lateral images of the main stem vessel which is seen superimposed with other vessels in the postero-anterior projection. When a single plane C-arm is employed, a second injection is therefore necessary to image the main stem vessel.

The right side of the heart is normally approached via catheterisation of an antecubital or femoral vein. A 6 or 7F NIH or Berman balloon catheter is selected and positioned in the right ventricle under fluoroscopic control.

Contrast is delivered by means of a pressure injector.

During the investigation the patient's ECG and blood pressure is monitored continuously.

### Indications

Abnormalities of the pulmonary arteries, pulmonary artery hypertension and confirmation of the location of a pulmonary embolism prior to surgery.

### Position of the patient and imaging modality

Postero-anterior projections of the thorax are taken with the patient supine and the image intensifier/film changer parallel to the imaging couch. Lateral images are acquired with the intensifier parallel to the sagittal plane to show the main stem vessel in the lateral plane. Anterior oblique images of either lung are acquired by rotating the X-ray tube towards the side under investigation.

### Imaging procedure

The tip of the NIH catheter is positioned in the main pulmonary artery or its major branches or alternatively a Berman balloon catheter is located in the right ventricle. A bolus of contrast is injected using a pressure injector, following which images are acquired during arrested respiration.

*Imaging parameters*

| *Images/s* | *Run time* | *Total images* |
|---|---|---|
| 2 | 10 s | 20 |

*Cine radiography*
50 frames/s for approximately 8 s.

## Lungs

### Ultrasound

Routine examination of the lung fields using diagnostic ultrasound is ruled out because ultrasound will not penetrate air-containing structures. When fluid or a mass occupies the pleura, however, ultrasound can be useful in detecting pathology. A combination of sector and linear scanning is employed, with either a 3.5 or 5 MHz transducer to provide both good penetration and good resolution. The sector transducer is used for access between the ribs, while the linear transducer allows both diaphragm and effusion to be viewed simultaneously. A recent chest radiograph will provide a guide when locating a pleural effusion.

**Indications**

Pleural effusion and pleural masses. To distinguish between a mass or fluid, as a loculated fluid pocket can be mistaken for a mass on a chest radiograph. The assessment of diaphragmatic movement (having the advantage that ionising radiation is not employed). The placement of pleural drains, in which case ultrasound is used to identify the appropriate entry point on the skin surface for the placement of the drain. As a guide to tissue biopsy.

**Position of patient and imaging modality**

The patient is positioned so that the pathology site is easily accessible and that the patient is comfortable enough not to move during the procedure. The patient is erect or seated on a stool without a back, thus affording ready access from all sides. As pleural effusions usually pool above the diaphragm in the pleural recess, which descends much further posteriorly than anteriorly, pleural effusions are often better viewed using a posterior approach. The transducer is applied directly to the area under investigation.

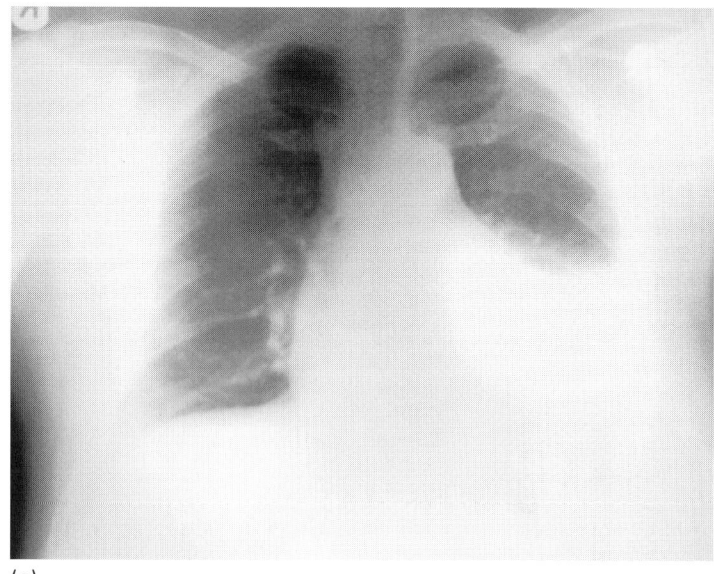

(a)

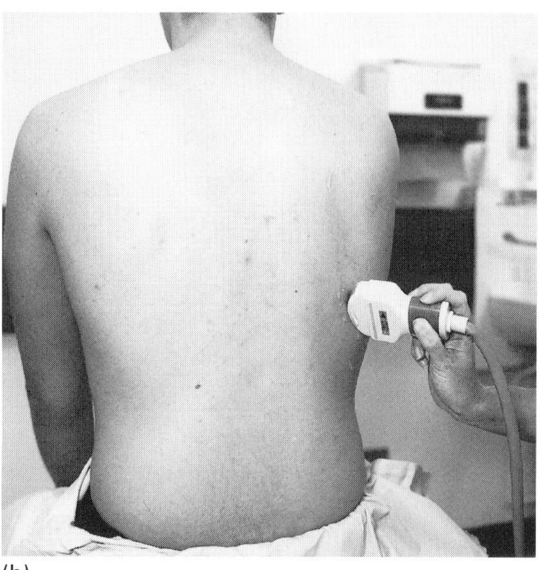

(b)

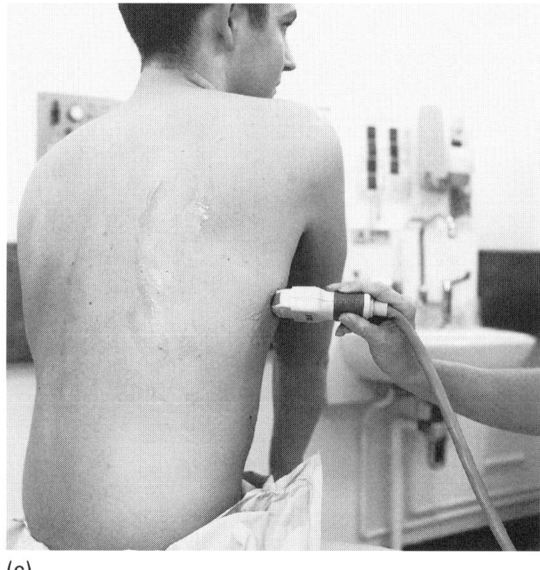

(c)

**Figure 4.21** (a) Chest radiograph showing pleural effusion; (b,c) positioning of ultrasound transducer

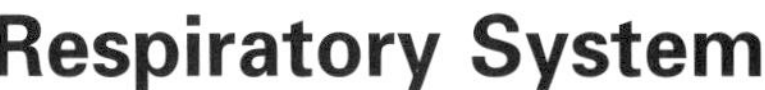


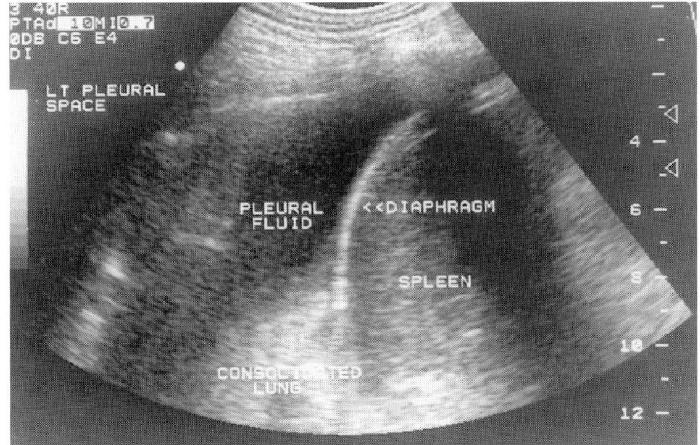


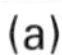
(a)

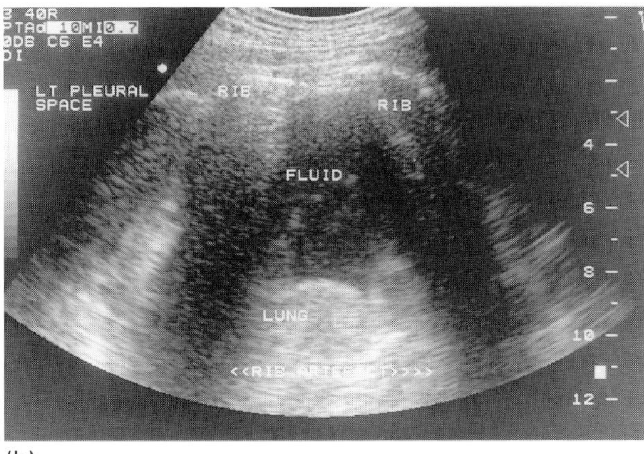

(b)

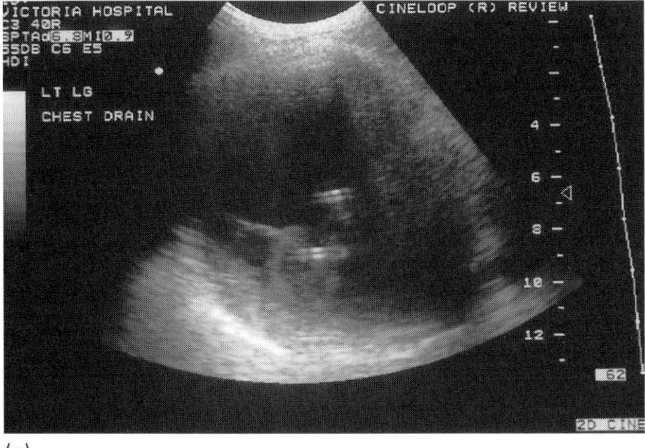


(c)

**Figure 4.22a–c** A series of ultrasound images of the left lung: (a,b) a pleural effusion; (c) a chest drain *in situ* (see chest radiograph opposite)

**Imaging procedure**

A recent chest radiograph is examined before the procedure to aid in the localisation of pathology.

When investigating pleural effusions it is usual to commence scanning with the sector transducer which provides a good lateral field of view with a small point of contact, making it ideal for intercostal scanning. With the patient erect, the transducer is held against the posterior aspect of the thorax near the midline at the intercostal space corresponding with the lower lobe and diaphragm. The transducer is moved along the intercostal space so that the pleura is examined from the posterior and lateral aspects. The transducer is moved higher to the next intercostal space, with the process repeated to trace the superior extent of an effusion or other pathology. During this procedure the patient is examined using arrested respiration following deep inspiration.

In order to assess the position of an effusion fully, the diaphragm must be demonstrated. Using a linear array probe, both the diaphragm and the effusion are viewed simultaneously.

The right dome and lung basal region are examined, with the right lobe of the liver used as an acoustic window. The left lung basal region is examined using the spleen as an acoustic window. For this procedure the transducer is positioned on the anterior abdominal wall just below the costal cartilages and rib cage on either side of the trunk. Multiple views are obtained using a combination of transverse, parasagittal and oblique sections, with the transducer angled cranially. The lungs are effectively examined using arrested respiration following deep inspiration.

When diaphragmatic movement is being assessed, the patient will be asked to take deep breaths, during which the extent of movement will be assessed visually on the ultrasound monitor.

## Bronchography

Bronchography is achieved by outlining part of the bronchial tree with a suitable contrast agent which ideally should be isotonic, cause no reaction to the lung tissues and be readily removed from the lungs.

This procedure was a common examination for many years for investigating abnormalities associated with the bronchi. However, modern bronchoscopy equipment, with the use of flexible fibreoptic endoscopes and the availability of CT, has made this procedure virtually redundant. Its role now is limited, when used with bronchoscopy, to assess a specific lung segment where the contrast agent used is confined to an isolated area of lung tissue.

For this procedure the patient is prepared as for bronchoscopy and the examination is performed on a conventional fluoroscopy couch. Because of the rapid flow of the contrast agent, image acquisition is by means of 100 mm film camera or digital imaging using a rapid exposure sequence.

### Indications

Bronchial stenosis and bronchiectasis in a specific lung segment.

### Imaging procedure

The bronchoscopy examination is carried out initially on the imaging couch, with the image intensifier positioned so that it does not obstruct the procedure. When the fibreoptic scope has been directed to the lung segment under investigation, the image intensifier is positioned over the thorax. Contrast is then delivered through the endoscope under fluoroscopic control and images are acquired immediately of the contrast-coated bronchi. The patient is positioned to allow postero-anterior, lateral or oblique projections of the lung segment or lobe under examination. After the procedure, suction is used via the bronchoscope to remove any contrast.

*Contrast medium and injection data*

| *Volume* | *Concentration* | *Flow rate* |
|---|---|---|
| 2–3 ml | 300 mg/ml | Hand injection |

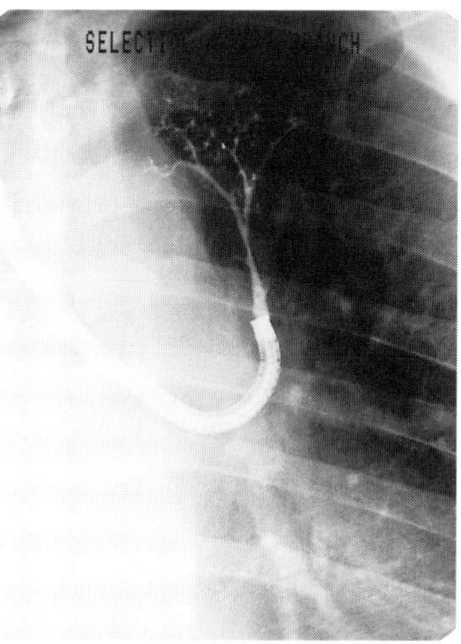

**Figure 4.23a** Image showing selective filling of the apical branch of the left lung

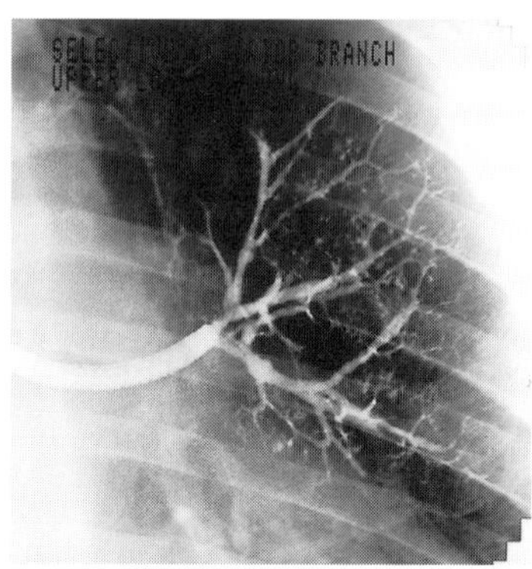

**Figure 4.23b** Image showing selective filling of the anterior branch of the upper lobe of the left lung

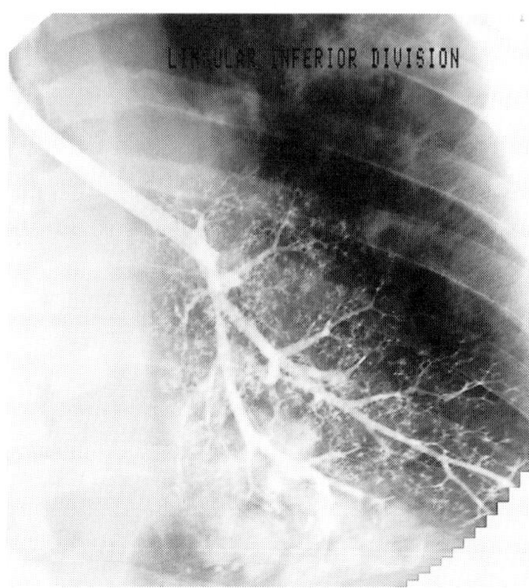

**Figure 4.23c** Image showing selective filling of the lingular inferior division of the left lung

# 5

# Alimentary System

## CONTENTS

# 5 Alimentary System

## Salivary Glands

There are three pairs of salivary glands: the parotid glands, the submandibular glands and the sublingual glands. They are situated adjacent to the oral cavity and secrete saliva, which contains a digestive enzyme called ptyalase, to aid digestion.

The parotid glands are the largest of the salivary glands and lie just below the zygomatic arch in front of, and below, the ear. The parotid duct (Stenson's duct) is about 5 cm in length and runs forwards over the masseter muscle opening on the surface of a small papilla on the inner surface of the cheek, opposite the second upper molar tooth.

The submandibular glands are paired and lie on either side of the neck, forming part of the soft tissues on the medial margin of the mandible, between the body of the mandible and the hyoid bone. The submandibular duct (Wharton's duct) is about 5 cm in length and runs forward, medially and upwards, beneath the mucous membrane of the floor of the mouth and opens at a small papilla at the base of the frenulum of the tongue.

The two sublingual glands are the smallest of the salivary glands and lie on the anterior part of the floor of the mouth, on the surface of the mylohyoid muscle. The glands secrete directly into the oral cavity through multiple ducts (ducts of Rivinus) which may open adjacent to the frenulum of the tongue, or may join to form a single duct (Bartholin's duct) which empties into the submandibular duct.

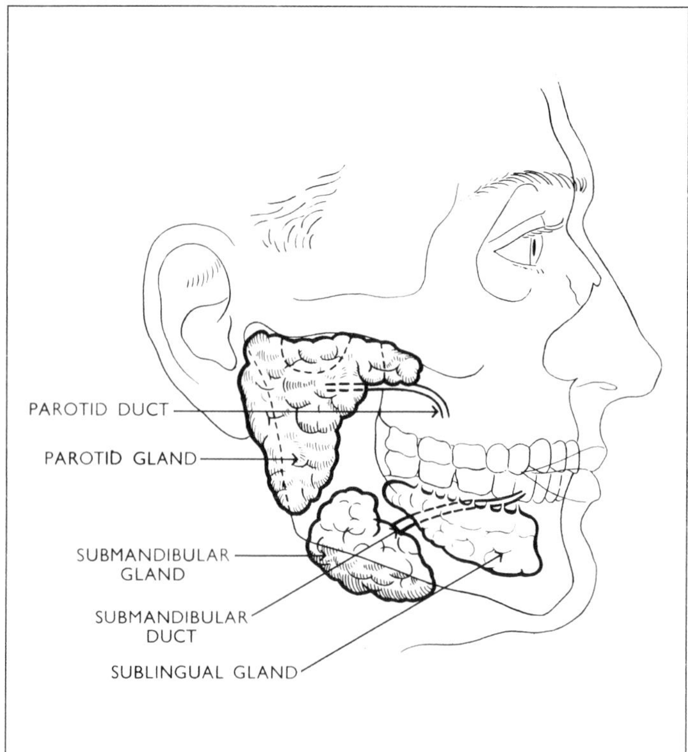


**Figure 5.1** Salivary glands and ducts – lateral aspect

### Recommended imaging procedures

Following plain radiography, similar to that for the mandible, the most common method used to investigate the parotid and submandibular glands is sialography. Computed tomography is used in cases of glandular enlargement and in the evaluation of parotid and submandibular tumours. Radionuclide imaging is employed to provide additional physiological information in cases of over- and under-secretion of saliva.

### Sialography

Sialography is the radiographic examination of the parotid and submandibular salivary glands and their ducts following the introduction of a contrast agent. The anatomy of the ducts from the sublingual glands, however, makes the investigation of these glands impossible.

It can be performed using conventional, an isocentric skull unit or orthopantomographic equipment or alternatively with the aid of fluoroscopic equipment. Prior to the procedure, plain standard films of the glands should be available.

#### Indications

It is performed in cases of pain, recurrent salivary gland enlargement, duct obstruction and changes secondary to trauma, or when plain radiography has failed to demonstrate conclusively the underlying cause of the patient's condition.

#### Contraindications

Sialography is contraindicated in cases of acute inflammation.

#### Imaging procedure

Control films, using standard projections with conventional equipment, are taken prior to commencement.

Both conventional and digital fluoroscopy imaging techniques using an overcouch tube are described for sialography.

The duct orifice is sprayed with a topical anaesthetic. If the duct is difficult to locate, the patient may be given citric acid (or a slice of lemon or lime to suck). This stimulates secretion of saliva and makes the orifice visible. A salivary duct dilator may be necessary prior to insertion of the cannula or sialography catheter. If a catheter is used it can be left in situ until the examination is complete.

Either an oil-based or a water-soluble iodinated contrast agent (240 mgI/ml concentration) can be used. The contrast is injected manually until the patient complains of discomfort. The precise quantity necessary to fill a particular duct may vary between 1 and 2 ml.

Images are acquired immediately after the injection is complete.

After the prescribed views are completed the patient may be given citric acid and delayed images acquired after 5 min to demonstrate residual contrast in the gland.

## Sialography

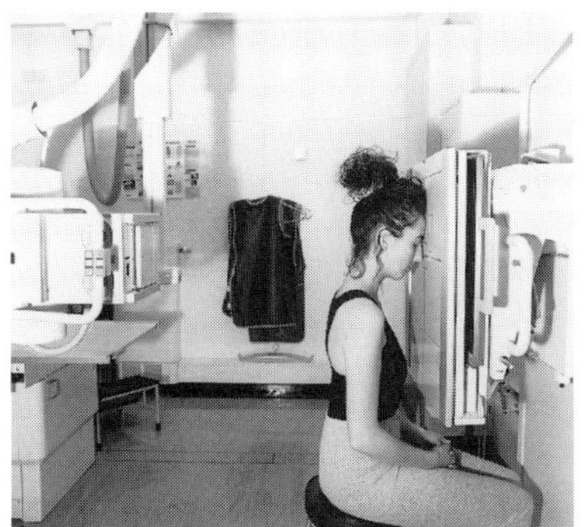

Figure 5.2a Equipment for PA projection

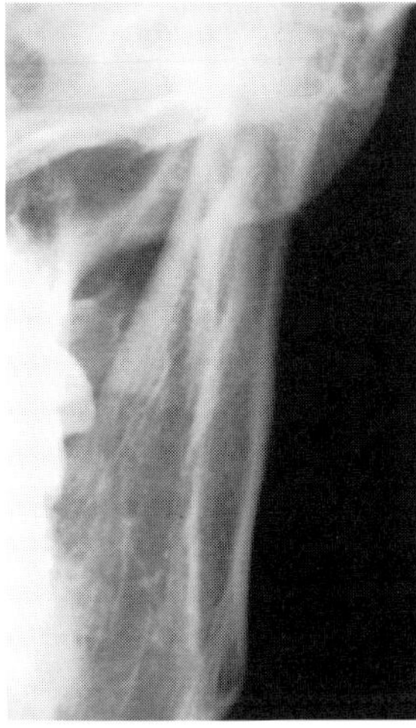

Figure 5.2b PA image with X-ray tube centred to the side under investigation (left parotid gland)

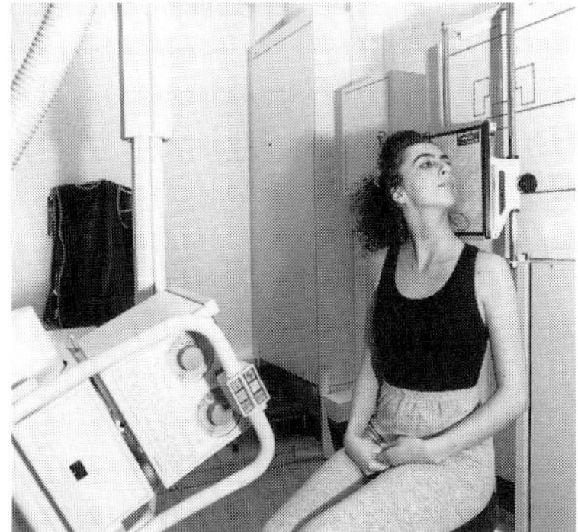

Figure 5.2c Equipment for lateral oblique projection

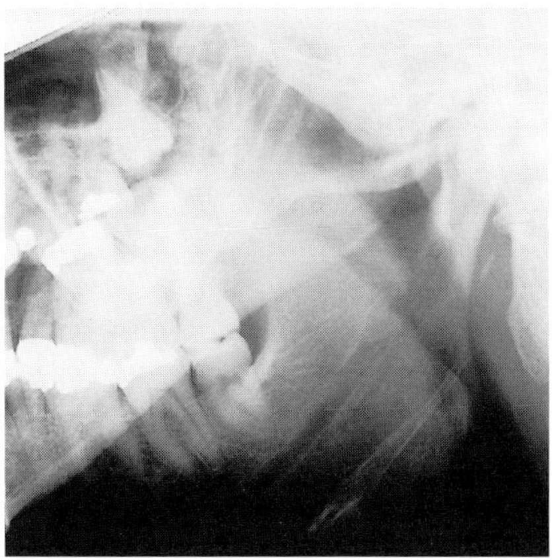

Figure 5.2d Lateral oblique image of mandible

**Parotid glands – control films**

Standard images of the mandible are acquired using postero-anterior, lateral and lateral oblique projections of the affected side.

A positioning technique with the patient erect is described; however, the patient may be examined on the Bucky table.

### Postero-anterior projection

This gives a profile view of the glands. Alternatively, for children an anteroposterior projection with the patient supine may be more acceptable.

The radiographic exposure is adjusted to demonstrate the superficial soft tissues containing the glands.

*Position of patient and imaging modality*

The patient sits facing the vertical Bucky or lies prone on the Bucky table if necessary. For both glands, the patient's nose and forehead are placed in contact with the midline of the Bucky and then the head adjusted to bring the orbitomeatal baseline and the median sagittal plane at right angles to the Bucky. An 18 × 24 cm cassette is placed longitudinally in the Bucky and is centred at the level of the angles of the mandible.

*Direction and centring of the X-ray beam*

The central ray is directed perpendicular to the film and centred in the midline at the level of the angles of the mandible or alternatively to the side under investigation.

### Lateral oblique projection

The parotid gland is shown in the best possible detail in this projection due to the separation of each side of the jaw. Image acquisition is made without the use of the Bucky.

*Position of patient and imaging modality*

Initially the patient sits erect, back to the Bucky table. The neck is allowed to move laterally toward the affected side until the parietal region is in contact with the cassette. In this position the patient's trunk is slightly rotated with the opposite shoulder raised. The head is adjusted into the lateral position so that the median sagittal plane is parallel and the interorbital line perpendicular to the film.

An 18 × 24 cm cassette is placed longitudinally in the cassette holder and positioned to include the whole of the mandible, with its lower edge 2 cm below the lower border of the mandible.

*Direction and centring of the X-ray beam*

The central ray is angled 25° cephalad and centred 1 cm below the angle of the mandible remote from the film.

## Sialography

### Lateral projection

This is used as an alternative to the lateral oblique projection with the angles of the mandible overshadowing each other. The parotid gland is demonstrated in the space between the mandible and the cervical spine.

The position of the patient is similar to that described for the lateral oblique projection or alternatively the patient may stand erect in the lateral position.

*Position of patient and imaging modality*
The neck is extended slightly to show as much as possible of the parotid gland between the mandible and cervical spine. An 18 × 24 cm cassette is placed longitudinally in the cassette holder and positioned to include the whole of the mandible, with its lower edge 2 cm below the lower border of the mandible.

*Direction and centring of the X-ray beam*
The horizontal central ray is centred over the angle of the mandible.

## Parotid glands – sialography images

Modified projections of the mandible are necessary to take account of the fact that the duct may still be cannulated and minimum disturbance of the patient is therefore necessary.

### Anteroposterior projection

For sialography, the anteroposterior projection is selected immediately following the injection of contrast medium. In the acquired image the main duct is projected across the mandible while the gland is free of overlying bone.

Two separate exposures may be necessary, adjusted to show the duct and gland.

*Position of patient and imaging modality*
With the patient supine, the head is raised on a small non-opaque pad, with the orbitomeatal line and median sagittal plane perpendicular to the image receptor.

For conventional radiography an 18 × 24 cm cassette is positioned longitudinally in the Bucky tray and is centred at the level of the angle of the mandible.

*Note*. A profile projection of the gland may be performed by rotating the head 5° away from the affected side.

*Direction and centring of the X-ray beam*
For conventional radiography the vertical central ray is directed in the midline along the upper occlusal plane. Centring over the midline will ensure that the oblique rays will project the gland free from overlying bone.

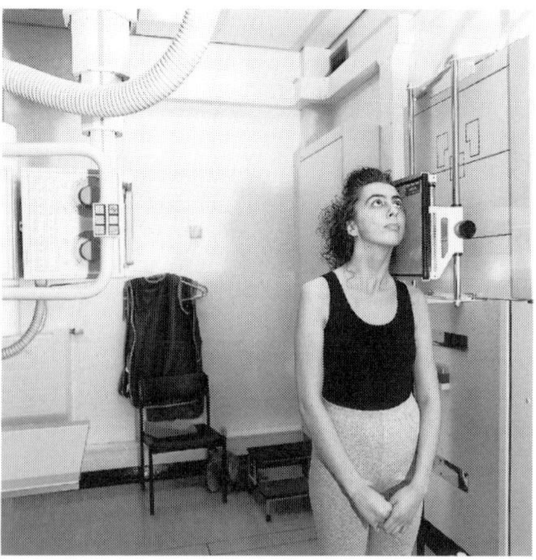
(a)

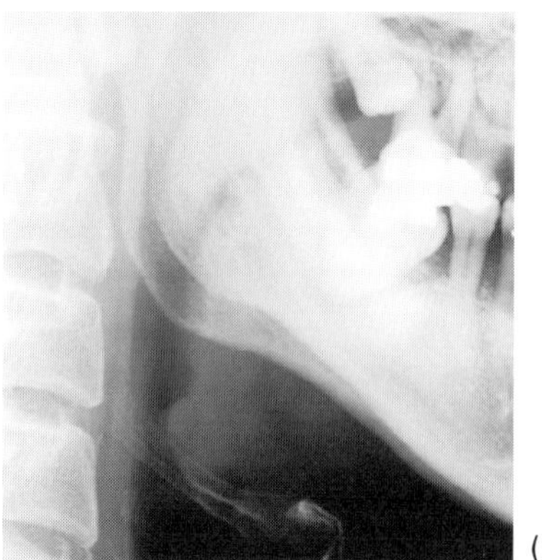
(b)

(c)

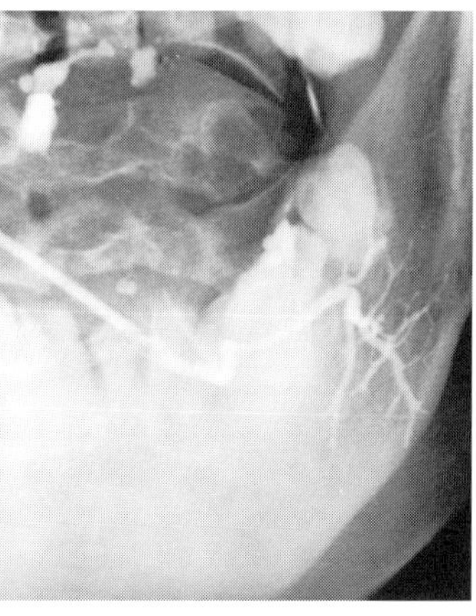
(d)

**Figure 5.3** (a,b) Equipment for lateral projection, and lateral image of mandible; (c,d) equipment for anteroposterior projection, and AP image of parotid gland

## Sialography

(a)

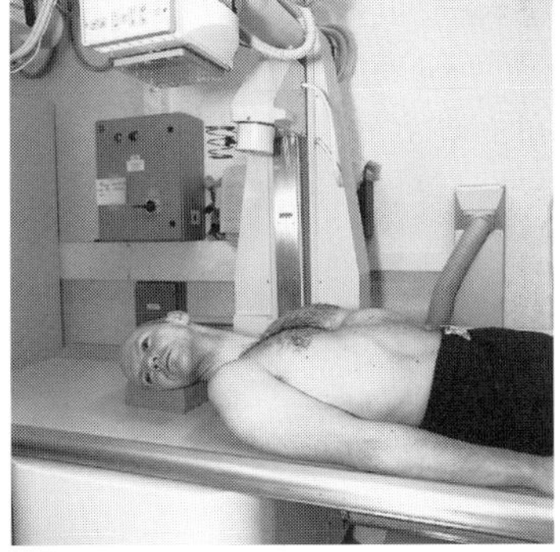

(b)

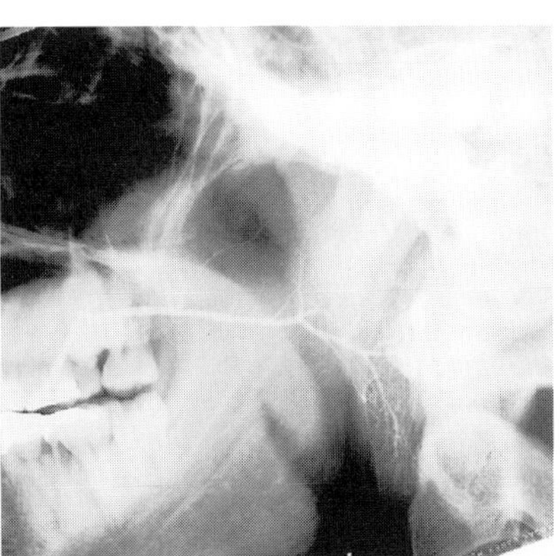

(c)

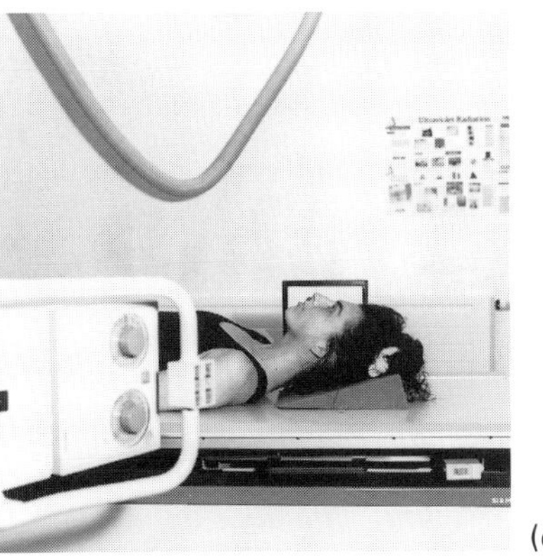

(d)

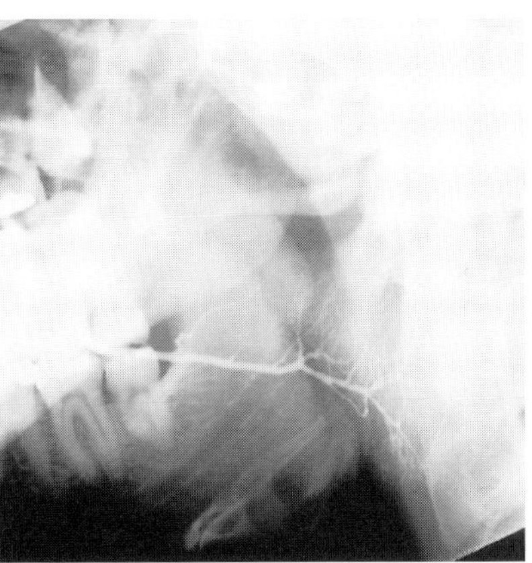

(e)

**Figure 5.4** (a) Equipment for lateral projection using over-couch tube and cassette, and (b) using image intensifier; (c) lateral image showing parotid gland; (d) equipment for lateral oblique projection using overcouch tube and cassette; (e) lateral oblique image showing parotid gland

### Lateral projection

This projection may be taken using a horizontal central ray, thereby minimising disturbance of the patient, or alternatively with digital fluorography equipment.

*Position of patient and imaging modality*

The patient lies supine on the Bucky table with the median sagittal plane at right angles to the table top. An 18 × 24 cm cassette is supported vertically in contact with the side of the face being examined, to include the whole of the mandible, with its lower edge 2 cm below the lower border of the mandible.

The median sagittal plane is brought parallel to the film by ensuring that the interorbital line is at right angles to the cassette, and the nasion and external occipital protuberance are equidistant from it.

When employing remote control equipment the patient is positioned supine and, with the aid of fluoroscopy, is rotated on to the affected side to bring the skull into the true lateral position.

*Direction and centring of the X-ray beam*

The horizontal central ray is centred over the angle of the mandible.

### Lateral oblique projection

*Position of patient and imaging modality*

The position of the patient and film is similar to that described above.

*Direction and centring of the X-ray beam*

Using a horizontal beam the central ray is angled 25° cranially and centred 1 cm inferiorly to the angle of the mandible remote from the film.

When employing remote control equipment the X-ray tube is angled, with the aid of fluoroscopy, to the required position to demonstrate the gland to best effect.

# 5 Salivary Glands

## Sialography

### Submandibular glands – control films

Standard images are acquired using inferosuperior (occlusal), inferosuperior (occlusal) with the head tilted away from the affected side, lateral and lateral oblique projections of the mandible. For the lateral the tongue is depressed to demonstrate the gland free from overlying bone.

The inferosuperior (occlusal) projections are necessary to demonstrate a calculus situated in the anterior part of the submandibular duct.

For sialography, lateral and/or lateral oblique projections, as described for the parotid glands, are taken.

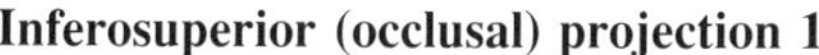

#### Inferosuperior (occlusal) projection 1

The occlusal films are best acquired using dedicated dental equipment.

*Position of patient and imaging modality*
The patient is seated with the neck well extended and supported on a head rest. An occlusal film is placed between the jaws, well over to the side examined and well back in the mouth, and is held lightly between the teeth.

*Direction and centring of the X-ray beam*
Centre from beneath the jaw, with the axial ray at right angles to the film.

#### Inferosuperior (occlusal) projection 2

This projection may be necessary to demonstrate a small calculus hidden by a tooth shadow at the posterior angle of the duct.

*Position of patient and imaging modality*
The position is similar to that described above, but with the chin raised and the head turned away from the affected side. The occlusal film is positioned diagonally in the mouth with the long edge along the jaw of the affected side, thus allowing it to be placed well back into the mouth. The film is held lightly between the teeth.

*Direction and centring of the X-ray beam*
Centre beyond the angle of the jaw at right angles to the film.

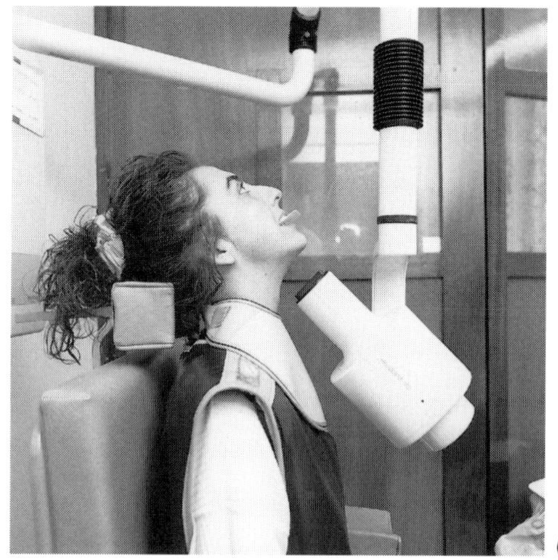

(a)

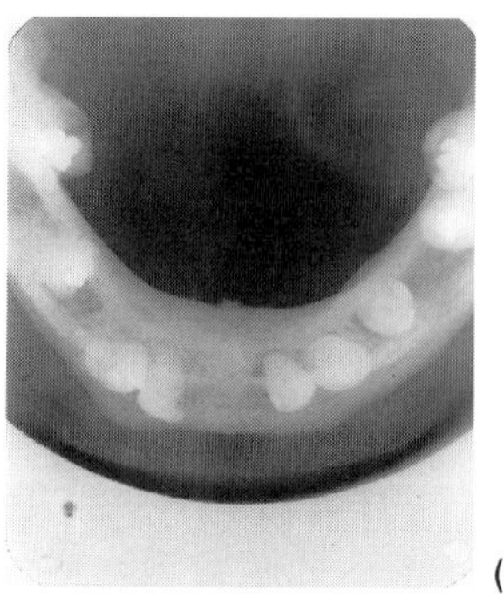

(b)

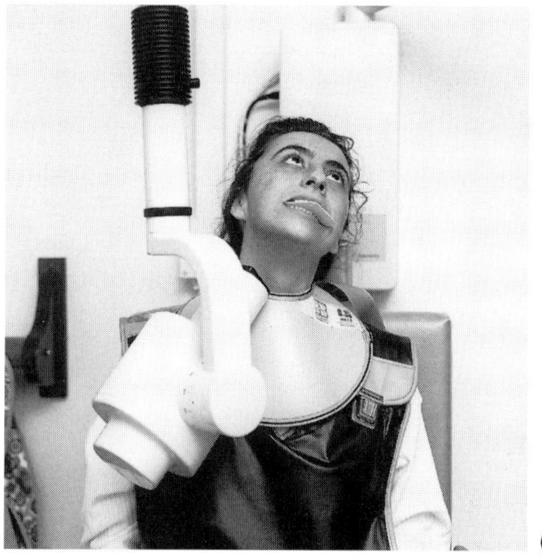

(c)

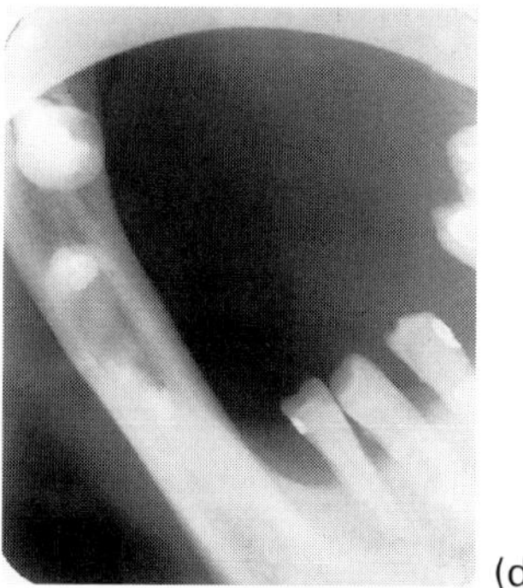

(d)

**Figure 5.5** (a) Occlusal projection using dental equipment, and (b) occlusal image of submandibular gland; (c) equipment for occlusal projection 2, and (d) occlusal image of submandibular gland

## Sialography

### Lateral projection

For the standard lateral projection the tongue is well depressed down with a spatula or the patient's finger to bring the soft tissues of the floor of the mouth below the level of mandible. Any opacity in the posterior two-thirds of the duct or in the gland will then become visible on the radiograph.

*Position of patient and imaging modality*
The patient stands sideways, with the affected side against the vertical Bucky. A comfortable position is secured with the feet slightly apart. The head is adjusted into the lateral position so that the median sagittal plane is parallel and the interorbital line perpendicular to the film.

The patient's tongue is well depressed down with a spatula or the patient's finger to bring the soft tissues of the floor of the mouth below the level of mandible.

An 18 × 24 cm cassette is placed longitudinally in the cassette holder and positioned to include the whole of the mandible, with its lower edge 2 cm below the lower border of the mandible.

*Direction and centring of the X-ray beam*
The horizontal central ray is directed to a point 2.5 cm below the angle of the mandible remote from the film.

## Submandibular glands – sialography images

### Lateral and lateral oblique projections

For sialography, lateral and lateral oblique projections are selected immediately following the injection of contrast medium. The acquired images demonstrate the main duct overlying the body of the mandible and the gland lying in the gap below the angle of the mandible and above the hyoid bone.

The radiographic technique for these projections is similar to the projections described for parotid glands on pages 139 and 140.

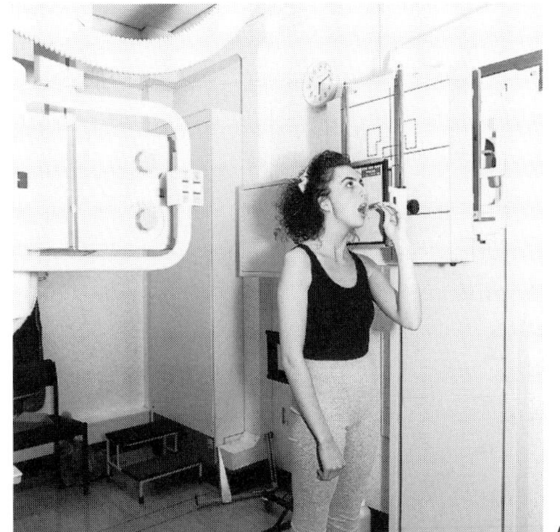

(a)

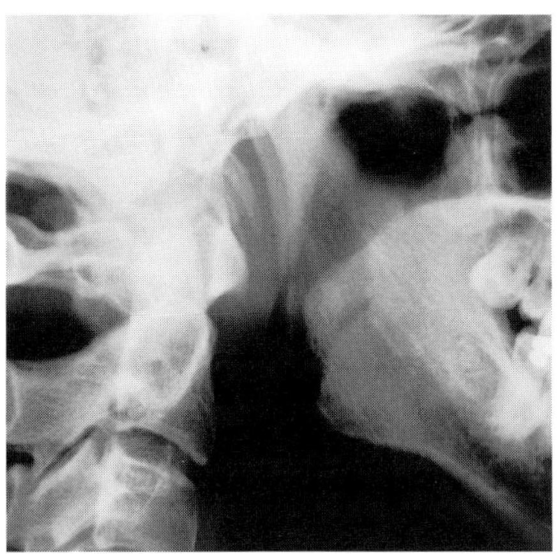
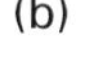
(b)

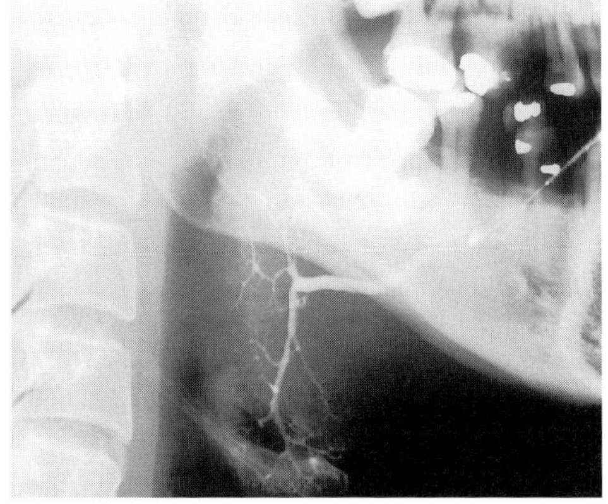
(c)

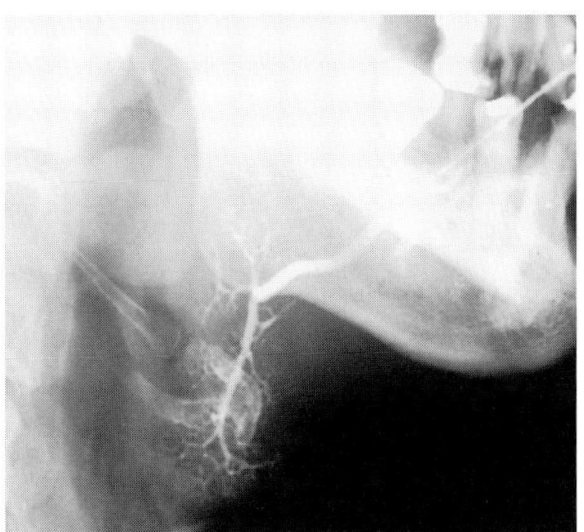
(d)

**Figure 5.6** (a) Equipment for lateral projection, and (b) lateral image of mandible; (c) lateral image of submandibular gland, and (d) lateral oblique image of submandibular gland

# 5 Salivary Glands

## Computed tomography

Transaxial plane imaging is undertaken pre-and post-injection of a water-soluble iodinated contrast agent. The patient is instructed not to swallow or move the tongue during scanning, to reduce movement artefacts.

### Indications

Computed tomography is used in the differential diagnosis of parotid and submandibular tumours. It is also employed as a preoperative assessment of tumour spread or to demonstrate recurrence following resection.

### Position of patient and imaging modality

The patient lies supine on the imaging couch, with the head resting in the transaxial head support. Positioning is aided by transaxial, coronal and sagittal alignment lights.

The anthropological baseline is positioned parallel to the scan plane and the median sagittal plane perpendicular to it. The patient is positioned in the scanner so that the scan reference point is at the level of the anthropological baseline.

### Imaging procedure

A postero-anterior or lateral scan projection radiograph is performed, commencing 10 cm above and ending 12 cm below the scan reference point.

From the scan projection radiograph, 10 mm sections are prescribed through the area of interest. These pre-contrast medium images are reviewed and the relevant area to be rescanned during the infusion of contrast medium is determined.

Either 3 or 5 mm contiguous sections are then prescribed dependent on the size of the lesion.

If spiral scanning options are available, these images may be acquired with a volume acquisition, using a 5 mm slice thickness and 5 mm table increments, but with a 3 mm reconstruction index to give overlapping sections.

A 40-second pre-scan delay is chosen, allowing 80 ml of contrast to be injected prior to commencement of scanning.

If a malignant tumour is suspected clinically, 10 mm contiguous sections will then be performed through the neck to assess any lymph node involvement.

*Contrast medium and injection data*

| *Volume* | *Concentration* | *Flow rate* |
|---|---|---|
| 100 ml | 300 mgI/ml | 2 ml/s |

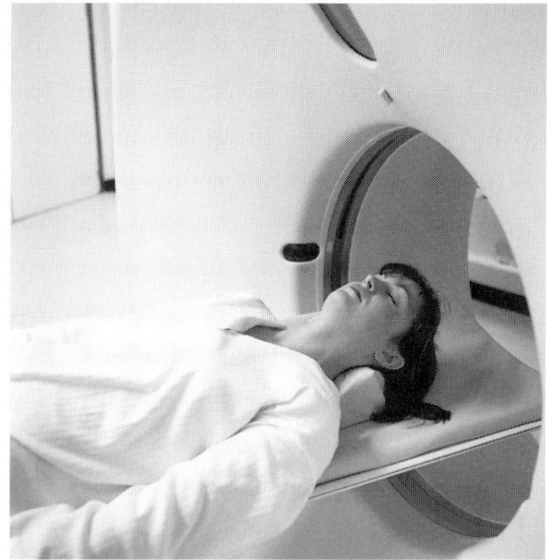

**Figure 5.7a** CT equipment

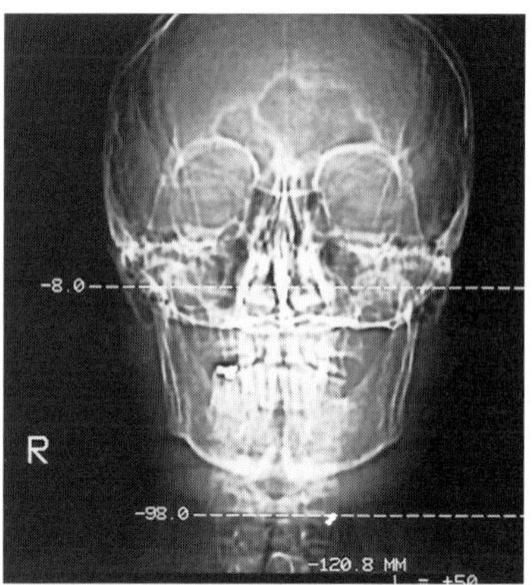


**Figure 5.7b** Postero-anterior scan projection radiograph showing start and end locations

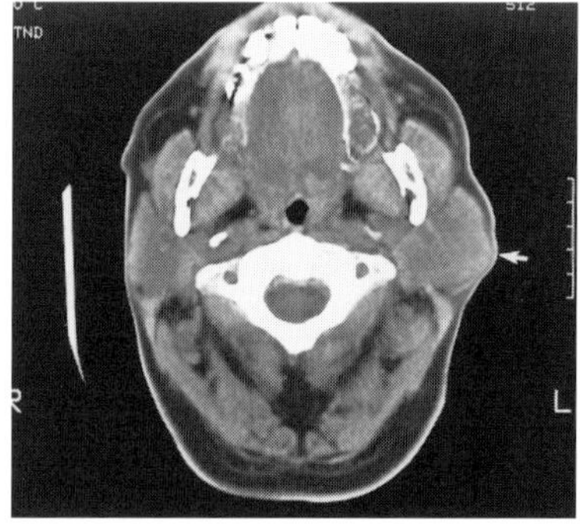


**Figure 5.7c** Pre-contrast transaxial image showing image left parotid tumour

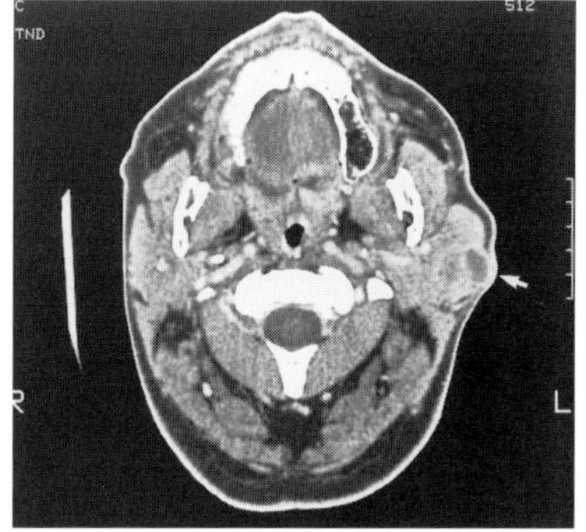


**Figure 5.7d** Post-contrast transaxial image showing left parotid tumour

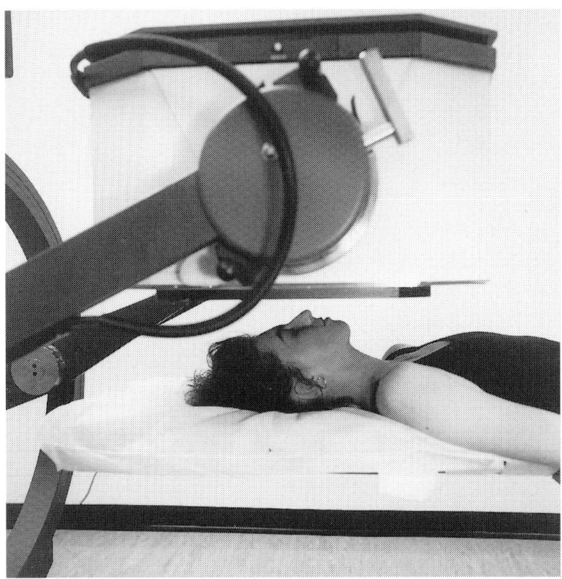

**Figure 5.8a** The gamma camera

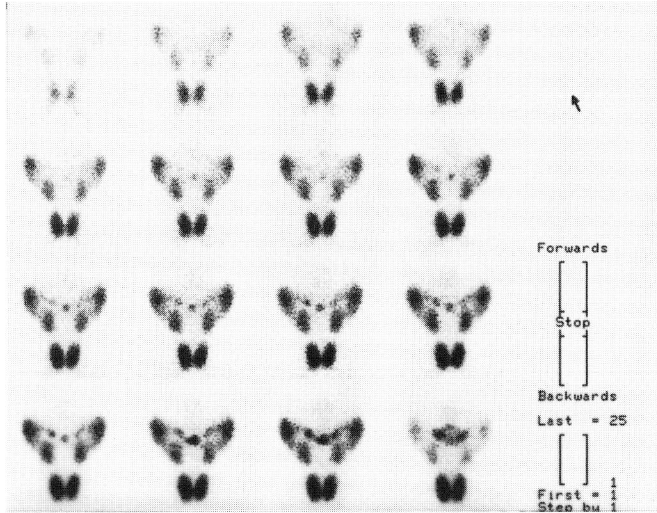


**Figure 5.8b** Series of dynamic images showing filling and emptying of the salivary glands

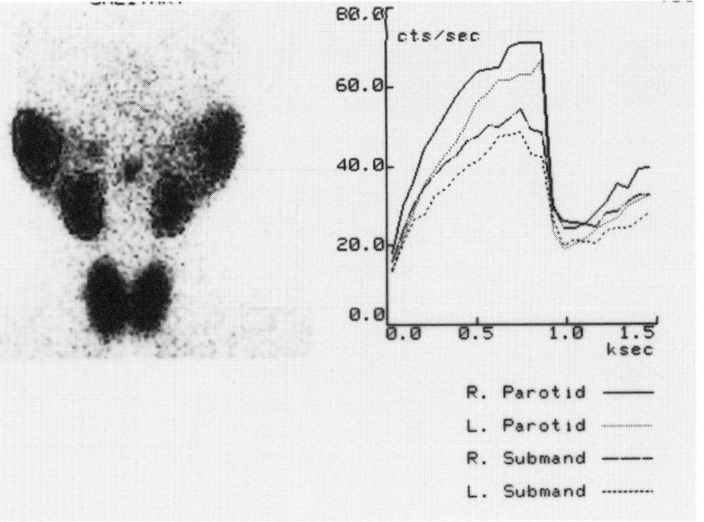


**Figure 5.8c** Image analysis with ROI drawn around each gland, with graphical representation of normal emptying pattern following lemon given to suck

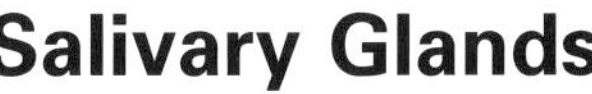

# Salivary Glands 5

## Radionuclide imaging

The anatomical detail which is available from radionuclide imaging is relatively poor. It has the advantage, however, of low patient dosage, and complications resulting from investigations are rare.

Dynamic scanning is used to assess physiological disorders, whereas static scans determine size, shape and position of the parotid and submandibular glands.

**Position of patient and imaging modality**

In the routine anterior view, the patient is seated in front of the gamma camera or lies supine on the imaging couch. The camera is placed as close as possible to the patient's face and centred over the mandible.

**Imaging procedure**

A high-sensitivity general-purpose collimator is used for dynamic scanning and zoomed to the area of interest.

An injection of technetium-99m pertechnetate ($^{99m}Tc\text{-}NaTcO_4$) is administered intravenously into the median cubital vein using a syringe fitted with a radiation guard. Image acquisition starts immediately after the injection is complete. Twenty-five 1-minute frames are collected and time–activity curves are drawn.

The patient is given a lemon to suck (or citric acid is placed on the tongue) after 15 min and image acquisition continues during gland secretion.

Static images in the anterior and right and left lateral positions may also be performed 25 min after injection, to assess size, shape, position and residual activity in the glands.

*Imaging and radiopharmaceutical parameters*

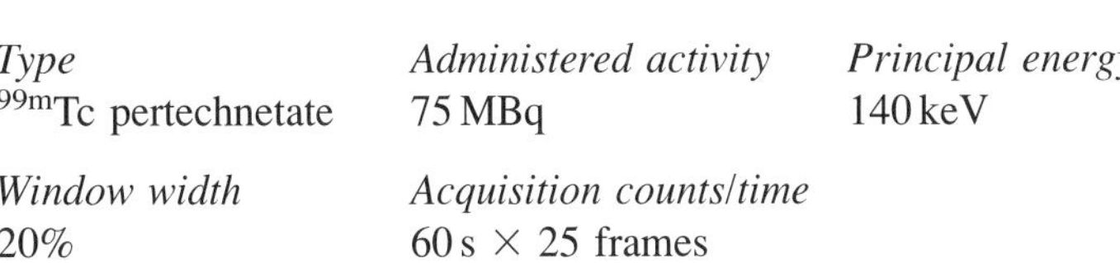

| *Type* | *Administered activity* | *Principal energy* |
|---|---|---|
| $^{99m}$Tc pertechnetate | 75 MBq | 140 keV |
| *Window width* | *Acquisition counts/time* | |
| 20% | 60 s × 25 frames | |

# 5 Salivary Glands

## Magnetic resonance imaging

The high inherent contrast, the direct multiplanar imaging capability and the non-invasive nature of the modality all combine to make MRI an excellent tool for evaluating lesions of the head and neck. Either a conventional head coil or a volume or quadrature neck coil may be used, depending on the patient's body size and pathology location.

**Indications**
Tumours of the salivary glands and surrounding structures.

**Position of patient and imaging modality**
The patient lies supine on the scanner table with the head resting in the head support, and positioning is aided by halogen alignment lights. The anthropological baseline is positioned parallel to the transaxial alignment light and the median sagittal plane is parallel to the sagittal alignment light. Either the head coil or the volume or quadrature neck coil is positioned around the area of interest, after which the patient and coils are driven into the centre of the magnet. The patient is instructed to remain as still as possible, with no tongue movements or swallowing during scans.

**Imaging procedure**
A sagittal pilot scan is performed to obtain reference points for other images. $T_1$ and $T_2$ weighted images are obtained in either the sagittal, coronal or transaxial plane through the region of interest. The choice of planes depends on the position of the tumour. The transaxial plane is used for the parotid region with others as necessary.

Spin-echo sequences are most commonly used.

$T_1$ weighted scans may be repeated following the administration of a suitable contrast agent.

Where available, fat suppression techniques may be used, particularly in the parotid region.

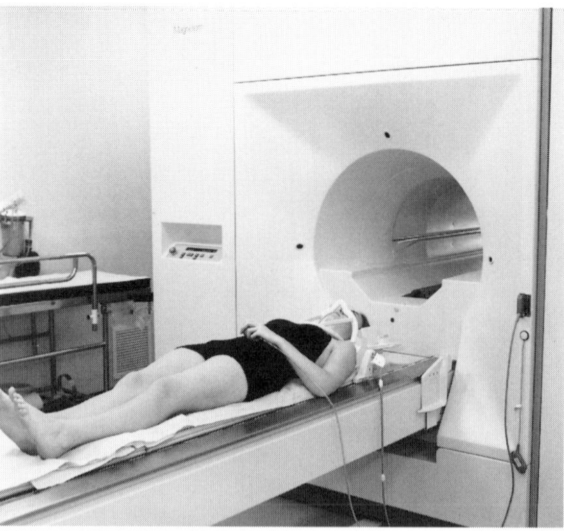

**Figure 5.9a** Neck coil in position

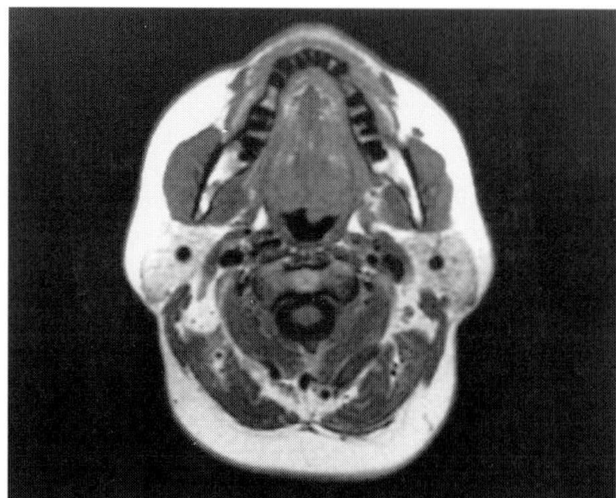

**Figure 5.9b** $T_1$ weighed transaxial image showing normal anatomy

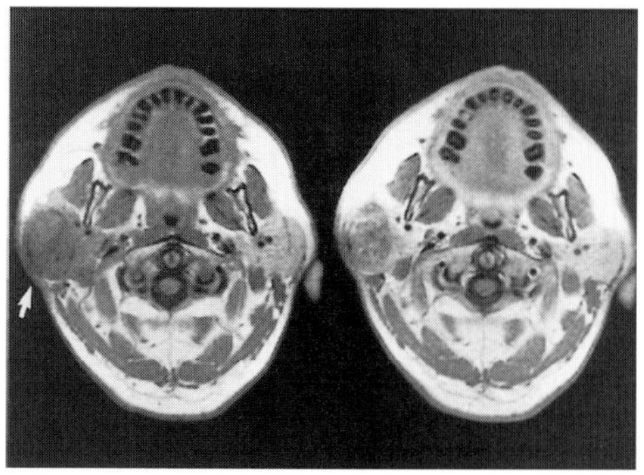

**Figure 5.9c** $T_1$ weighted transaxial images – pre- and post-contrast enhancement showing right parotid tumour

**Table 5.1 Imaging parameters**

| *Imaging sequence* | *TR* | *TE* | *Field of view* (cm) | *No. of NEX* | *Slice width/ gap* (mm) | *Matrix (horizontal–vertical)* |
|---|---|---|---|---|---|---|
| Spin-echo $T_1$ weighted | 500 | 20 | 25 | 2–4 | 3–5/1–2 | 192 × 256 |
| Fast spin-echo $T_2$ weighted (echo train length –6) | 4000 | 100 | 25 | 2–3 | 3–5/1–2 | 192 × 256 |
| STIR | 1500 | 25/114 | 25 | 2 | 5/1 | 192 × 256 |

## Pharynx and Oesophagus

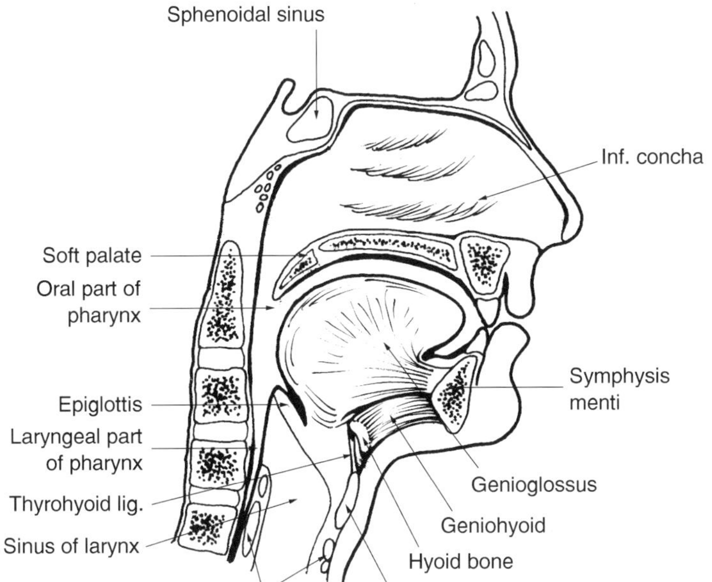


**Figure 5.10a** Pharynx – sagittal section

The pharynx or throat cavity lies between the mouth and the oesophagus, extending from the base of the skull to the sixth thoracic vertebra. Only the lower part (oropharynx) below the level of the soft palate serves as a passage for food. The part above the soft palate is the nasopharynx lying behind the nasal cavity. The oropharynx lies below the soft palate in front of the prevertebral soft tissues and extends from the first cervical vertebra to the sixth cervical vertebra, below the nasopharynx.

The oesophagus extends from the termination of the pharynx at the lower border of the cricoid cartilage, usually at the level of the sixth cervical vertebra, to the cardiac sphincter lying between the oesophagus and the stomach at the level of the 11th thoracic vertebra. The oesophagus passes through a hole in the diaphragm called the oesophageal hiatus which is situated at the level of the 10th thoracic vertebra.

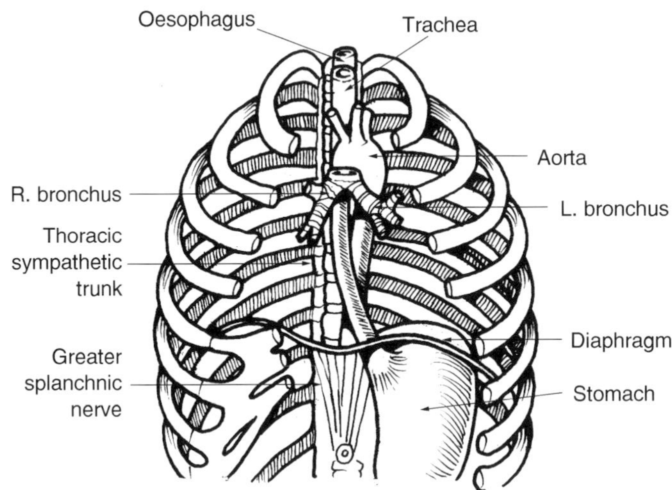


**Figure 5.10b** Oesophagus showing relations

### Recommended imaging procedures

The posterior relationship of the thoracic spine to the oesophagus and its proximity to other structures within the mediastinum make visualisation by plain films difficult. With the exception of foreign body localisation, they are often of little value.

Erect soft tissue exposures of the neck, however, may assist in the diagnosis of oesophageal perforation since the presence of air in the adult oesophagus is almost always associated with oesophageal pathology.

Barium examinations and/or endoscopy are the most common technique for examination of the oesophagus.

Radionuclide imaging can be used to assess gastro-oesophageal reflux, while CT and MRI are used to determine the extent of oesophageal carcinoma and for radiotherapy planning.

Magnetic resonance imaging is employed for tumours in the pharynx region. The protocol is similar to that for the salivary glands (see page 146).

Procedures specific to pharyngeal function are incorporated into the section entitled ‘Respiratory system’ (page 113).

# 5 Alimentary System

## Pharynx and Oesophagus

### Barium swallow

Both single and double contrast techniques are employed in the examination of the oesophagus. Double contrast offers improved visualisation of fine mucosal detail, but single contrast is still employed for compression, displacement and motility disorders.

No special patient preparation is required unless the examination is likely to include a barium examination of the stomach.

It can be performed using conventional undercouch fluoroscopy equipment; however, remote control equipment incorporating undercouch image intensification and 100/105 mm camera is desirable to provide rapid repetition and a reduction in patient dose.

Digital fluoroscopic equipment which is becoming more widely available is the equipment of choice, offering advantages in image quality through real-time image processing, and reduced dose.

Videotape recording is usefully employed, especially in the diagnosis of motility disorders, but lacks the facility for hard copy images.

#### Indications

Dysphagia is the most common condition requiring examination by barium swallow. Carcinoma of the oesophagus or associated structures, oesophageal strictures, varices and ulceration are common causes of dysphagia.

Hiatus hernia and oesophageal reflux are also investigated using barium techniques.

#### Contraindications

Oesophageal perforation resulting in leakage into the mediastinal, pleural or peritoneal cavities contraindicates the initial use of a barium compound. In such cases it is normal to commence the examination using a water-based non-ionic contrast agent.

#### Imaging procedure (single contrast)

In practice, precise patient positioning is achieved under fluoroscopic control using remote control equipment. The position of the patient as described here should be seen as a guide.

The fluoroscopy table is placed in the vertical position and the patient stands facing the X-ray tube, with back against the table top. The patient is rotated into the left posterior oblique position, with the right side of the body raised. In this position the oesophagus is projected clear of the spine.

The patient swallows a good mouthful of barium on direction, which is observed under fluoroscopic control until it enters the stomach. This procedure is repeated until the entire oesophagus has been visualised satisfactorily.

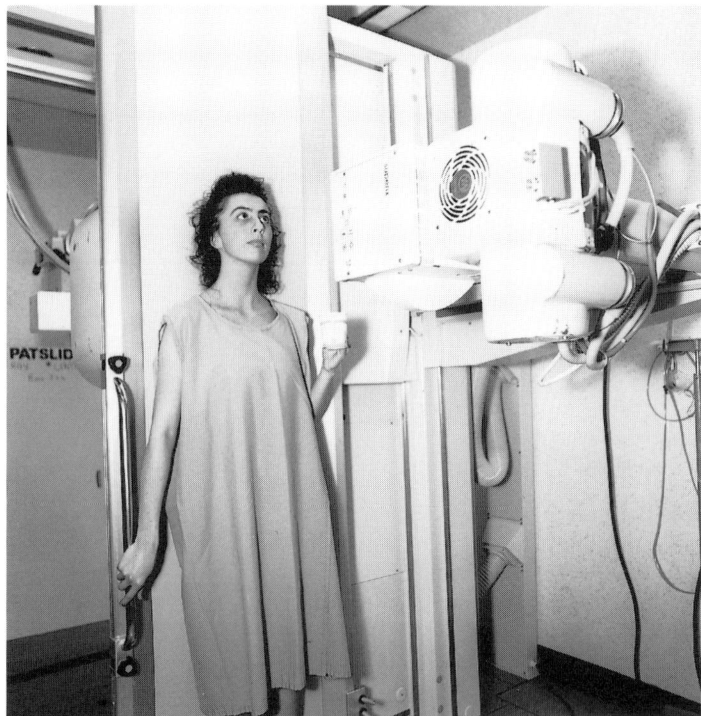


**Figure 5.11a** Patient positioned for anteroposterior projection

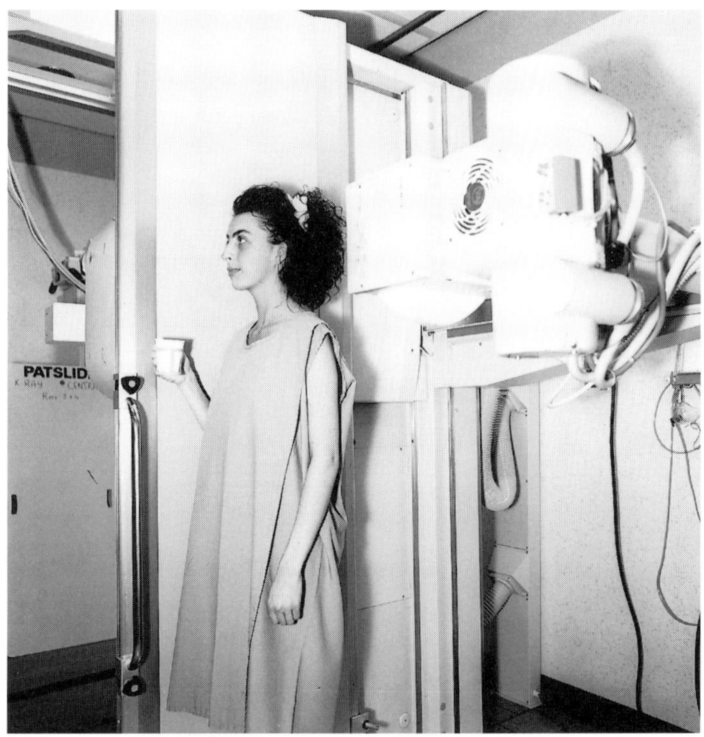


**Figure 5.11b** Patient positioned for lateral projection

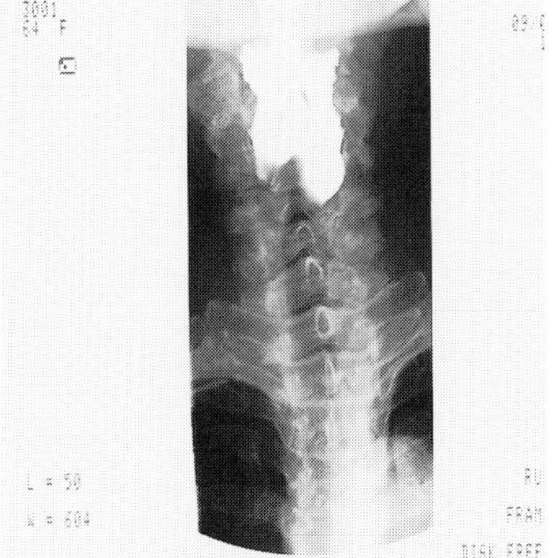

**Figure 5.12a** Anteroposterior image – early swallowing phase barium seen in the oropharynx

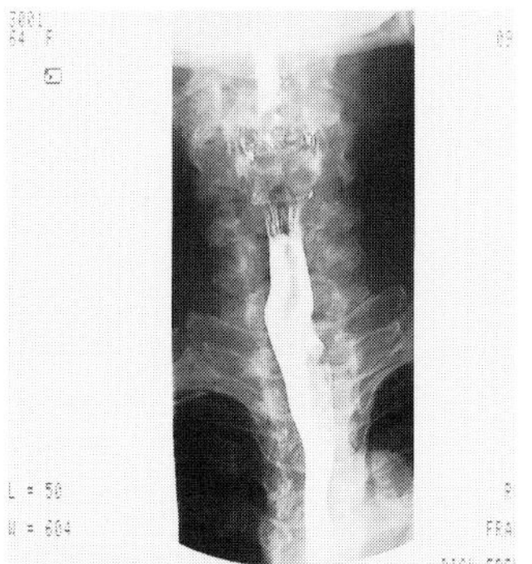

**Figure 5.12b** Anteroposterior image showing barium in the upper oesophagus

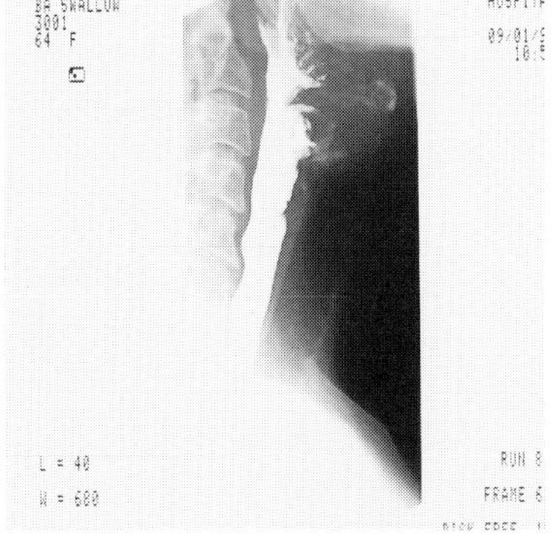

**Figure 5.12c** Lateral image – barium filling upper oesophagus

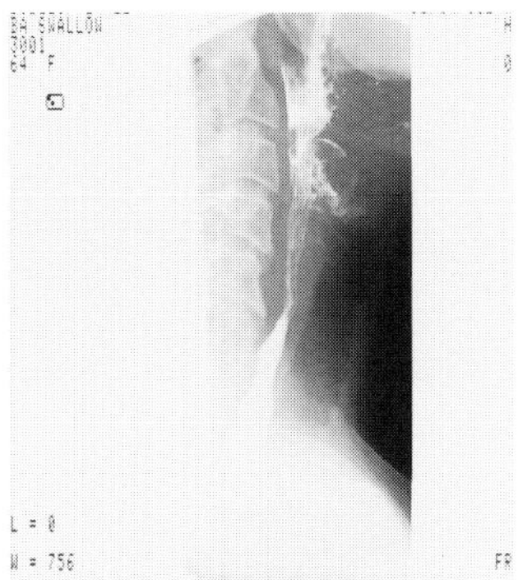

**Figure 5.12d** Lateral image – same position as above with barium emptying from upper oesophagus

# Pharynx and Oesophagus 5

## Barium swallow

**Imaging procedure (single contrast)**
The table is returned to the horizontal position and the patient is then turned prone and placed in the right anterior oblique position with a bolster under the rib cage. The patient is observed drinking barium through a straw to demonstrate the presence of hiatus hernia.

**Imaging procedure (double contrast)**
The imaging technique for a double contrast barium swallow is similar to that of a single contrast study, except that the patient is given an effervescent agent prior to the administration of the barium compound. An intravenous hypotonic agent may also be given.

The patient is then instructed to drink several mouthfuls of barium rapidly and is examined using a similar protocol to that for the single contrast technique.

### Anteroposterior projection (neck)

*Position of patient and imaging modality*
The patient stands erect with back against the fluoroscopy table and the median sagittal plane perpendicular to the film. The chin is elevated slightly and images are recorded as the patient swallows a mouthful of barium using digital acquisition, or a split 24 cm × 30 cm film or a 100/105 mm camera.

*Direction and centring of the X-ray beam*
The horizontal central ray is centred in the midline at the level of the fifth cervical vertebra.

### Lateral projection (neck)

*Position of patient and imaging modality*
The patient is rotated 90° so that the median sagittal plane is parallel to the table top. The chin is elevated slightly and the shoulders are depressed to permit maximum visualisation of the soft tissues above the shoulder.

Images are recorded using either digital acquisition, split 24 cm × 30 cm film or a 100/105 mm camera.

*Direction and centring of the X-ray beam*
The horizontal central ray is centred at the mid-cervical region.

## Barium swallow

### Left posterior oblique projection

*Position of patient and imaging modality*
From the erect, anteroposterior position the patient is rotated 20–30° onto the left side under fluoroscopic control until the oesophagus is projected clear of the spine.

*Direction and centring of the X-ray beam*
Using a horizontal central ray, images are recorded using either a split 35 cm × 35 cm film or a 100/105 mm camera to demonstrate the entire length of the oesophagus.

### Right or left posterior oblique projections (supine)

These projections are used as an alternative to those taken with the patient erect when non-ambulant or non-weight-bearing patients present for examination.

The right posterior oblique projection can also be selected to demonstrate reflux from the fundus of the stomach into the oesophagus as the patient rotates onto the right side from the supine position.

*Position of patient and imaging modality*
The fluoroscopy table is placed in the horizontal position and the patient is rotated 20–30° onto the right or left side under fluoroscopic control until the oesophagus is projected clear of the spine. The patient is supported with the aid of foam pads.

*Direction and centring of the X-ray beam*
For the non-ambulant patient, images are recorded using a vertical central ray to demonstrate the entire length of the oesophagus. When the projection is used to demonstrate oesophageal reflux, the central ray is directed at the level of the eighth thoracic vertebrae to include the lower end of the oesophagus and diaphragm.

*Contrast medium and injection data*

| *Volume* | *Concentration* | *Flow rate* |
|---|---|---|
| 70–100 ml | 250% w/v | Oral |

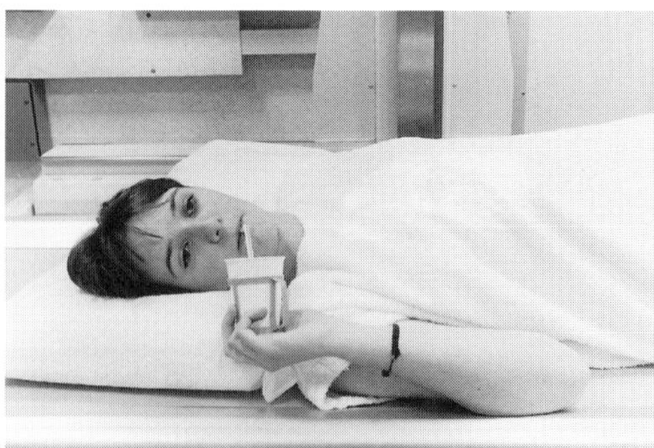

**Figure 5.13c** Patient positioned for right posterior oblique projection – table horizontal

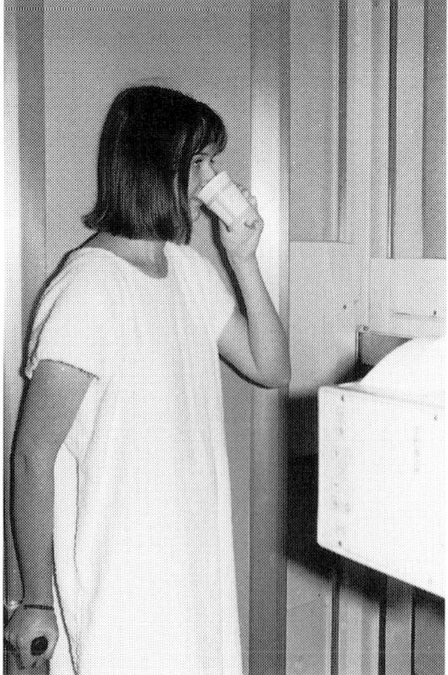

**Figure 5.13a** Patient positioned for left posterior oblique projection

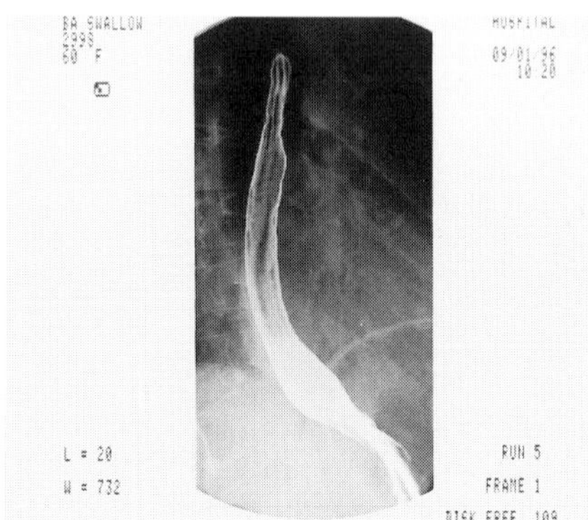


**Figure 5.13b** Left posterior oblique image – barium flowing through oesophagus into the stomach

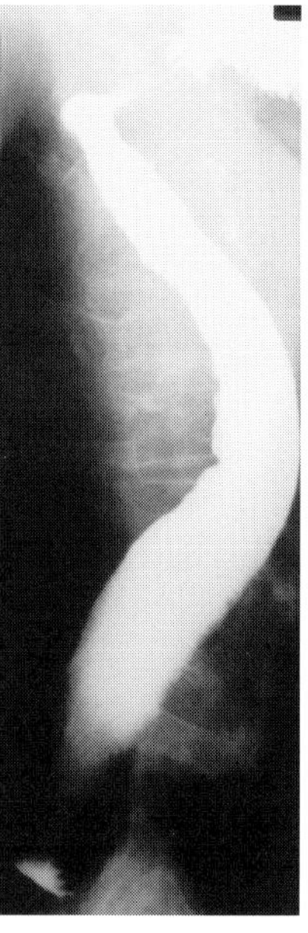

**Figure 5.13d** Series of images with the table horizontal showing barium flowing through oesophagus into the stomach

## Computed tomography

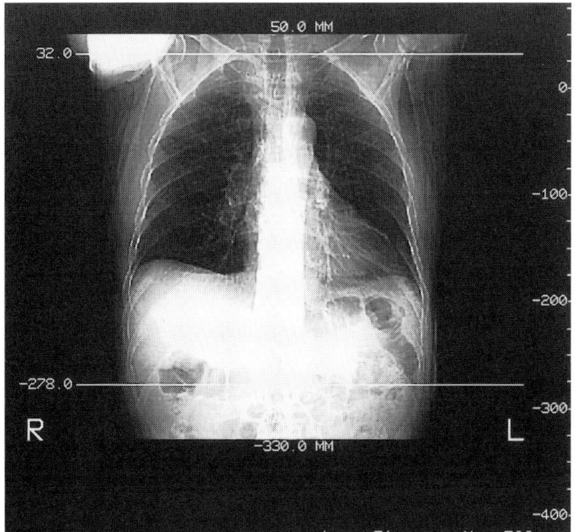


**Figure 5.14a** Scan projection radiograph showing start and end locations

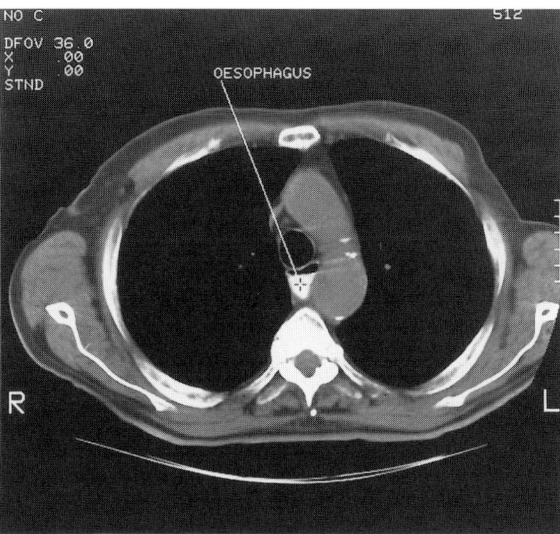


**Figure 5.14b** Transaxial image showing pooling of contrast in the oesophagus above a tumour

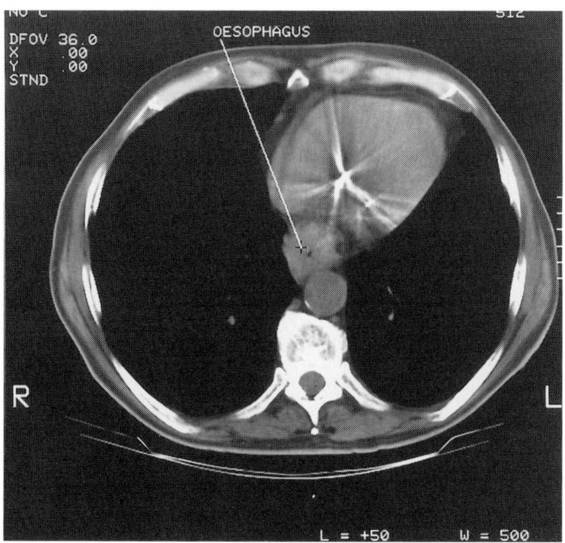


**Figure 5.14c** Transaxial image showing a tumour in the oesophagus

Transaxial CT can be used to assess the extent of disease in patients with oesophageal carcinoma. The results can be used to determine treatment, e.g. resection or accurate radiotherapy planning.

Ideally, oral contrast in the form of dilute Gastrografin or barium should be administered 10 min prior to scanning to outline the stomach and oesophagus.

Transaxial images are initially obtained through the lesion.

After review, contrast enhanced images may be required of surrounding structures, including the liver, to assess the extent of any metastatic spread and mediastinal lymph node involvement.

**Indications**

Oesophageal carcinoma or carcinoma of associated structures.

**Position of patient and imaging modality**

The patient lies supine, head first on the scanner table. Arms are raised and placed behind the patient's head, out of the scan plane. Positioning is aided by transaxial, coronal and sagittal alignment lights. The median sagittal plane is adjusted so that it is perpendicular to the centre of the table top and the coronal plane parallel to it. The scan plane is perpendicular to the long axis of the body to enable transaxial imaging to be undertaken. The scanner table height is adjusted to ensure that the coronal plane alignment light is at the level of the mid-axillary line. The patient is now moved into the scanner until the scan reference point is at the level of the sternal notch.

**Imaging procedure**

A postero-anterior scan projection radiograph is obtained, commencing at the level of the sternal notch and ending 28 cm below this point. From this image, 10 mm contiguous sections are prescribed through the affected area. Scanning is performed on arrested respiration. These pre-contrast images are reviewed, following which the same area may be rescanned during the infusion of the contrast agent using the same imaging protocol. Scanning commences after 40 ml of the contrast agent has been administered. If required 10 mm contiguous sections are performed through the liver to assess the extent of the disease.

If spiral scanning options are available, post-contrast enhanced scans may also be acquired through the area of abnormality with a volume acquisition, using a 10 mm slice thickness and 10 mm table increments, but with a 5 mm reconstruction index to give overlapping sections.

*Contrast media and injection data*

| *Volume* | *Concentration* | *Flow rate* |
|---|---|---|
| 100 ml | 240 mgI/ml | 2 ml/s |

# 5 Pharynx and Oesophagus

## Radionuclide imaging – oesophageal transit and reflux tests

Gastro-oesophageal imaging is a non-invasive technique for investigating motility and reflux. It is claimed to be more accurate than barium swallow examinations which can produce reflux in asymptomatic patients. This may take the form of a combined study with the reflux test following the transit study. To ensure that the stomach is empty, the patient fasts from midnight the previous evening and is asked to refrain from smoking for 4 h prior to the test. A drink in the form of a sulphur colloid labelled with $^{99m}$Tc and mixed with fruit juice can be used for these tests.

Normally up to six consecutive swallows are performed to determine a comprehensive average transit time average.

**Indications**

Oesophagitis, dysphagia, odynophagia and atypical chest pain.

**Position of patient and imaging modality**

The patient is usually supine, but can be seated erect when oesophageal clearance is prolonged. Anterior views are acquired, with the gamma camera parallel to the imaging couch and positioned to include the oesophagus and fundus of the stomach.

**Imaging procedure – transit time**

A low-energy general-purpose collimator is selected. Just as the patient is about to swallow a mouthful of the preparation, an image acquisition protocol is initiated comprising 120 × 0.25 s frames for a period of 30 s. With the mouth empty the patient is asked to attempt swallowing about three times during the acquisition sequence to aid motility. If a delay in transit is detected, the last three swallows are carried out with the patient supine.

Using the software package, all the frames are summed up to form one image. Regions of interest are drawn around upper, middle and lower oesophagus and stomach to produce time–activity curves, from which the data can be manipulated to produce a functional image progressing the craniocaudal movement of a bolus from mouth to stomach.

**Reflux test**

This may be done independently or as a follow-up if clinically indicated after a transit test, to assess the frequency and duration of any reflux episodes after the stomach is filled with 500 ml of a suitable labelled drink. Before the test the patient is encouraged to drink more fruit juice to fill the stomach and clear the oesophagus of any activity. Image acquisition with the patient supine spans up to 40 min, with images acquired of one frame per 20 s. Any reflux is detected from time–activity curves which are produced from regions of interest drawn over the stomach and oesophagus. The test may be performed with the use of a pressure cuff placed around the patient's abdomen. By increasing the pressure in 20 mmHg steps from 0 to 100 mmHg, and acquiring an image at each stage, any reflux will be detected by an increase in activity in the oesophagus.

*Imaging and radiopharmaceutical parameters*

| *Type* | *Principal energy* | *Window width* |
|---|---|---|
| $^{99m}$Tc colloid | 140 keV | 20% |

*Administered activity*
Transit test – 10 MBq per swallow
Reflux test – 20 MBq

*Acquisition counts/time* – as above

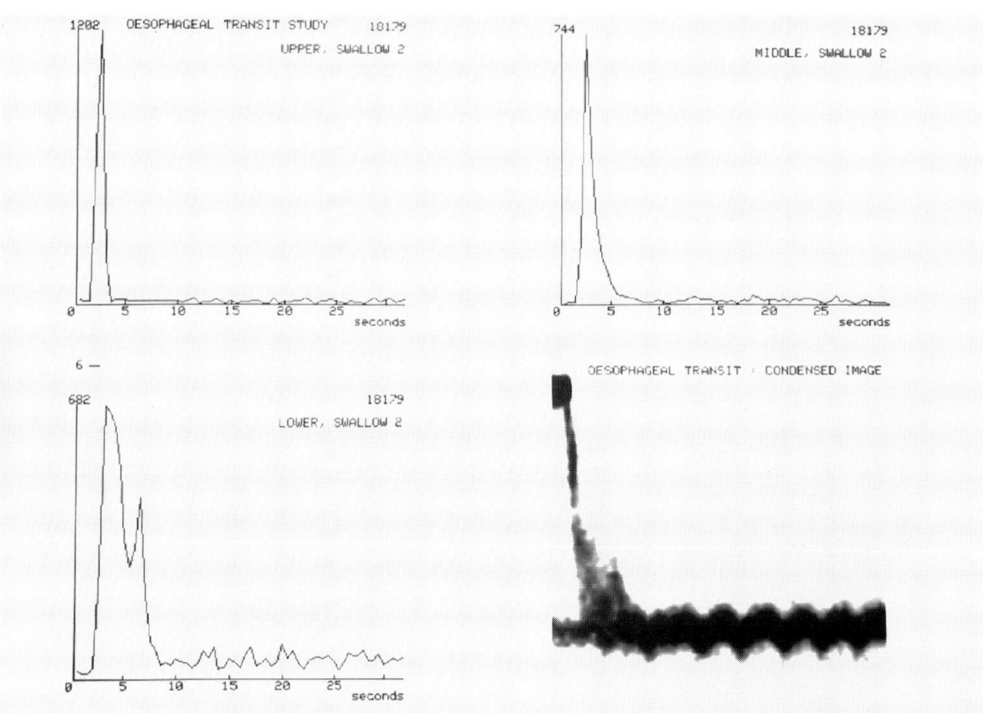


**Figure 5.15** Typical transit study showing time–activity curves for three regions of interest and a summed image showing transit of activity down the oesophagus as a function of time

## Stomach and Small Bowel

The stomach is the widest part of the alimentary tract, acting as a reservoir for food and drink. It has a capacity of between 1000 and 1500 ml. It lies between the oesophagus and the small intestine, mostly to the left of the spine, but varies in position, particularly with different subject types. In thin subjects (asthenic) and in the elderly the lower part of the stomach may reach below the iliac crest. The stomach is extremely mobile, and changes its position with different positions of the body, especially erect and supine.

Food enters the stomach through the cardiac orifice and leaves the pyloric canal, to go into the duodenum. The medial margin of the stomach is known as the lesser curvature and the lateral and inferior margin as the greater curvature. The fundus lies beneath the left hemidiaphragm and the antrum immediately adjacent to the pyloric canal with the body of the stomach between the fundus and the gastric antrum. The fundus actually lies above the level of the entry of the oesophagus into the stomach, being closely approximated to the inferior surface of the curved left hemidiaphragm.

Gas collects in the fundus of the stomach in the erect position, but lies in the gastric antrum when the patient is supine, with food or barium then moving into the fundus.

The small intestine is approximately 6.5 m in length and between 2 and 4 cm in diameter. It is divided into three parts: the duodenum (30 cm), the jejunum (2.5 m) and the ileum (4 m). Immediately after the pyloric canal the duodenum opens out into a triangular shape called the duodenum cap. It then passes posteriorly and inferiorly on the right side of the upper lumbar spine before crossing to the left side of the abdomen at the level of the second lumbar vertebra. It then passes upwards and to the left posterior to the stomach, to form the duodenal–jejunal flexure at the ligament of Treitz.

The jejunum lies between the duodenum and the ileum below the level of the stomach within the margins of the colon. The ileum is frequently found in the pelvic cavity, particularly when the bladder is empty. A full bladder will displace the ileum out of the pelvic cavity.

### Recommended imaging procedures

Barium studies are still widely used for the examination of the stomach and small intestine. The barium meal is used to investigate the stomach and the proximal portion of the small bowel. Hypotonic duodenography can provide additional information where lesions of the duodenogram are suspected, including lesions of the head of pancreas.

The small bowel enema and the barium follow-through are used to examine the small bowel in its entirety.

Fibreoptic endoscopy plays an important role in the examination of the upper gastrointestinal tract and has resulted in significantly reducing the number of barium studies being performed. It is used particularly in the assessment of the gastric wall and associated viscera.

Radionuclide imaging is most commonly used to assess the rate of gastric emptying. It can also be used in other conditions including Mickel's diverticulum and inflammatory bowel disease.

Angiography is useful in the examination of acute bleeding.

Computed tomography has limited application as a first-line imaging modality. It may be used to investigate mass lesions of associated structures such as the pancreas.

Ultrasound also has limited application in the small bowel because of the problems associated with gas interface. It can be used in cases of pyloric stenosis to measure the antral wall thickness, but it is not the modality of choice, except in neonates.

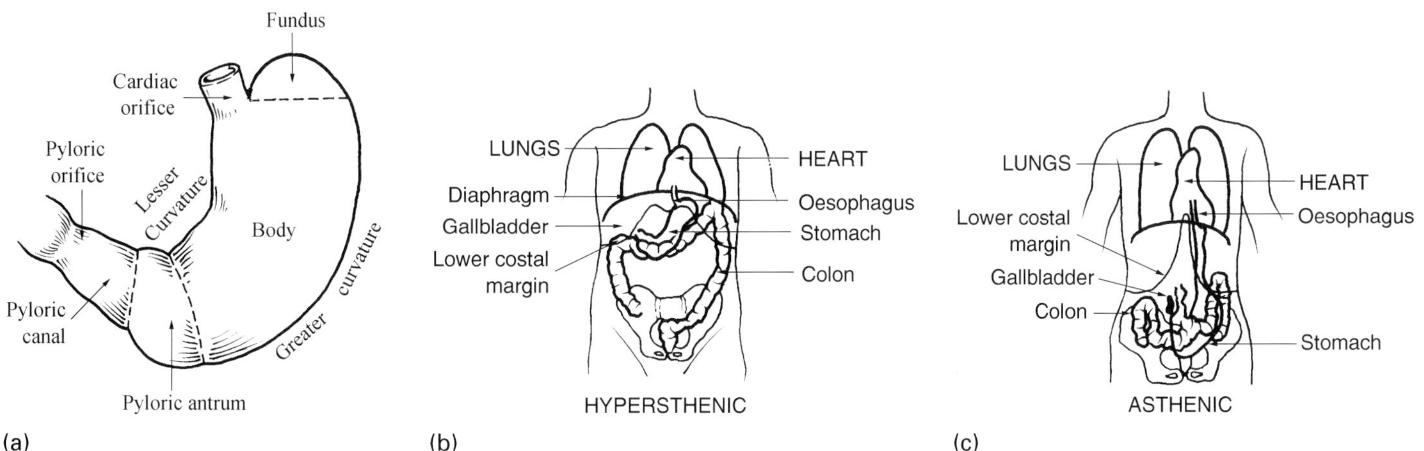


**Figure 5.16** (a) Anterior aspect of stomach showing regions; (b,c) variations in position of abdominal contents in different subject types

# 5 Stomach and Small Bowel

## Barium meal

The double contrast barium meal has now replaced the traditional single contrast technique employed for many years. It provides superior visualisation of the gastric mucosa and consequently is invaluable in the early detection of carcinoma and ulceration. It is usually performed with the minimum amount of barium (70 ml) and 250–500 ml of $CO_2$ used for optimum distension of the stomach and coating the gastric mucosa with barium.

A smooth muscle relaxant may be administered intravenously to overcome peristalsis and spasm. The type prescribed is dependent on the departmental protocol and the patient's medical history where there may be specified contraindications.

The examination can be performed using conventional over-couch fluoroscopy equipment or remote control equipment incorporating undercouch image intensification. Digital fluoroscopic imaging is preferred as it offers advantages in image quality through real-time image processing and reduced dose. However, permanent images may be acquired using 100/105 mm camera or with a cassette/film screen combination. Because of the dynamic nature of the examination, the equipment must be capable of rapid serial radiography in order to acquire a particular phase of gastric emptying.

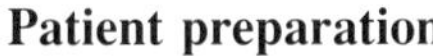

### Patient preparation

The patient is not allowed to eat or drink for at least 5 h before the examination and smoking should be discouraged. Non-essential radio-opaque medication should also be withheld.

### Indications

Gastric or associated carcinoma, dyspepsia, suspected gastric and duodenal ulcers, hiatus hernia, pyloric stenosis and unexplained sudden weight loss, anorexia and iron deficiency are indications for barium meal examination.

### Contraindications

Suspected perforation of the oesophagus, stomach or small intestine, and obstruction, contraindicate the use of a barium suspension.

In such cases a non-ionic water-soluble contrast agent may be used.

*Contrast medium and injection data*

| *Volume* | *Concentration* | *Flow rate* |
|---|---|---|
| 70–150 ml | Low-viscous/high-density 250% w/v barium suspension | Oral |
| 250–500 ml | $CO_2$ | |

Produced by a combination of sodium bicarbonate granules and citric acid solution.

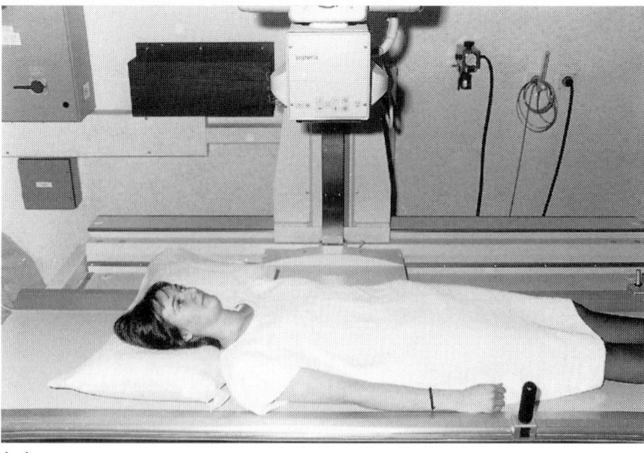

(a)

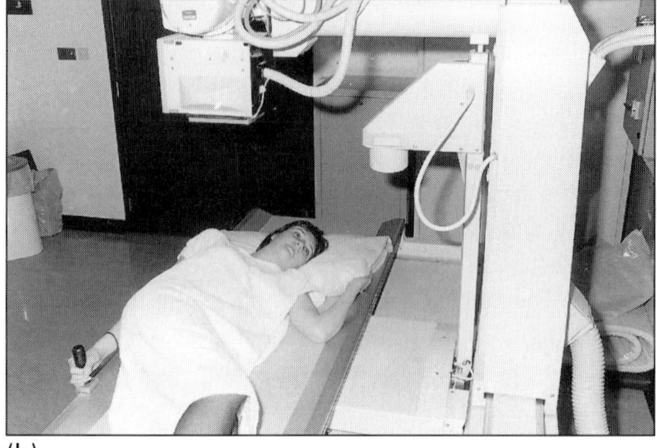

(b)

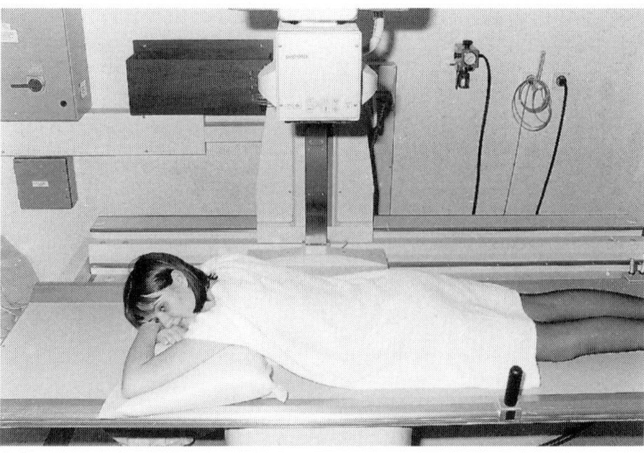

(c)

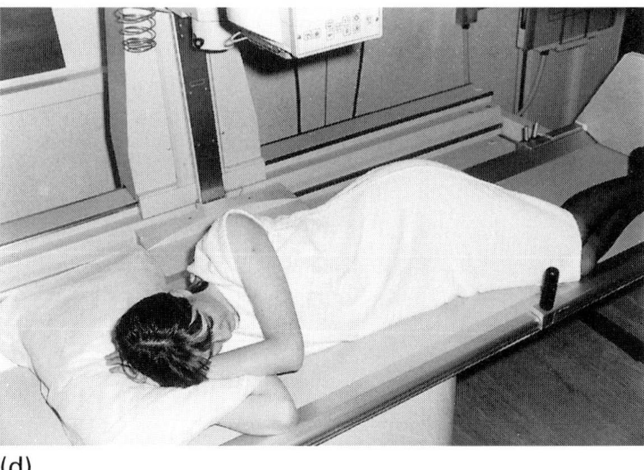

(d)

**Figure 5.17** (a) Patient supine for AP image; (b) left posterior oblique steep angle for duodenal cap; (c) patient prone for PA image; (d) right lateral position

# Stomach and Small Bowel



## Barium meal

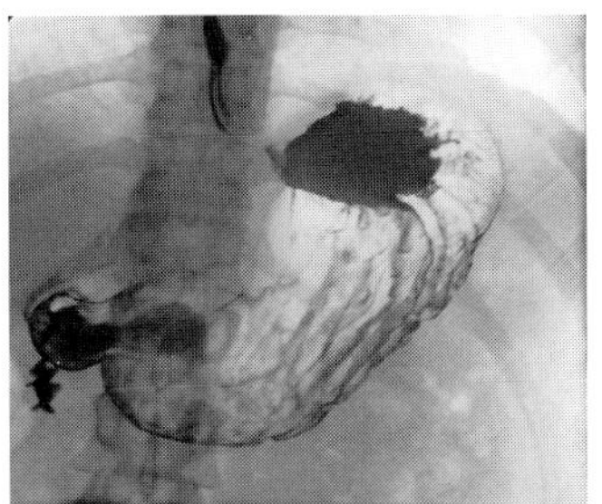

**Figure 5.18a** Supine

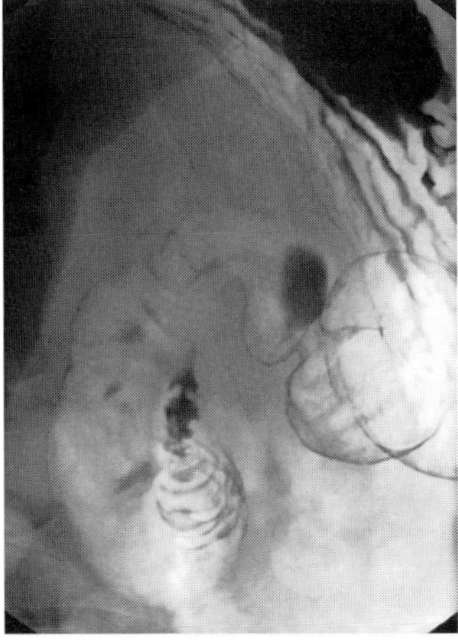

**Figure 5.18b** Left posterior oblique (steep angle)

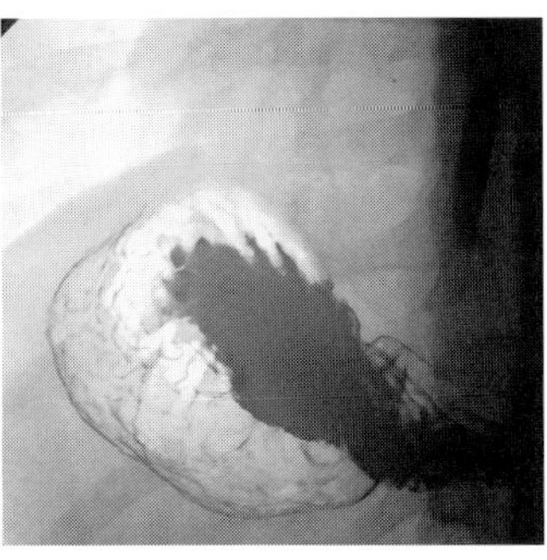

**Figure 5.18c** Prone

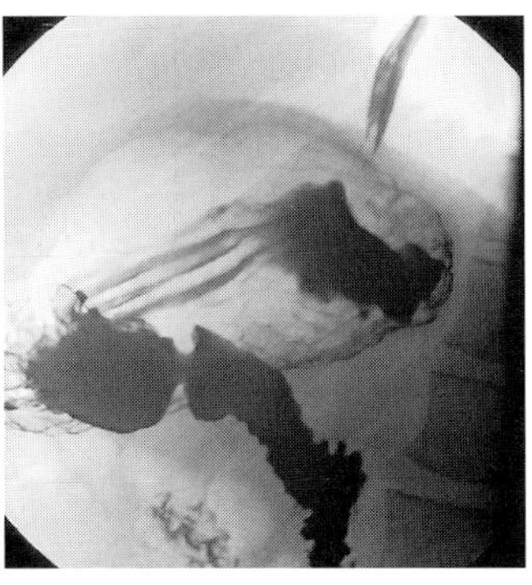

**Figure 5.18d** Right lateral

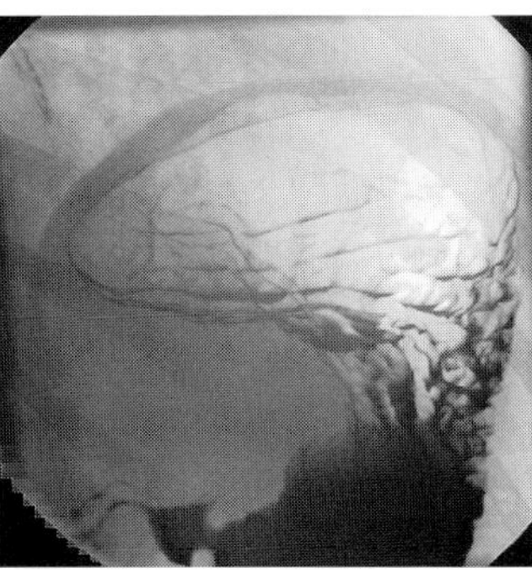

**Figure 5.18e** Left posterior oblique (erect)

### Imaging procedure

The technique used varies considerably, depending on the condition of the patient and the preference of the individual radiologist. The examination, however, will consist of a standard imaging protocol, with images acquired in a specific sequence in predetermined positions, in order that the whole of the stomach mucosa is visualised in double contrast effect. In practice, precise patient positioning is achieved under fluoroscopic control and the sequence and positions described here should be only seen as a guide. If prescribed, an intravenous injection of a smooth muscle relaxant is administered during the procedure.

The technique and positioning assumes the use of undercouch image intensification equipment.

Immediately prior to the start of the procedure the patient is asked to swallow an effervescent agent together with 10 ml of a gas-releasing solution to produce $CO_2$ gas. This takes immediate effect and the patient is warned not to expel the gas.

The fluoroscopy table is placed in the vertical position and the patient stands initially with back to the table (facing the X-ray tube).

Image acquisition is made in the following manner. The patient is rotated 20–30° onto the left side to assume the left posterior oblique position. The patient is asked to swallow 70 ml of barium suspension in two or three large mouthfuls in order to form a bolus which distends the oesophagus. The barium is observed by fluoroscopy as it passes down the oesophagus and images are usually recorded showing the oesophagus filled with barium as it enters the stomach at the cardiac orifice.

The table is then placed in the horizontal position and the patient is rotated through 360° (left side down → prone → right side down → supine) to coat the gastric mucosa.

In the supine position an anteroposterior image is acquired, demonstrating the body of the stomach with its lesser and greater curvatures coated with barium.

The patient is turned onto the left side in the left posterior oblique position, at a steep angle, so that images may be acquired showing double contrast views of the duodenal cap and loop. (It may be advantageous to bring the patient semi-erect to assist dilatation of the duodenal cap with air.)

With the table horizontal the patient is turned prone for postero-anterior images showing the fundus of the stomach filled with barium, and any gastro-oesophageal reflux and single contrast views of the duodenal cap.

The patient is then turned into the right lateral position for an image of the lesser curvature the stomach *en face*.

Finally, the table is moved into the erect position and a left posterior oblique projection is taken to demonstrate the fundus of the stomach filled with gas.

# 5 Stomach and Small Bowel

## Hypotonic duodenography

Hypotonic duodenography is the examination of the duodenum in its flaccid state. It provides additional information of the duodenal loop, but the procedure has been largely replaced by endoscopy combined with conventional CT of the pancreas.

It is usually performed as part of a conventional double contrast barium meal, but if required the patient may be intubated and barium placed directly into the duodenum. This can result in improved visualisation of the duodenum unobstructed by the overlying barium-filled stomach.

The patient is not allowed to eat or drink for 5 h before the examination.

The examination must be performed under fluoroscopic control with equipment similar to that described for the double contrast barium meal.

### Indications

Duodenal lesions, lesions of the head of the pancreas and evaluation of superior mesenteric artery syndrome.

### Imaging procedure

*Double contrast barium meal method*

Barium suspension and $CO_2$ gas is given as described for the double contrast barium meal on page 155. However, to overcome peristalsis the smooth muscle relaxant is administered intravenously when the duodenum is full of barium.

At this stage the imaging couch is brought to the horizontal and the patient turned from the supine position into the left posterior oblique position. This allows barium to drain from the second part of the duodenum which fills with gas to produce the double contrast effect. With the aid of fluoroscopy, images are acquired at different degrees of rotation.

*Intubation method*

A duodenal catheter is passed through the nose and directed through the stomach into the lower part of the duodenum. Approximately 50 ml of barium suspension is introduced through the catheter.

The patient is given the intravenous smooth muscle relaxant. Air is injected through the catheter and images are acquired in the supine, left posterior and prone positions.

*Contrast medium and injection data*

| *Volume* | *Concentration* | *Flow rate* |
|---|---|---|
| 70–150 ml | Low-viscous/high-density 250% w/v barium suspension | Oral |

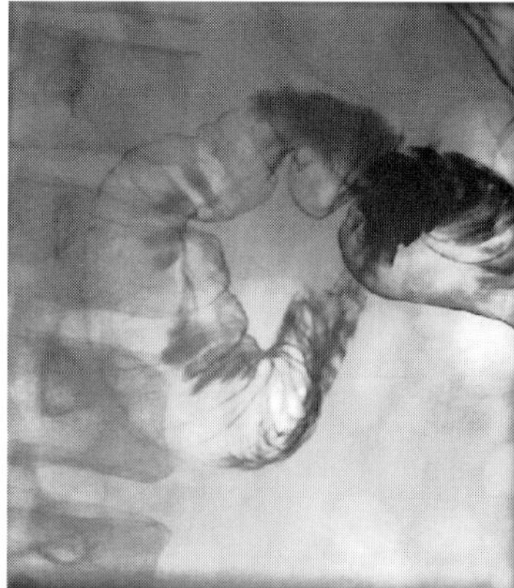

**Figure 5.19a** Duodenal loop demonstrated as part of a double contrast barium meal

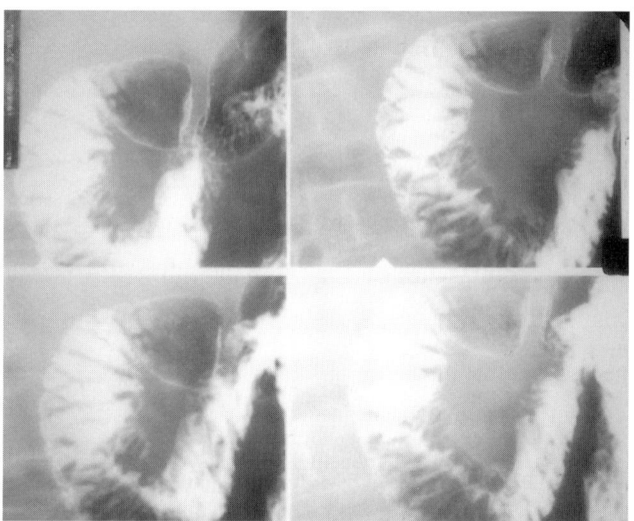

**Figure 5.19b** Composite image showing duodenal cap and loop

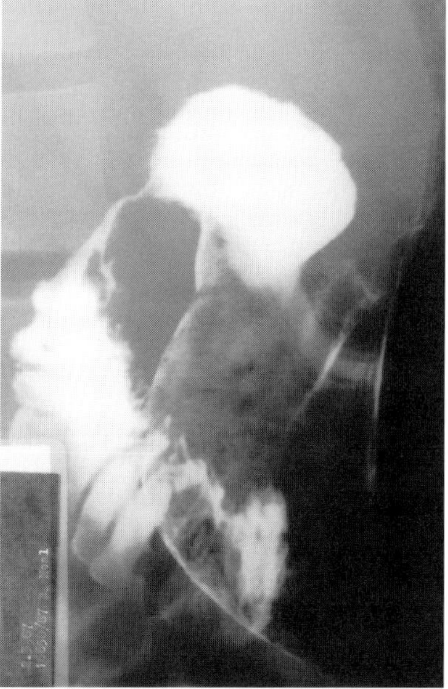

**Figure 5.19c** Duodenal loop showing stricture

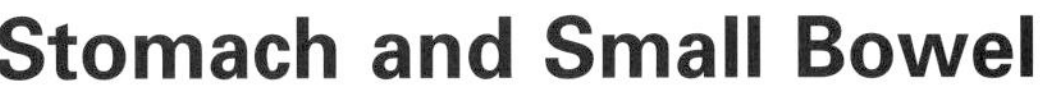


## Barium follow-through

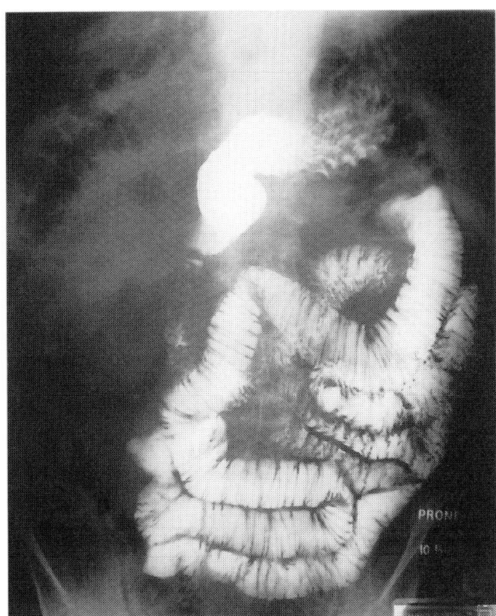

**Figure 5.20a** Ten-minute post-contrast image showing stomach, duodenum and proximal filling of the jejunum

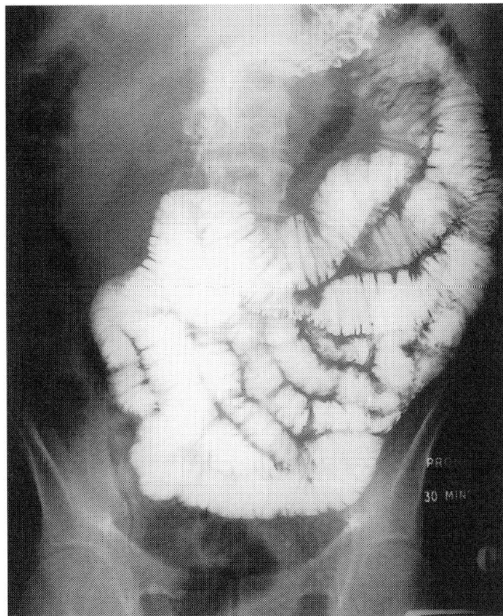

**Figure 5.20b** Thirty-minute post-contrast image showing mid-filling of the jejunum

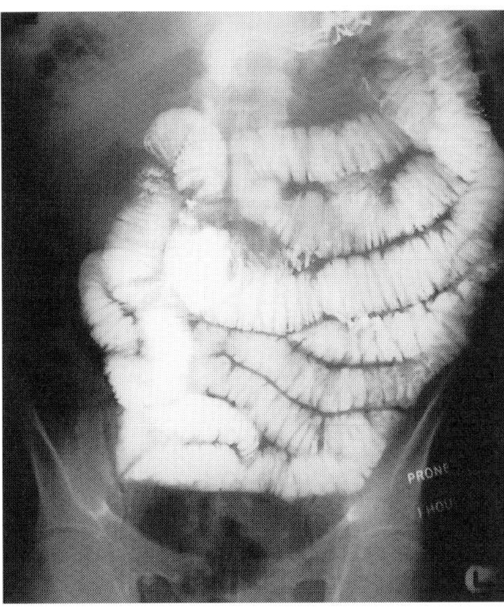

**Figure 5.20c** One-hour post-contrast image showing proximal filling of the ileum

**(a)–(c) Barium follow-through examination showing normal distribution of barium with no flocculation and normal mucosal folds**

The barium follow-through, as the name suggests, is used to demonstrate the whole of the small intestine.

A double contrast technique is normally adopted and the procedure employs both fluoroscopy and permanent image recording.

The patient is not allowed to eat or drink for at least 5 h before the examination and is warned that the examination may require their attendance in the imaging department for most of the day.

### Indications

Crohn's disease is perhaps the most common indication for undertaking a barium follow-through. Other lesions which have proved difficult to diagnose by other techniques, such as strictures, neoplasms and Meckel's diverticulum, may also benefit from this study.

### Contraindications

Suspected or actual perforation of the gastrointestinal tract and in cases of distal large bowel obstruction.

### Imaging procedure

The barium follow-through may accompany a barium meal examination or may be undertaken as a stand-alone procedure.

For the stand-alone procedure a 250–300 ml drink is prepared, consisting of a suspension of barium sulphate, water and an effervescent agent. The actual quantities of each constituent will depend on the local protocol.

Some centres use a canned carbonated barium suspension agent diluted 50/50 with water and added Gastrografin which acts as an accelerator.

Following the drink the patient may lie in the right lateral decubitus position to promote gastric emptying.

A high kVp technique increases the range of densities visualised on the radiograph, as well as reducing exposure time and minimising patient dose.

A series of conventional overcouch radiographs of the abdomen, with the patient normally in the prone position, are taken until the barium reaches the terminal ileum. The actual time varies considerably between patients.

The first radiograph is taken 10 min following the drink, with the second image at the 30 min stage. Radiographs are then taken at 30 min intervals until the barium has reached the terminal ileum.

Once the barium has reached the terminal ileum, fluoroscopic examination of the ileocaecal area is necessary to complete the procedure.

Fluoroscopy may also be necessary at any stage during the procedure, with compression employed to acquire optimum images at specific sites along the small bowel.

# 5 Stomach and Small Bowel

## Barium follow-through

### Postero-anterior projection (prone)

A series of postero-anterior radiographs of the abdomen are required to image the small bowel in its entirety as the barium and gas mixture progresses through the bowel from the stomach to the terminal ileum.

Radiographs showing the terminal ilium are taken with a non-opaque pad pressed firmly into the right iliac fossa to improve visualisation of this region. Alternatively, fluoroscopy and the use of compression is used to visualise the ileocaecal valve. Permanent images are then recorded either digitally on laser film, on 100/105 mm camera film or with film/cassette systems using rare earth screens.

*Position of patient and imaging modality*

The patient lies prone on the X-ray table and is adjusted so that the median sagittal plane is perpendicular to the table top.

A 35 × 45 cm cassette is positioned longitudinally in the cassette tray to include the diaphragm superiorly. This position is adjusted downwards as the examination progresses.

*Direction and centring of the X-ray beam*

The vertical central ray is centred in the midline at the level of the lower costal margin. This centring point is adjusted downwards as the examination progresses.

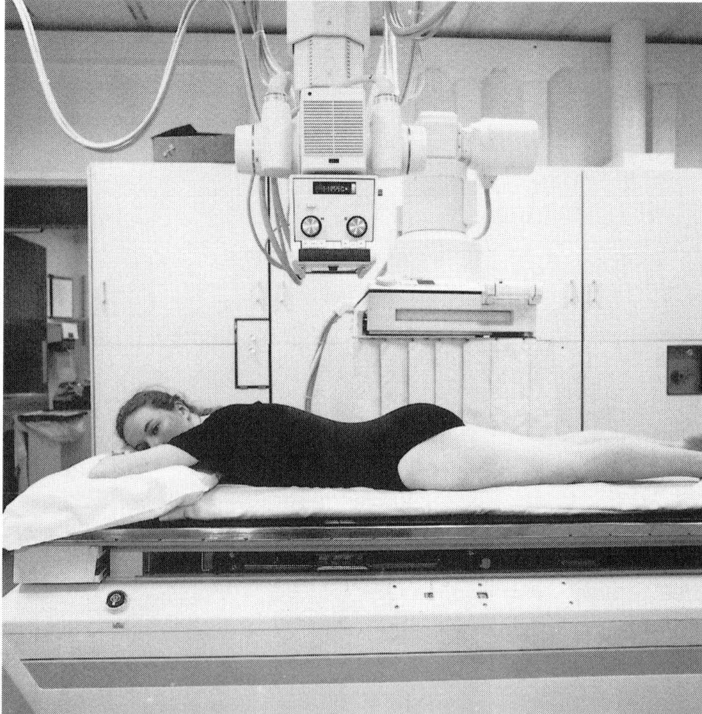

**Figure 5.21a** Patient in prone position

### Postero-anterior (terminal ileum)

*Position of patient and imaging modality*

The patient lies prone on the X-ray table and is adjusted so that the mid-clavicular line on the right side corresponds to the centre of the cassette. A non-opaque pad is pressed firmly into the right iliac fossa to improve visualisation of the terminal ileum.

A 24 × 30 cm cassette is positioned longitudinally in the cassette tray and centred on the iliac crest.

It may be necessary to place the patient in the left anterior oblique position, but this can only be assessed following fluoroscopy or once the prone radiograph has been studied.

*Direction and centring of the X-ray beam*

The vertical central ray is centred in the mid-clavicular line on the right side at the level of the iliac crest.

*Contrast medium and injection data*

| *Volume* | *Concentration* | *Flow rate* |
|---|---|---|
| 250–300 ml | 70% w/v | Oral |

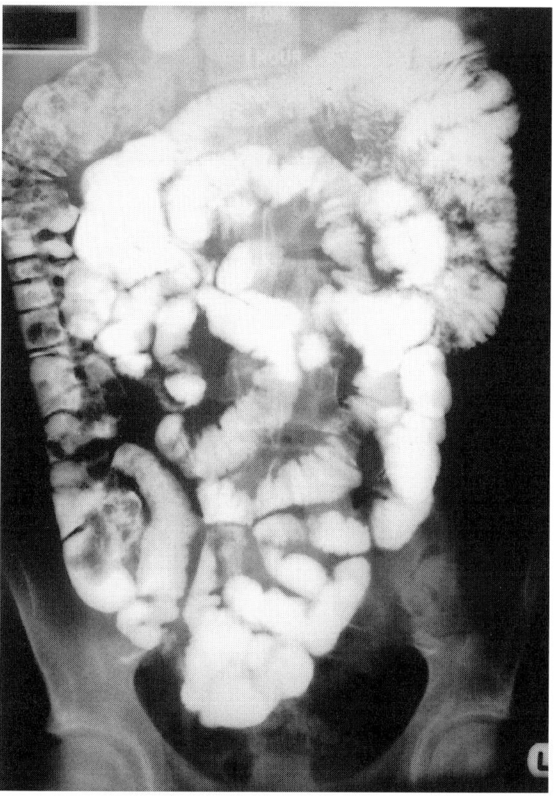



**Figure 5.21b** Prone radiograph taken 1 h after contrast administration showing barium in the terminal ileum

## Small bowel enema

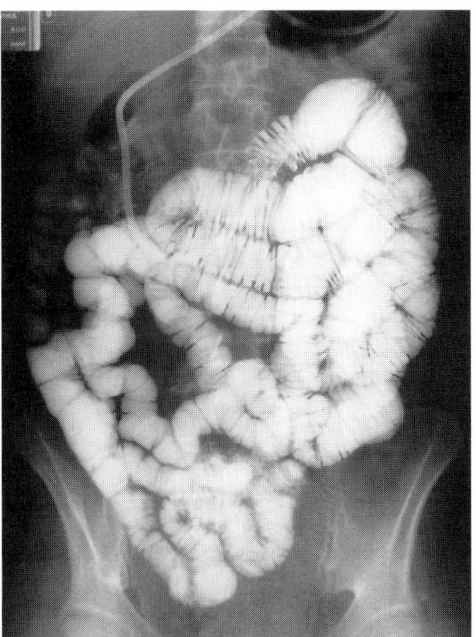

**Figure 5.22a** Enteroclysis (single contrast) small bowel enema

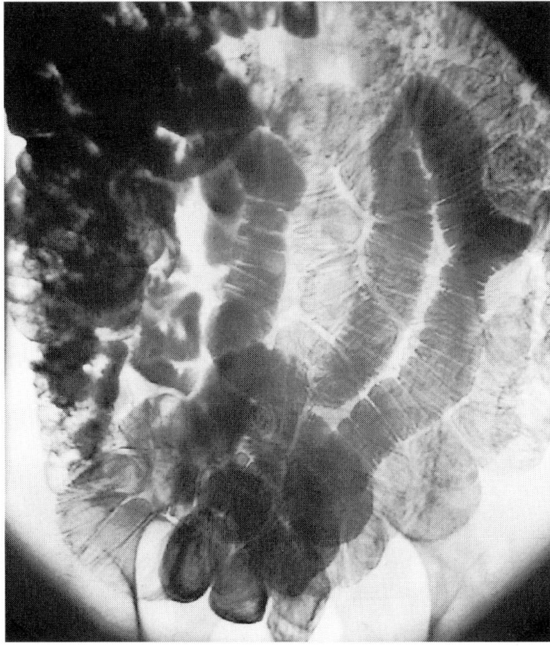

**Figure 5.22b** Normal double contrast small bowel barium enema showing a column of barium filling the distal bowel and methylcellulose filling the proximal bowel, producing a double contrast effect. Bowel loops are well demonstrated and there is no mucosal thickening

The small bowel enema is arguably the ideal method for investigating the small bowel. It is, however, both invasive and time consuming.

The small bowel is demonstrated following duodenal intubation rather than by oral administration of contrast as in the barium follow-through. This results in improved visualisation of the small bowel, unobstructed by the overlying barium-filled stomach and duodenum.

Either a single contrast (enteroclysis) or double contrast method using methylcellulose may be employed.

### Indications

Suspected small bowel disease, e.g. Crohn's disease. Recurrent or chronic small bowel obstruction. Recurrent or chronic intestinal blood loss.

### Patient preparation

The patient is starved for 8–12 h prior to the examination to ensure that the flow of barium is not retarded by residual remnants of food in the ileum. Laxatives are administered to ensure a clean colon.

### Imaging procedure

For the single contrast method, approximately 1000 ml of dilute cool barium (10°C) is mixed in an administration set and suspended from a drip stand. For the double contrast method, 150–200 ml of barium is administered, followed by up to 2 litres of a 0.5% solution of methylcellulose.

The patient lies supine on the X-ray table and a duodenal catheter or nasogastric tube is inserted under fluoroscopic control until the tip is in the duodenojejunal flexure.

The barium suspension is then infused by gravity. With the single contrast method this may be followed by a similar quantity of cold water to accelerate the passage of the barium towards the terminal ileum. With the double contrast method a methylcellulose solution is infused at the rate of 100 ml/min until the terminal ileum is shown in double contrast.

Fluoroscopy is performed during the infusion and images are recorded using digital acquisition, 100/105 mm film or full-size radiographs as required.

The patient is turned prone once the column of barium has reached the terminal ileum, and fluoroscopy/radiographs are taken using the same technique described in the barium follow-through.

Following the single contrast method, air may be introduced via the catheter once the barium has reached the caecum to provide a double contrast effect.

Patients are warned that they may suffer from diarrhoea following the examination.

*Contrast medium and injection data*

| | *Volume* | *Concentration* | *Flow rate* |
|---|---|---|---|
| Single Contrast | 1000 ml | 19% w/v | 75 ml/min |
| Double Contrast | 150–200 ml | 150% w/v | 100 ml/min |

Followed by up to 2 litres of a 0.5% solution of methylcellulose infused at the rate of 100 ml/min.

# Angiography

Angiography is used to demonstrate the blood supply to the stomach, small and large bowel by selective catheterisation of the coeliac axis, and superior and inferior mesenteric arteries.

The coeliac axis arises from the anterior aspect of the abdominal aorta at the level of the 12th thoracic vertebra, just below the diaphragm. It is 1.25 cm long and divides into the left gastric, hepatic and splenic arteries.

The superior mesenteric artery arises from the anterior aspect of the abdominal aorta about 1 cm below the coeliac trunk at the level of the transpyloric plane. It supplies the whole of the small intestine (except the superior part of the duodenum), the caecum, the ascending colon and most of the transverse colon.

The inferior mesenteric artery is smaller than the superior mesenteric and arises from the abdominal aorta 3–4 cm above its bifurcation. It supplies the left third of the transverse colon, the descending colon, the sigmoid colon and the rectum.

Angiography is best performed using dedicated angiography equipment together with digital imaging or a 35 × 35 cm rapid film changer.

A non-ionic water-soluble contrast agent is used.

### Indications

Angiography is used primarily to investigate gastrointestinal bleeding or ischaemia. It may also be used to demonstrate tumour circulation.

### Imaging procedure

A flush aortogram may be performed before selective catheterisation of the appropriate artery.

A Seldinger technique is used to introduce a straight or pigtail catheter (size 5F). The tip is positioned under fluoroscopic control until it is situated just above the coeliac axis.

A bolus of contrast is injected using a pressure injector and the resultant films processed.

Selective catheterisation of the coeliac axis, and superior and inferior mesenteric arteries, is performed using a sidewinder, cobra or headhunter catheter, depending on local anatomy.

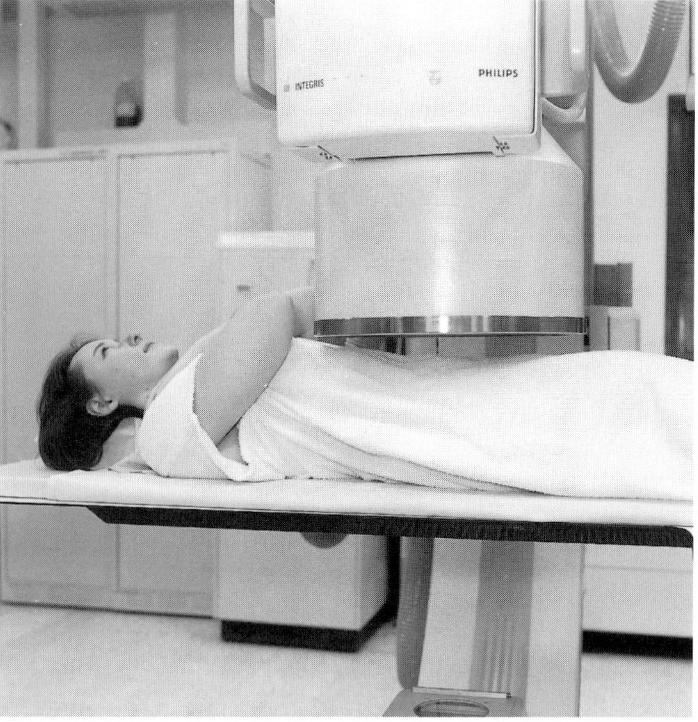


**Figure 5.23a** The angiography table

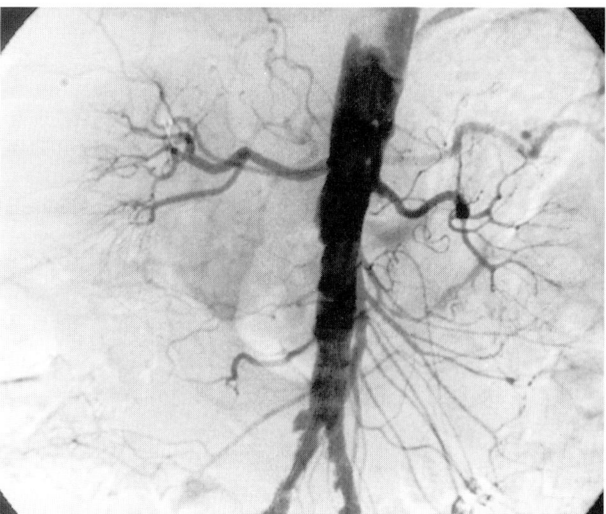

**Figure 5.23b** Flush aortogram

## Angiography

Figure 5.24a Coeliac axis arteriogram

Figure 5.24b Superior mesenteric arteriogram

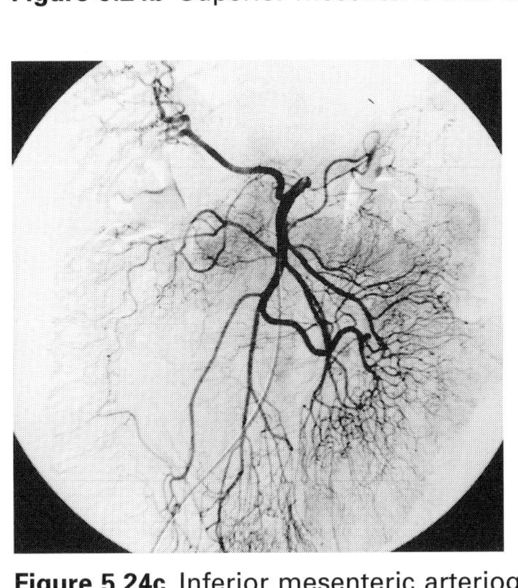

Figure 5.24c Inferior mesenteric arteriogram

### Coeliac axis arteriography

| *Image/s* | *Run time* | *Total images* |
|---|---|---|
| 2 | 3 s | 6 |
| 0.5 | 4 s | 2 |

Exposure delay 0.5 s.

*Contrast medium and injection data*

| *Volume* | *Concentration* | *Flow rate* |
|---|---|---|
| 25–30 ml | 300 mgI/ml | 10 ml/s |

In DSA the concentration may be reduced.

*Position of patient and imaging modality*

The patient lies supine in the centre of the imaging table. The X-ray tube and image intensifier are positioned under fluoroscopic control at the level of the transpyloric plane or lower if a selective inferior mesenteric arteriogram is performed. Once the catheter is in position, imaging commences. For rapid serial radiography using a film changer on a C-arm system the equipment is rotated into position, or if conventional angiography equipment is being used the patient and tube are moved into position over the 35 × 35 cm rapid film changer.

*Direction and centring of the X-ray beam*

A vertical central ray is centred in the midline at the level of the lower costal margin for the coeliac and superior mesenteric arteriogram or at the level of the transcrestal line for an inferior mesenteric.

The patient may be adjusted 8 cm to the left or right for selective gastric catheterisation.

*Imaging parameters*

Image sequences are controlled by the speed of blood flow observed during fluoroscopy and by the preference of individual radiologists. The following protocols should be seen as a guide.

### Inferior mesenteric arteriogram

| *Image/s* | *Run time* | *Total images* |
|---|---|---|
| 2 | 4 s | 8 |
| 1 | 4 s | 4 |

Exposure delay 2 s.

*Contrast medium and injection data*

| *Volume* | *Concentration* | *Flow rate* |
|---|---|---|
| 12 ml | 300 mg/Iml | 3 ml/s |

### Superior mesenteric arteriogram

| *Image/s* | *Run time* | *Total images* |
|---|---|---|
| 2 | 3 s | 6 |
| 0.5 | 4 s | 2 |

Exposure delay 1 s.

*Contrast medium and injection data*

| *Volume* | *Concentration* | *Flow rate* |
|---|---|---|
| 25 ml | 300 mg/Iml | 5 ml/s |

In DSA the concentration may be reduced.

# 5 Stomach and Small Bowel

## Radionuclide imaging – gastric emptying

Radionuclide imaging offers an excellent means of studying gastric emptying following a liquid, solid or semi-solid meal which has been labelled with a radioactive isotope. When studying liquid emptying, a drink in the form of a $^{99m}$Tc tin colloid mixed in warm milk or fruit juice is prepared. For solid food a meal such as $^{99m}$Tc tin colloid in scrambled egg or $^{99m}$Tc bran is prepared. Semi-solid food is prepared using either a milk and food mixture, porridge or soup mixed with a $^{99m}$Tc tin colloid. To study liquid and solid gastric emptying simultaneously, it is necessary to label the liquid and solid components with different radionuclides, with different characteristic energies.

Patients are required to fast for 4 h prior to the procedure, avoid smoking as this promotes gastric emptying, and to stop any drugs prescribed to promote gastric motility or emptying.

Imaging using liquid, semi-solid or solid food, or a combination of liquid and solid foods, can be performed using one of a number of acquisition protocols. A plain dynamic acquisition is commonly used, but the measurement of emptying rate will be inaccurate because of changes in attenuation effects due to the forward movement of the meal in the abdomen as the stomach empties. This effect is quite marked for a low-energy radionuclide such as $^{99m}$Tc. Dynamic acquisitions can have attenuation correction applied to compensate for changing attenuation. Alternatively, multiple anterior and posterior static image pairs can be acquired, and the data combined to remove attenuation effects.

If a dual-headed camera is available, anterior and posterior dynamic or static images can be acquired simultaneously.

### Indications

Abnormalities following gastric surgery such as dumping syndrome, diarrhoea and gastric stasis. Additionally, it is also indicated following certain drug medication, obesity and diet control associated with diabetics.

### Position of patient and imaging modality

*Plain dynamic image acquisition*

Dynamic images are acquired most frequently from the anterior side, with the patient in a sitting, standing or in a semi-recumbent position. The height of the camera head is adjusted to centralise the stomach in the field of view.

When investigating dumping syndrome, the study is performed with the patient prone, to allow the stomach to move forwards, which is the ideal position following vagotomy.

*Dynamic image acquisition with attenuation correction*

Dynamic images are acquired most frequently from the anterior side, with the patient in a sitting, standing or semi-recumbent position. The height of the camera head is adjusted to centralise the stomach in the field of view. A left lateral static view with the patient in the same position as for the dynamic image, and with the left side against the collimator, is also taken as part of the imaging protocol. In this position the left arm is positioned across the chest with the left hand gripping the right shoulder and the patient adjusted to ensure that the stomach and the anterior or posterior skin surface through which the dynamic images were acquired are both within the camera field of view.

*Multiple alternate anterior and posterior static images*

Anterior and posterior static images may be performed with the patient standing or sitting. For the anterior view the patient faces the camera and for the posterior view is positioned with back to the camera. Again the camera height is adjusted to centralise the stomach in the field of view.

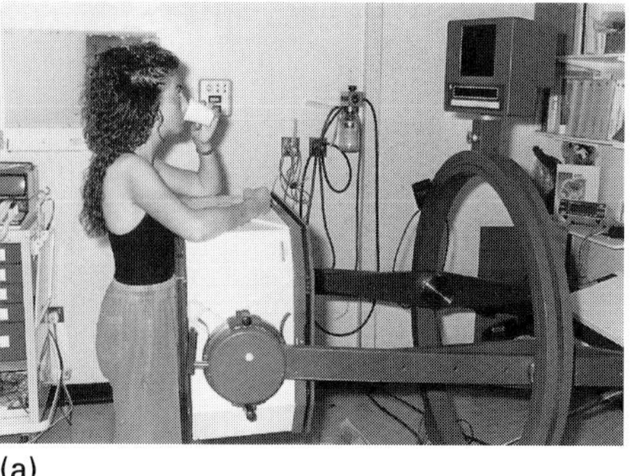

(a)

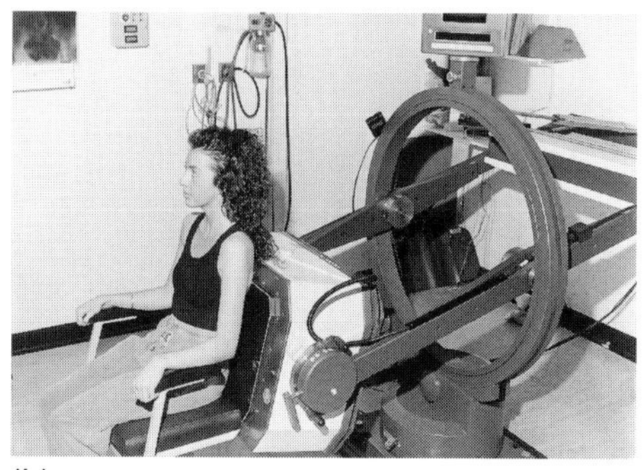

(b)

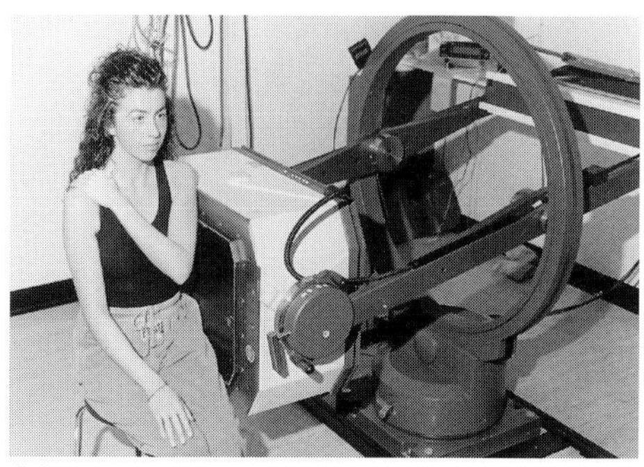

(c)

 **Figure 5.25** (a)–(c) Radionuclide imaging equipment postioned for (a) anterior, (b) posterior and (c) lateral views

### Imaging procedure

A single-headed gamma camera protocol is described using a low-energy general-purpose collimator.

*Plain dynamic image acquisition*

The patient is positioned in front of the camera and asked to drink or swallow the prepared liquid or food labelled with $^{99m}$Tc, as quickly as is comfortable. Image acquisition is initiated as the patient begins to consume the test meal. The dynamic imaging protocol is divided into two phases, the first consisting of 30 frames in rapid succession, with each frame acquired over a 10-second period, and a second phase of 1-minute frames for a period up to 2 h, terminated at any time if emptying is observed to be complete.

*Dynamic image acquisition with attenuation correction*

This is divided into two phases, a 'dynamic phase' to study gastric emptying and a 'static phase' at the end of the dynamic phase to acquire a static lateral image of the stomach. This is used to calculate attenuation factors for the emptying study. The dynamic phase is acquired as for the plain dynamic study.

Following the dynamic study a left lateral static image of the stomach is acquired after the patient has swallowed 200 ml of water mixed with tin colloid labelled with $^{99m}$Tc. During the 300 s acquisition a $^{99m}$Tc marker source is traced down the skin surface to delineate the position of the skin relative to the stomach so that it can clearly be seen on the image.

*Multiple alternate anterior and posterior static images*

After the patient has swallowed the prepared drink or meal they are positioned for anterior and posterior paired views of the stomach at 5–10 min intervals during the emptying phase. Each image acquisition is set for 1 min.

### Image analysis

The purpose of the procedure is to determine the half-time ($t_{1/2}$) of emptying which is achieved in computer software. For dynamic acquisitions the software sums the frames required for delineation of the stomach region of interest (ROI) and after attenuation correction, if applicable, produces a gastric emptying curve plotting counts/s against time. For static image acquisition, ROIs are drawn around the stomach on each anterior and posterior image pair in order to calculate the geometric mean count rate for the stomach. This is repeated for each image pair over the period of emptying.

Gastric emptying rates are affected by the volume, calorific value and composition of the meal. For comparable results it is important that a constant technique is established and a normal range determined. As an example, for a meal consisting of porridge it is suggested that a half emptying time of less than 30 min is abnormally rapid, while a half emptying time of more than 60 min is strongly suggestive of abnormal emptying and that of 90 min or over being certainly abnormal.

*Imaging and radiopharmaceutical parameters*

| *Liquid/Type* | *Administered activity* | *Principal energy* |
|---|---|---|
| $^{99m}$Tc tin colloid in 200 ml warm milk | 10 MBq | 140 keV |
| *Window width* | *Acquisition counts/time* | |
| 20% | As above | |

*Solid and semi-solid*

| *Type* | *Administered activity* | *Principal energy* |
|---|---|---|
| $^{99m}$Tc tin colloid in test meal | 10 MBq | 140 keV |
| *Window width* | *Acquisition counts/time* | |
| 20% | As above | |

*Left lateral static image for attenuation correction*

$^{99m}$Tc tin colloid in 200 ml water (3 MBq, 140 keV)

(a)

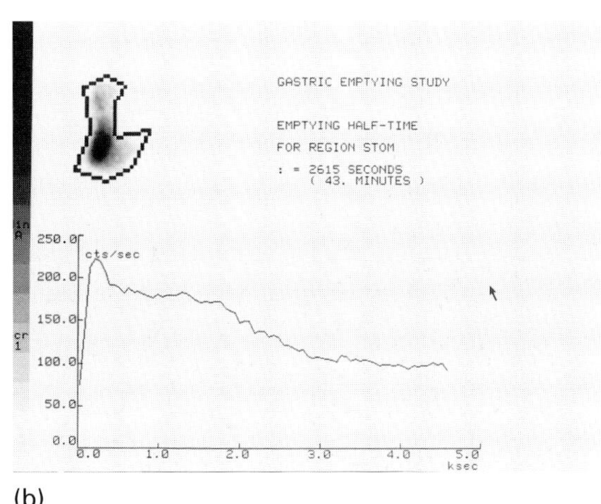


(b)

**Figure 5.26** (a,b) Gastric emptying study showing selection of frames from a dynamic acquisition and a gastric emptying curve

# 5 Alimentary System

## Large Bowel

The large bowel comprises the colon and rectum. It is approximately 150 cm in length and its diameter varies between 3 and 9 cm.

The caecum, or blind end of the colon, lies in the right iliac fossa extending slightly, 6 cm below the ileocaecal valve.

The appendix, which is a blind-ended tube 3–12 cm long, projects from the inferior and medial end of the caecum.

The ascending colon passes upwards from the ileocaecal valve to the under-surface of the liver, where it bends to form the hepatic flexure. It continues as the transverse colon, passing across the upper abdomen from the right to the left side along the under-surface of the liver.

On the left side the transverse colon passes upwards and backwards towards the left hemidiaphragm to form the splenic flexure which then bends downwards, becoming the descending colon.

The descending colon passes downwards on the left side of the abdomen to the iliac crest where it bends towards the midline to form the sigmoid colon.

The sigmoid colon is S-shaped and curves posteriorly in front of the sacrum, ending in the rectum.

The rectum is a slightly dilated portion of the colon and is approximately 13 cm long. It leads from the sigmoid colon and terminates at the anus.

The transverse and sigmoid colons have mesenteries, but the ascending and descending colons are fixed to the posterior abdominal wall.

### Recommended imaging procedures

Following plain abdominal radiography, the double contrast barium enema examination is the radiological examination of choice.

Angiography may be used in cases of acute bleeding. Details of mesenteric angiography will be found in the previous section on stomach and small bowel.

Computed tomography is useful in certain recurrent carcinomas and the investigation of acute diverticulitis, but is not the first-line investigation.

Ultrasound suffers from the problem of gas–tissue interface and is hence not the modality of choice. It may, however, be used in cases of tumour to assess bowel wall thickness (doughnut sign) or in cases of suspected abscess.

Radionuclide imaging can be used to locate gastrointestinal bleeding and Meckel's diverticulum.

Radiolabelled leucocyte imaging can also be used in cases of intra-abdominal infection (see Chapter 11). At the time of writing, MRI has so far found little application in the investigation of the large bowel.

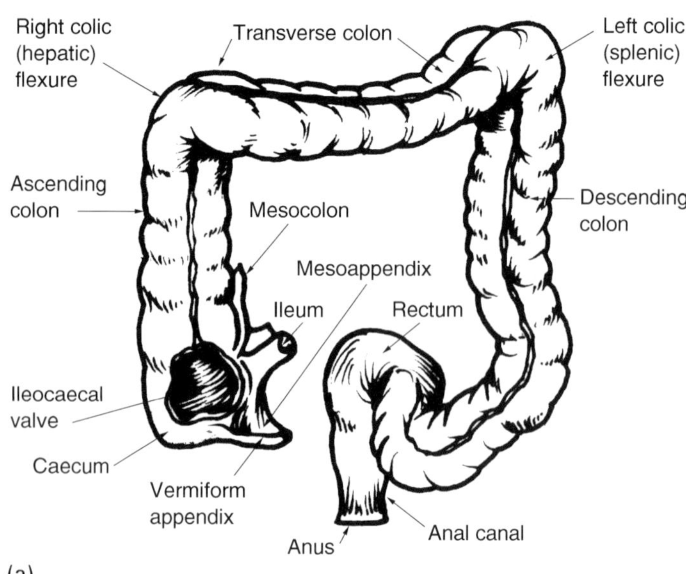


(a)

(b)

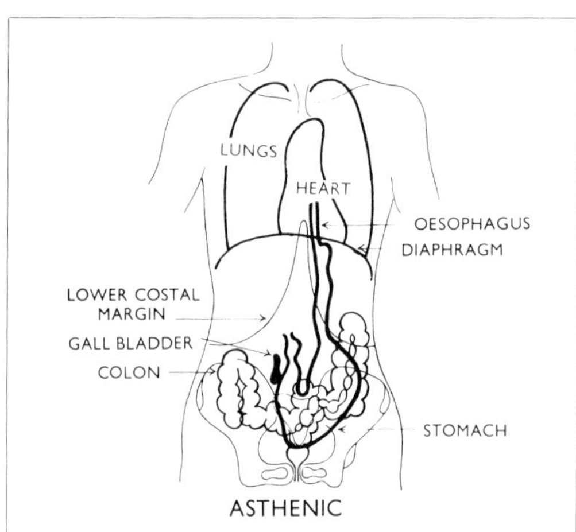


(c)

**Figure 5.27** (a) Large bowel – anterior aspect; (b,c) variation in position of abdominal content in different subject types

## Double contrast barium enema

The large bowel is visualised by fluoroscopy and images taken at intervals following the administration of barium via the rectum. The double contrast barium enema has superseded the single contrast barium enema as the routine method for the examination of the colon.

Modern digital fluoroscopic equipment is the equipment of choice, offering advantages in larger field of view, improved image quality and reduced dose. A conventional or remote control screening table is employed. Alternatively, conventional image intensification with 100/105 mm camera or film/cassettes are used to record permanent images of the bowel. Additionally, following fluoroscopy images may also be recorded using large film/cassette combinations and a standard ceiling tube suspension system.

For the decubitus projections, a wedge-shaped filter, attached to the light beam diaphragm, may be employed to overcome the differences in abdominal thickness and density when the patient is turned on to the side. The thickest part of the wedge will absorb some of the radiation which would have been incident on the least dense uppermost half of the abdomen. This has the effect of increasing the range of tissue densities that may be recorded within the useful density range of the film. Additionally, use of a high kVp for the decubitus projections increases the range of densities visualised on the radiograph.

### Patient preparation

Sigmoid- or colonoscopy should be performed before a barium enema, as it provides direct viewing of the mucosa. It may demonstrate evidence of colitis, thus obviating the need for full bowel preparation. Sigmoidoscopy is the examination of choice for lesions of the rectosigmoid, which has the highest incidence of adenomatous cancers and polyps.

The type of bowel preparation for the barium enema will vary considerably, dependent on the clinician's preference and the condition of the patient. In certain cases, e.g. ulcerative colitis, the barium enema may be performed with no preparation at all, although it is generally recognised that a good bowel preparation resulting in an 'empty bowel' is important. Most methods rely on a combination of dietary restriction and laxatives. Cleansing water enemas may be used to ensure a completely clean colon. Some fluid restriction in the hours immediately preceding the examination may improve coating because the mucosa will be drier.

Immediately prior to the examination the patient is given elbow pads to wear to reduce the risk of skin damage while being moved into many positions. The examination is also carefully explained and the patient encouraged to hold on to the barium while it is administered.

### Indications

Change of bowel habit, lower abdominal pain, rectal bleeding and palpable masses in the abdomen are all indications for barium enema examinations. Paediatric referrals include suspected intussusception and volvulus.

### Contraindications

In the examination of patients with suspected bowel perforation or fistula, demonstration with barium is contraindicated and a non-ionic water-soluble contrast agent is recommended.

### Administration technique

A high-density low-viscosity suspension of barium sulphate is used. Barium enema administration kits are available which comprise a polythene container for the barium suspension, connecting tubing and control valve, and a rectal catheter.

Warm water must be added to the barium powder/liquid in the polythene container to provide a suspension of suitable specific gravity. This varies, depending on the manufacturer and the clinician's requirements, but is usually between 400 and 600 ml. The administration kit also provides the facility for air insufflation. The polythene container is suspended from a dripstand approximately 1 m above the patient.

An intravenous smooth muscle relaxant may be administered to reduce spasm.

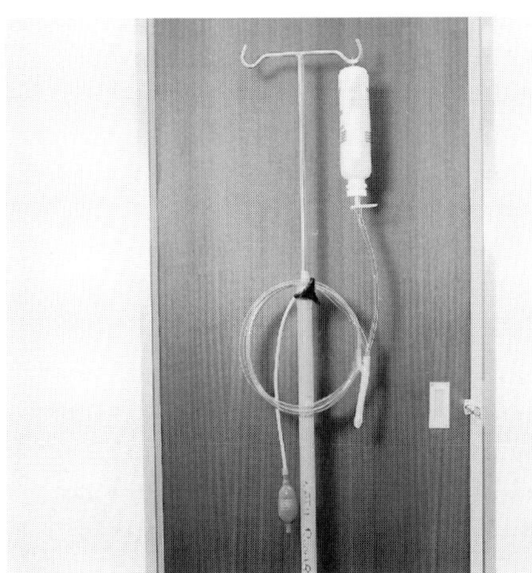

**Figure 5.28a** Typical barium enema administration set

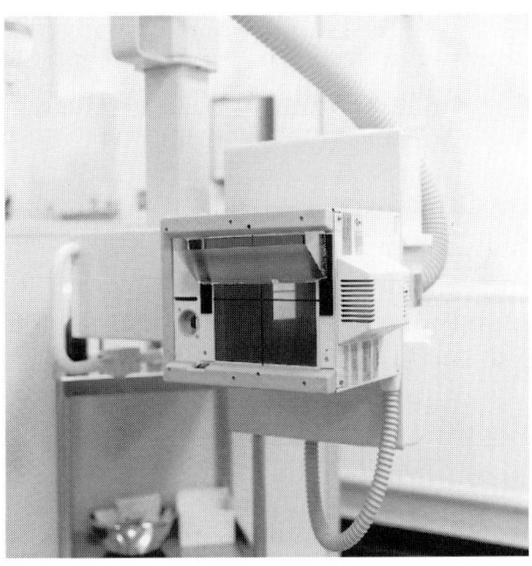

**Figure 5.28b** Wedge filter attached to light beam diaphragm

## Double contrast barium enema

**Imaging procedure**
The procedure may be divided into two phases:

- Fluorography phase, during which barium and air is administered to coat and outline the colon. Permanent images are recorded with the aid of fluoroscopy.
- Conventional radiography phase, during which additional full-size radiographs are taken to complete the examination.

*Fluorography phase*
The procedure assumes use of a conventional screening table and, if selected, 24 × 30 cm cassettes. The patient lies on the left side with the knees and hips flexed and a lubricated catheter is inserted approximately 4 cm into the rectum. (In the lateral position, the location of the catheter in female patients is confirmed under fluoroscopic control by administering a small quantity of barium to ensure that the catheter is seen in the rectum and not the vagina.)

The patient is turned prone, following which the barium suspension is run in slowly under fluoroscopic control until half of the transverse colon is well filled. At this stage the tubing is clamped and the patient is turned back on to the left side, with the head of the table raised so that the patient is approximately 20° head up. The barium container is then placed on the floor and the clamp removed. This allows excess barium to be drained from the colon. Air is now gently insufflated into the rectum to fill the colon.

The following sequence of projections is taken using fluoroscopy to ensure that the patient is in the optimum position to show the appropriate section of colon:

- **Right lateral** of the pelvic region, with the patient turned on the left side. This shows the rectum.
- **Right anterior oblique** of the pelvic region, with the patient first supine and then with the right side raised approximately 30°. This demonstrates the sigmoid.
- **Left posterior oblique** of the pelvic region, after the patient is first turned from the RAO position onto the right side and then prone. From the prone position the left side is raised approximately 30°. This demonstrates sections of the sigmoid not outlined with air in the RAO projection.
- **Left anterior oblique** of the left upper abdomen, with the head of the table raised so that the patient is almost erect. The patient stands with back to the table and with the left side raised approximately 30°. This demonstrates the splenic flexure.
- **Right anterior oblique** of the right upper abdomen, again with the patient almost erect, with the patient's back to the table but with the right side raised approximately 30°. This demonstrates the hepatic flexure.

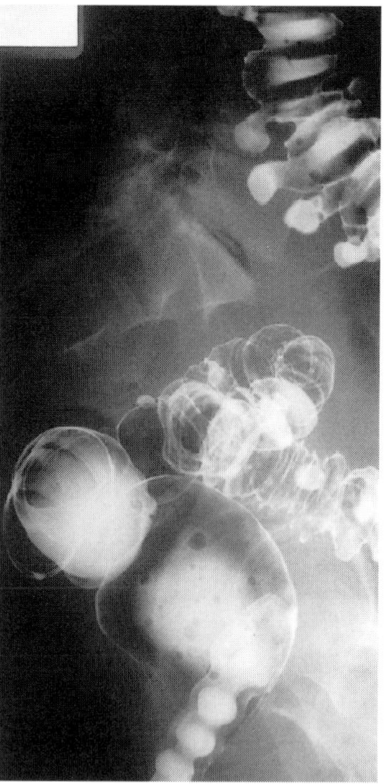

**Figure 5.29a** Right lateral image of rectum

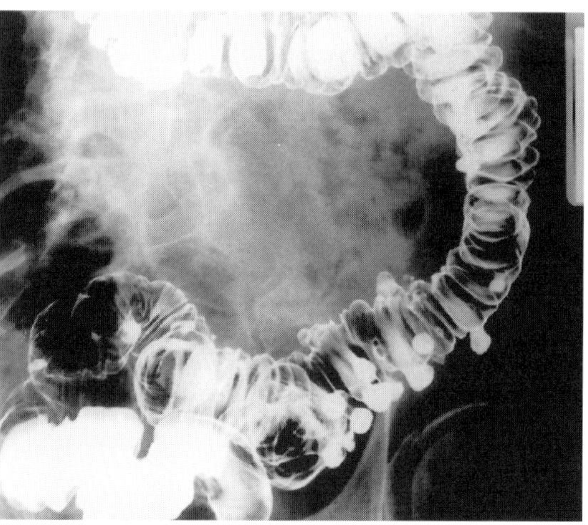

**Figure 5.29b** Right anterior oblique showing sigmoid (patient supine – right side raised)

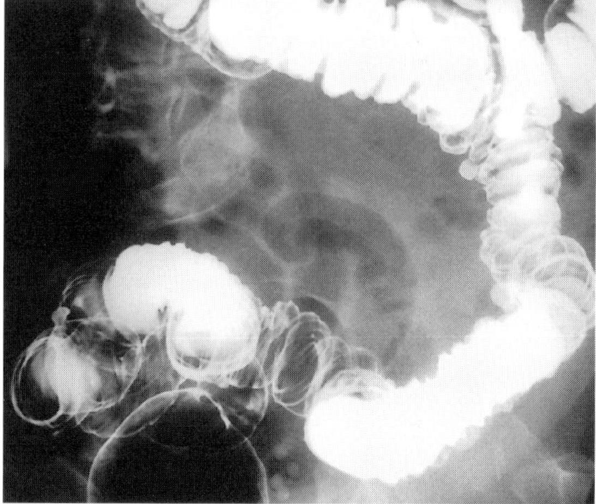

**Figure 5.29c** Left posterior oblique showing sigmoid (patient prone – left side raised)

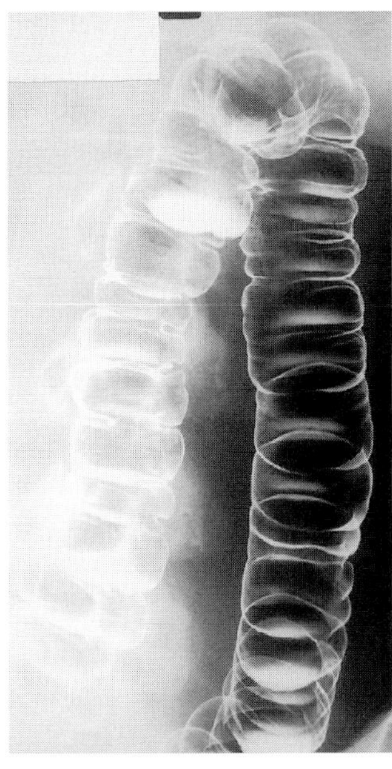

**Figure 5.30a** Left anterior oblique showing splenic flexure

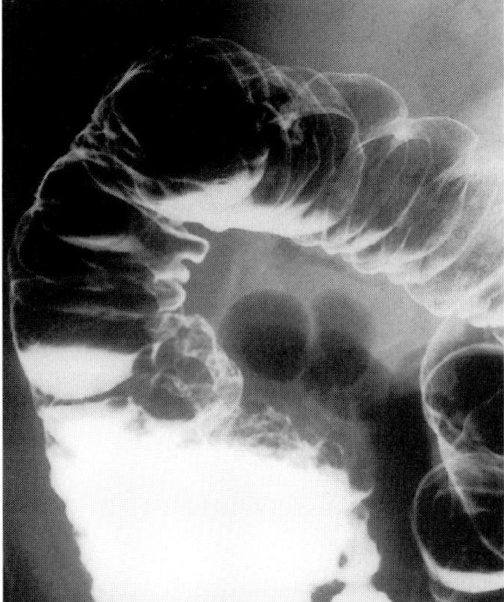

**Figure 5.30b** Right anterior oblique showing hepatic flexure

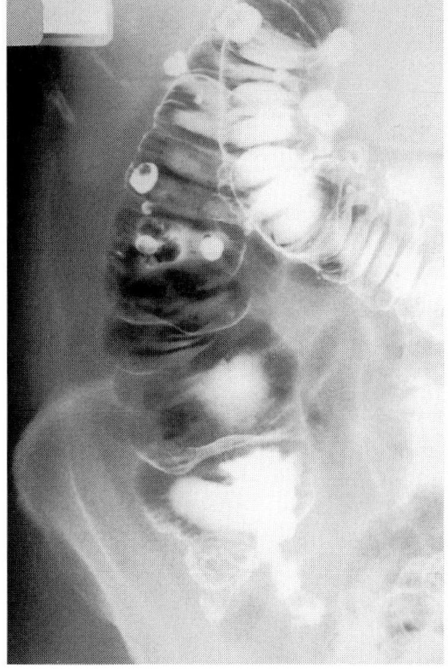

**Figure 5.30c** Right anterior oblique showing ileocaecal junction

### Ileocaecal junction

A projection of the caecum and the ileocaecal junction, filled with barium, is taken to complete the fluorography phase.

**Right anterior oblique** of the right abdominal region, with the patient positioned supine on the screening couch and the head end of the table lowered so that the patient is approximately 5–12° head down. This position displaces any excessive barium filling the caecum which would otherwise obscure the ileocaecal junction. The patient's right side is then raised until the junction is seen in profile. Alternatively, if there is difficulty in demonstrating the junction the patient is positioned prone and the left side raised. To ensure patient safety, grab handles are positioned on the table sides for the patient's use.

*Note*. Although the caecum can be difficult to demonstrate it is essential that the barium is observed in the caecum and appendix and particularly the ileocaecal junction to complete the examination.

Additional air insufflation may be required during the fluorography phase to ensure that all sections of the colon are demonstrated in double contrast relief.

### Conventional radiography phase

To complete examination of the colon, full-size radiographs of the abdomen are acquired using conventional overcouch equipment. For the decubitus projections, 35 × 43 cm grid cassettes are employed.

The projections which are described on the following pages include:

- **anteroposterior**
- **postero-anterior 30° caudad**
- **Left lateral decubitus**
- **Right lateral decubitus.**

Following inspection of both series of images, additional images may be required if the various sections are not adequately demonstrated.

### After-care

Following completion of the examination the catheter is carefully removed from the rectum and the patient escorted to the toilet.

Before the patient leaves the department at the end of the examination, they should be advised of the need to drink plenty of fluids and of the possibility of constipation. If a muscle relaxant has been used, the patient should be warned of the possibility of blurred vision.

## Double contrast barium enema

### Anteroposterior projection (supine)

This projection is used to demonstrate a general outline of the colon.

*Position of patient and imaging modality*
The patient lies supine on the fluoroscopy table with the median sagittal plane of the body at right angles to and in the midline of the table. Check that the anterior iliac spines are equidistant from the couch. The hands may be placed high on the chest or the arms may be by the patient's side, slightly away from the trunk. A 35 × 43 cm cassette is placed longitudinally in the Bucky tray and positioned to include the symphysis pubis, bearing in mind that the fact that the oblique rays will project the symphysis pubis downwards. The centre of the cassette will be almost at the level of the iliac crests in the mid-axillary line.

*Direction and centring of the X-ray beam*
The vertical central ray is directed to the centre of the film and the exposure is made on arrested expiration.

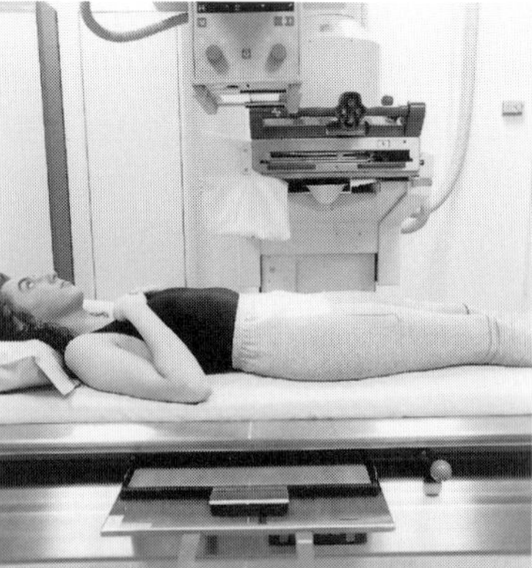

**Figure 5.31a** Patient in position for AP projection of abdomen

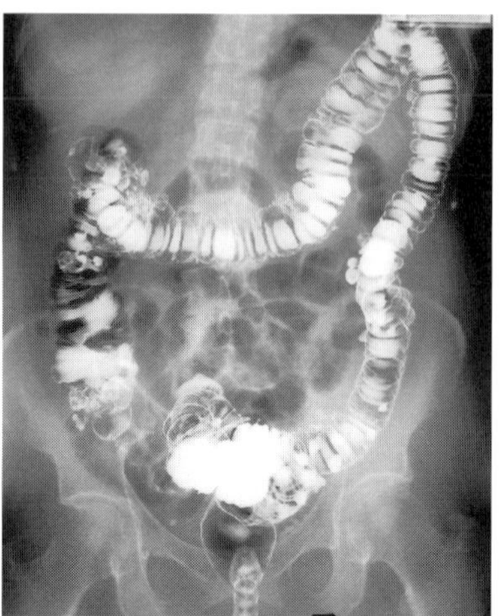

**Figure 5.31b** Anteroposterior radiograph showing double contrast barium enema

### Postero-anterior 30° caudad projection (prone)

This projection is used to demonstrate the rectosigmoid region, with the oblique rays unfolding the sigmoid loops.

*Position of patient and imaging modality*
The patient lies prone on the fluoroscopy table, with the median sagittal table perpendicular and coincident with the centre of the table. The pelvis is adjusted so that the anterior superior iliac spines are equidistant from the table top.

A 35 × 35 cm cassette is placed in the Bucky tray, with the upper border placed level with the iliac crests.

*Direction and centring of the X-ray beam*
The central ray is angled 30° caudally and directed to the centre of the film. The exposure is made on arrested respiration.

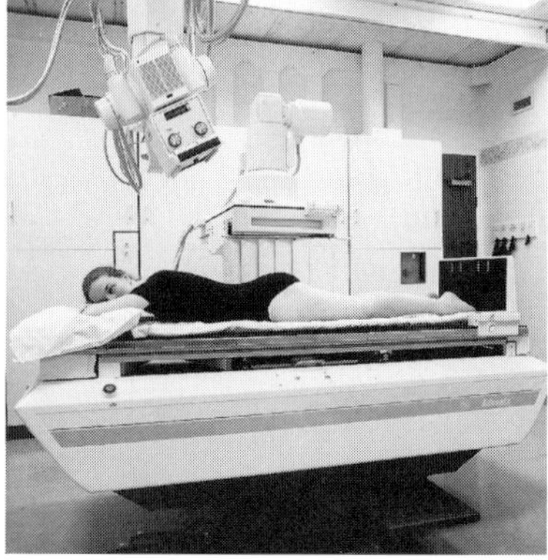

**Figure 5.31c** Patient in position for postero-anterior projection

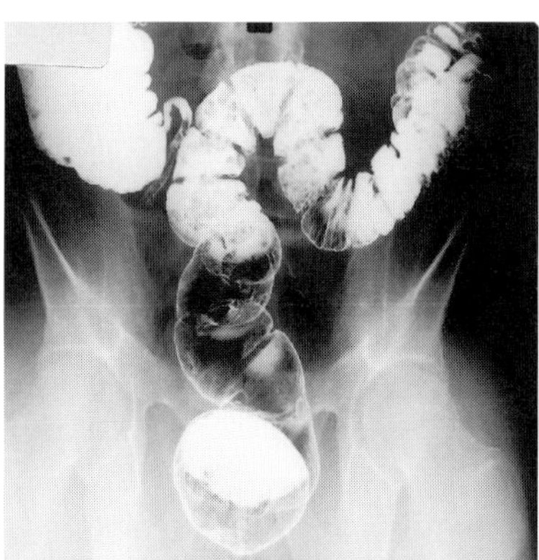

**Figure 5.31d** Postero-anterior 30° caudad projection

## Left lateral decubitus projection

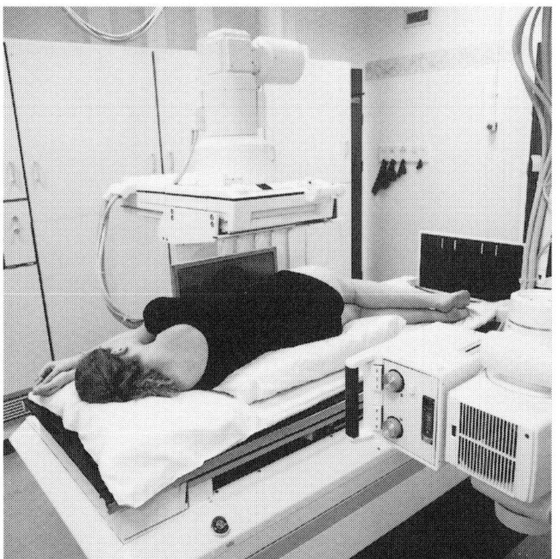
**Figure 5.32a** Anteroposterior (left lateral decubitus)

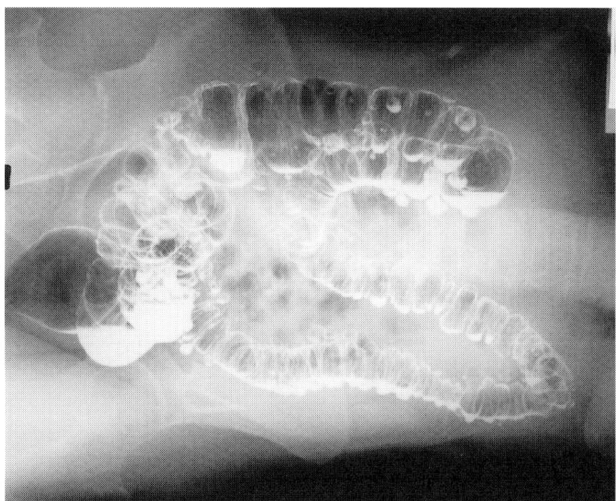
**Figure 5.32b** Left lateral decubitus

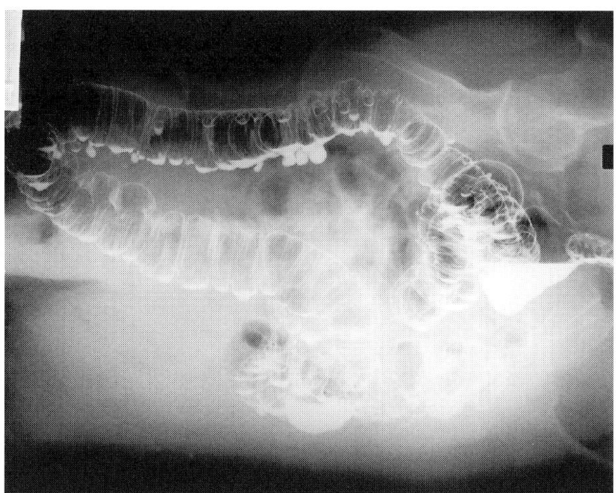
**Figure 5.32c** Right lateral decubitus

This projection demonstrates the lateral wall of the ascending colon and caecum, hepatic flexure and superior and inferior walls of the transverse colon, medial wall of the descending colon, sigmoid and rectum outlined with barium and distended by gas.

A wedge-shaped filter attached to the light beam diaphragm, as described on page 167, may be employed for the decubitus projections.

*Position of patient and imaging modality*

The patient lies on the left side, raised up on a foam pad. Arms are extended above the head, knees together and flexed. The median sagittal plane should be parallel and the coronal plane at right angles to the table top. A 35 × 43 gridded cassette is supported vertically in a lateral cassette holder and positioned against the abdominal wall to include the rectum.

*Note*. When including the rectum on these projections it is not always possible to visualise the splenic flexure; however, this area has usually been demonstrated on the LAO upper abdomen projection taken during the fluorography phase.

*Direction and centring of the X-ray beam*

The horizontal central ray is centred in the midline at the level of the iliac crests, with the exposure made on arrested respiration.

### Right lateral decubitus projection

This projection demonstrates the lateral wall of the descending colon, sigmoid and rectum, splenic flexure and superior and inferior walls of the transverse colon, medial wall of ascending colon and caecum outlined with barium and distended by gas.

The procedure for the right lateral decubitus is identical to the left lateral decubitus except that the patient lies on the right side facing the X-ray tube, back against the cassette.

*Variations on routine technique*

The use of a water-soluble contrast agent is indicated in cases of suspected bowel perforation or to demonstrate the site of recent bowel anastomosis.

In ileostomy and colostomy patients, the proximal bowel can be examined using a soft Foley catheter either inserted into the stoma and then gently inflated with up to 10 ml of air or by inflating the balloon and holding it against the external opening on the anterior abdominal wall.

*Contrast medium and injection data*

| *Volume* | *Concentration* | *Flow rate* |
| --- | --- | --- |
| 750 ml | 81% w/v | Gravity |

Volume includes 350 ml of hot water and 1 ml of bubble breaker added to 400 ml of concentrated barium suspension.

# 5 Alimentary System

## Radionuclide imaging – gastrointestinal bleeding

Localisation of a GI bleed by means of radionuclide imaging is normally performed when endoscopy and barium investigation have failed to localise the site of bleeding. This non-invasive procedure involves the injection of a suitable radiopharmaceutical into the blood stream, following which any bleeding into the GI tract can be detected over a period of time, dependent on the rate of bleeding. One method is to label autologous red cells with technetium *in vivo* or *in vitro*. For the *in vivo* method, two injections are necessary. The patient is first given an intravenous injection of a stannous salt for *in vivo* loading of erythrocytes with stannous ion. Then after a period of 20–30 min $^{99m}$Tc pertechnetate is injected into the blood stream where it becomes bound to the stannous ion in the red blood cells. This technetium-labelling method allows immediate image acquisition, with the procedure being best performed when the patient presents with symptoms of bleeding.

### Indications

Haematemesis and melaena when endoscopy and barium procedures have failed to localise the site of bleeding. As an alternative to arteriography and to prove that bleeding has stopped. It is also indicated when endoscopy is contraindicated, e.g. immediately following GI surgery.

### Position of patient and imaging modality

The patient is usually supine. Anterior views are acquired, with the gamma camera parallel to the imaging couch and positioned to include the abdomen and pelvis. Lateral views, with the gamma camera rotated through 90°, may also be acquired to localise the site of any bleeding. In this case the camera is positioned adjacent to the side nearest the site of the bleeding.

### Imaging procedure

A low-energy general-purpose collimator is selected. Immediately following the $^{99m}$Tc pertechnetate injection a dynamic sequence of images are acquired at the rate of 3 frames/s for 2 min to show the descending aorta and major vessels and any blushing indicative of a major bleed. This is immediately followed by a further series of up to 30 images over a 90-minute period, with an image acquisition time of 3 min per view to show any bleeding. If no bleeding is localised, further images may be obtained up to 24 h post-injection.

*Imaging and radiopharmaceutical parameters*

| *Type* | *Administered activity* | *Principal energy* |
|---|---|---|
| $^{99m}$Tc pertechnetate | 400 MBq | 140 keV |
| *Window width* | *Acquisition counts/time* | |
| 20% | As above | |

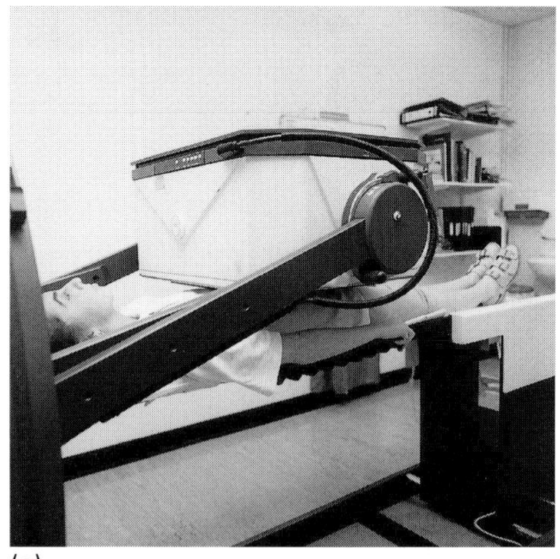

(a)

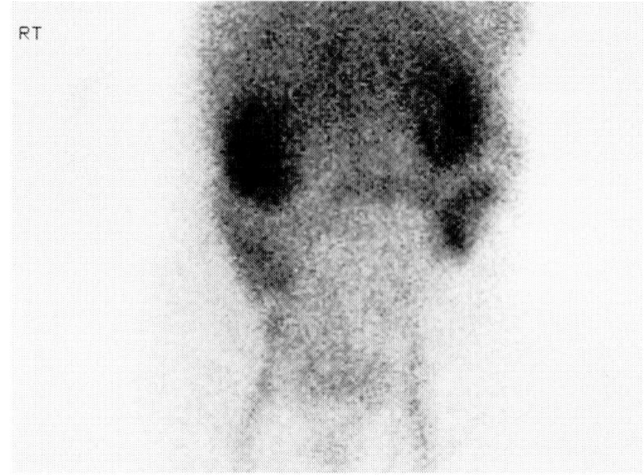


(b)

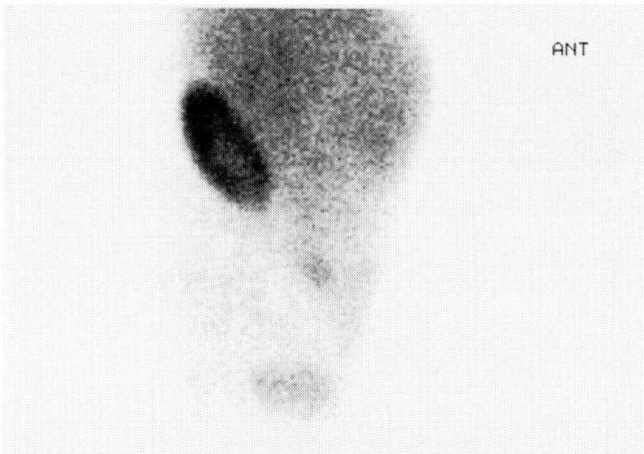


(c)

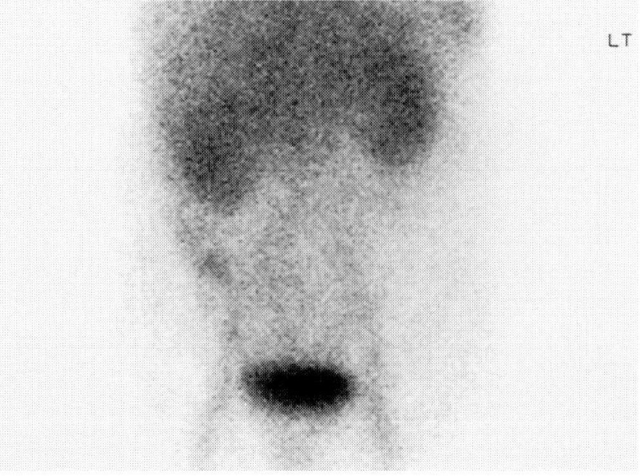


(d)

**Figure 5.33** (a) The gamma camera; (b) anterior and (c) right lateral images 5 h post-injection showing bleeding into the lumen of the GI tract in the right iliac fossa; (d) anterior image 24 h post-injection showing caecal bleeding and distribution of the isotope in the large bowel

## Radionuclide imaging – Meckel's diverticulum

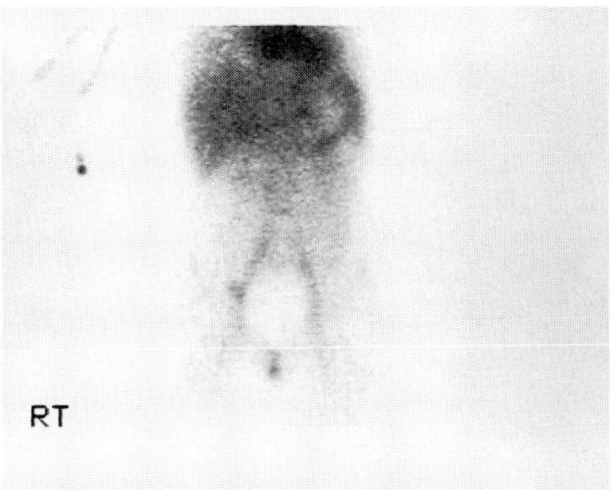


**Figure 5.34a** One minute post-injection

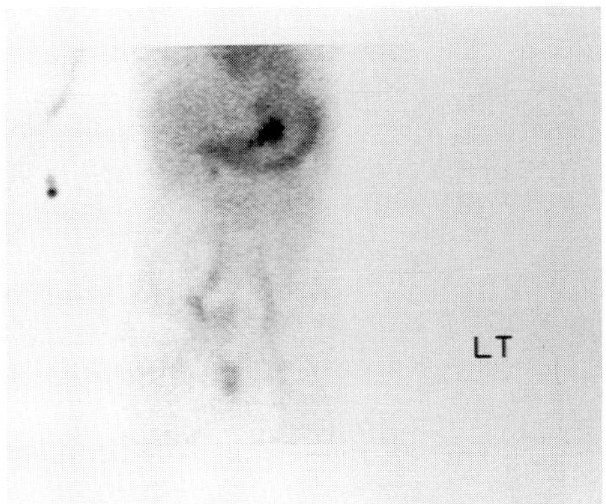


**Figure 5.34b** Five minutes post-injection

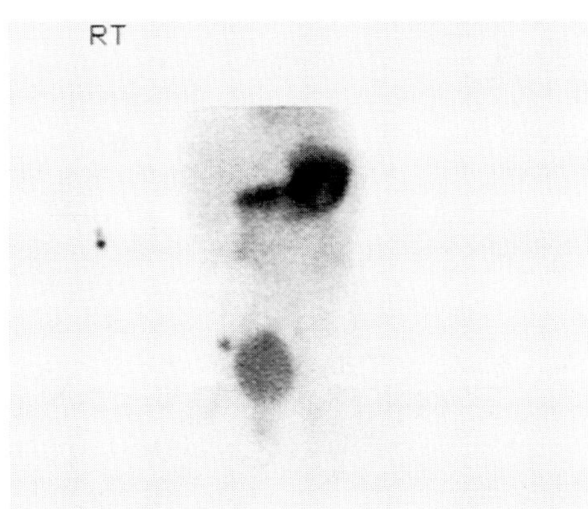


**Figure 5.34c** Thirty minutes post-injection

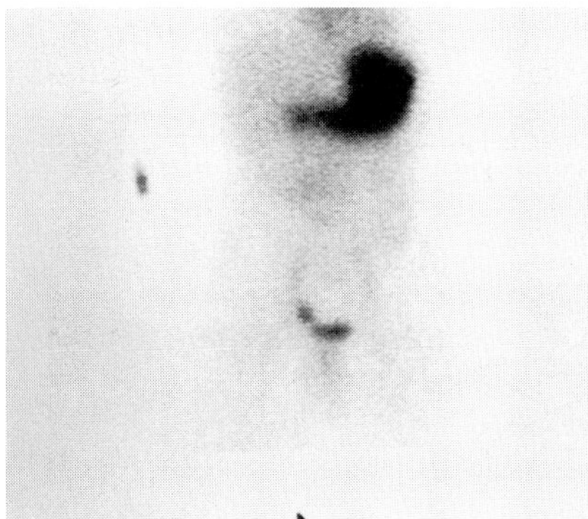

**Figure 5.34d** Forty minutes post-injection – after micturation

**Selection of images from a series showing gradual uptake of pertechnetate in the gastric mucosa and Meckel's diverticulum**

Meckel's diverticulum is a fibrous tube or cord located usually about 50 cm above the ileocaecal valve and is found in about 2% of the population. As the diverticulum may contain active ectopic gastric mucosa, it can be localised following an intravenous injection of a radiopharmaceutical such as $^{99m}$Tc pertechnetate which will also at the same time outline the stomach.

Patients are required to fast for 4 h prior to the procedure. In some departments drugs are given to enhance visualisation by blocking the release of pertechnetate into the lumen or bowel, thereby increasing the uptake of pertechnetate in the gastric mucosa and by preventing peristalsis of the bowel.

**Indications**

Rectal bleeding or inflammation of the bowel due to suspected Meckel's diverticulum.

**Position of patient and imaging modality**

The patient is usually supine. Anterior views are acquired with the gamma camera parallel to the imaging couch and positioned to include the lower abdomen and pelvis, to demonstrate the ileum and ileocaecal valve.

**Imaging procedure**

A low-energy general-purpose collimator is selected. Following intravenous injection of the radiopharmaceutical, an imaging protocol is initiated consisting of a dynamic sequence of up to 30 images over a 90-minute period, with an image acquisition time of 3 min per image.

Because the kidneys excrete the pertechnetate the patient is asked to micturate at the end of the protocol to obtain an additional view of the pelvis with an empty bladder.

A right lateral image may also be acquired at the end of the procedure to distinguish between any activity in the posterior abdomen associated with the urinary tract and a diverticulum in the alimentary tract.

During image acquisition any uptake in activity in a Meckel's diverticulum will be associated with a corresponding uptake of activity in the gastric mucosa.

*Imaging and radiopharmaceutical parameters*

| *Type* | *Administered activity* | *Principal energy* |
|---|---|---|
| $^{99m}$Tc pertechnetate | 200 MBq | 140 keV |
| *Window width* | *Acquisition counts/time* | |
| 20% | 600 K counts per view | |

# 5 Alimentary System

## Liver

The liver is the largest gland in the body. It weighs approximately 1.5 kg and is situated under the diaphragm occupying most of the right hypochondrium, part of the epigastrium and extending across the midline into the left hypochondrium.

It is divided into the right and left lobes by the falciform ligament and then each lobe further divides into segments.

The right lobe is considerably larger than the left and is further divided into the right, caudate and quadrate lobes.

The portal fissure, where various vessels enter and leave the liver, is situated on the posterior surface of the gland. These vessels include: the portal vein (which carries blood from the stomach, small and large intestine, pancreas and spleen), the hepatic artery (which usually arises from the coeliac axis), sympathetic and parasympathetic nerve fibres, right and left hepatic ducts (carrying bile from the liver to the gallbladder), and lymph vessels.

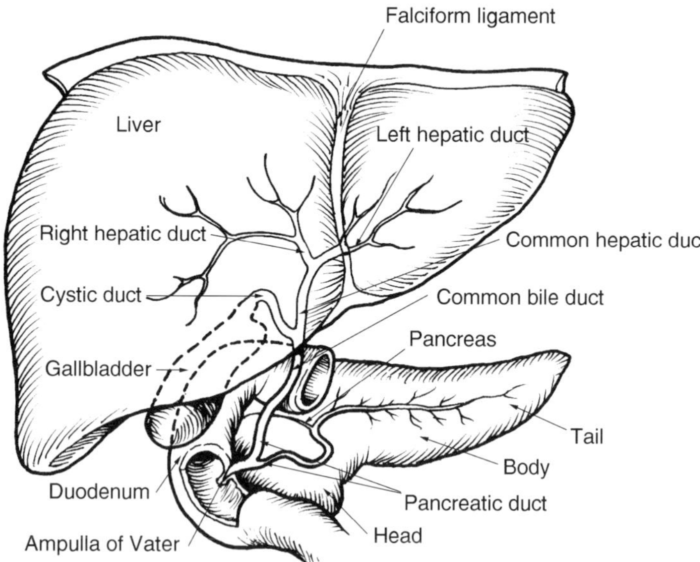


**Figure 5.35a** Liver and pancreas – anterior aspect

### Recommended imaging procedures

Plain radiography is of little value in the investigation of the liver. Preliminary radiographs may demonstrate enlargement and calcifications, but these may be difficult to differentiate from biliary calculi, renal calculi or calcification in the costal cartilages. The structure and position of the liver is such that normally a combination of imaging modalities are employed in its investigation.

Ultrasound is a useful first-line imaging modality and can differentiate cystic and solid lesions. It is also useful for the demonstration of hepatic vessels and can be used to guide needle biopsy.

The liver is well suited to examination by radionuclide imaging. Technetium-99m sulphur colloid liver scanning is a method widely used to assess function of the cells of the reticulo-endothelial system.

Computed tomography is also widely used in the diagnosis of focal and diffuse liver lesions and plays an important role in assessing the patency of the portal vein. It is often performed as an adjunct to ultrasound examination if results of the former are inconclusive.

Magnetic resonance imaging is playing an increasingly important role in liver imaging. With the recent improvements in ultrasound, CT and MRI, angiography because of its invasive nature is less frequently used. However, selective coeliac axis arteriography is still used to demonstrate vascular lesions within the liver and can be combined with CT in CT angiographic studies.

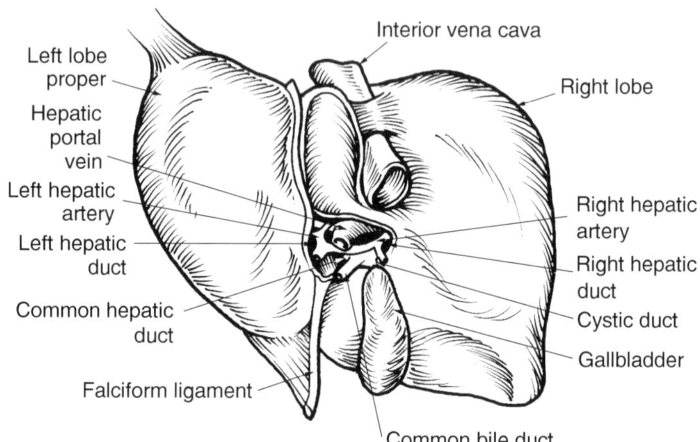


**Figure 5.35b** Inferior aspect of liver

## Ultrasound

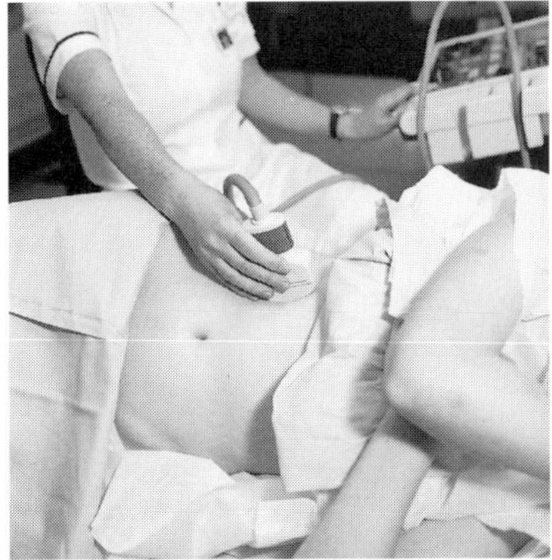

**Figure 5.36a** The transducer

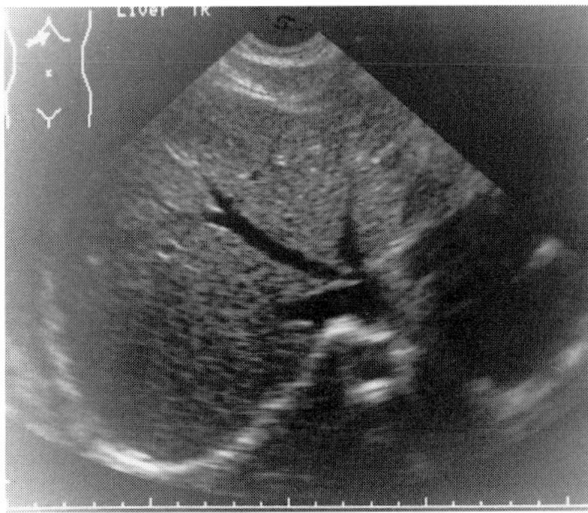

**Figure 5.36b** Transverse oblique image demonstrating hepatic veins and enlarged IVC

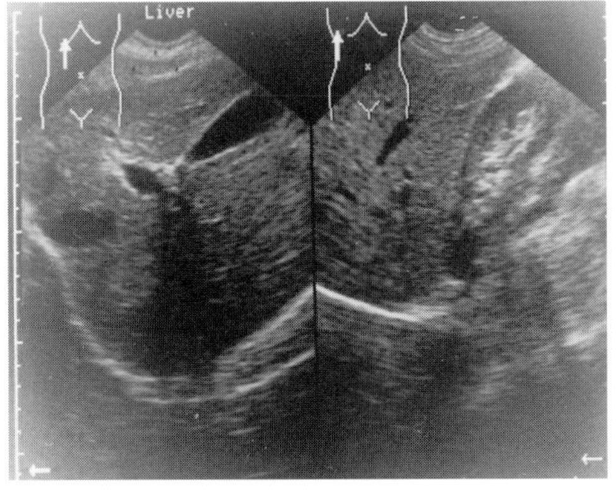

(i) (ii)

**Figure 5.36c** Parasaggital scans through right lobe of liver showing (i) gallbladder, and (ii) right kidney

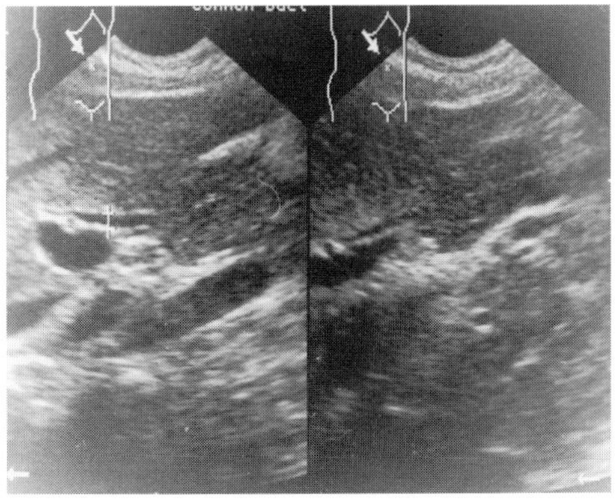

(i) (ii)

**Figure 5.36d** Oblique scans of the right upper quadrant of the liver demonstrating in (i) the common bile duct (identified by calipers), and (ii) the hepatic artery running between the common bile duct and the portal vein

Ultrasound is particularly useful in differentiating solid and cystic lesions in the liver. Its non-invasive nature makes it an ideal first-line imaging modality.

Scans are usually performed on deep arrested inspiration to move the liver downwards with respect to the overlying ribs.

### Indications

Ultrasound is used to examine known or suspected focal lesions and to investigate diffuse liver disease and its complications.

### Patient preparation

Nil by mouth for 6–12 h prior to the examination of the liver. If interventional procedures (biopsy) are planned, blood clotting studies must be carried out prior to the examination.

### Imaging procedure

The patient lies supine on the imaging couch. The choice of probe may vary according to the subject type. A 3.5 MHz probe is normally used because of the thickness of the right lobe of the liver, but on slim patients a 5 MHz probe may be used.

Using real-time equipment the liver is scanned in longitudinal, transverse and oblique planes. Depending upon morphology, the scans can be obtained subcostally in suspended respiration, intercostally or both. In addition, scans may be obtained with the patient rotated onto the left side.

The hepatic and portal vein should be examined individually. Vessel patency can be assessed using colour flow or spectral Doppler. Normal blood flow direction in the hepatic veins is hepatofugal (away from the liver) and hepatopetal (towards the liver) in the portal vein. The diameter of the portal vein should be measured as it crosses the inferior vena cava. The normal diameter is less than 14 mm.

Biopsy using either a fine needle (20–22 gauge) or a cutting needle (14–18 gauge) can be performed under ultrasound guidance. Fine needle is preferred for focal lesions and cutting needle for diffuse lesions.

Further interventional procedures undertaken with ultrasound guidance include cyst and abscess drainage and tumour ablation by alcohol or laser.

# 5 Liver

## Radionuclide imaging

Radionuclide imaging tends to be used as a complementary technique to ultrasound and CT, providing useful functional information.

The $^{99m}$Tc sulphur or stannous colloid scan is commonly used to assess function of the cells of the reticulo-endothelial system. This gives valuable information on both the liver and spleen in distinguishing between focal and diffuse pathology.

### Indications

Hepatic metastases, parenchymal liver disease and trauma.

### Position of patient and imaging modality

The patient lies supine on the imaging couch. For the anterior view the camera is positioned parallel to the imaging couch and situated as close as possible to the surface of the patient over the upper abdomen. Further views are obtained by rotating the camera into the posterior and right and left lateral positions.

### Imaging procedure

A high-resolution collimator is used for static scanning.

An intravenous injection of a $^{99m}$Tc-labelled tin or sulphur colloid is administered into the median cubital vein. The patient is then positioned supine on the imaging table.

The positions of the lower costal margin and xiphisternum (or mass if is palpable) are marked using radioactive markers or a flexible lead strip.

Static images are obtained in the anterior, posterior, right and left lateral positions, commencing 10–15 min after injection.

SPECT may be employed using a circular tomograph.

*Imaging and radiopharmaceutical parameters*

| *Type* | *Administered activity* | *Principal energy* |
|---|---|---|
| $^{99m}$Tc sulphur colloid | 75 MBq | 140 keV |
| *Window width* | *Acquisition counts/time* | |
| 20% | 400 K counts per image | |

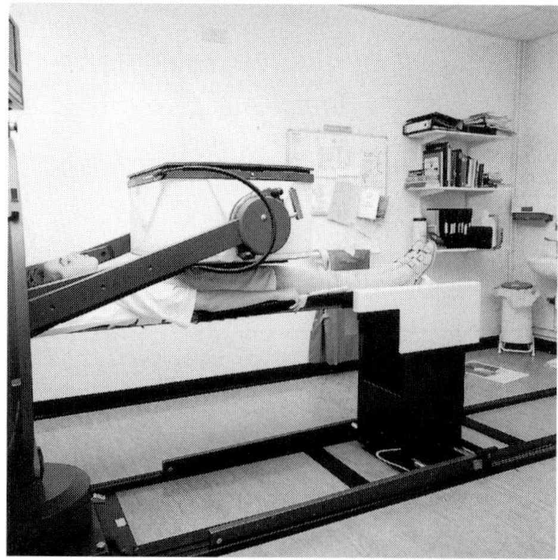

**Figure 5.37a** Radionuclide imaging camera

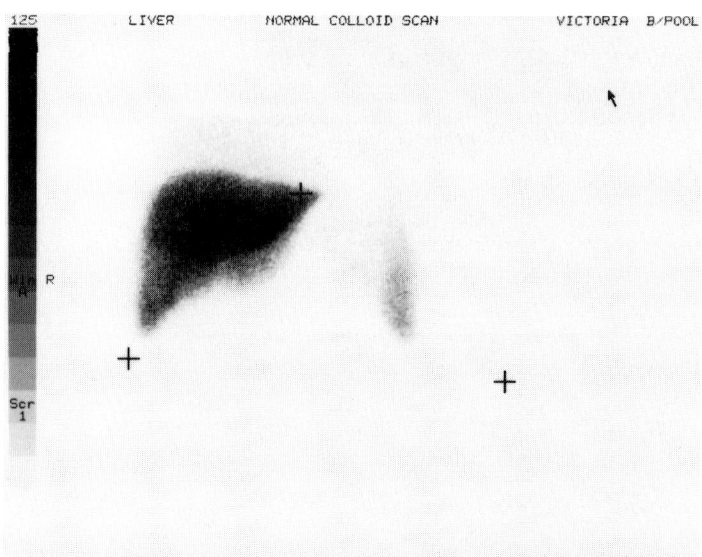


**Figure 5.37b** Normal anterior view showing costal markers

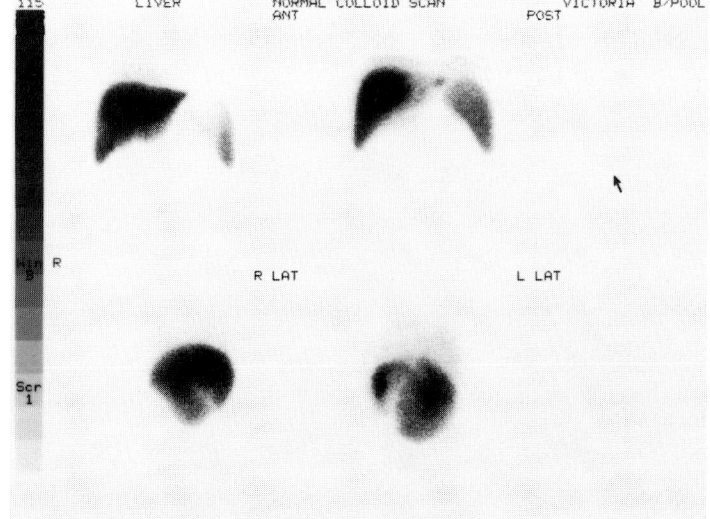


**Figure 5.37c** Routine image set showing anterior, posterior, right and left lateral views of a normal liver

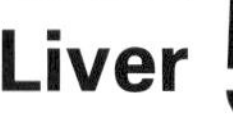

# Computed tomography

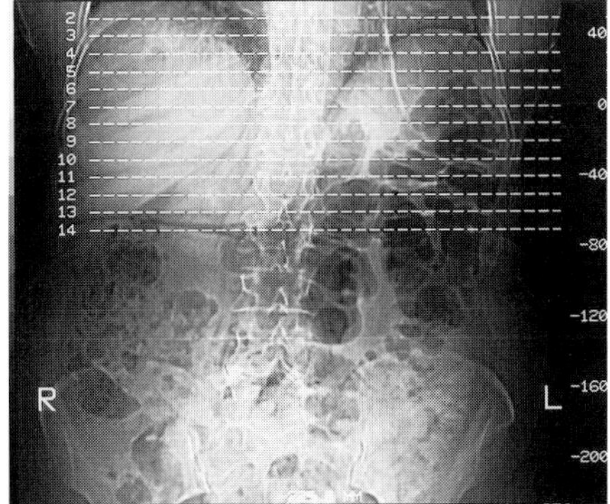

**Figure 5.38a** Scan projection radiograph showing prescribed scanning locations

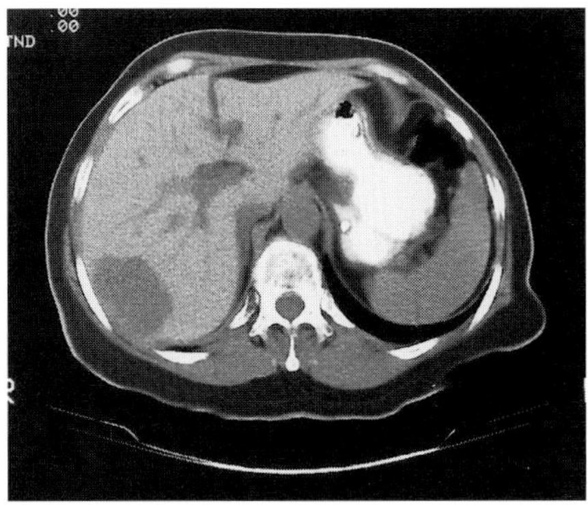

**Figure 5.38b** Pre-contrast transaxial image showing a well-defined low-attenuation area in the posterior aspect of the right lobe of the liver

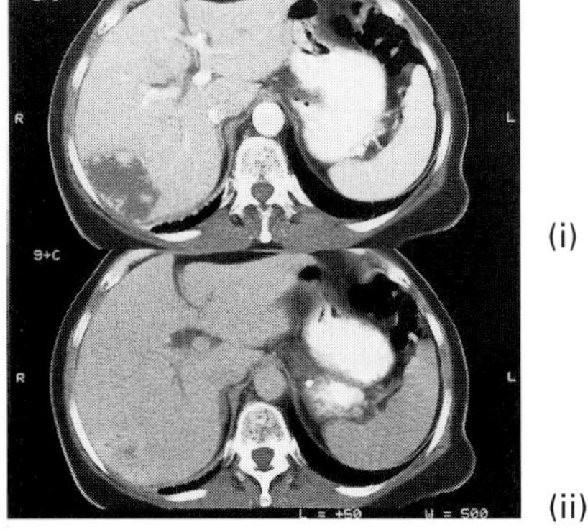

(i)

(ii)

**Figure 5.38c** Post-contrast images (i) during infusion of contrast showing slight enhancement of tumour, and (ii) 10 min post-contrast image showing lesion now with similar attenuation to surrounding normal liver

*Contrast medium and injection data*

**Standard protocol**

| *Volume* | *Concentration* | *Flow rate* |
|---|---|---|
| 100 ml | 300 mgI/ml | 2 ml/s |

Scanning commences 50 s after start of injection.

**Dual phase**

| *Volume* | *Concentration* | *Flow rate* |
|---|---|---|
| 100 ml | 300 mgI/ml | 4 ml/s |

Scanning commences 15 s after start of injection with a 15-second interscan delay between phases.

Computed tomography is frequently used following ultrasound examination to confirm the presence of a solitary lesion prior to surgery, or to identify the extent of disease within the gland. Modern scanners capable of rapid serial scanning have increased the information that can be obtained with contrast medium studies. Imaging is undertaken pre- and post-injection of a water-soluble contrast agent. It is also necessary to opacify the small bowel using dilute Gastrografin given orally 30 min and 15 min prior to scanning.

**Indications**

Diagnosis of focal liver lesions and staging of neoplasms.

**Position of patient and imaging modality**

The patient lies supine, feet first on the scanner table. The arms are raised and placed behind the patient's head, out of the scan plane. The median sagittal plane is perpendicular to the centre of the table top and the coronal plane parallel to it. The scanner table height is adjusted to ensure that the coronal plane alignment light is at the level of the mid-axillary line. The patient is moved until the scan reference point is at the level of the xiphisternum.

**Imaging procedure**

A postero-anterior scan projection image is performed commencing 5 cm above and ending 25 cm below the scan reference point. From this image, 10 mm contiguous sections are prescribed through the entire liver/pancreas from the dome of the diaphragm to the middle of the third lumbar vertebra (typically 15 sections). After review, the sections are rescanned during the infusion of a contrast medium.

If spiral scanning options are available these images may be acquired with a volume acquisition, using a 10 mm slice thickness and 10 mm table increments, but with a 5 mm reconstruction index to give overlapping sections.

A dual phase scanning protocol may also be prescribed, enabling imaging of the arterial and portal venous phases of the liver using one contrast injection. Using the same imaging parameters for spiral scanning, post-contrast image data are acquired first caudally (arterial phase) and after a 15-second delay, in reverse, cranially (portal phase).

Contrast medium enhanced CT sections may enable characterisation of focal lesions. Cysts are of low attenuation (CT value 0–10) and fail to enhance. Abscesses, although of low attenuation, will show peripheral enhancement. Therefore delayed slices should be performed to confirm a diagnosis. Metastases can show a range of appearances and can show a variable response to contrast. The most frequent appearance is of an ill-defined low-attenuation lesion enhancing heterogeneously with contrast. Contrast medium enhancement is also of value in assessing portohepatic veins and in the demonstration of varices commonly seen in chronic liver disease.

# 5 Liver

## Magnetic resonance imaging

Up to the time of writing, MRI of the liver is used mainly to characterise focal and diffuse abnormalities. Because of the anatomical relationship of the liver to the diaphragm, heart and great vessels, image quality is degraded by movement artefact. Although both respiratory and cardiac gating facilities are widely available, both can result in an unacceptable increase in the scan time and in repetition time incompatible with lesion detection. A successful way to reduce movement artefact is by using a compression band across the upper abdomen. Faster scanning techniques, such as gradient echo sequences, have very short imaging times and allow data acquisition during breath holding, thus eliminating respiratory movement artefacts. Presaturation pulses applied to the anterior abdominal wall and to the tissue above and below that being imaged will reduce artefacts from subcutaneous fat and from arterial and venous blood flowing into the imaging area.

The use of contrast agents in liver imaging is currently being evaluated. Paramagnetic contrast agents by altering the $T_1$ relaxation time can be used to characterise tumours further by assessment of their vascularity. Rapid image acquisition using either gradient-echo or fast spin-echo sequences is necessary with paramagnetic agents to achieve maximum contrast between normal and abnormal areas. Superparamagnetic agents are taken up by the reticulo-endothelial cells of the liver. These shorten the $T_2$ relaxation of the normal liver which is then of lower signal intensity, increasing the contrast between normal and abnormal areas and thus the sensitivity of tumour detection. The contrast agent is retained within the liver and imaging can be performed several hours after administration.

Either spin-echo or gradient-echo sequences can be selected, the latter being more sensitive to the effects of contrast. It is important that the decibel level set for the contrast enhanced scans is identical to that of the initial pre-contrast scans.

### Indications

To examine known or suspected focal lesions and to investigate diffuse liver disease.

### Position of patient and imaging modality

The patient lies supine, head first on the scanner table, with the median sagittal plane perpendicular to the centre of the table and compression is applied if required. Using the external alignment lights the external reference point is obtained at the level of the xiphisternum. From this position the patient is moved the fixed distance into the isocentre of the magnet which is also the centre of the radiofrequency coil.

### Imaging procedure

An initial coronal localiser is performed. From this image, transaxial $T_1$ weighted, $T_2$ weighted and proton density sequences are prescribed through the liver, including at least one sequence obtained during suspended respiration. Because of the variation in signal intensity from structures within the liver, additional sequences may be required in the coronal plane to identify blood vessels and bile ducts further and to define the relationship between the liver and adjacent organs.

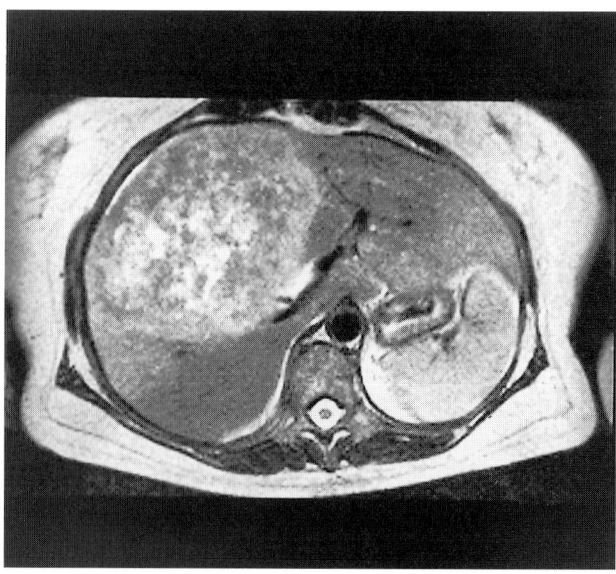

 **Figure 5.39a** Pre-contrast $T_2$ weighted image of the liver

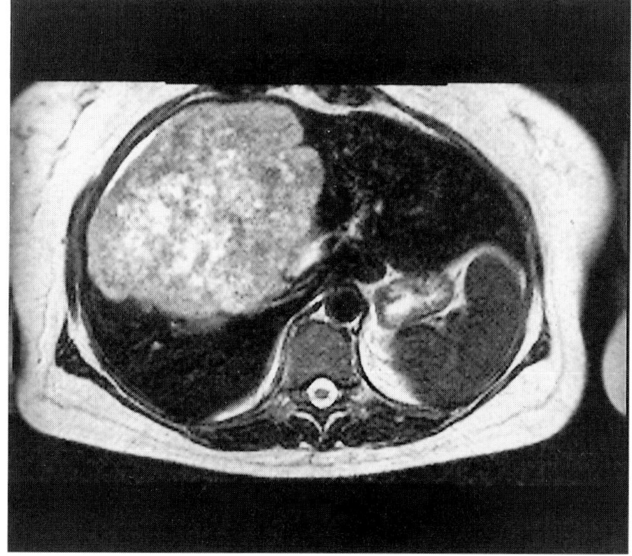

**Figure 5.39b** Post-contrast $T_2$ weighted image of the liver

## Angiography

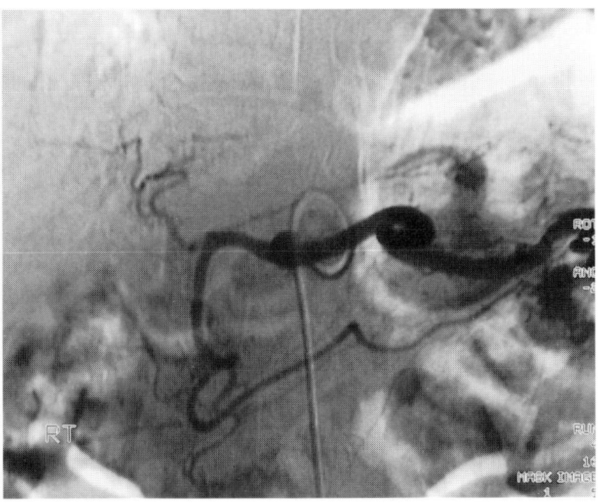


Figure 5.40a Angiography image showing hepatic artery

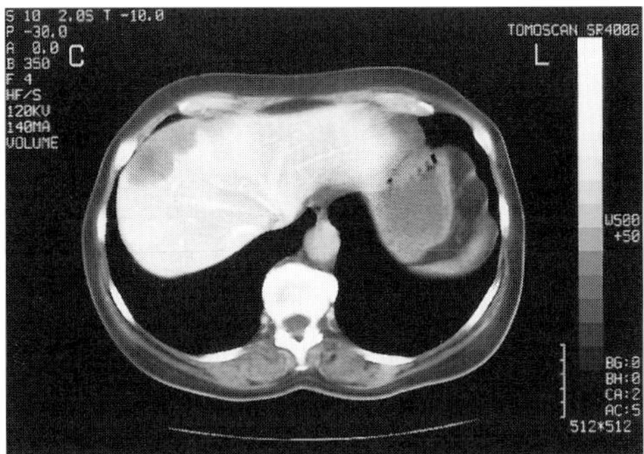


Figure 5.40b CT image showing hepatic veins

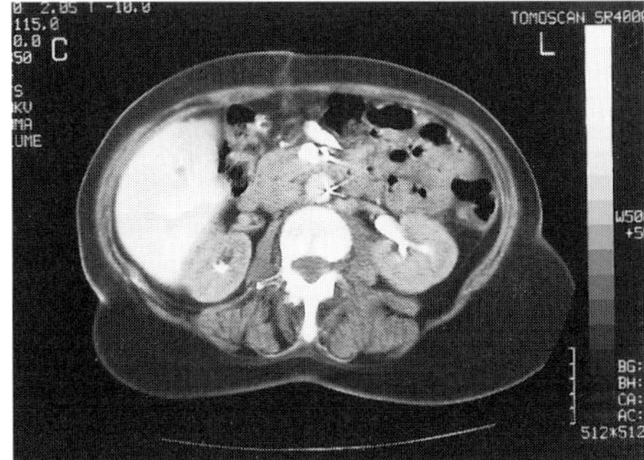


Figure 5.40c CT image showing small focal lesions

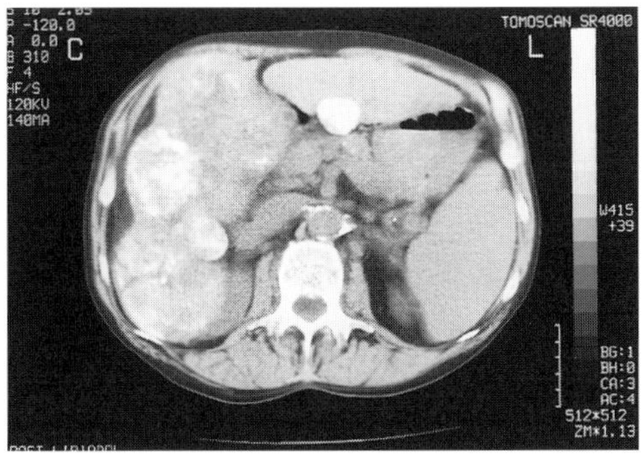


Figure 5.40d CT image 10 days after Lipiodol contrast injection

The improvements in ultrasound and radionuclide imaging have to some extent reduced the need for splenoportography. Selective coeliac axis arteriography, however, remains an essential complementary diagnostic investigation in many conditions.

Digital subtraction angiography is playing an increasingly important role as equipment becomes more readily available. It offers advantages of reduced volume requirement of contrast agent and high-quality images capable of post-processing.

When digital subtraction is not available, conventional photographic subtraction is valuable in removing overlying structures.

### Indications

Angiography is useful in cases of portal hypertension, invasive neoplasms and as a precursor to embolisation.

### Imaging procedure

The imaging procedure is identical to that for selective mesenteric angiography (see page 161).

The image acquisition or film sequence is extended at a slower rate up to 30 s to allow time for the portal vein to fill with contrast.

An oily medium may be injected during the angiographic procedure which is selectively taken up by primary liver tumours, thus facilitating their detection on subsequent CT examinations which are usually performed 7–10 days later.

## CT angiography and portography

Computed tomography angiography is extremely sensitive in assessing small focal lesions and is performed following fluoroscopy for selective catheterisation of the coeliac axis or preferably the hepatic artery. In this technique, metastatic lesions are shown as peripherally enhancing hyperdense lesions.

CT portography relies on the fact that no tumours are fed by the portal vein. A catheter is placed in the superior mesenteric artery and following the contrast injection focal lesions will appear as hypodense areas compared to the hyperdense hepatic tissue.

### Imaging procedure

An anteroposterior scan projection radiograph of the upper abdomen is performed to identify the position of the liver. From this image, 10 mm sections, with 10 mm table increments, of the liver are prescribed during the infusion of a 140 mgI/ml non-ionic strength contrast agent. A total of 150 ml is injected at the rate of 3 ml/s, with scanning commencing following a 30-second delay.

# 5 Alimentary System

## Gallbladder and Biliary Ducts

The gallbladder is a hollow pear-shaped structure, lying anterior and inferior to the lower margin of the liver, and contains bile which is manufactured in the liver. It is divided into the fundus, body and neck and is normally 7–10 cm in length and approximately 3 cm wide at the level of the fundus. It has a capacity of 30–50 ml. The neck of the gallbladder communicates with the cystic duct through the valve of Heister. Bile is secreted by the liver and then passes into the biliary system, collecting in the right and left hepatic ducts which join to form the common hepatic duct. The cystic duct joins the common hepatic duct to form the common bile duct which passes behind the first part of the duodenum and along the lateral margin of the head of the pancreas close to the medial wall of the second part of the duodenum. It finally joins the pancreatic duct at the ampulla of Vater and empties into the duodenum through a small papilla at the sphincter of Oddie.

There is considerable variation in the size, position and shape of the gallbladder. In the majority of cases it lies close to the lower margin of the liver. Its position can vary however from the level of the 11th rib, to the level of the first sacral segment, and from close to the lateral abdominal wall to the vertebral column. Occasionally it is situated on the left side of the abdomen.

Similarly, its depth can vary from the level of the anterior margin of the vertebral body to the anterior abdominal wall. There is also considerable postural variation of the gallbladder position, particularly in elderly patients.

The hepatic flexure of the colon frequently overlies the gallbladder and can result in superimposition of gas and faecal matter. This may necessitate modification of patient positioning or technique to image the gallbladder and ducts adequately.

The physique of the patient is the most important factor in determining the position of the gallbladder. In sthenic and hyposthenic patients the gallbladder appears pear shaped and is situated at the level of the third lumbar vertebra approximately 5 cm from the spinous process on the right side of the abdomen.

In hypersthenic subjects the gallbladder lies horizontally and appears circular. It lies at the level of the first lumbar vertebra and is situated closer to the lateral abdominal wall. In asthenic subjects the gallbladder is elongated and is situated at the level of the fourth or fifth lumbar vertebra close to the midline.

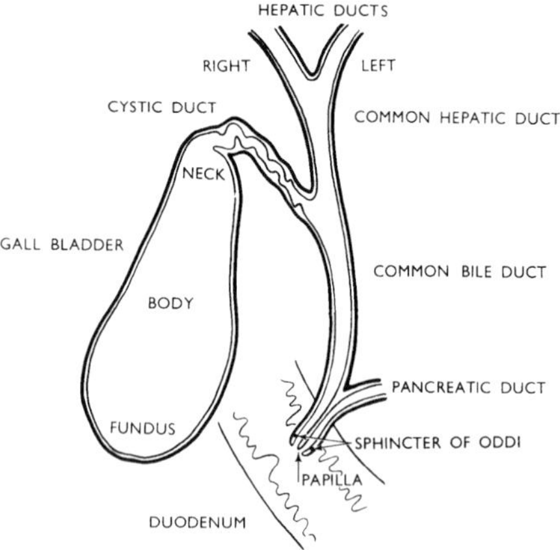


**Figure 5.41a** Gallbladder and bile ducts – anterior aspect

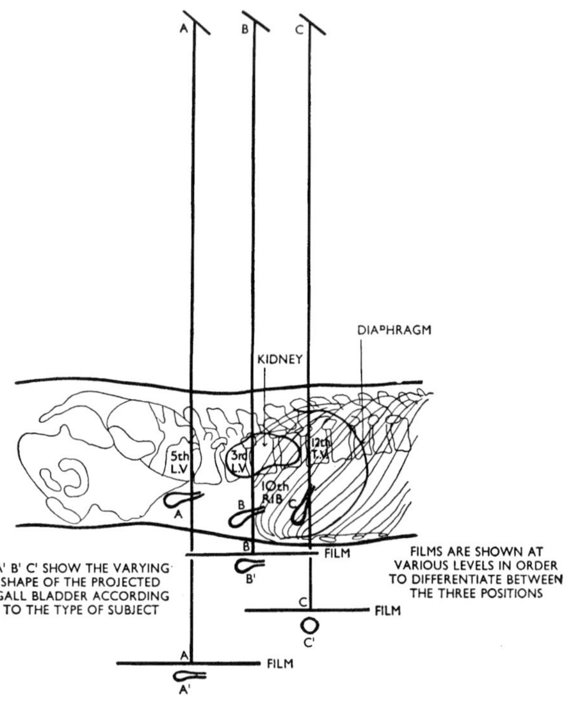


**Figure 5.41b** Varying position of X-ray tube according to subject type

## Recommended imaging procedures

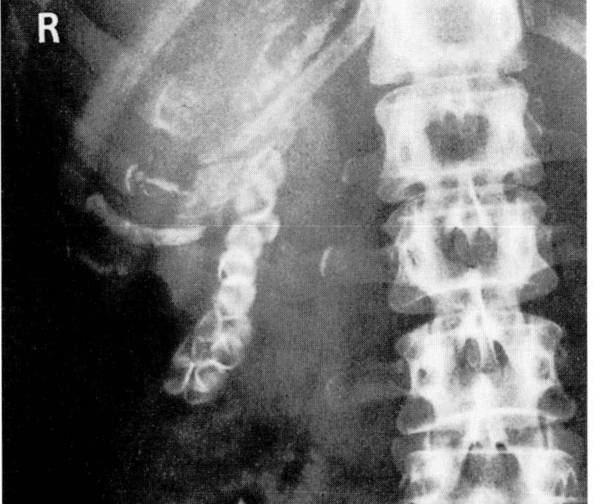


**Figure 5.42a** Plain radiograph (left anterior oblique) demonstrating multiple opaque gallstones

A plain radiograph of the abdomen or left anterior oblique projection in the prone position is frequently taken prior to any other imaging procedure. It remains a useful technique for demonstrating radio-opaque gallstones, air in the biliary tree and pancreatic calcifications.

Ultrasound is the primary imaging procedure in the investigation of the gallbladder and ducts. It has largely replaced the oral cholecystogram in the detection of gallstones and the identification of the ducts in the jaundiced patient. Oral cholecystography may, however, still be performed if ultrasound has failed to demonstrate conclusively the presence of gallstones in the gallbladder.

In cases of obstructive jaundice and duct dilatation, endoscopic retrograde cholangiopancreatography (ERCP) or percutaneous cholangiography (PTC) may be used to demonstrate ductal anatomy to supplement the information obtained by ultrasound.

ERCP offers the facility to image both the biliary and pancreatic ducts by direct contrast medium injection as well as offering the potential for interventional techniques such as stone extraction dilatation and stent insertion.

Computed tomography is a useful adjunct to ultrasound, particularly in obese patients and in the detection of tumours.

Radionuclide imaging produces valuable information on gall-bladder function and is the examination of choice in cases of acute cholecystitis.

Postoperative cholangiography may be performed following cholecystectomy to demonstrate duct patency or residual stones.

Peroperative cholangiography, which is employed during open surgery to demonstrate biliary duct anatomy and to demonstrate the flow of bile into the duodenum, is described in Section 17 – Theatre Radiography of the eleventh edition of *Clark's Positioning in Radiography*.

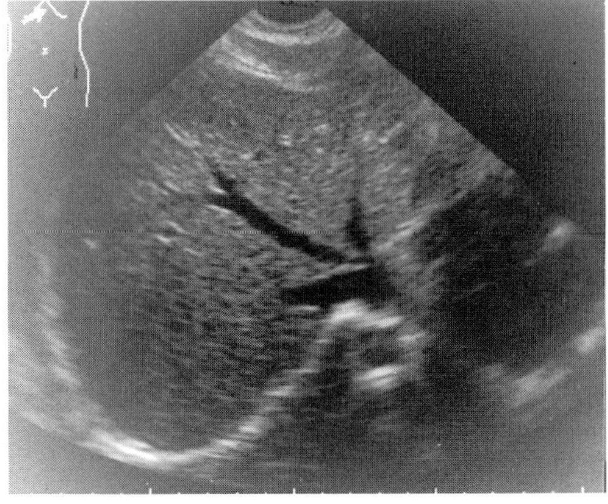

**Figure 5.42b** Ultrasound image demonstrating hepatic ducts

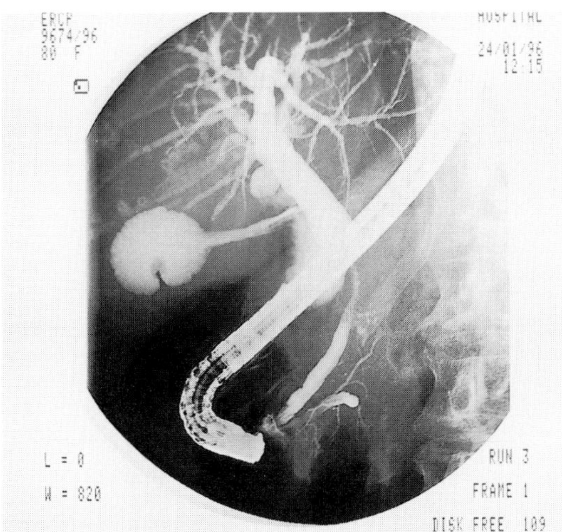


**Figure 5.42c** ERCP image showing dilated hepatic ducts and gallbladder

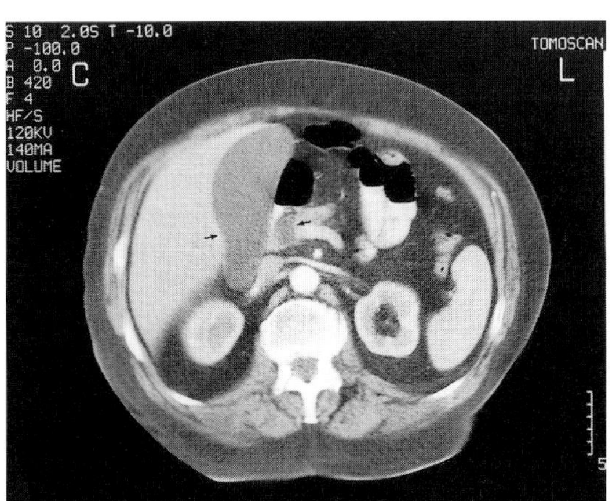


**Figure 5.42d** Post-contrast enhanced CT image showing distended gallbladder and dilated common bile duct

# 5 Gallbladder and Biliary Ducts

## Ultrasound

Ultrasound is the imaging modality of choice in the examination of the gallbladder and ducts. It is non-invasive and has largely replaced the oral cholecystogram.

The whole length of the common duct may be demonstrated, from the porta hepatis to the junction of the pancreatic duct. Ultrasound may also demonstrate thickening of the wall of the gallbladder in acute cholecystitis.

Doppler techniques have the ability to distinguish dilated intra- and extrahepatic ducts from vascular structures. Colour Doppler imaging allows real-time assessment of blood flow.

Scans are performed on arrested deep inspiration so that the gallbladder can be examined subcostally.

### Indications

Ultrasound is used to investigate right upper quadrant pain, medical and surgical jaundice, fatty food intolerance and biliary obstruction.

### Patient preparation

The patient should be starved for 6–12 h prior to the examination to ensure that the gallbladder is full.

### Imaging procedure

The technique for the ultrasound examination of the intrahepatic ducts is described in the ultrasound section on the liver (page 173).

For gallbladder imaging the patient lies supine on the imaging couch. A 5 Mhz probe is used, as it offers improved resolution and aids the detection of small stones.

Using real-time equipment the gallbladder is scanned in the longitudinal, transverse and oblique planes. Subcostal and/or intercostal scans may be performed, depending on the exact position of the gallbladder.

Additional scans may be performed with the patient rotated obliquely onto the left side, with the right arm raised above the head.

The patient may also be scanned lying on the left side or erect to demonstrate movement of stones or to dislodge stones from the neck of the gallbladder.

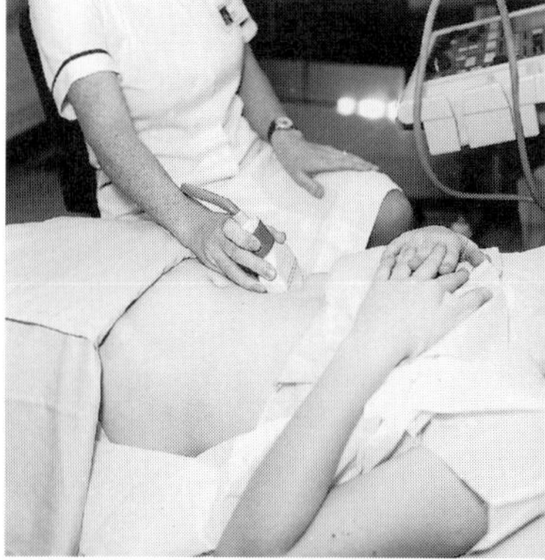

**Figure 5.43a** Patient undergoing ultrasound scan

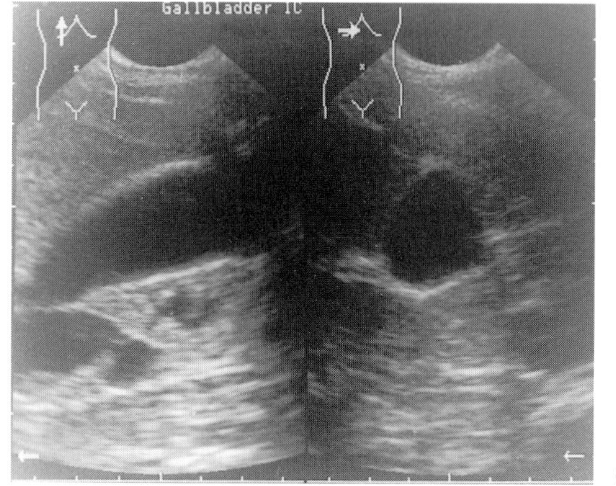


**Figure 5.43b** Scans of the upper abdomen showing the gallbladder: (i) in longitudinal section, and (ii) in transverse section

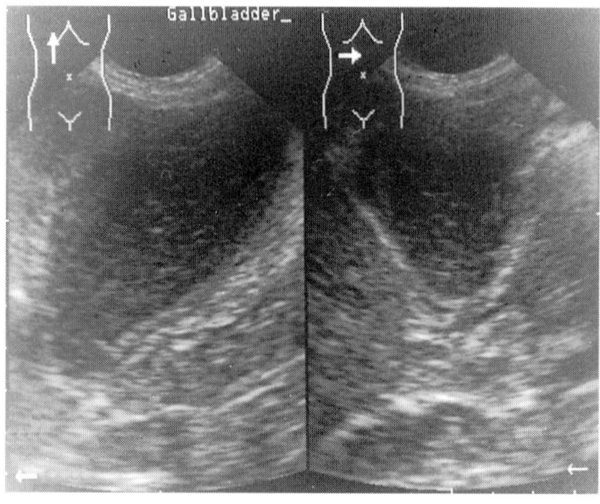


**Figure 5.43c** Scans of the upper quadrant of the abdomen: (i) right parasagittal showing longitudinal section of the gallbladder with oedematous wall and biliary sludge, and (ii) transverse scan of same patient

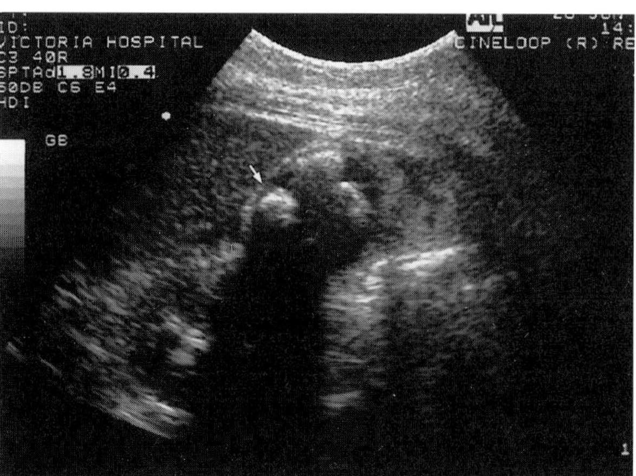


**Figure 5.43d** Scan showing acoustic shadowing from gallstones

## Endoscopic retrograde cholangiopancreatography (ERCP)

Endoscopic retrograde cholangiopancreatography is the radiographic examination of the biliary and/or pancreatic ducts following intubation of the papilla of the ampulla of Vater via a fibreoptic endoscope.

In addition to facilitating contrast examination of the biliary and pancreatic ducts by direct injection of a contrast agent, it offers opportunities for performing biopsies and potential for therapeutic techniques.

The examination is performed under fluoroscopic control.

### Indications

Suspected biliary or pancreatic disease including obstructive jaundice in post-cholecystectomy patients.

### Contraindications

Oesophageal strictures and pyloric stenosis are contraindications in that they may render the examination very difficult to perform.

### Patient preparation

The patient is starved for 6 h and an intravenous smooth muscle relaxant is administered 10 min prior to the investigation. Local anaesthetic lozenges may be given 30 min before the investigation and a topical anaesthetic sprayed onto the tongue immediately before intubation.

Sedation may also be given as required.

### Imaging procedure

The patient lies on the left side on a fluoroscopy table. The fibreoptic endoscope is introduced via the mouth and passes through the stomach and duodenum. When the tip of the endoscope reaches the second stage of the duodenum the papilla of the ampulla of Vater is identified. The patient may then be turned prone to assist in selective cannulation of the biliary duct and a catheter filled with contrast agent is introduced via the endoscope, through the ampulla into the lower end of the biliary duct. Contrast is injected slowly under fluoroscopic control and a series of spot films are taken as required when duct filling is complete. Further radiographs are taken immediately after removal of the endoscope. In addition to fluoroscopy, images may be recorded from direct viewing via the endoscope by videotape or 35 mm attachments.

### After-care

Nil by mouth for 4 h until the anaesthetic has worn off. Blood pressure and pulse are recorded every 15 min for the first 4 h and then 4 hourly for the next 24 h.

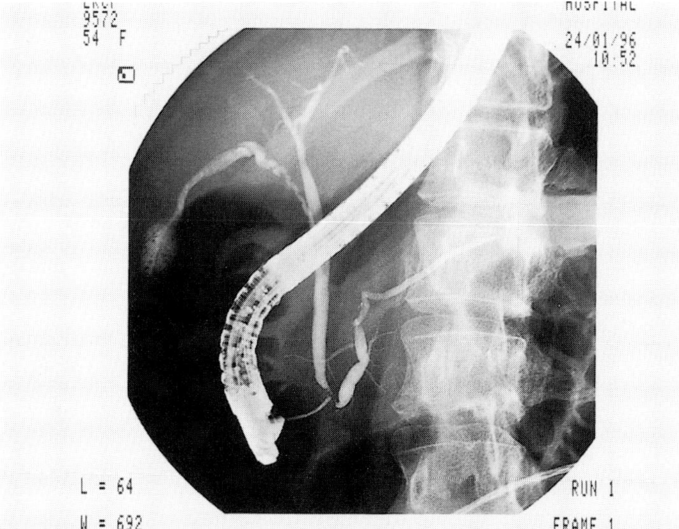


**Figure 5.44a** ERCP image showing early filling of the biliary tree and pancreatic duct with opacities visualised in the gallbladder and cystic duct

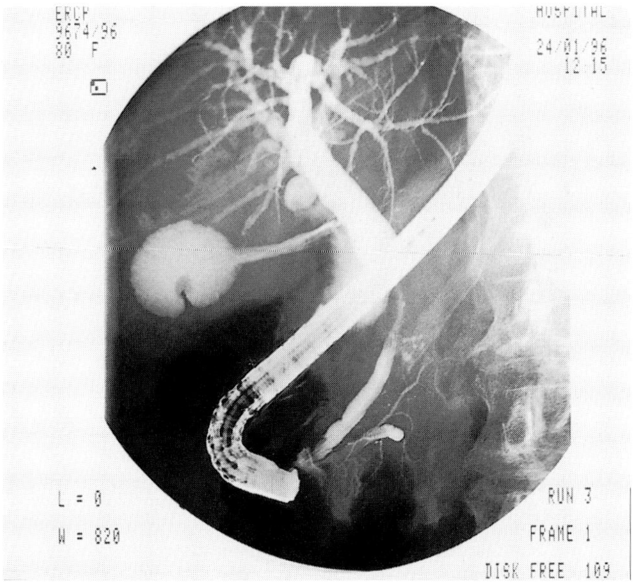


**Figure 5.44b** ERCP image showing dilated biliary system due to stricture in the common bile duct (note filling of abnormal gallbladder)

*Contrast medium and injection data*

| *Volume* | *Concentration* | *Flow rate* |
|---|---|---|
| 20–60 ml | 320 mgI/ml | Hand injection |

Contrast is diluted to 50% strength with normal saline for biliary ducts. Additional contrast may be employed during therapeutic procedures.

# 5 Gallbladder and Biliary Ducts

## Percutaneous transhepatic cholangiography (PTC)

Percutaneous transhepatic cholangiography is the radiographic examination of the biliary system by direct percutaneous injection of contrast agent into one of the hepatic ducts.

It is frequently performed preoperatively on patients with obstructive jaundice to assess the site and extent of the lesion. The success rate of the examination is improved where duct dilatation is present.

The examination is ideally performed using dedicated angiographic equipment similar to that described for abdominal angiography.

### Indications

To differentiate between extrahepatic obstructive biliary obstruction and intrahepatic cholestasis, and to assess the extent of a lesion preoperatively. It may also be used to facilitate internal or external bilary drainage and insertion of a biliary stent in the common bile duct.

### Contraindications

The examination is contraindicated in patients with a tendency to bleed.

### Patient preparation

The patient fasts for 6–8 h and prophylactic antibiotic cover is given commencing 24 h before the investigation and continuing for 3 days afterwards.

Coagulation studies are performed and vitamin K is administered if prothrombin times are excessive. Sedation may be administered if appropriate.

*Contrast media and injection data*

| *Volume* | *Concentration* | *Flow rate* |
|---|---|---|
| 20 ml per injection | 140–180 mgI/ml | Hand injection |

### Imaging procedure

The patient lies supine on the imaging couch. A control (postero-anterior) image may be taken to determine the presence of gas shadows or opaque calculi.

The injection site is identified under fluoroscopic control and is marked on the skin surface.

The examination is performed under strict aseptic conditions. The skin surface of the right upper quadrant of the abdomen is prepared using a suitable antiseptic solution and sterile towels are draped over the area. Local anaesthetic is administered at the injection site.

The patient is instructed to arrest respiration at mid-phase. This reduces the risk of damage to the liver substance when respiration recommences. A Chiba needle is inserted into the liver. The trocar/stylet is withdrawn and the patient may recommence gentle respiration.

A syringe and extension tubing are fitted to the Chiba needle and the needle is withdrawn slowly until bile is aspirated through the tubing.

Water-soluble contrast agent is injected under fluoroscopic control and images are acquired as the biliary tree is opacified. The quantity of contrast agent required will depend on the degree of distension of the biliary tree.

Contrast and bile are aspirated at the end of the examination to reduce intrabiliary pressure and the needle is removed.

Further postero-anterior images are taken with the patient supine and, if required, oblique and lateral images acquired by rotating the C-arm system.

Finally a sterile dressing is applied over the injection site.

Where duct dilatation is not present, positioning of the needle in a duct may be facilitated by the gradual introduction of a contrast agent as the needle is slowly withdrawn.

### After-care

The patient must be observed for 48 h following the examination for signs of haemorrhage, leakage of bile or peritonitis. Temperature and blood pressure are checked every 15 min for 4 h and then every 4 h for the next 24 h. Antibiotic cover is continued for 3 days.

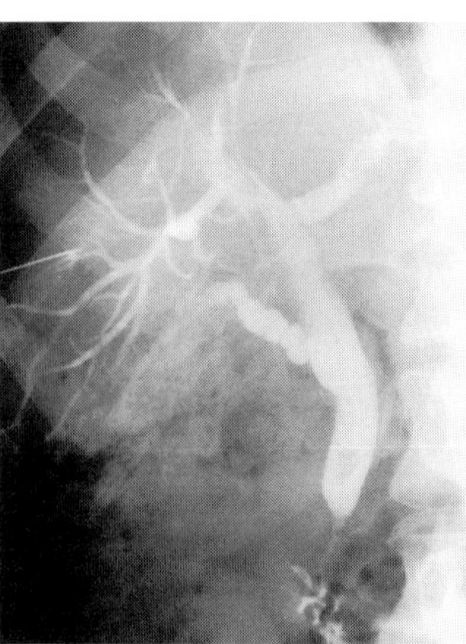

**Figure 5.45a** PTC image showing a stone above a distal common bile duct stricture

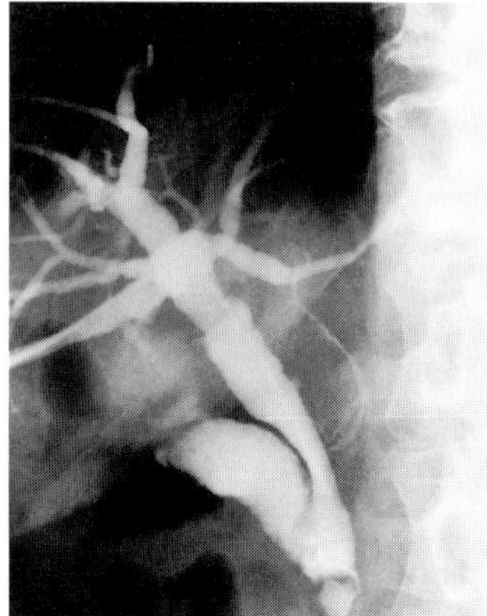

**Figure 5.45b** PTC image taken during a stenting procedure showing a catheter in situ in the distal duct

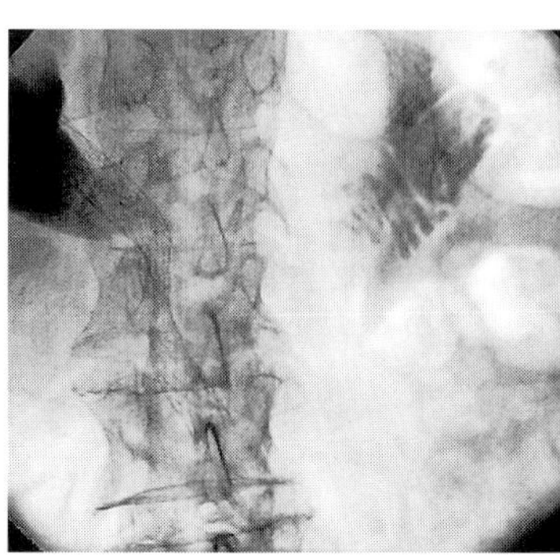

**Figure 5.45c** Stent in the common bile duct

## T-tube cholangiography

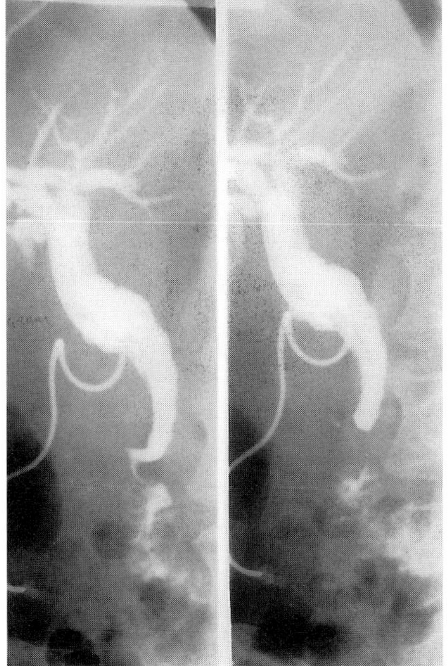


**Figure 5.46a** T-tube procedure showing: (i) clear passage of contrast into the duodenum, and (ii) some spasm at the lower end of the CBD

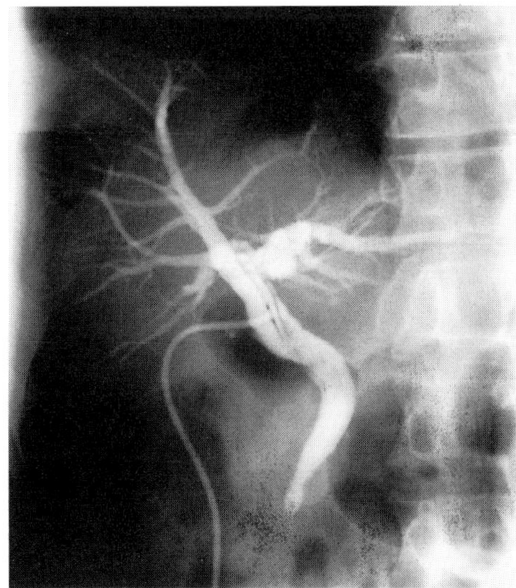

**Figure 5.46b** T-tube procedure showing a small residual stone in the distal end of the common bile duct

T-tube cholangiography is the contrast examination of the biliary ducts postoperatively. A T-tube is placed in the common bile duct at cholecystectomy and a cholangiogram is performed 7–10 days later. The T-tube also acts as postoperative bile drainage. If excessive bile drains through the T-tube it can be indicative of a lack of free drainage into the duodenum.

A contrast agent of low concentration is selected so that small calculi are not obscured by the contrast.

The examination is performed under fluoroscopic control.

### Indications

To confirm patency of the ducts and to assess free drainage of bile into the duodenum.

### Position of patient and imaging modality

The patient lies supine on the fluoroscopy table and the progress of contrast is observed until it passes into the duodenum.

It may be necessary to rotate the patient up to 20° into the right posterior oblique position to show the junction of the common bile duct with the duodenum and to project the duct clear of the vertebral column and bowel loops. This can be assessed by fluoroscopy.

### Imaging procedure

A control film may be taken prior to the introduction of contrast agent.

Excessive bile may be aspirated to reduce the risk of pressure build-up. The T-tube is clamped off, approximately 30 cm from the skin, and swabbed with antiseptic solution.

The contrast agent is injected, via a 21-gauge needle, directly into the lumen of the tube, under fluoroscopic control. Care is taken to avoid introducing air bubbles which could be confused with filling defects due to non-opaque stones.

Images are obtained as required to demonstrate free flow of contrast into the duodenum.

*Contrast medium and injection data*

| *Volume* | *Concentration* | *Flow rate* |
|---|---|---|
| 20 ml | 280 mgI/ml | Hand injection |

# 5 Gallbladder and Biliary Ducts

## Oral cholecystography

Prior to the advances in ultrasound, oral cholecystography was the primary imaging technique for demonstrating the gallbladder. Its role is now limited to patients with non-acute gallbladder disease in whom ultrasound has proved inconclusive.

### Indications

Non-acute gallbladder disease and to confirm gallbladder function in patients selected for stone dissolution therapy prior to commencement of treatment.

### Patient preparation

When the patient attends for an appointment, a control film of the right upper quadrant of the abdomen is performed in the left anterior oblique position. The film should include the right hemidiaphragm, vertebral column and right iliac crest. General abdominal preparation in the form of a mild laxative is administered on the two evenings prior to the administration of the contrast agent. At lunchtime on the day prior to the examination the patient takes a fatty meal which has the effect of emptying the gallbladder. This is followed by a light fat-free meal taken in the early evening of the same day. Laxatives and any food likely to produce flatulence should be avoided.

### Imaging procedure

The patient takes 3 g of sodium ipodate (or calcium ipodate) in water, 14 h before the examination. After this the patient is encouraged to drink plenty of water or clear fluids (at least 1 litre) to reduce nephrotoxicity. No further food is permitted and smoking should be avoided. A further dose of contrast (3 g) may be taken early in the morning of the examination in an attempt to opacify the ducts.

Radiographs are taken with the patient prone in the left anterior oblique (LAO) position to project the gallbladder clear of the vertebral column. Compression may be applied to reduce scatter radiation and exposure factors are chosen to optimise image contrast. An additional radiograph is taken with the patient erect, to clarify the nature of any filling defect.

Alternative or additional projections, e.g. supine, right posterior oblique, right lateral decubitus or cranial/caudal tube angulation or tomography, may be necessary where overlying gas shadows are present. Some centres use fluoroscopy to achieve optimum visualisation with respect to overlying gas shadows and the vertebral column.

A fatty meal is administered to the patient to assess gallbladder function. A LAO radiograph taken 30 min later should demonstrate a contracted gallbladder, cystic duct and common bile duct. If contraction is not shown, a delayed film should be taken after 1 h.

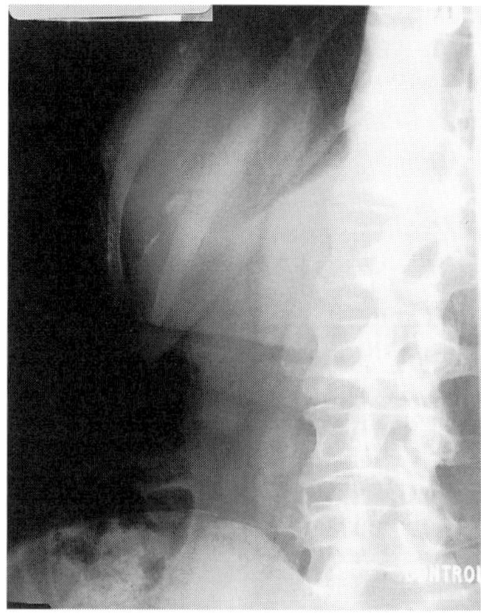

**Figure 5.47a** Preliminary image left anterior oblique (prone)

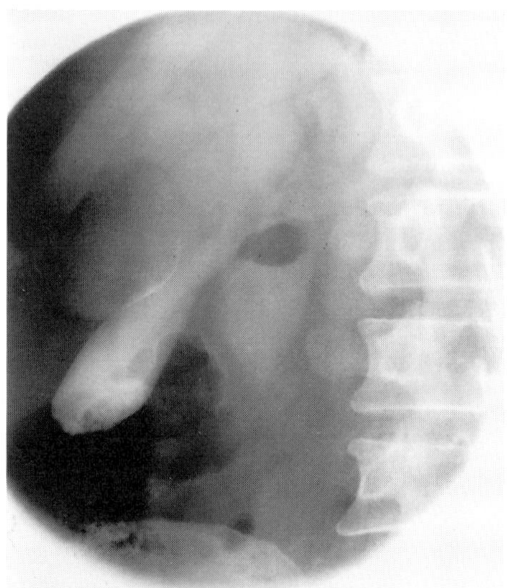

**Figure 5.47b** Fourteen-hour post-contrast image – left anterior oblique (prone) projection showing opacified gallbladder and adjacent calcified renal cyst

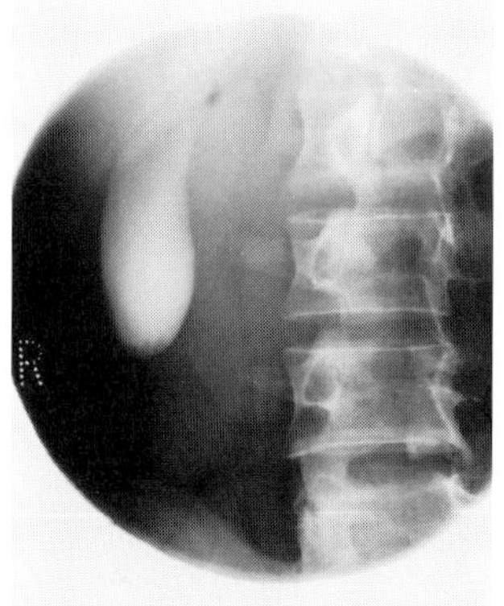


**Figure 5.47c** Fourteen-hour post-contrast image – left anterior oblique (erect) projection showing multiple small gallstones in the fundus of the gallbladder

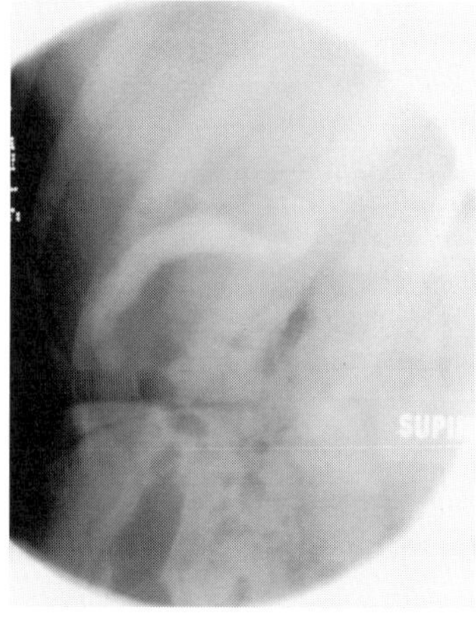

**Figure 5.47d** Thirty minutes AFM image showing gallbladder contraction

## Oral cholecystography

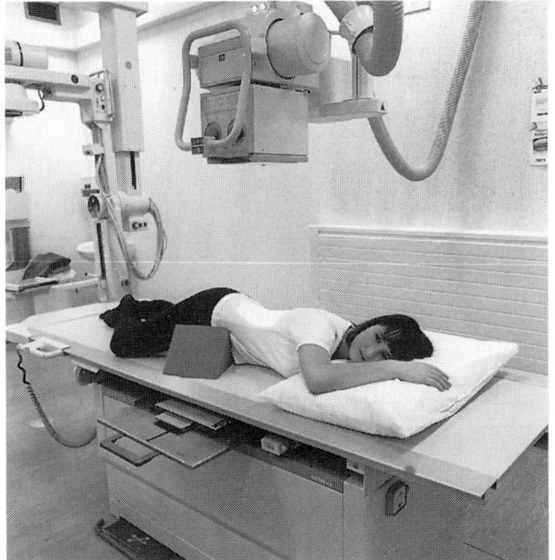
(a)

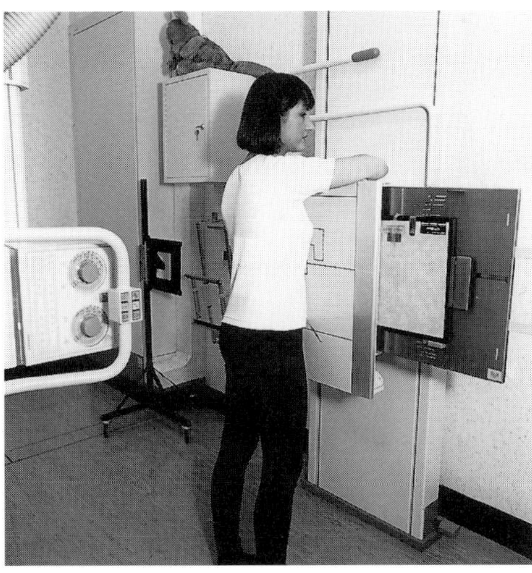
(b)

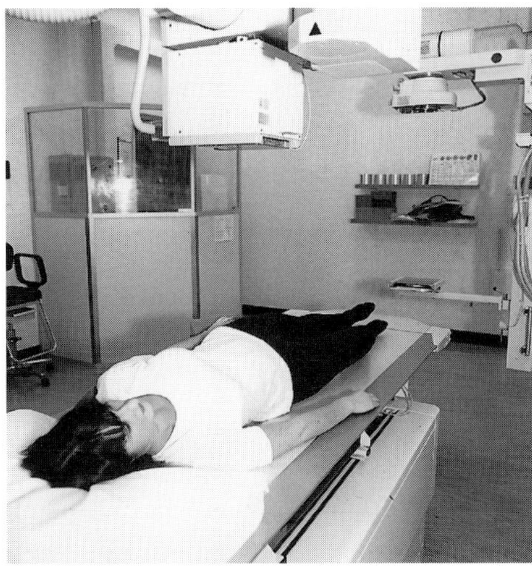
(c)

**Figure 5.48a–c** Positioning of patient for LAO (prone), LAO (erect) and RPO (supine) projections

### Left anterior oblique (prone) projection

*Position of patient and imaging modality*
The patient lies prone on the Bucky table. The right side is raised approximately 20° into the LAO position to project the gallbladder clear of the vertebral column. The degree of obliquity will depend on physique: asthenic patients will require greater rotation, hyposthenic patients proportionally less.

A 23 × 30 cm cassette is placed longitudinally in the Bucky tray and is positioned to include the 11th rib superiorly and iliac crest inferiorly.

*Direction and centring of the X-ray beam*
The vertical central ray is centred 8 cm to the right of the spinous process and approximately 5 cm above the lower costal margin. This may be adjusted as indicated by the patient's physique. The centring point should be marked on the patient, so that any necessary adjustments may be effected for subsequent projections.

### Left anterior oblique (erect) projection

*Position of patient and imaging modality*
The patient is positioned erect facing the erect Bucky. The positioning is identical to that for the prone projection, except that the cassette is displaced approximately 5 cm caudally.

*Direction and centring of the X-ray beam*
The horizontal central ray is centred in a similar way to that described above. The centring point is displaced approximately 5 cm caudally.

### Right posterior oblique (supine) projection

This projection may be employed when bowel gas is overlying the gallbladder in the routine LAO projection.

*Position of patient and imaging modality*
The patient lies supine on the Bucky table, with the left side raised approximately 20–30° and supported by foam pads. The 23 × 30 cm cassette is placed longitudinally in the Bucky tray and is positioned to include the 11th rib superiorly and iliac crest inferiorly.

*Direction and centring of the X-ray beam*
The vertical central ray is centred just below the costal margin along the mid-clavicular line.

# 5 Gallbladder and Biliary Ducts

## Computed tomography

The main disadvantage of CT compared with ultrasound is the use of ionising radiation. It is, however, a useful modality for differentiating between obstructive and non-obstructive jaundice. It can also demonstrate both the location and cause of obstruction.

It is particularly useful in patients in whom ultrasound examination has proved difficult, e.g. obese patients and those with excessive bowel gas.

### Indications

Obstructive jaundice in obese patients and obstruction due to suspected mass in the head of pancreas.

### Position of patient and imaging modality

The patient lies feet first on the scanner table. The arms are raised and placed behind the patient's head, out of the scan plane. Positioning is aided by transaxial, coronal and sagittal alignment lights.

The median sagittal plane is perpendicular and the coronal plane parallel to the scanner table. The scan plane is now perpendicular to the long axis of the body to enable transaxial cross-sectional imaging to be undertaken. The scanner height is adjusted to ensure that the coronal plane alignment light is at the mid-axillary line. The patient is then moved into the scanner until the scan reference point is at the level of the xiphisternum.

### Imaging procedure

An anteroposterior scan projection radiograph is performed, commencing 5 cm above and ending 25 cm below the scan reference point. From this image, 10 mm contiguous sections are prescribed through the entire liver/pancreas, from the dome of the diaphragm to the middle of the third lumbar vertebra.

After review, the sections are rescanned during an infusion of a non-ionic contrast agent. Scanning commences after 60 ml of contrast medium has been administered.

If spiral scanning options are available, these images may be acquired with a volume acquisition, using a 10 mm slice thickness and 10 mm table increments, but with a 5 mm reconstruction index to give overlapping sections.

Contrast medium enhanced CT sections may enable characterisation of focal lesions. Gallstones can represent a variety of appearances, depending on their constitution. Most gallstones have an attenuation coefficient higher than that of surrounding bile, but pure cholesterol stones can also be detected as areas of reduced attenuation.

*Contrast medium and injection data*

| *Volume* | *Concentration* | *Flow rate* |
|---|---|---|
| 100 ml | 300 mgI/ml | 2 ml/s |

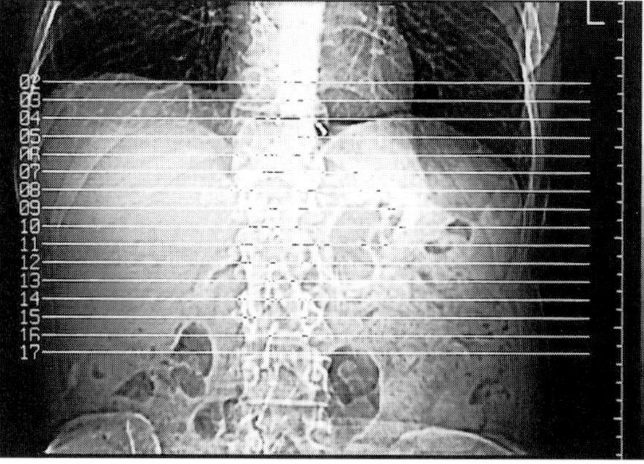

**Figure 5.49a** Scan projection radiograph showing prescribed sections

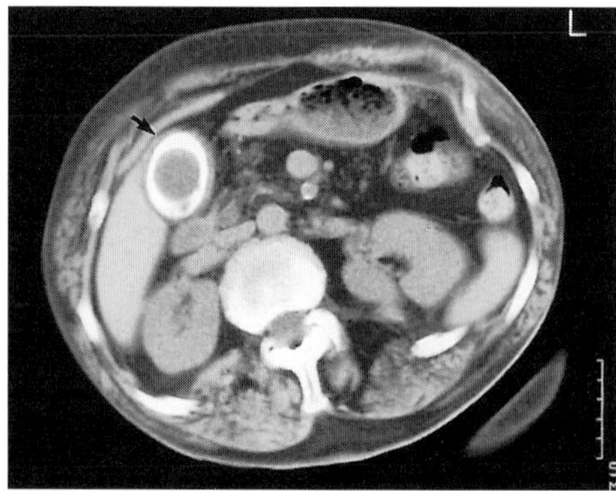

**Figure 5.49b** Transaxial section through the liver showing a large stone occupying the gallbladder

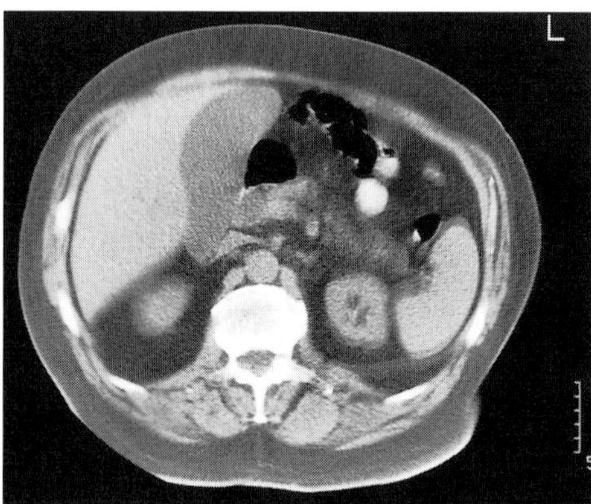

**Figure 5.49c** Pre-contrast enhancement section showing distended gallbladder

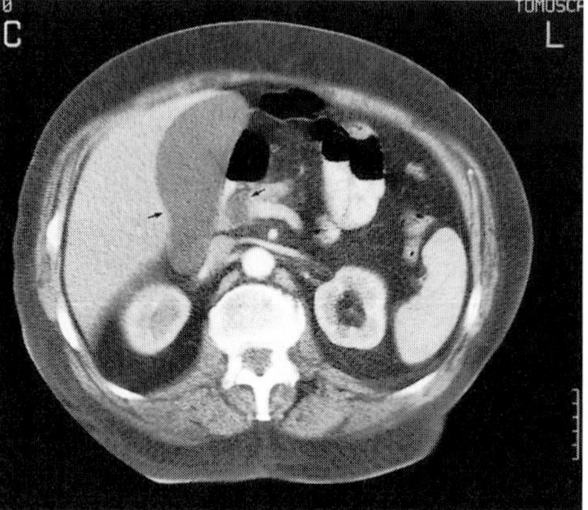

**Figure 5.49d** Post-contrast enhancement section showing dilated common bile duct

## Radionuclide imaging

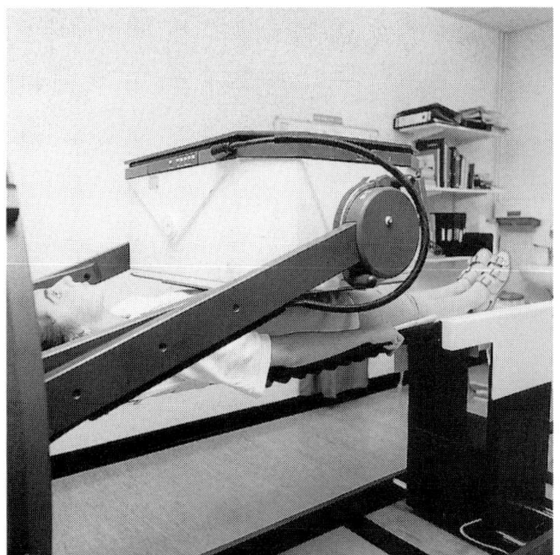

**Figure 5.50a** Patient in position for anterior imaging

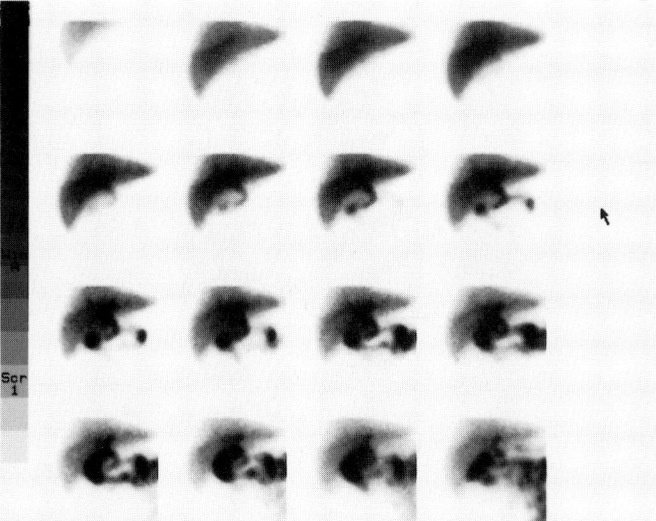

**Figure 5.50b** Sequential set of images following intravenous injection of radiopharmaceutical

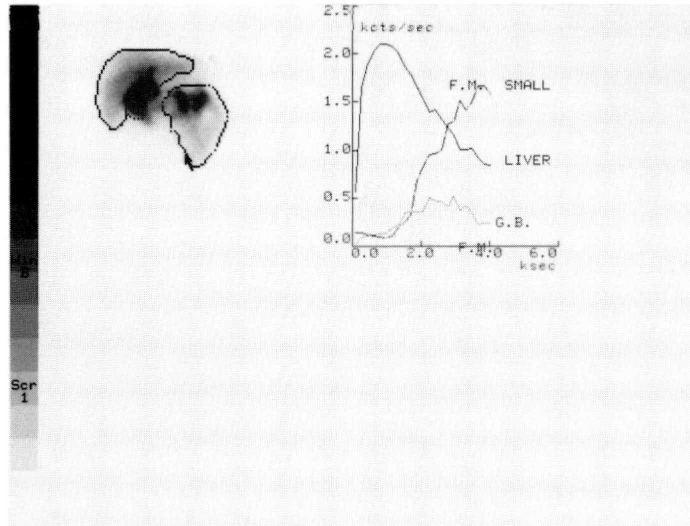


**Figure 5.50c** Graph showing filling and emptying of the gallbladder following fatty meal

$^{99m}$Technetium-labelled iminodiacetic acid compounds ($^{99m}$Tc-HIDA) allow quantifiable studies of biliary function. Following intravenous administration they are cleared rapidly from the blood pool and excreted into the bile.

During image acquisition the liver is seen to function and fill the gallbladder. Following a fatty meal the gallbladder should be seen to empty, with subsequent filling of the small bowel. Analysis of gallbladder filling and emptying is aided by the production of graphical time–activity curves.

### Indications

Acute cholecystitis and gallbladder function. Biliary leakage (post-surgery or interventional procedure), biliary atresia and bile reflux.

### Patient preparation

The patient fasts for 4–6 h (or overnight).

### Position of patient and imaging modality

The patient lies supine on the imaging couch to facilitate anterior imaging of the abdomen. The camera is positioned above the patient, parallel to the imaging couch, over the anterior surface of the upper abdomen and as close as possible to the skin surface.

### Imaging procedure

A high-resolution collimator is employed. The patient is made comfortable on the imaging couch and, following a bolus intravenous injection of the radiopharmaceutical, sequential 3-minute images are acquired over a period of approximately 60 min up to a maximum of 90 min after the injection. At 30 min, provided that the gallbladder has filled, the patient is given a fatty meal or alternatively a glass of milk.

### Image analysis

Following review of the images acquired, a composite image is produced on which regions of interest are drawn around the liver, gallbladder and the small bowel. Time–activity curves are subsequently produced to quantify hepatobiliary function.

Non-visualisation of the gallbladder 60 min after injection in cases with supporting clinical findings is suggestive of acute cholecystitis. Delayed visualisation up to 3 h post-injection is indicative of chronic cholecystitis.

Delayed or absent visualisation of gallbladder, bile ducts and intestine is indicative of obstructive jaundice or diffuse liver disease.

Biliary reflux can be diagnosed by observing if activity is present in the stomach.

*Imaging and radiopharmaceutical parameters*

| *Type* | *Administered activity* | *Principal energy* |
|---|---|---|
| $^{99m}$Tc-HIDA | 75–150 MBq | 140 keV |
| *Window width* | *Acquisition counts/time* | |
| 20% | 3 min/frame × 20 frames | |

# 5 Alimentary System

## Pancreas

The pancreas lies retroperitoneally and is situated in the epigastric and left hypochondriac regions of the abdomen. It is between 12 and 15 cm long and comprises a broad head which lies in the curve of the duodenum, a body behind the stomach, and a tail which reaches the spleen. Its posterior relations include the aorta and inferior vena cava.

The gland is divided into lobules, the walls of which are lined with secretory cells. These drain by a series of ducts into the main pancreatic duct which extends the length of the pancreas before joining with the bile duct at the ampulla of Vater. This opens into the second stage of the duodenum through a small papilla controlled by the sphincter of Oddie.

Distributed throughout the body and tail of the pancreas are collections of endocrine tissue known as the islets of Langerhans. These secrete insulin and glucagon directly into the blood stream. The pancreas receives its blood supply from the splenic and mesenteric arteries and drains via pancreatic and splenic veins.

### Recommended imaging procedures

Plain radiographs of the abdomen do not demonstrate the normal pancreas. It is only since the introduction of ultrasound and CT that successful imaging of the gland has been possible.

Ultrasound can provide detailed information on the structure of the gland and its vasculature. However, the depth of the gland, particularly the tail, may mean it is not possible to visualise the entire gland in obese patients or patients with excessive bowel gas.

Computed tomography is the modality of choice in the investigation of acute pancreatitis and suspected tumour.

Endoscopic retrograde cholangiopancreatography permits good visualisation of the pancreatic duct and its major branches and is the examination of choice in suspected chronic pancreatitis or when interventional techniques are planned.

Angiography may be performed prior to surgery or to demonstrate small adenomas.

With the advent of respiratory gating, MRI of the pancreas may provide useful information to support the findings of CT.

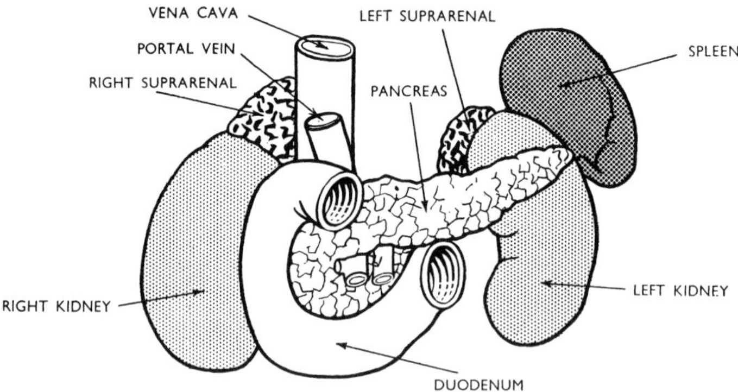


**Figure 5.51a** Relationship of the pancreas to surrounding anatomical structures

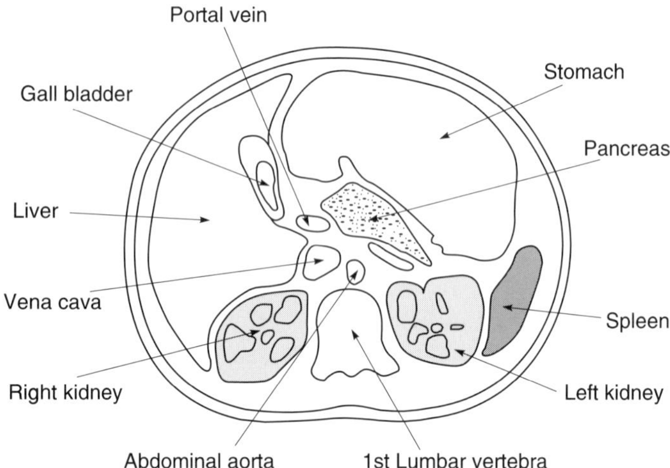


**Figure 5.51b** Transaxial section at level of first lumbar vertebra

## Ultrasound

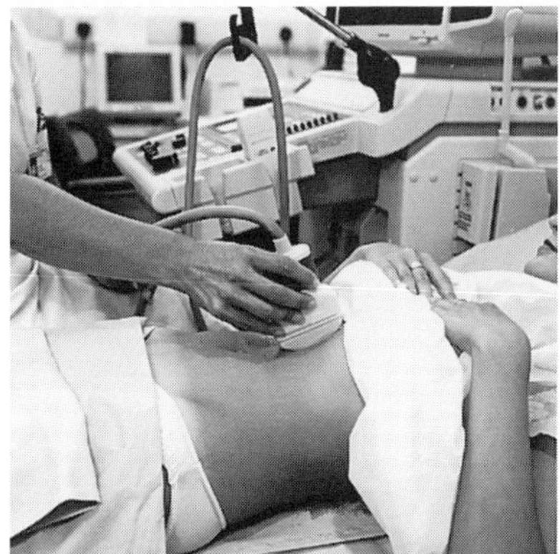

**Figure 5.52a** Transducer positioned for longitudinal scan

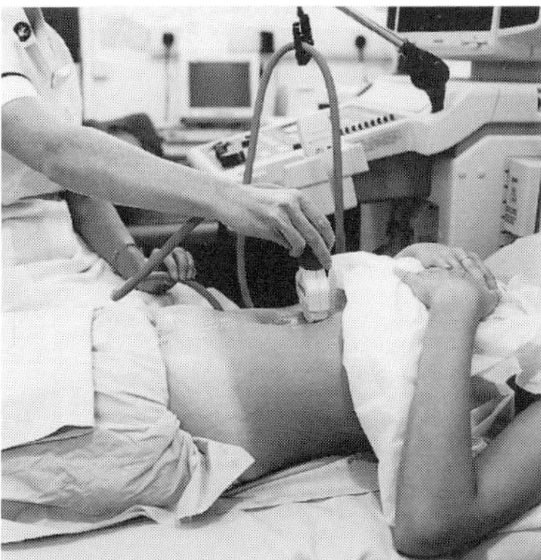

**Figure 5.52b** Transducer positioned for transverse scan

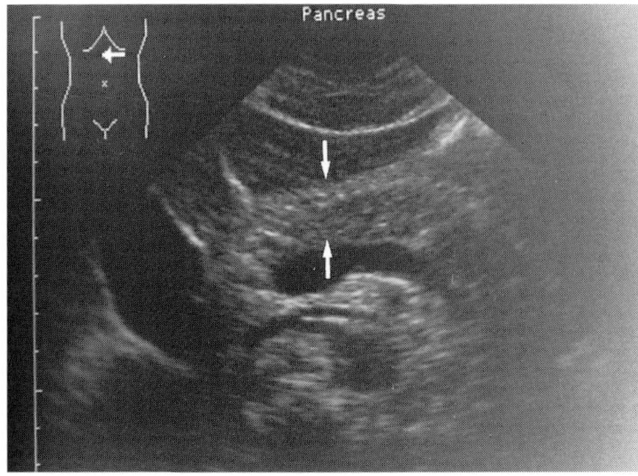


**Figure 5.52c** Transverse scan with caudal angulation showing normal pancreas

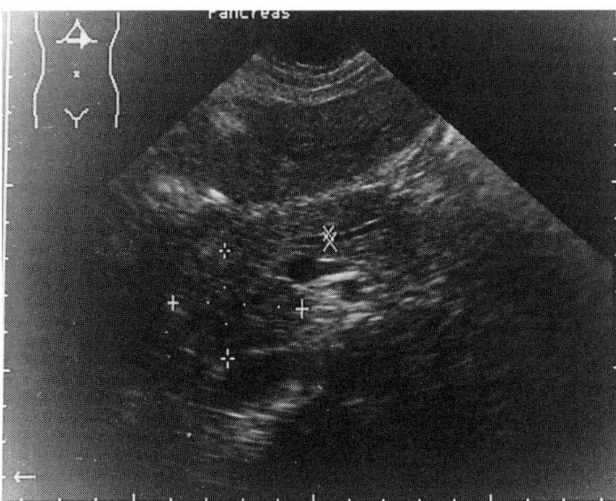

**Figure 5.52d** Transverse scan of abdomen with caudal angulation showing calipers positioned around a bulky head of pancreas and pancreatic duct

Ultrasound provides a painless, simple, non-invasive method of examining the pancreatic anatomy in patients of normal physique. To be successful, however, the examination requires minimal intestinal gas and small difference in echo structure of the retroperitoneal fat tissue to successfully examine the whole of the pancreas. It also has the advantage of not employing ionising radiation.

A real-time scanner is selected for accurate assessment of the pancreas and surrounding organs and any pathology. A sector or curvilinear probe provides a large field of view and excellent access to the abdominal organs. A 3.5 MHz probe provides the high frequency required for good resolution and good penetration. A 5 MHz probe will offer improved resolution in slimmer patients. Machine settings are varied, depending on the region of interest, to reduce power, i.e. patient dose, and at the same time to maintain good penetration and quality of image.

### Indications

Inflammatory or neoplastic disease of the pancreas and pseudocysts. In jaundice cases it is also used to distinguish between biliary tree dilatation caused by carcinoma of the head of pancreas and that caused by large stones in the biliary tree.

### Patient preparation

Fasting for up to 6 h is advisable to reduce gas and food residue in the stomach and bowel and is necessary when it is planned to include investigation of the biliary system, for maximum dilatation of the gallbladder.

### Imaging procedure

With the patient supine the transducer is initially placed 2 cm to the left of the midline below the xiphisternum, so that a longitudinal section of the left lobe of the liver and aorta is obtained. The pancreas is located by identifying the upper abdominal vasculature and is seen as a more echogenic structure compared to the liver. In cross-section the body of the pancreas should be seen anterior to the superior mesenteric artery and posterior to the liver.

At this stage, general examination of the upper abdomen is usually performed using parasagittal sections to assess the liver and other structures, as well as examining the pancreas longitudinally. During this process the obliquity of the pancreatic lie is assessed. The transducer is rotated in a transverse position and angled slightly to obtain long axis views of the pancreas. The transducer is further rotated to identify the pancreatic tail and head. All views are obtained with the patient performing quiet breathing and, if necessary, with the patient asked to arrest respiration or gently push forward the anterior abdominal wall.

# 5 Pancreas

## Computed tomography

Computed tomography provides valuable information on the pancreas and adjacent structures. Transaxial scanning is undertaken pre- and post-intravenous injection of a water-soluble contrast agent. It is necessary to opacify the bowel using dilute Gastrografin/barium given orally 30 and 15 min prior to scanning.

**Indications**
Carcinoma of the pancreas, insulinomas, radiotherapy planning, cysts and pseudocysts.

**Imaging procedure**
An anteroposterior scan projection radiograph is performed, commencing 5 cm above and ending 25 cm below the scan reference point. From this image, 10 mm contiguous scans are performed to include the liver and the pancreas. The pancreas area is rescanned during the infusion of contrast medium, using 5 mm table increments and a 5 mm slice width, to demonstrate the pancreatic parenchyma and major vascular structures. If spiral scanning options are available, these images may be acquired with a volume acquisition, using a 5 mm slice thickness and 5 mm table increments, but with a 3 mm reconstruction index to give overlapping sections.

Scanning may commence after 60–80 ml of contrast medium has been administered.

*Contrast medium and injection data*

| *Volume* | *Concentration* | *Flow rate* |
|---|---|---|
| 100 ml | 300 mgI/ml | 2 ml/s |

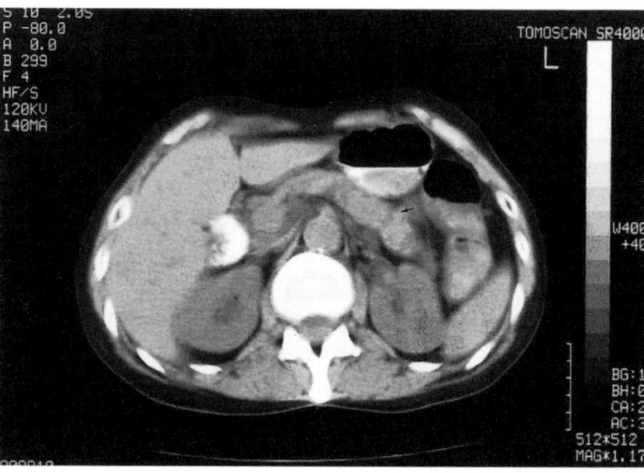

**Figure 5.53a** Transaxial pre-contrast enhancement image of the pancreas

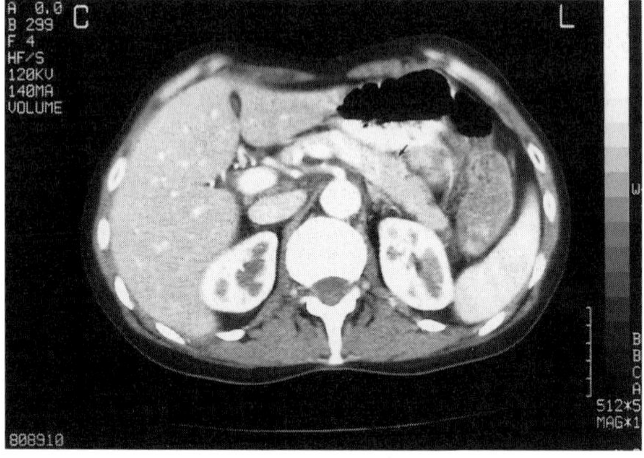

**Figure 5.53b** Transaxial post-contrast enhancement image of the pancreas

## Endoscopic retrograde cholangiopancreatography (ERCP)

Endoscopic retrograde cholangiopancreatography is the ideal modality for the investigation of chronic pancreatic disease and for duct visualisation. It also facilitates interventional procedures such as duct dilatation and stent insertion. The technique is similar to that described for endoscopic examination of the biliary ducts (see page 179), except that the catheter is inserted into the pancreatic duct.

## Angiography

Selective superior mesenteric and coeliac axis arteriography can be performed to demonstrate the blood supply to the pancreas prior to surgery. It is useful in demonstrating small pancreatic tumours and can assist in differentiating inflammatory and neoplastic disease where CT has failed. The technique is described under the small bowel (see page 160).

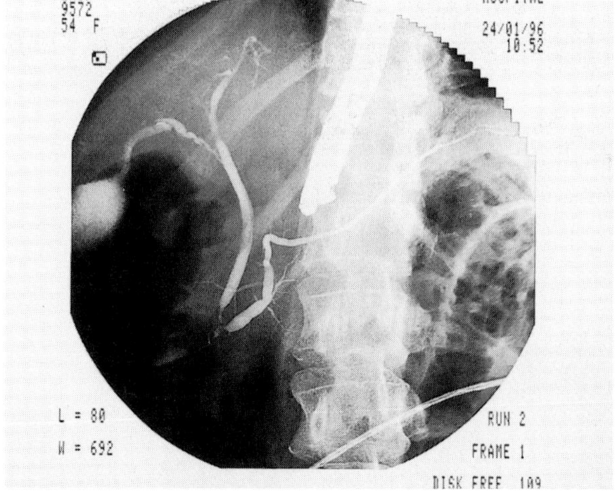

**Figure 5.53c** Pancreatic duct demonstrated on ERCP

## Magnetic resonance imaging

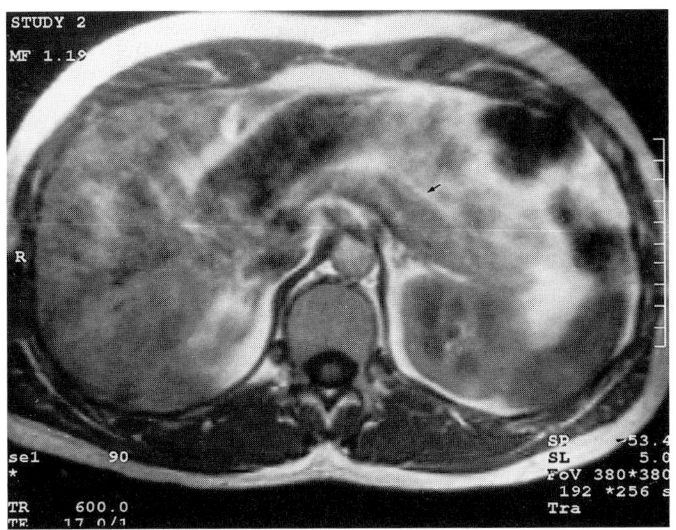


Figure 5.54a Transaxial $T_1$ weighted spin-echo image

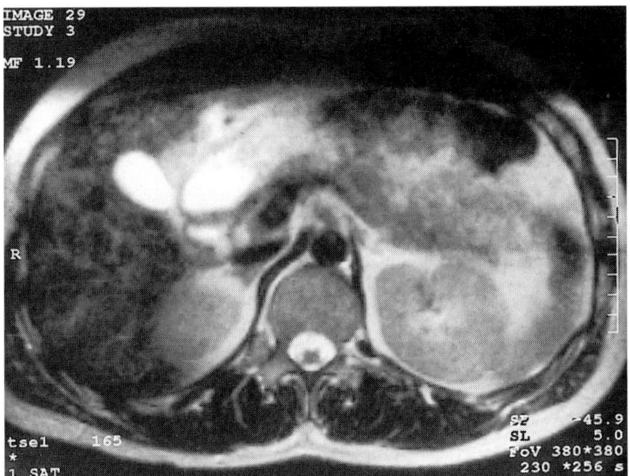


Figure 5.54b Transaxial $T_2$ weighted spin-echo sequence

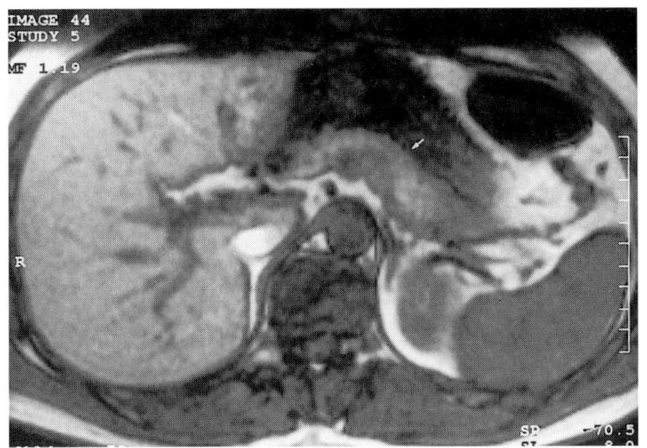


Figure 5.54c Transaxial gradient-echo image with breath hold

Up to the time of writing, MRI of the pancreas has been made difficult due to relatively slow scan times with associated respiratory, bowel and vascular motion artefacts. Currently, however, faster scanning techniques are being developed, such as echo-planar imaging (EPI) associated with the use of phased array coils, giving better signal-to-noise, with anatomy demonstrated more clearly. The use of MRI to demonstrate the biliary and pancreatic ducts (MR cholangiography) is still a matter of research.

*Indications*

Acute and chronic pancreatitis, adenocarcinoma, solid and papillary epithelial neoplasms of the pancreas, islet cell tumours and cystic neoplasms.

*Position of patient and imaging modality*

The patient and modality are positioned in a similar way to that described for the liver on page 176.

*Imaging procedure*

An initial coronal localiser is performed. From this image transaxial $T_1$ weighted and fast spin-echo $T_2$ sequences are prescribed through the pancreas, followed by a series of fat-suppressed $T_1$ weighted images and a series of breath-hold rapid fat-suppressed, gadolinium-enhanced fast multiplanar spoiled gradient recalled (FMPSPGR) images. This sequence may be done before, immediately after and 1 min after a bolus injection of gadolinium contrast. A further series of post-contrast $T_1$ and fat-suppressed $T_1$ weighted images are also obtained. Slices are 6–8 mm thick, with a 1–2 mm gap. Motion artefacts are suppressed, with respiratory ordered phase encoding and spatial presaturation for spin-echo images and flow compensation for $T_2$ weighted images. Glucagon is administered intramuscularly for bowel movement peristalsis.

*Image analysis*

On fat-suppressed $T_1$ weighted images the pancreas is hypertense to liver due to aqueous protein in the pancreas granular elements. If there is a low-signal abnormality on $T_1$ fat saturation images, this may be due to cancer or pancreatitis. On pre-contrast FMPSPGR images the páncreas appears low signal, but immediately after contrast enhances uniformly with higher signal intensity than the liver and surrounding fat.

# 5 Spleen

## Introduction

The spleen is situated principally in the left hypochondriac region of the abdomen, lying behind the fundus of the stomach and the diaphragm. It is ovoid in shape and its size and weight varies significantly with age and between individuals. It is related closely to the diaphragm superiorly and the visceral surface has gastric, renal, pancreatic and colic impressions. The hilum is situated on the visceral surface and permits passage of vessels, including the splenic artery, splenic vein, lymphatic vessel and nerves. The spleen is covered on its visceral surface by peritoneum, under which is a fibroelastic capsule. The bulk of the organ is composed of lymphoid tissue and blood capillaries, known collectively as the splenic pulp. The function of the spleen is to act as a reservoir for blood and the destruction of red blood cells.

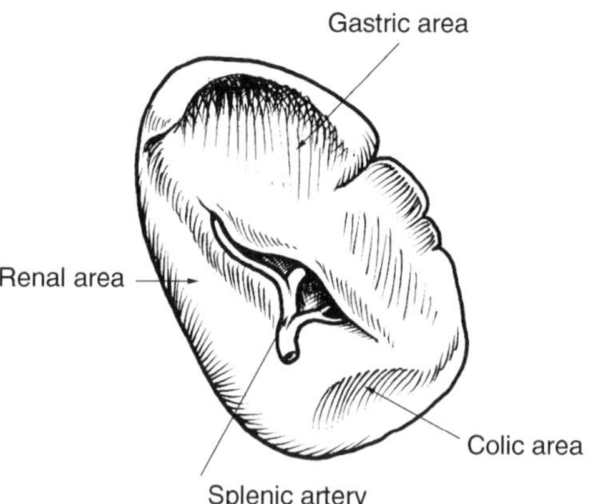


**Figure 5.55a** Schematic diagram of spleen showing indentations

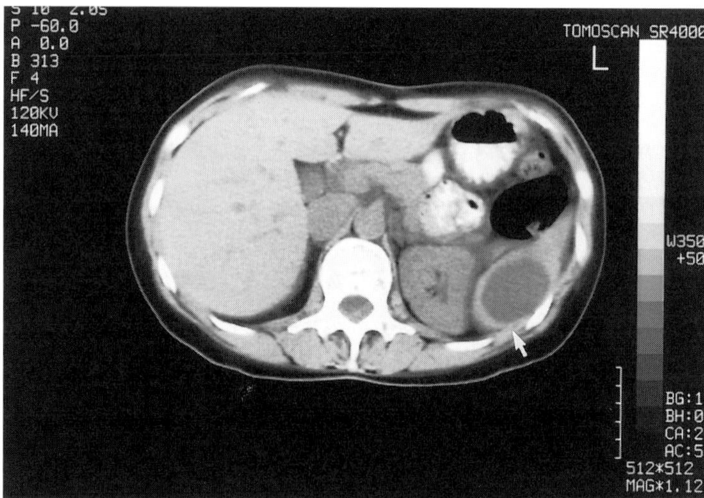


**Figure 5.55b** Pre-contrast enhancement CT image showing a splenic cyst

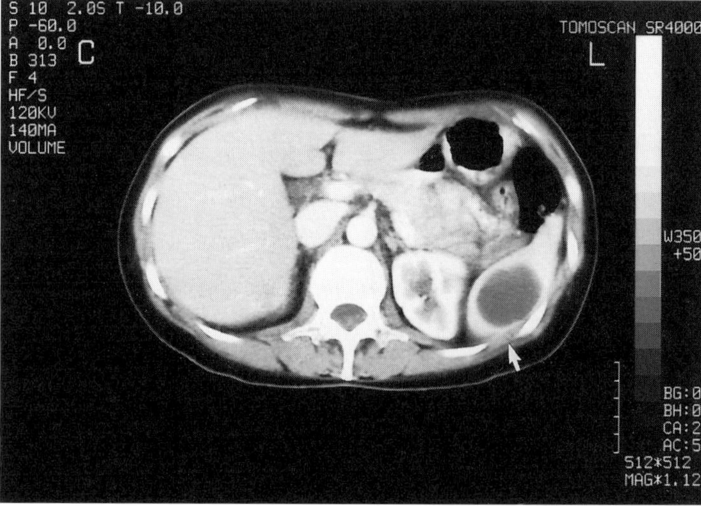


**Figure 5.55c** Post-contrast enhancement CT image of splenic cyst

### Recommended imaging procedures

Plain radiographs of the abdomen do not demonstrate the normal spleen; however, fluid levels as a result of haemorrhage from the spleen may be demonstrated by a combination of erect and supine radiographs of the chest and abdomen. Ultrasound, which is widely available, enables detailed demonstration of splenic anatomy and is the modality of choice in the diagnosis of splenic haematomas, lacerations and other masses (e.g. tumours). Ultrasound, however, has its limitations as interference from rib shadows, gas in the bowel and air in the lung may hinder proper visualisation. The spleen may be difficult to examine after trauma as the patient is usually acutely tender in the region of interest.

The organ may be demonstrated by CT and MRI in a similar fashion to those procedures described for the liver. Radionuclide imaging using a colloid as described for RNI of the liver (see page 174) also demonstrates the spleen. Another RNI examination to demonstrate the spleen uses labelled denatured red blood cells which are sequestrated by the organ.

### Ultrasound

A real-time scanner is used for rapid interrogation of the organ, visualisation of the diaphragmatic movement and visualisation of any effusions which may have been the cause of pain. A sector scanner provides a small coupling surface, producing a wedge-shaped beam, enabling access to the organs subcostally and intercostally. A 3.5 MHz transducer frequency provides maximum penetration with good resolution of all abdominal structures. Power and receiver gain is adjusted to provide maximum penetration and optimum amplification of the echoes from the splenic parenchyma. Colour flow Doppler can also be performed to identify the origin of a continual fresh bleed.

## Ultrasound

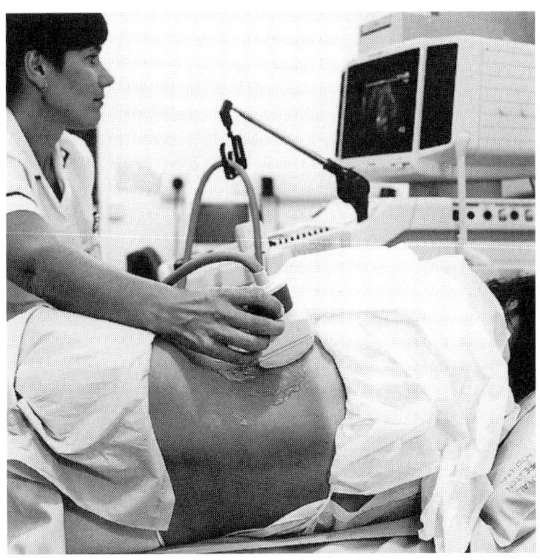
**Figure 5.56a** Patient in right lateral position with transducer held for a longitudinal scan

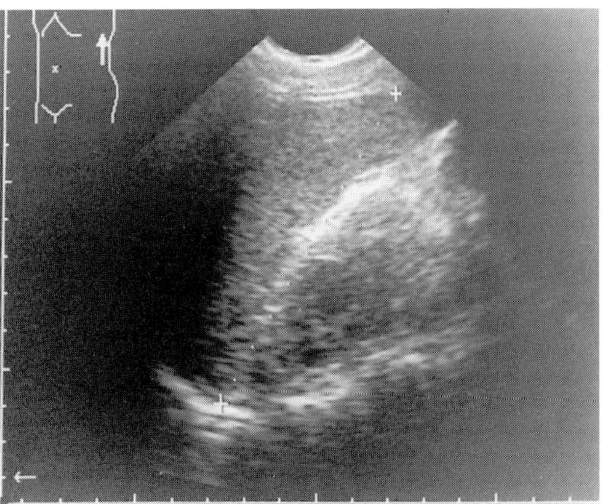
**Figure 5.56b** Coronal image of normal spleen

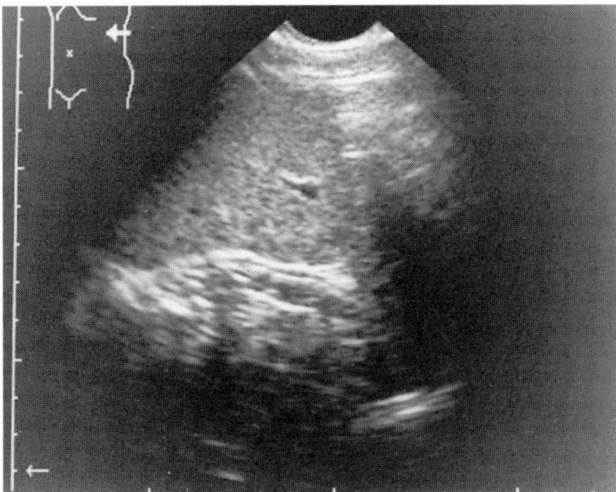
**Figure 5.56c** Transverse image of spleen – note shadowing from ribs due to intercostal positioning of transducer

### Indications

Identification and demonstration of progressive signs of splenic haemorrhage, ranging from early subcapsular haematoma to the build-up of peritoneal bleeding resulting from blunt abdominal trauma. Abscesses developed from unresolved haematomas, splenomegaly, acute or chronic inflammation, congestive disease or primary hepatic disease.

### Patient preparation

Fasting for up to 6 h is advisable to reduce intestinal gas and food residue in the stomach and bowel.

### Position of patient and imaging modality

The patient is asked to lie on the right side or is rotated obliquely 45° from the supine position, towards the right, with the left side raised. The left arm is raised above the patient's head. The 10th intercostal space is the preferred position for the transducer. The transducer is angled obliquely so that the beam passes between the ribs. If this does not provide a suitable acoustic window the ninth or 11th spaces may be tried. Placing a pillow under the patient may improve access.

The patient may also be positioned supine and scanned with the transducer held horizontally to overcome any problems of overlying lung.

### Imaging procedure

The spleen is examined on arrested inspiration or gentle respiration, depending on the access between left lung and overlying bowel gas. The procedure normally includes examination of the adjacent left kidney, the left crus of the diaphragm to eliminate the presence of a subphrenic abscess or left pleural effusion, liver and other abdominal structures.

Initially, longitudinal scans are performed along the 10th intercostal space until the maximum length of the spleen is visualised on one image. From this position the transducer is gently moved anteriorly and posteriorly to obtain a series of coronal sections through the organ.

To examine the spleen in transverse sections, the transducer is rotated through 90° and placed intercostally. The transducer is then angled both cranially and caudally while the patient uses a combination of quiet breathing manoeuvres and arrested respiration.

# 6

## Urinary System

### CONTENTS

# 6 Urinary System

## Introduction

The urinary system extends from the kidneys to the urethral meatus, and is comprised of the kidneys, the ureters, the bladder and the urethra.

The kidneys, which excrete urine, are situated in the lumbar region either side of the vertebral column, between the 12th thoracic and third lumbar vertebrae and are behind the peritoneum. The precise position varies slightly according to the build of the subject. Both are oblique in position, with their upper poles nearest the vertebrae and the lower poles more anterior than the upper poles. They are approximately 10 cm in length, the left usually slightly longer and narrower than the right. The right is normally positioned 1 cm lower in the abdomen.

Each kidney consists of an outer cortex and an inner medulla containing the complex filtering system and minute blood vessels. Urine flows into a collecting system consisting of small cavities called calyces which drain into the renal pelvis and then into the bladder via the ureters.

The ureters are approximately 25–30 cm in length and extend downward from the renal pelvis at the level of the second lumbar vertebra, usually overlying the tips of the transverse processes, to the pelvis. Here they sweep anteriorly around the pelvic sidewall, finally approaching the midline to terminate in the ureteric orifices, 2.5 cm apart in the posterior wall of the bladder.

The bladder is situated in the anterior part of the pelvic cavity, behind and just above the symphysis pubis. Its exact position depends on the degree of distension. When full it dilates to form an ovoid shape with the fundus rising to the level of the sacroiliac joints.

The urethra starts at the neck of the bladder, 2.5 cm from the ureteric orifices, with the three apertures forming a triangle named the trigone. It extends to the urethral meatus, and is 18–20 cm in length in males and 4 cm in length in females.

In the male the urethra traverses the prostate gland which lies below and adjacent to the bladder.

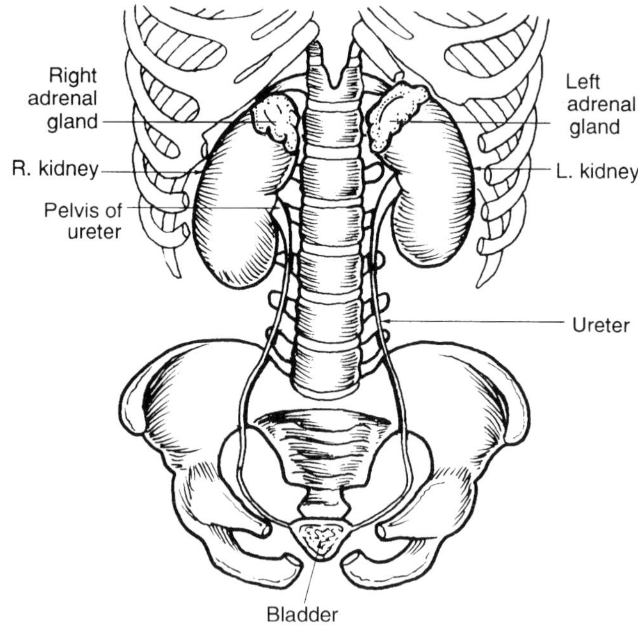


**Figure 6.1a** Urinary system – anterior aspect

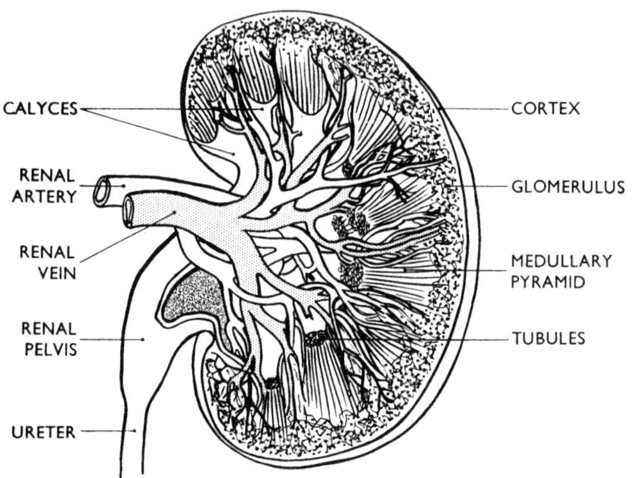


**Figure 6.1b** Coronal section through the left kidney

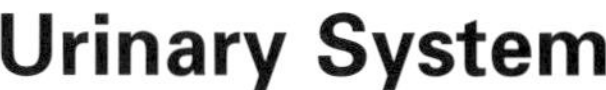

## Recommended imaging procedures

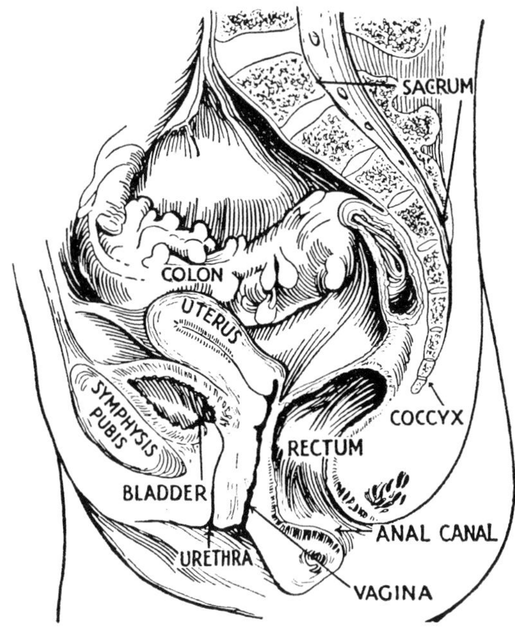


**Figure 6.2a** A median sagittal section through the female pelvis

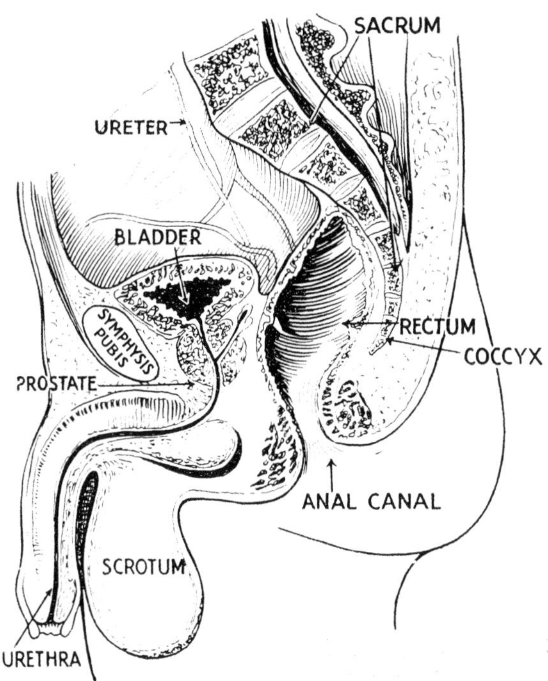


**Figure 6.2b** A median sagittal section through the male pelvis

Plain radiography of the abdomen and pelvic cavity is frequently carried out to demonstrate opacities in the kidneys, ureters and bladder and is routinely performed prior to intravenous urography. Other imaging modalities may also be employed to show the nature and extent of disease.

Intravenous urography is an invaluable tool in demonstrating the renal parenchyma and the filling and drainage of the collecting system. It readily shows the cause and effects of ureteric obstruction and is used to demonstrate transitional cell tumours in the pelvicalyceal system and ureters.

Retrograde pyelography and antegrade pyelography can also be used to show the renal pelvis and ureter in more detail.

Cystography and urethrography can be performed for bladder and urethra investigations.

Ultrasound plays an important primary role in assessing renal size and shape as well as demonstrating blood vessels and the internal renal structure, where it is sensitive in showing a minor degree of dilatation of the collecting system and any mass lesions. It is also used in the diagnosis of prostatic disease as well as measuring the post-micturition capacity of the bladder.

Radionuclide imaging is used to assess split renal function, vascularity and drainage and to confirm non-functioning tissue.

Computed tomography can be used following intravenous urography to evaluate the extent and nature of renal and bladder masses, as well as ascertaining the cause of extrinsic ureteric obstruction.

Renal angiography is generally restricted to the diagnosis of renal artery stenosis and occasionally for the diagnosis of difficult space-occupying lesions. It may also be employed in conjunction with renal artery embolization of inoperable renal tumours to control bleeding and superselective embolisation for severe bleeding following trauma if appropriate, e.g. post-renal biopsy. Magnetic resonance imaging may have a role in the future but at the time of writing has not been fully assessed.

Fluoroscopy or ultrasound is used during interventional procedures such as nephrostomy tube insertion, percutaneous nephrolithotomy (PCNL) and lithotripsy.

# 6 Urinary System

## Intravenous Urography

### Introduction

Intravenous urography (IVU) is the examination of the urinary tract following the introduction of a water-soluble iodine contrast medium through a vein in the arm. The contrast medium is excreted by the kidneys, rendering the urine opaque to X-rays and allowing visualisation of the renal parenchyma together with the calyces, renal pelvis, ureters and bladder.

Abdominal preparation is normally necessary, but is abandoned if the examination is carried out as an emergency procedure.

The examination is normally carried out using conventional overcouch radiography equipment capable of performing tomography. A suitable film/screen system is selected to give optimum image resolution.

Use of abdominal compression is employed in many centres to delay drainage and promote filling of the renal pelvis/calyceal system.

#### Indications

Haematuria, suspected transitional cell carcinoma, renal calculi, ureteric obstruction, trauma and prostatic disease.

#### Contraindications

Renal failure, myeloma and known contrast sensitivity with a risk of severe reaction. As contrast is excreted by a similar mechanism to creatinine, a serum creatinine level above 200 μmol/l would indicate a patient who would be unlikely to excrete contrast satisfactorily. Caution should be exercised in diabetics and patients with severe disturbances of the liver and kidneys.

#### Contrast medium and injection data

Ionic and non-ionic agents are available, both of which are excreted by different mechanisms. The ionic group is excreted mainly by glomerular filtration causing a peak concentration of iodine in the renal cortex much faster compared to the non-ionic group which is excreted mainly in the proximal tubules. The timing of the first radiograph to demonstrate the parenchymal phase of the examination best will therefore differ. For ionic agents this will normally be at 1–2 min and for non-ionic agents 4–5 min post-injection. The low-osmolar non-ionic agents are better tolerated than the high-osmolar ionic agents and are recommended for patients at risk, e.g. those with known asthma, diabetes, allergies, sickle cell disease and those with renal or cardiac problems.

The contrast medium is injected at body temperature into a suitable vein, normally the antecubital.

**The examination described uses 50 ml of a non-ionic agent with a concentration of 350–370 mgI/ml.**

#### Patient preparation

Bowel preparation is an important consideration, as the abdomen should ideally be free of radio opaque faecal matter and gas. The type and dose of medication prescribed will vary, dependent on the radiologist's preference and the condition of the patient. Most methods, however, rely on a combination of dietary restrictions and laxatives to ensure an 'empty bowel'. Current medication habits are checked to ensure the exclusion of possible opaque drugs such as bismuth.

Fluid restriction, with its effect on the patient's electrolytic balance and the concentration of the contrast medium in the renal parenchyma and the pelvicalyceal system, is an important consideration. In the majority of cases this entails restriction of fluids for 2–3 h prior to the examination.

Dehydration should not be carried out in patients with renal failure or diabetes mellitus, or in infants.

Immediately prior to the commencement of the examination the patient is asked to empty the bladder.

#### Radiation protection

The 'pregnancy rule' should be observed unless permission has been given to ignore it in cases of emergency.

If the whole of the renal tract is to be visualised, no gonad shielding is possible for females, but for males the testes can be protected by placing a lead rubber sheet over the upper thighs below the lower edge of the symphysis pubis.

When the bladder and lower ureters are not to be included on the radiograph, females can also be given gonad protection by placing a sheet of lead rubber over the lower abdomen to protect the ovaries.

#### Identification of radiographs

Identification of the patient, right or left side, date and time of each image acquisition following the intravenous injection of the contrast medium are imperative details to be noted on each radiograph.

A timing device, having a clock-like face with an X-ray opaque movable arm and opaque timing indicators from zero onwards at 5-minute intervals, is placed on the cassette. The arm is moved to the required setting for each exposure to record the actual time sequence on the radiograph following the injection of the contrast medium. Alternatively, a set of individual X-ray opaque legends, each indicating a specific time sequence, can be used for the procedure.

### Abdominal compression

Abdominal compression is used to promote filling of the pelvicalyceal system. The type of apparatus used is designed so that when it is positioned correctly over the anterior abdominal wall it has the effect of compressing the ureters where they pass over the pelvic brim, thus causing a temporary obstruction which facilitates optimum filling of the minor calyces.

It is normally placed in position in readiness for immediate use before the contrast injection and is applied properly immediately after the first radiograph is taken. It is released following radiography of the renal areas, and just before the full-length film, to show the ureters and bladder. It is not used in circumstances involving an abdominal mass, renal trauma or renal or ureteric calculi and should be discontinued if the patient complains of pain.

A variety of devices are available. One simple device uses the Bucky compression band normally supplied with the X-ray table and two tennis balls which are secured in position, one either side of the midline at the level of the anterior superior iliac spines. Compression of the ureters is achieved by careful adjustment of the ratchet tension control.

Alternatively, another more elaborate device consists of a plastic plaque placed over an inflatable bag. The plastic plaque is secured in position at the level of the anterior superior iliac spines with strapping which is wrapped around the patient. The compression bag is inflated in accordance with the patient's condition. This type of device allows the patient to move more easily for minor adjustment of patient positioning.

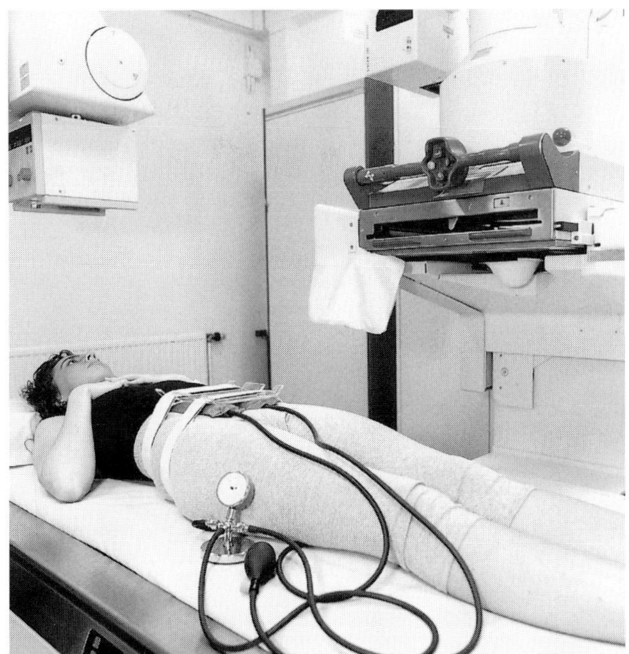

**Figure 6.3** X-ray table showing compression device

A typical standard imaging protocol, using a non-ionic contrast medium, is described consisting of the following:

- preliminary film – full-length abdomen
- contrast medium injected
- 4-min post-injection – renal areas
- compression applied
- 10-min post-injection – renal areas
- 20-min release film – full-length abdomen
- localised full bladder (only if not filled adequately on release film)
- post-micturition bladder.

This protocol, however, may vary from hospital to hospital and may be subject to variation, as it is essential to tailor each IVU to the particular patient and to the clinical problem involved.

The preliminary anteroposterior radiograph of the abdomen should include both kidneys, bladder and the prostatic urethra in males. This film will act as a reference when comparing opacities demonstrated on contrast-filled images of the urinary system as well as checking the effectiveness of abdominal preparation. It is essential for the contrast medium injection to be given with the patient already in position on the X-ray table, and there should be no movement of the patient after the preliminary film until the examination is complete, unless renal function is unduly delayed or additional films are required with the patient oblique or erect. The rest of the anteroposterior radiographs, taken in sequential order, show the renal parenchyma and collecting system, the ureters, and the bladder filled with contrast medium and empty, immediately following micturition.

Exposures are taken on arrested expiration. The timing sequence of this protocol will be modified to demonstrate kidney filling and excretion. Delayed radiographs, some with the patient prone, may be required to identify the site of an obstruction. In cases of hypertension an immediate series of three films at 1-, 3- and 5-minute intervals are taken to compare the excretion of each kidney. Tomography may also be selected as a matter of routine when imaging the renal areas or confined to cases when these areas are obscured by bowel contents. Additional projections with the patient oblique, erect or taken supine on suspended inspiration may be necessary to confirm the relationship of an opacity to the urinary tract.

When the preparation of a child is unsatisfactory the kidneys may be examined after the child swallows a fizzy drink to inflate the stomach. The gas shadow usually extends across both kidneys.

# 6 Intravenous Urography

## Standard imaging protocol

### Preliminary – anteroposterior abdomen

This plain film is used to demonstrate the urinary tract prior to the administration of contrast medium.

*Position of patient and imaging modality*

The patient lies supine on the imaging table with the median sagittal plane at right angles and coincident with the midline of the table.

The pelvis is adjusted so that the anterior superior iliac spines are equidistant from the table top. A 35 × 43 cm cassette is placed longitudinally in the cassette tray and positioned so that the symphysis pubis is included on the lower part of the film, bearing in mind that the oblique rays will project the symphysis pubis downwards. The centre of the cassette will be approximately at the level of the lower costal margin in the mid-axillary line.

*Direction and centring of the X-ray beam*

The vertical central ray is directed to the centre of the cassette in the midline at the level of the lower costal margin in the mid-axillary line.

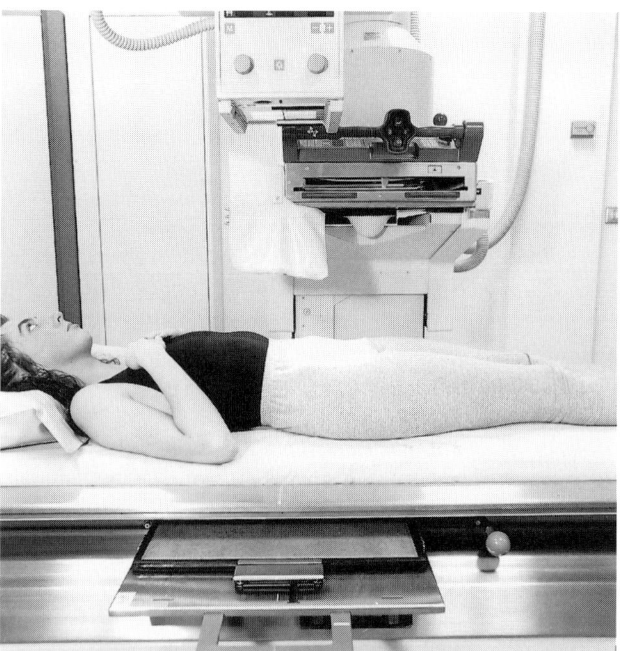

Figure 6.4b Patient and cassette

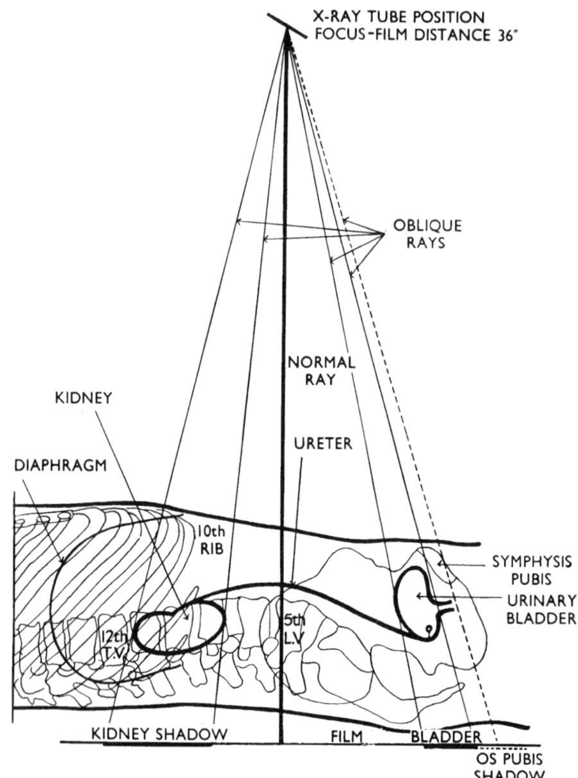


Figure 6.4a Use of oblique rays to project symphysis downwards

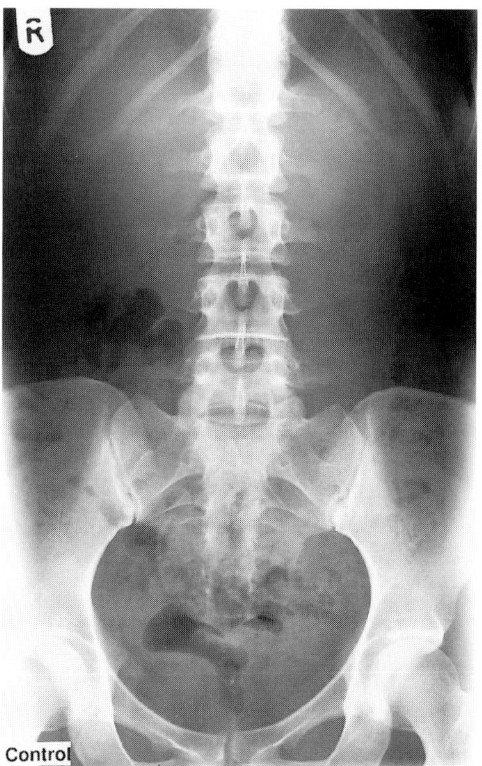


Figure 6.4c Radiograph of abdomen

## Standard imaging protocol

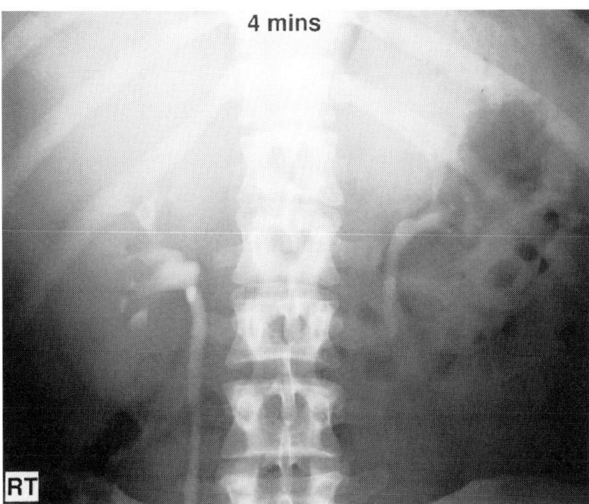

**Figure 6.5a** Four minutes post-injection

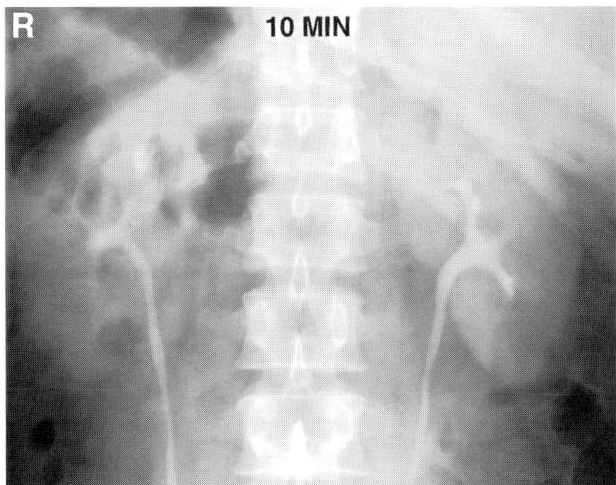

**Figure 6.5b** Ten minutes post-injection

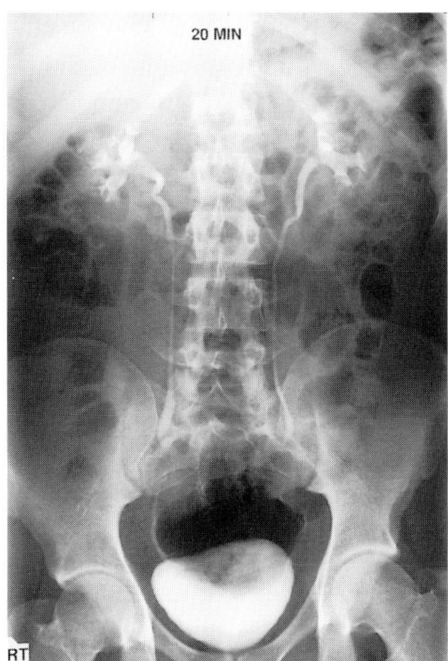

**Figure 6.5c** Twenty minutes post-injection with compression released

### 4-min post-injection – anteroposterior

This film is taken 4 min following the injection of contrast medium and shows the renal parenchyma during the nephrogram phase of the examination.

**Immediately after this film, compression is applied.**

*Position of patient and imaging modality*

The patient lies in a similar position to that described for the preliminary anteroposterior projection. A 24 × 30 cm cassette is placed transversely in the cassette tray, with the centre of the cassette at a level to include the whole of the renal area which is determined by reference to the preliminary film.

*Direction and centring of the X-ray beam*

The vertical central ray is directed to the centre of the cassette.

### 10-min post-injection – anteroposterior

The procedure for the 10-min post-injection film is identical to that described for the 4-min film.

This film should demonstrate optimum filling of the renal pelvis, calyces and pelvi-ureteric junction of each kidney. It gives good assessment of any difference in the comparative rate of opacification of the collecting system. With compression applied correctly, better filling of the minor calyces is achieved, with the result that small abnormalities involving the minor calyces are more likely to be demonstrated compared with abdominal compression not being used.

### 20-min post-injection compression release – anteroposterior

The procedure for the 20-min post-injection film is identical for the preliminary anteroposterior projection, with the exposure made immediately following the release of compression.

This film should demonstrate the renal pelvis, calyces and the full extent of the ureter of each kidney. The bladder should also be shown filled with contrast.

A localised full-bladder film similar to the projection described for the post-micturition film may be necessary if the bladder is not adequately filled following the release of compression.

# 6 Intravenous Urography

## Standard imaging protocol

### Post-micturition bladder – anteroposterior 15° caudad

This film gives an indication of fluid residue in the bladder immediately after micturition.

*Position of patient and imaging modality*
The patient lies supine on the imaging table, with the median sagittal plane at right angles to and coincident with the midline of the table. An 18 × 24 cm cassette is placed longitudinally in the cassette tray, with its lower border 5 cm below the symphysis pubis to ensure that the symphysis is not projected off the film.

*Direction and centring of the X-ray beam*
The central ray is directed 15° caudally and centred 5 cm above the upper border of the symphysis pubis in the midline.

*Contrast medium and injection data*

| *Volume* | *Concentration* | *Flow rate* |
|---|---|---|
| 50 ml | 350–370 mgI/ml | Hand injection |

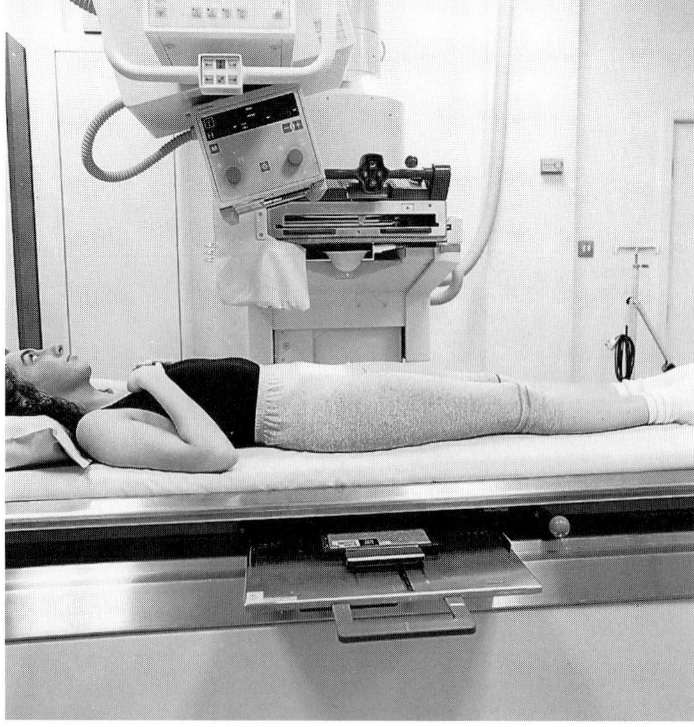

**Figure 6.6b** Patient and cassette

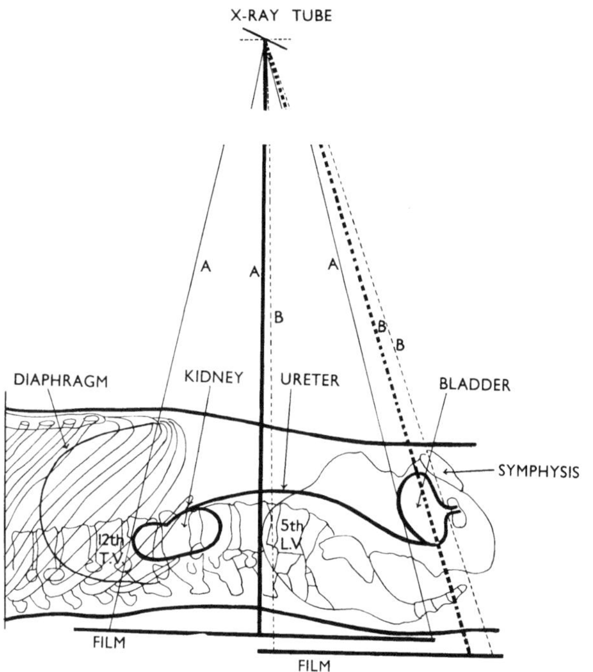


**Figure 6.6a** Use of X-ray tube angulation to project symphysis downwards

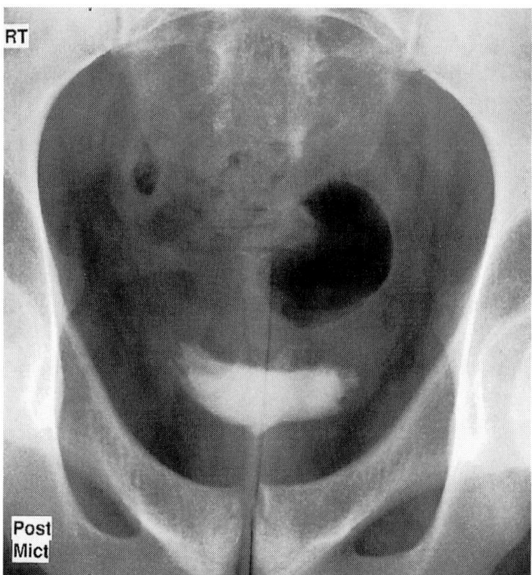


**Figure 6.6c** Radiograph of bladder

## Non-routine projections

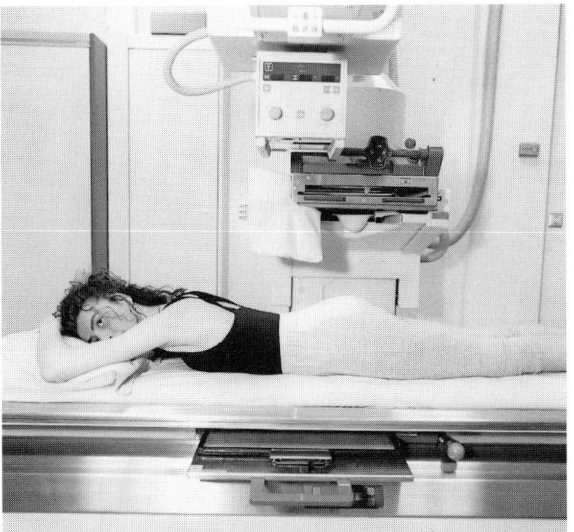

**Figure 6.7a** Patient lying prone

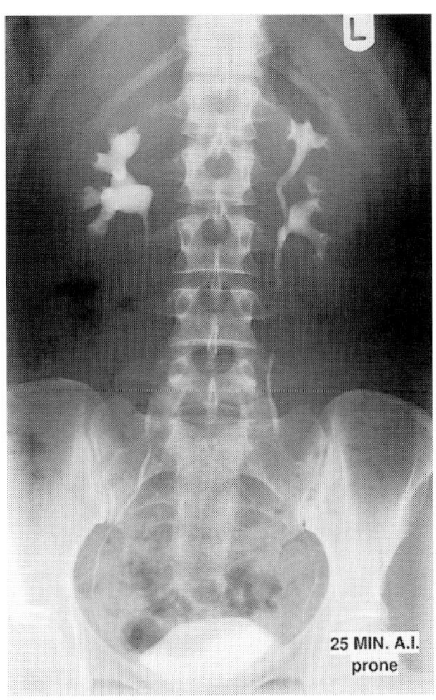

**Figure 6.7b** Prone projection showing duplex left kidney

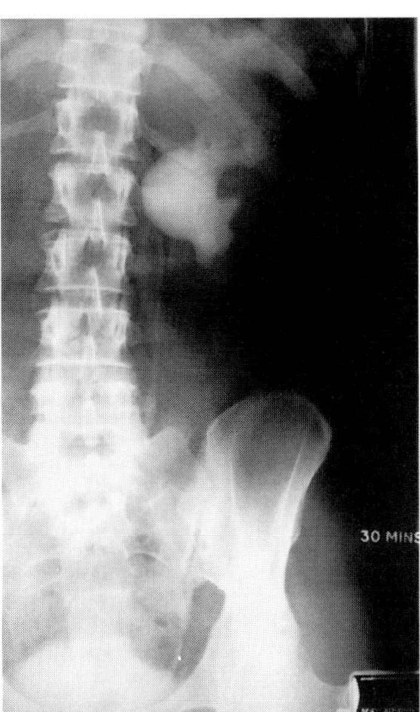

**Figure 6.7c** Prone projection showing hydronephrotic left kidney with X-ray beam centred to the left of the midline

In a number of cases, additional or modified projections may be required. Abnormal opacities shown overlying the urinary tract require further projections to determine their exact location. In cases of delayed filling or emptying of a kidney, films may be taken up to 24 h after the initial procedure, with some in the prone position to show the site of an obstruction.

### Postero-anterior (prone) – abdomen

This projection is often used to promote emptying of contrast from the pelvicalyceal system into the ureter. It can also be used in an attempt to show the site of an obstruction of the ureter in cases where delayed emptying can continue up to several hours following the initial examination. The projection is also employed when the upper poles of the kidneys are not adequately demonstrated on the anteroposterior projection. In the anteroposterior projection, the kidneys are at a slight angle in relationship to the film, with the upper poles of the kidneys at a deeper level than the lower poles. As a result the kidneys appear a little foreshortened. Using the postero-anterior position, the relationship is reversed and the kidneys appear with some enlargement.

*Position of patient and imaging modality*

The patient lies prone and central to the imaging couch, with the pelvis adjusted so that the anterior superior iliac spines are equidistant from the table top.

A 35 × 43 cassette is placed longitudinally in the cassette tray and centred at the level of the lower costal margin.

The timing of the exposure is important and is usually taken approximately 30 s after having turned the patient prone and after the patient has taken several deep breaths. This will hopefully promote emptying of the kidney and filling of the ureter which will be best seen at this stage.

*Direction and centring of the X-ray beam*

The vertical beam is centred over the midline at the level of the lower costal margin.

## Right or left posterior oblique

These projections may be employed to show the relationship of opacities to the kidneys, ureters and bladder. The right oblique, described below, is useful in distinguishing between renal or biliary stones. In these projections the image of either kidney is seen in profile.

*Position of patient and imaging modality*
From the supine position the patient is rotated 20–30° on to the right side. The patient is then moved across the couch until the spine is to the left of the centre of the couch and the patient is immobilised in this position. For the kidney area a 24 × 30 cm cassette is placed longitudinally in the cassette tray and centred to include both poles of the kidney which is determined from the contrast-filled film showing the opacity. Although rarely requested, the whole of the renal tract can be demonstrated using a 35 × 43 cm cassette which is centred at the level of the lower costal margin.

*Direction and centring of the X-ray beam*
The vertical central ray is directed to the centre of the cassette.

## Lateral

This projection may be used as an alternative to the oblique projection in determining the relative position of opacities near to or in the kidneys. Opacities in the kidneys will overshadow, or be very near, the vertebrae. Opacities outside the kidneys are usually shown anterior to the vertebrae.

*Position of patient and imaging modality*
The patient is turned onto the affected side and supported with the median sagittal plane parallel to the table.

*Direction and centring of the X-ray beam*
The vertical central ray is directed over the first/second lumbar vertebra about 5 cm superior to the lower costal margin.

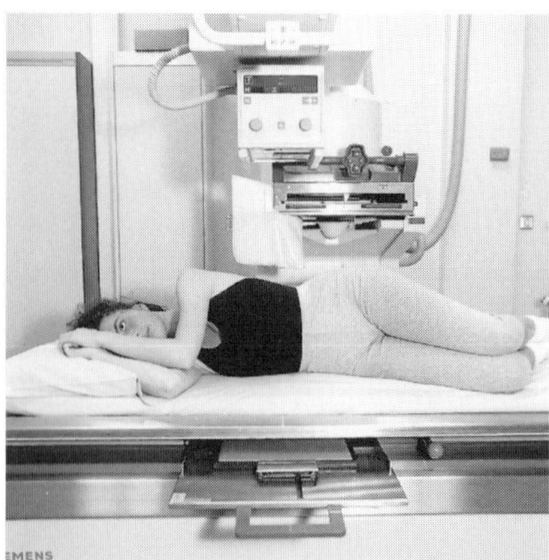

**Figure 6.8a** Position of patient for right lateral projection of abdomen

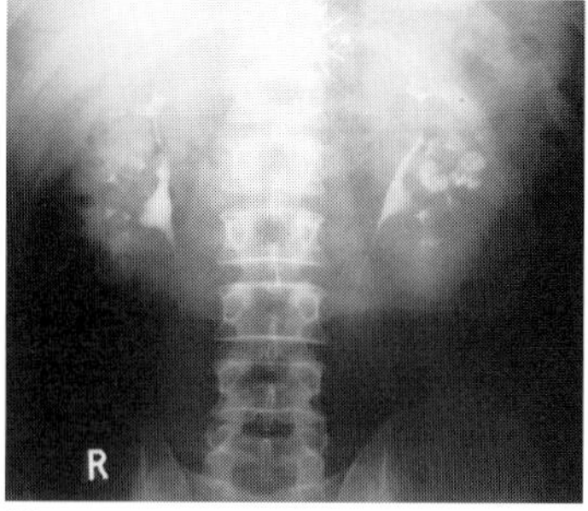


(i)

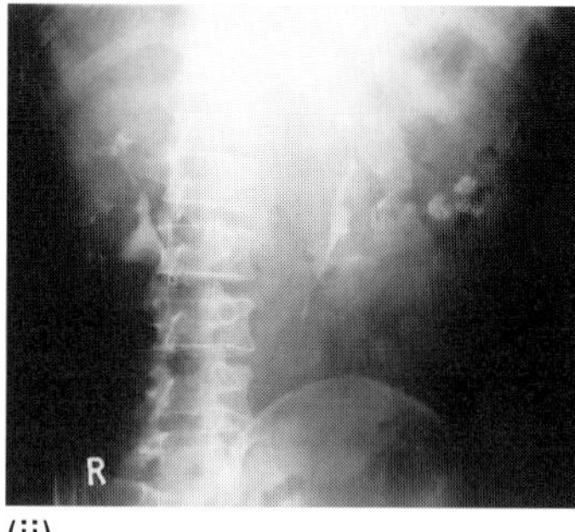


(ii)

**Figure 6.8b** (i, ii) AP and LAO projections taken at 10 min post-injection. Oblique image confirming that opacities lie anterior to left kidney

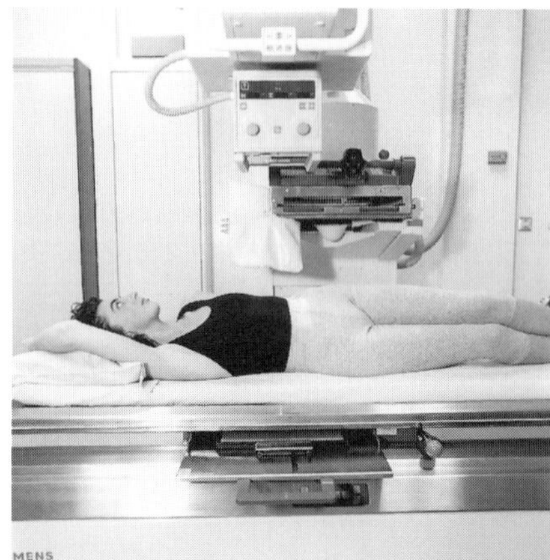

**Figure 6.8c** Position of patient for RAO of abdomen

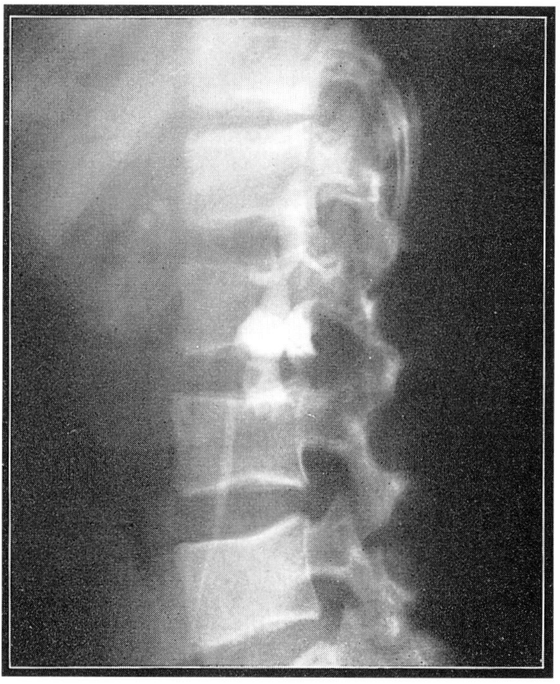

**Figure 6.8d** Lateral projection of a single kidney showing relative size and position in relation to the lumbar vertebrae

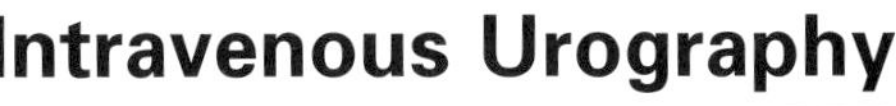


## Non-routine projections

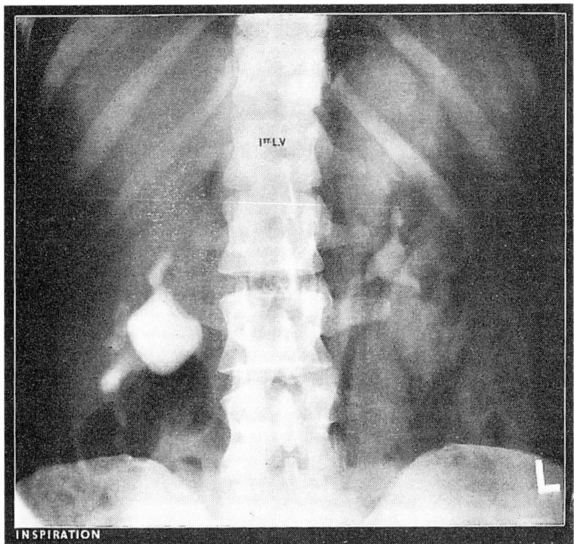


Figure 6.9a IVU – inspiration

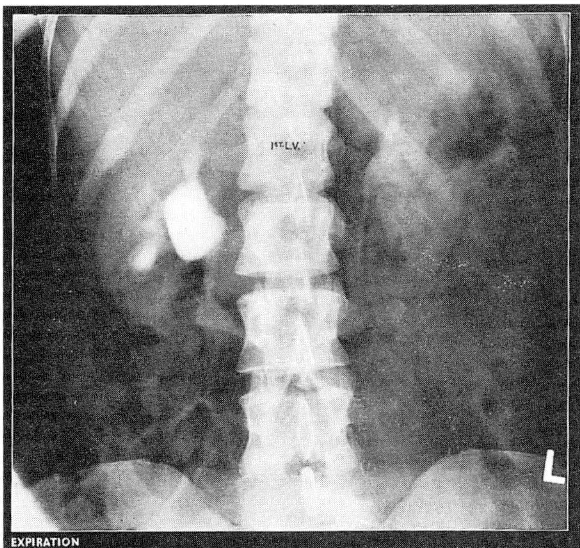


Figure 6.9b IVU – exspiration

Figure 6.9a,b AP images showing extent of kidney movement as the result of respiration. Shadows outside the kidneys move in varying degree during breathing, in relationship to the kidney outline

### Anteroposterior – inspiration

This projection may be taken at the control stage or at the same time as the 5- or 10-min post-contrast films when opacities may appear to be within the kidney substance.

The procedure is identical to these projections, except that the exposure is made on arrested respiration after full inspiration. The image might show a difference in direction and extent of movement of the kidney and calcification lying outside the kidney.

### Tomography – anteroposterior

Zonography may be employed at the same time as the 5- or 10-min post-contrast films to diffuse gas shadows which overlie the renal areas to show renal outlines and/or detail of the pelvicalyceal system.

*Position of patient and imaging modality*
The patient lies supine on the imaging table, with the median sagittal plane at right angles to and in the midline of the table.

*Imaging procedure*
The patient is positioned so that the renal areas are included on a 24 × 30 cm cassette which is placed transversely in the cassette tray. A linear 8–10° tomographic movement is selected, using an 8–11 cm pivot height. The exact location of the beam as it swings into the vertical is determined from the contrast-filled film showing the kidneys.

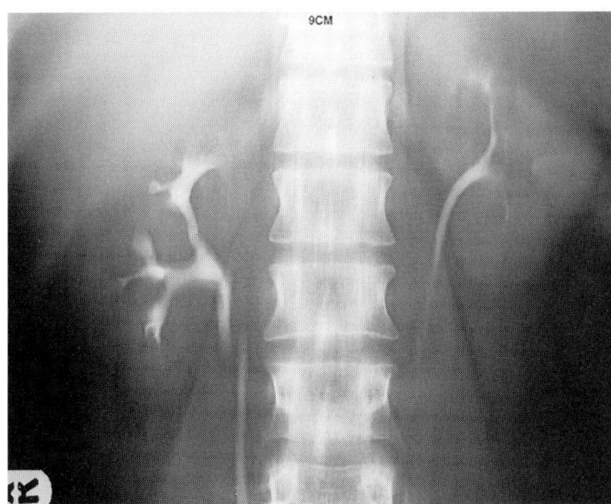


Figure 6.9c Tomograph of normal kidneys

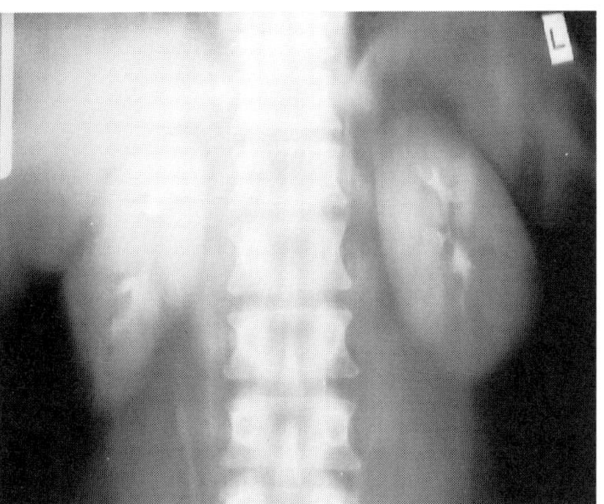


Figure 6.9d Tomograph demonstrating calcified right renal cyst

# 6 Urinary System

## Ultrasound

Ultrasound examination of the urinary system is normally confined to the kidneys and bladder using real-time B-mode imaging with a 3.5 MHz sector or phased array transducer. This provides a large field of view despite a small area of contact. A 5 MHz transducer can be used in children and small adults. A specialised transrectal probe (TRUS) allows more detailed examination of the prostate, seminal vesicles and bladder wall and the procedure is described in more detail in Chapter 7 (see page 258).

The ureters are normally not visualised, except when dilated.

Colour flow Doppler can be used to demonstrate the renal blood flow and may be used to assess renal artery stenosis. This procedure is particularly useful in the assessment of the post-transplant kidney. In the bladder it can be used to localise the ureteric orifices.

The patient may be fasted to reduce bowel gas and is given half a litre of water to drink 1 h prior to the examination to allow visualisation of the bladder.

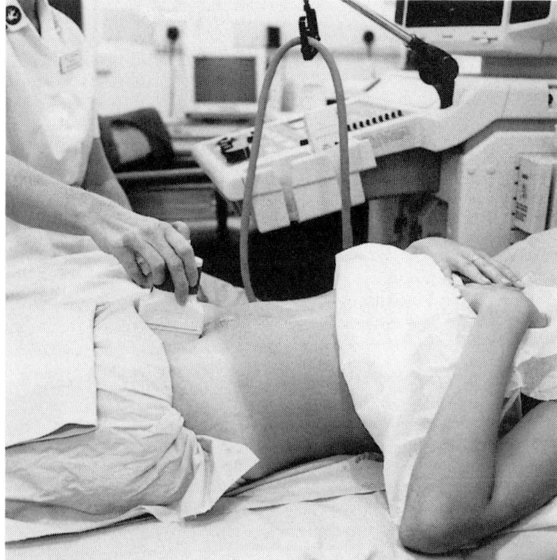

**Figure 6.10a** Transducer held for midline sagittal scan of bladder

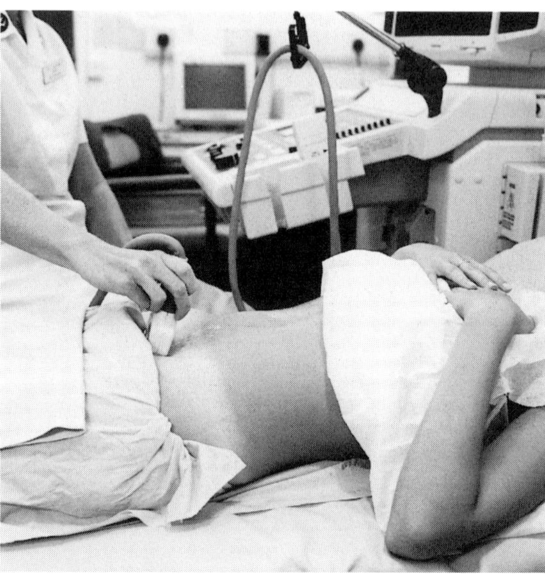

**Figure 6.10b** Transducer held for transverse scan of bladder

### Indications

**Kidneys**

Renal failure, hypertension, abdominal pain, suspected renal obstruction and hydronephrosis. Recurrent kidney infection caused by ureteric reflux. Non-opacified kidney on IVU. Tumours and cystic lesions of the kidneys and suspected perinephric abscess and fluid collections.

Obstruction of the ureters by a pelvic mass, e.g. fibroid uterus, ovarian cyst, etc.

In the transplanted kidney to identify causes of dysfunction, hydonephrosis, rejection, perinephric collection and for localization prior to percutaneous biopsy.

Doppler interrogation of the transplanted kidney is used to detect vascular complication, including renal artery stenosis and venous occlusion.

**Bladder**

Tumours, diverticula, bladder wall thickness, ureteroceles, calculi and intravesical filling defects.

Bladder volume and post-micturition residual volume. Prostatic size and disease.

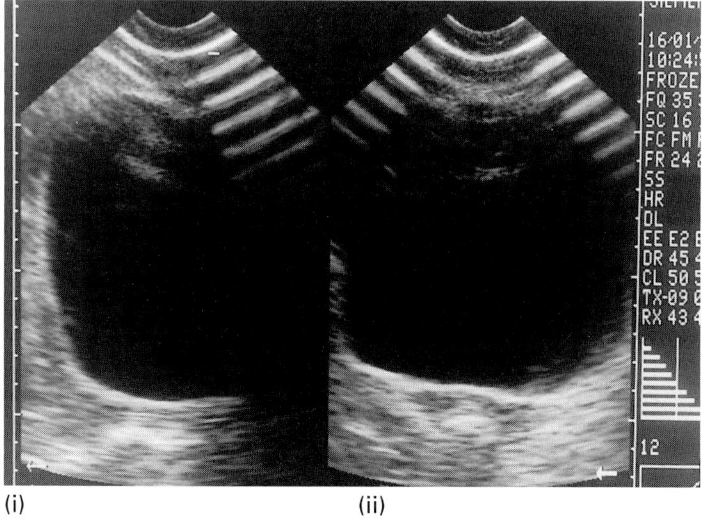


(i) (ii)

**Figure 6.10c** Composite image of bladder: (i) sagittal section; (ii) transverse section

## Bladder

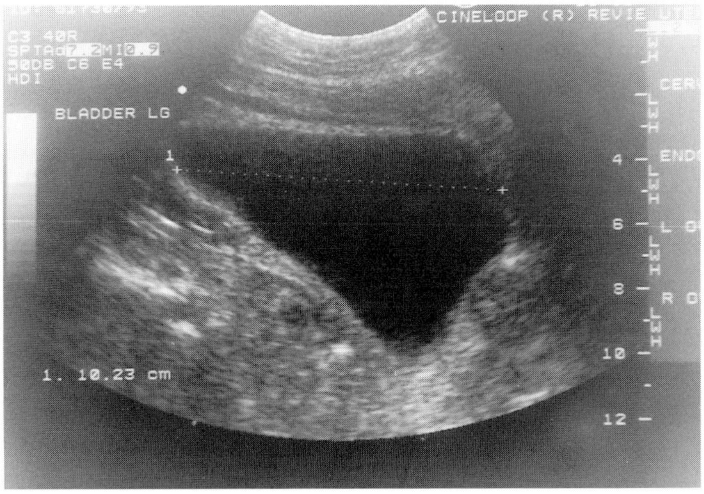

Figure 6.11a Midline sagittal image of full bladder with a maximum length dimension of 10.23 cm

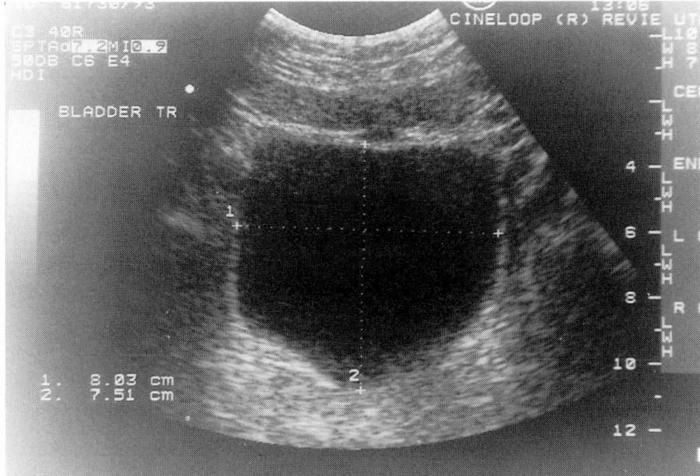


**Figure 6.11b** Transverse image of full bladder with a maximum width dimension of 8.03 cm and maximum height of 7.51 cm

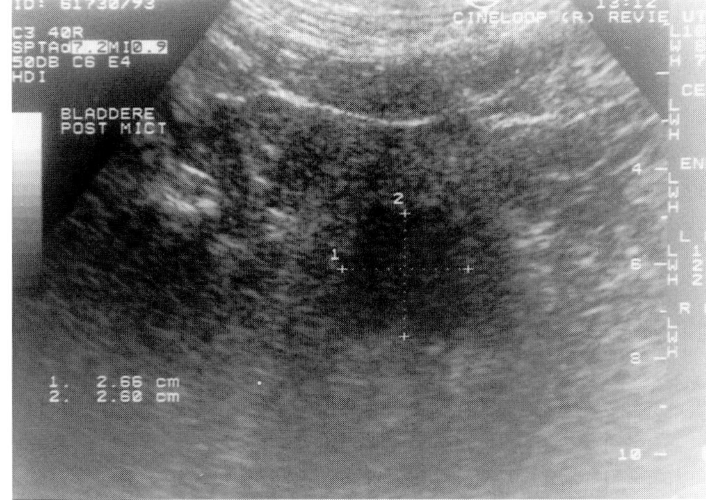


**Figure 6.11c** Transverse image of bladder, following micturation, with a maximum width of 2.66 cm and a maximum height of 2.60 cm

The following is a description of suprapubic transabdominal ultrasound with the bladder full.

### Position of patient and imaging modality

The bladder is examined with the patient supine. The transducer is held against the abdomen above the symphysis pubis to facilitate a combination of parasagittal and transverse scans of the bladder.

### Imaging procedure

A series of longitudinal scans are acquired, with the transducer initially placed in the midline above the symphysis pubis to obtain a median sagittal section scan. Parasagittal scans of the whole of the bladder are then performed by moving and angling the transducer to each iliac fossa in turn. The transducer is then rotated through 90° and positioned in the midline above the symphysis pubis. From this position transverse scans are made by angling the transducer caudally, posterior to the symphysis pubis, and then by moving and angling it cranially towards the umbilicus until the whole of the bladder is imaged. After the procedure the patient is asked to micturate, following which the bladder is rescanned to measure any residual volume. The full bladder can also be examined using colour flow Doppler to identify flow resulting from ureteric emptying. The frequency and position of these jets can provide information on the anatomy and function of the vesico-ureteric junction.

### Image analysis

On the transverse scans the full bladder appears oblong, while on the longitudinal scans it appears triangular and echo free. The normal wall thickness when full is 3 mm. The prostate may be visualised as a rounded echogenic structure at the base of the bladder. Bladder volume is normally calculated automatically following a set routine, but can be calculated manually by using the technique described by Poston:

$$\text{Volume (in ml)} = 0.7\,HDW$$

where $H$ = maximum diameter in the sagittal plane, $D$ = depth in sagittal plane, $W$ = maximum transverse diameter in the transverse diameter, with all measurements taken in cm.

# 6 Urinary System

## Kidneys

**Position of patient and imaging modality**

Positioning of the transducer to acquire both longitudinal and transverse images of the kidneys requires a combination of compound oblique scans.

Positioning of the transducer is determined by the fact that the longitudinal axis of either kidney is approximately 20° to that of the spine, with the transverse axis of each kidney also approximately 45° to the sagittal plane of the body. The lower pole is further away from the spine and also more anterior.

The transducer is also positioned to acquire images of the kidneys, unobscured if possible by paraspinal muscles and gas in the bowel.

**Right kidney**

The right kidney is examined with the patient either in the supine position or turned 45° onto the left side with the right side uppermost.

**Left kidney**

The left kidney can also be examined with the patient supine but more usually in a lateral position. For the lateral position the patient is turned onto the right side over a support pad or pillow, with the left arm raised over the head in an attempt to open up the acoustic window between the ribs and iliac crest.

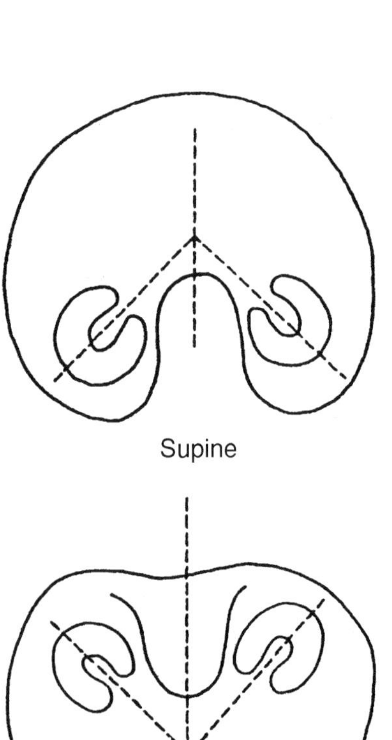


**Figure 6.12a** Relationship of short axis of kidneys (axial section)

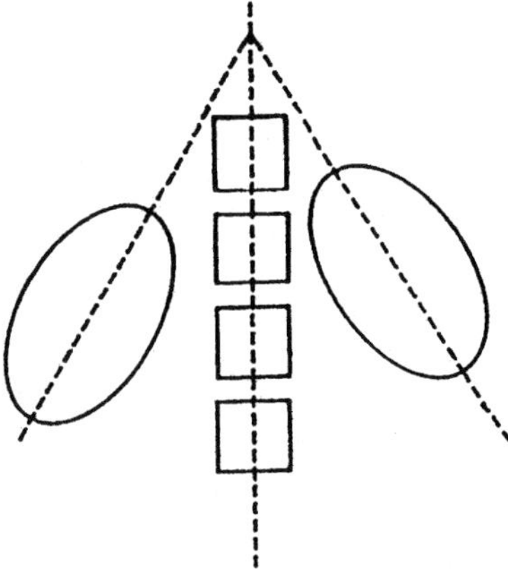

**Figure 6.12b** Relationship of long axis of kidneys (anterior aspect)

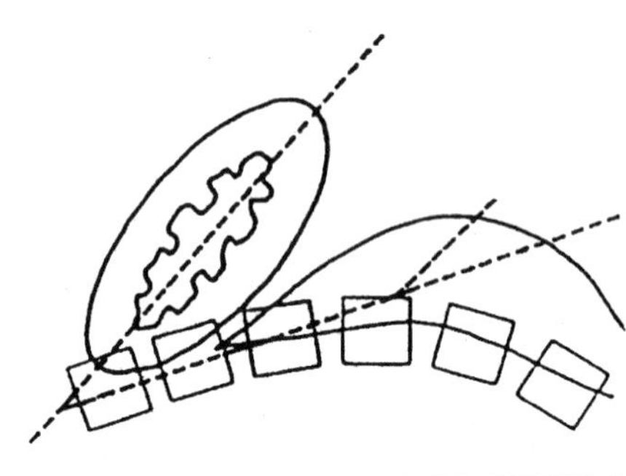

**Figure 6.12c** Relationship of long axis of kidneys (lateral aspect)

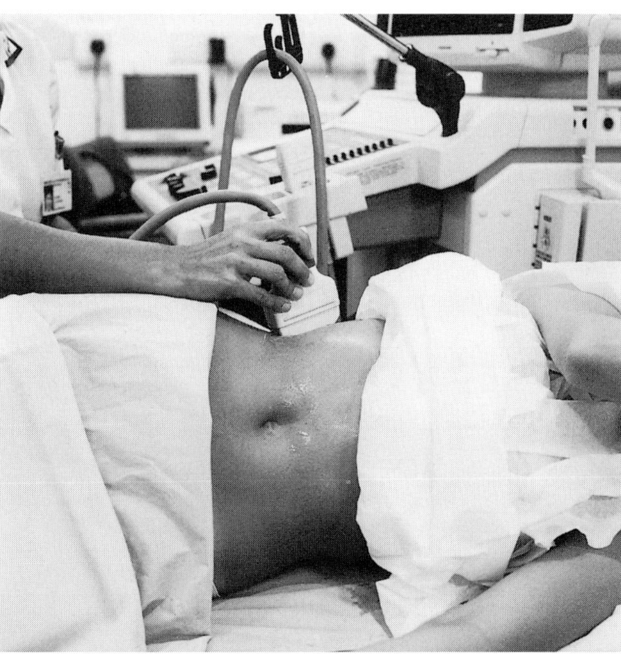

**Figure 6.12d** Patient and transducer positioned for right kidney scan (long axis view)

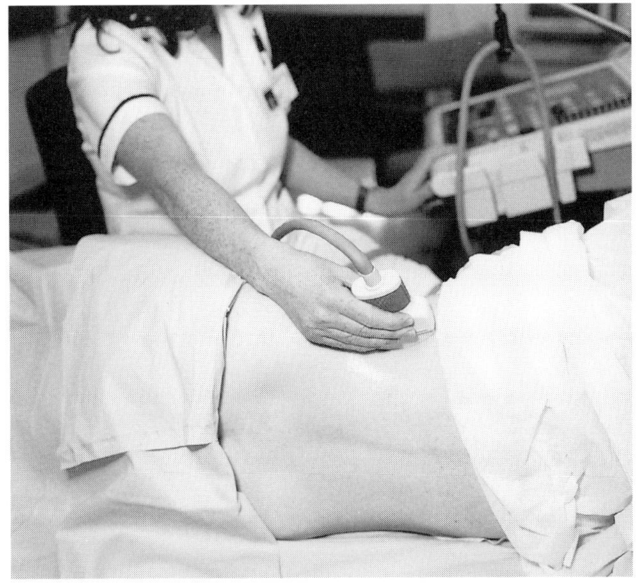

Figure 6.13a Patient and transducer positioned for left kidney scan (long axis view)

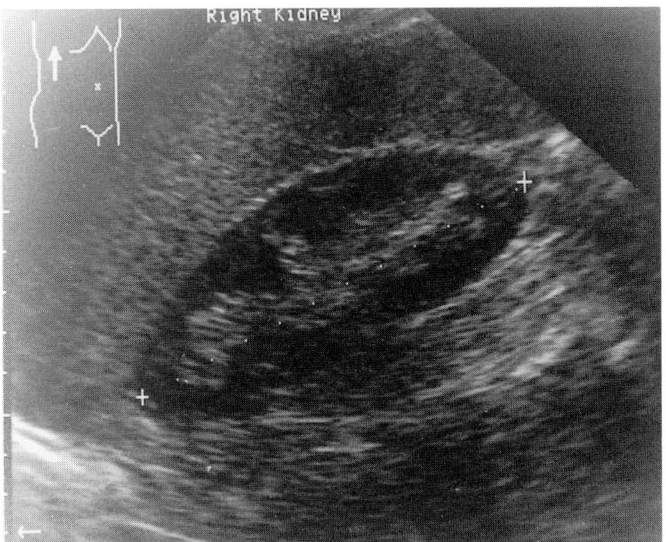


Figure 6.13b Longitudinal scan of right kidney with calipers indicating the maximum long axis dimension

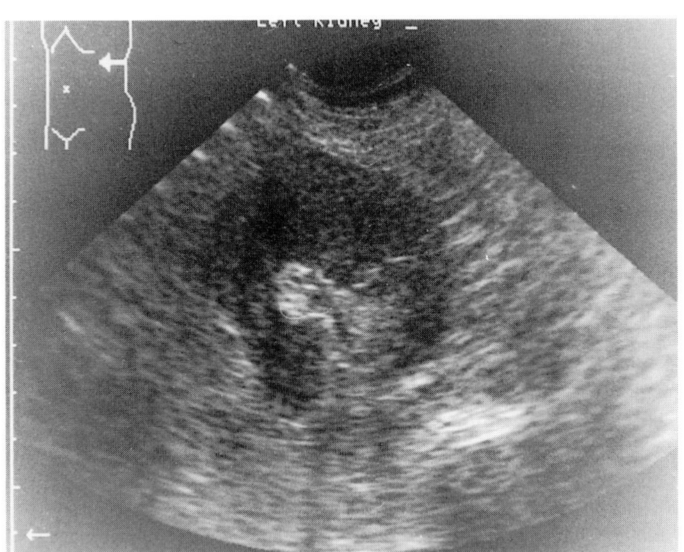

Figure 6.13c Transverse scan of the left kidney

### Imaging procedure

*Right kidney*
The liver is used as an acoustic window. The transducer is placed in a right parasagittal or coronal position either intercostally or subcostally on the mid-axillary line to locate the kidney. Once located, the transducer is rotated and positioned to scan along the long axis of the kidney to obtain a mid cross-sectional longitudinal image showing both lateral and medial borders. The transducer is further moved anteriorly and posteriorly to examine the entire kidney in longitudinal sections showing the renal cortex, medulla and collecting system. The transducer is then rotated through 90° and moved both cranially and caudally to examine the entire kidney in transverse sections.

*Left kidney*
Scans of the left kidney are obtained using an intercostal approach. The spleen is used as an acoustic window. The transducer is positioned between the ribs and angled to obtain a longitudinal scan. Longitudinal and transverse sectional scans are then made in a similar way to that of the right kidney.

Examination of either kidney may be facilitated by requesting the patient to hold on deep arrested inspiration. This displaces the kidney caudally, moving it away from overlying ribs.

### Image analysis

The kidneys appear ovoid on the longitudinal scans and rounded on the transverse scans. The renal parenchyma is observed for any abnormalities. In the normal kidney few echoes are seen in the parenchyma, with a cluster of high echoes seen centrally in the renal sinus from fat and collecting system interfaces. Measurements of the maximum long-axis dimensions of each kidney are acquired from the frozen real-time long-axis scans of either kidney and compared with standard nomograms. The normal adult kidney is 10–12 cm in length.

Colour flow Doppler can be used to identify the renal arteries and provide spectral analysis of following blood, thus demonstrating the presence of renal artery stenosis (see Plate 2).

# 6 Urinary System

## Radionuclide Imaging

Radionuclide imaging is used to study the renal vascular supply, function and drainage, as well as providing a means of observing gross anatomical details. By selecting the appropriate combination of radionuclide and pharmaceutical, quantitative analysis of renal function can be obtained from a processed time–activity curve. This is normally referred to as a renogram and is a graphical representation of the amount of radioactivity in the kidneys over a period of time. The kidneys are also seen to be functioning and emptying urine via the ureters to the bladder. The bladder can also be examined by this method of imaging, with the benefit that this offers an indirect, non-interventional method of performing a micturating cystogram. Depending on the radiopharmaceutical selected, static images of the kidneys can also be obtained to demonstrate the renal parenchyma in greater detail and with the acquired data relative renal function can also be calculated. A gamma camera linked to a computer system is essential for these procedures.

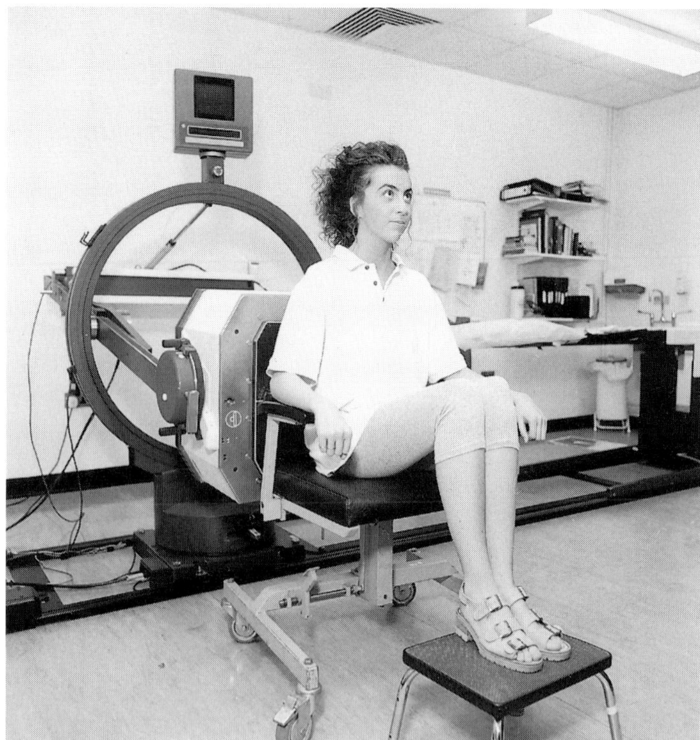

**Figure 6.14a** RNI – patient and camera, erect position

## Renogram

### Indications

Renal/ureteric calculi for complete or partial obstruction and relative functions. Pelvi-ureteric obstruction, hypertension and investigation of renal artery stenosis. Assessment of renal function, repeated urinary tract infections and vesico-ureteric reflux. Trauma, renal failure and assessment of bladder function. The investigation is also used as an alternative to intravenous urography when organic iodine contrast agents are contraindicated.

### Position of patient and imaging modality

The patient may be examined in the erect position, with the back resting against the gamma camera. This position is also adopted for the indirect micturating cystogram, with the patient seated on a disposable bed pan to enable imaging while the patient voids. Alternatively, the patient can be examined lying supine on the imaging couch, with the gamma camera positioned under and parallel to the couch to include the region of interest. This method is useful when the patient is unable to remain still in the erect position.

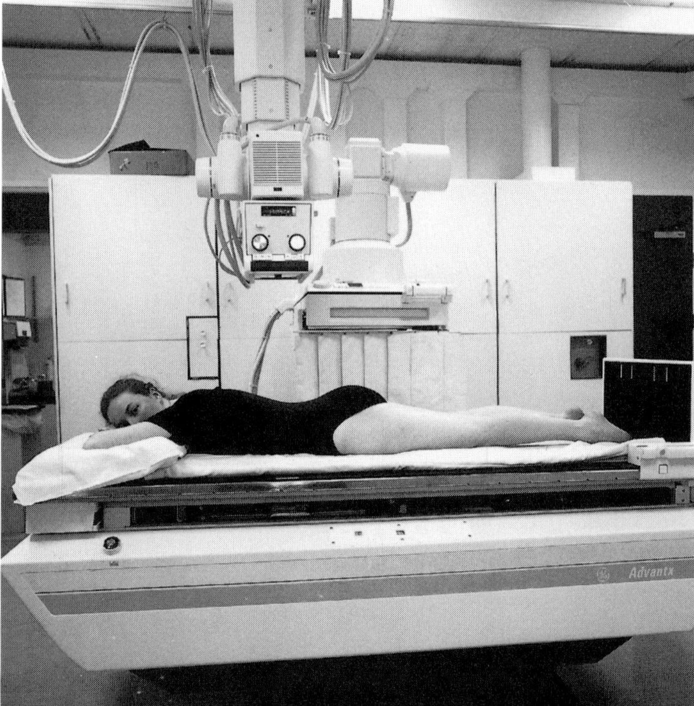


**Figure 6.14b** RNI – patient and camera, supine position

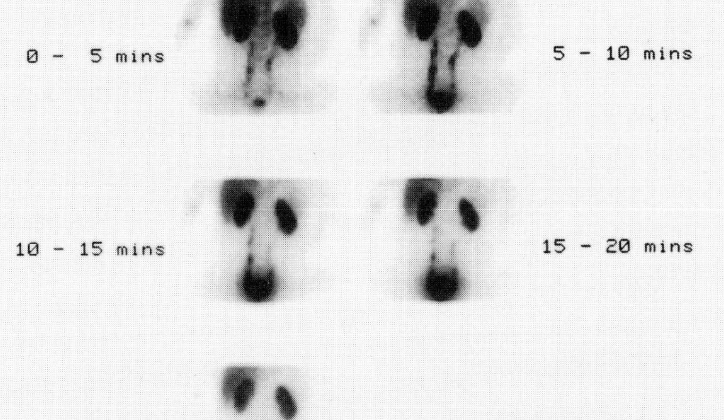


**Figure 6.15a** Summed renogram images showing normal kidney function

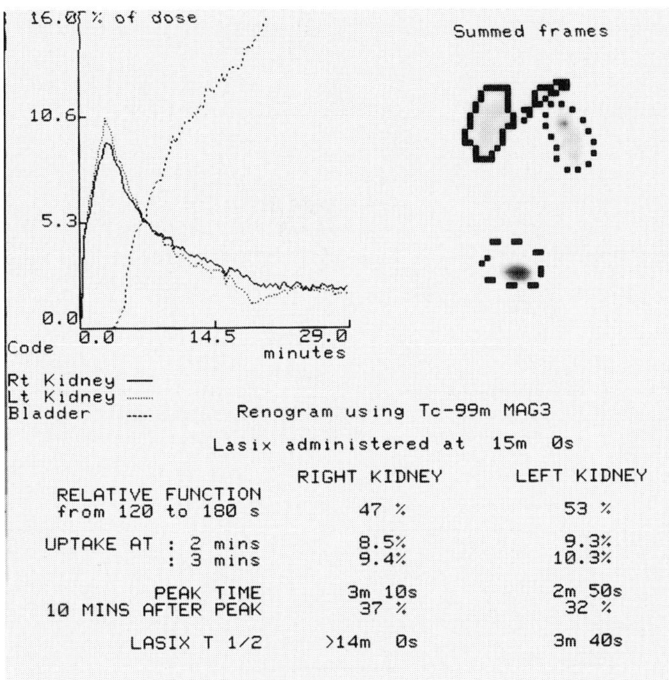


**Figure 6.15b** Normal renogram showing summed frames for both kidneys and bladder and associated time–activity curves

*Imaging and radiopharmaceutical parameters*

| *Type* | *Administered activity* | *Principal energy* |
|---|---|---|
| $^{99m}$Tc DTPA | 100–300 MBq | 140 keV |
| $^{99m}$Tc MAG-3 | 40–400 MBq | 140 keV |
| $^{123}$I Hippuran | 20 MBq | 159 keV |

| *Window width* | *Acquisition counts/time* |
|---|---|
| 20% | Frame time 20 s |
| | Total frames 120 |

A low-energy general-purpose collimator is selected. The patient is normally well hydrated and required to empty the bladder immediately before the commencement of the procedure.

Radiopharmaceuticals such as $^{99m}$Tc DTPA (diethylenetriamine pentaacetic acid) or $^{99m}$Tc MAG-3 (mercaptoacetyltriglycine), both give an accurate measurement of differential renal function and an assessment of urinary drainage from the kidneys. $^{99m}$TC MAG-3 is mainly eliminated via tubular secretion whilst $^{99m}$Tc DTPA is excreted by glomerular filtration. $^{99m}$Tc DTPA, therefore, can also be used to assess glomerular filtration rate.

$^{123}$I hippuran, which may require a medium-energy collimator, can also be used in cases of reduced renal function.

**Imaging procedure**

With the patient positioned for the procedure, a rapid bolus injection is made into an antecubital vein. The image acquisition protocol is immediately implemented and data acquired for up to 40 min. If a pelvi-ureteric obstruction is suspected the patient is injected with a diuretic at the 15–20 min stage of the image acquisition. This technique will distinguish between a true obstruction or a baggy pelvis which can hold back urine. In the case of a baggy pelvis, the diuretic effect will promote a washout of the affected kidney corresponding to an immediate drop of activity in the kidney.

**Image analysis**

Time activity curves are obtained using image processing software. ROIs are drawn around each kidney and the bladder. A further ROI is drawn in the area between the kidneys in order to determine the background activity. From these ROIs the programme will subtract the background activity and calculate the variation in activity in the kidneys and bladder during the course of the study. This gives an indication of relative renal function and shows emptying of the kidneys and filling of the bladder. The initial sharp rise of the graph (first phase) occurs as the radioactive tracer is extracted from the blood into the kidney. The peak of the curve (second phase) shows maximum uptake of the tracer in the kidney just prior to the excretion phase. The downard slope of the graph (third phase) shows the excretion of the tracer from the kidney to the bladder via the ureters.

Differential renal function is obtained from analysis of the first phase over a narrow range of time (e.g. from between 60 and 150 sec). At this stage the tracer has finished mixing with the bloodpool (i.e. the plasma concentration of the tracer is no longer rapidly changing) but the kidneys have yet to start excreting the tracer.

Further information on perfusion can be obtained from a different curve analysis using an aortic ROI, or by subjective viewing of the fast frame images acquired after a high dose injection of the radiopharmaceutical (200–400 MBq).

# 6 Urinary System

## Micturating cystogram

A micturating cystogram is normally performed using an indirect approach and is usually preceded by an isotope renogram, as described on the previous page. The procedure is carried out to investigate vesico-ureteral reflux, mainly in paediatric patients, and has the advantage of being less invasive than a conventional micturating cystogram. The procedure is explained to the patient to gain their full co-operation.

### Imaging procedure

With the bladder already full with urine containing radioactivity, the patient sits erect on a bed pan with back against the gamma camera fitted with a low-energy general-purpose collimator. If the patient has no urgency to micturate, he/she is given drinks and then returned to the imaging room.

The camera is adjusted to include the kidneys and bladder and provided the kidneys are empty the image acquisition protocol can commence. The first 20–30 frames are acquired with the patient straining but not actually micturating. The patient is then asked to micturate and data are acquired during micturation until the bladder is completely empty and then for a further 20–30 frames.

### Image analysis

Using the software package, all the frames that have been acquired are summed to form one image. Regions of interest are drawn around both kidneys and bladder, following which, time–activity curves are produced. Any marked peaks in the kidneys will suggest ureteric reflux. The bladder can also be seen emptying in playback using the cine mode.

*Imaging and radiopharmaceutical parameters*

| *Type* | *Administered activity* | *Principal energy* |
|---|---|---|
| $^{99m}$Tc DTPA | 40–200 MBq | 140 keV |
| $^{99m}$Tc MAG-3 | 40–200 MBq | 140 keV |

| *Window width* | *Acquisition counts/time* |
|---|---|
| 20% | Frame time 2 s |
| | Total frames 120 |

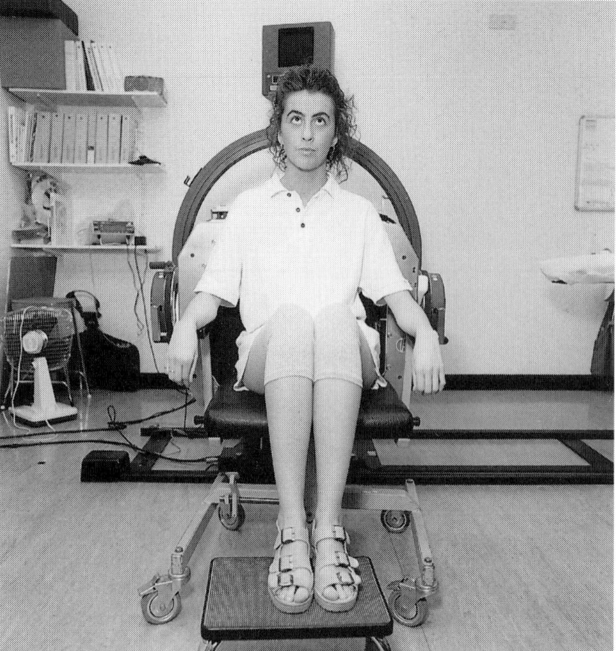

**Figure 6.16a** Patient in typical seated position for micturating cystogram

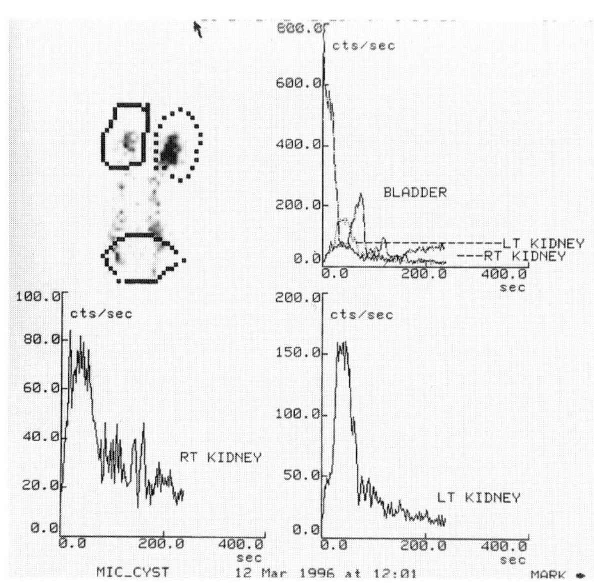


**Figure 6.16b** Analysis of dynamic image with ROI over kidneys and bladder, with corresponding time–activity curves, demonstrating bilateral reflux from bladder to each kidney

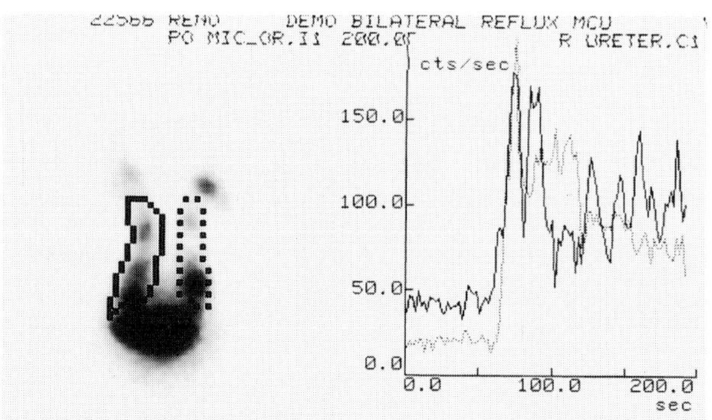


**Figure 6.16c** Time–activity curves showing reflux in both ureters

## Static imaging

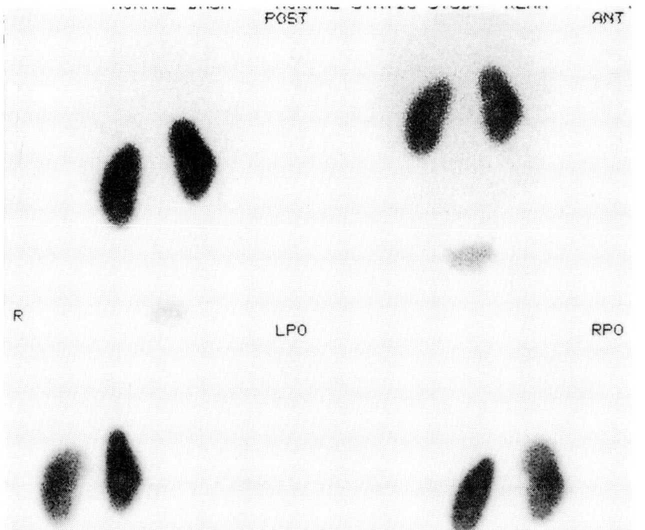


**Figure 6.17a** Normal static study showing posterior, anterior, left and right posterior views of both kidneys

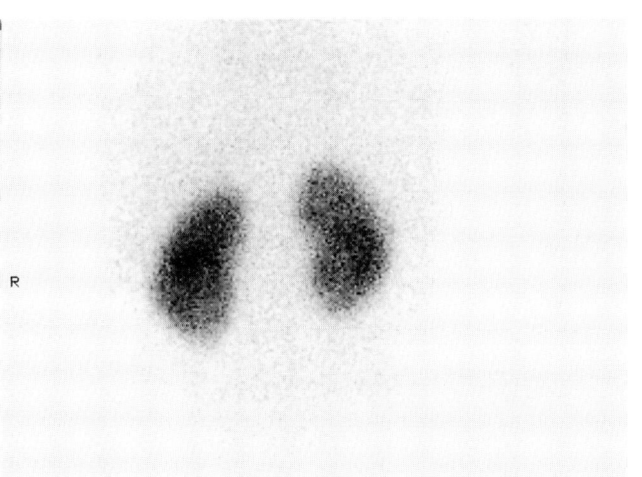


**Figure 6.17b** Anterior view of both kidneys with normal contours and no evidence of renal scarring. Percentage renal function of kidneys: right 55%, left 45%

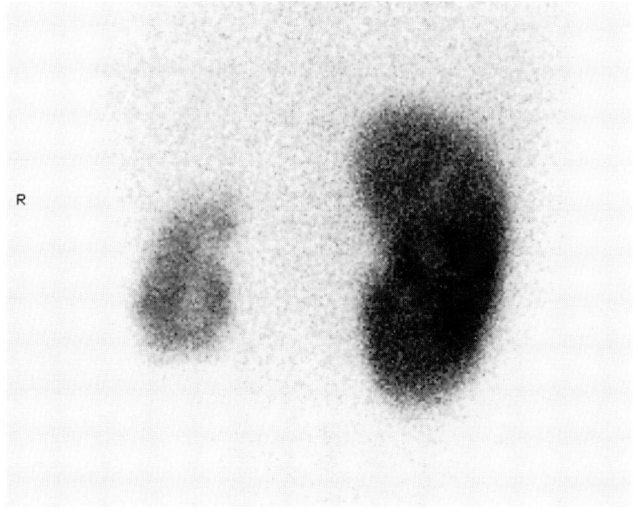


**Figure 6.17c** Abnormal study showing hypertrophied left kidney with 87.2% relative function and a small and scarred right kidney with 12.8% relative renal function

Static imaging is performed using $^{99m}$Tc DMSA (2,3-dimercapto-succinic acid) to demonstrate the renal parenchyma. This accumulates in the renal cortex as it is cleared from the blood by renal tubular absorption and is used to demonstrate renal scarring, narrowing of the cortex and pseudo-tumours. A high-resolution collimator is selected for maximum detail.

There is no particular preparation for this procedure, except that sedation is recommended for small children.

### Imaging procedure

Imaging commences approximately 2 h after the patient has been injected with the radiopharmaceutical.

The patient lies supine on the imaging couch, with the camera positioned parallel to the couch first above and then below to enable anterior and posterior views of the renal areas to be obtained. Right and left posterior oblique views are then obtained by rotating the camera 30° from its position below the patient towards the appropriate side or turning the patient into the oblique position.

### Image analysis

Qualitative visual assessment is carried out to assess cortical scarring and lesion involvement.

Quantitative assessment is done to give an indication of relative renal function using computer software analysis. The process includes background subtraction and adding together counts of radioactivity acquired from regions of interest drawn round each kidney on both the anterior and posterior views of the renal areas. Normally there is a 50% distribution of activity between either kidney, with an acceptable standard deviation of ∓ 5%. The formulae are seen below.

*Imaging and radiopharmaceutical parameters*

| *Type* | *Administered activity* | *Principal energy* |
|---|---|---|
| $^{99m}$Tc DMSA | 80 MBq | 140 keV |
| *Window width* | *Acquisition counts/time* | |
| 20% | Anterior and posterior 500 K counts<br>Posterior obliques 300 K counts | |

$$\textbf{Relative function (right kidney)} = \frac{\text{Counts in right kidney}}{\text{Counts in right and left kidneys}} \times 100$$

$$\textbf{Relative function (left kidney)} = \frac{\text{Counts in left kidney}}{\text{Counts in left and right kidneys}} \times 100$$

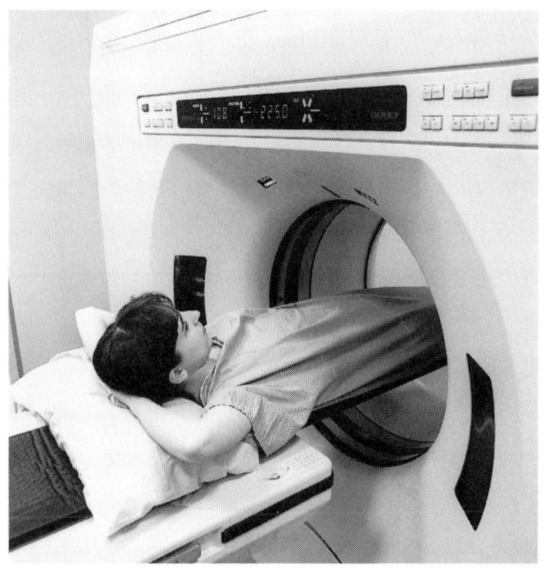

(a)

### Kidneys

Transaxial images are obtained prior to and during the infusion of a non-ionic contrast agent to determine the size, vascularity and anatomical relationship of a space-occupying lesion.

An oral contrast agent in the form of 300 ml of dilute (2%) Gastrografin or dilute barium sulphate suspension is required to outline the stomach and small bowel.

#### Indications

Renal tumours, unusual renal cysts, masses adjacent to the kidneys and filling defects detected on intravenous urography.

#### Position of patient and imaging modality

The patient lies supine, feet first on the scanner table. Arms are raised and placed behind the patient's head, out of the scan plane. Positioning is aided by transaxial, coronal and sagittal alignment lights. The median sagittal plane is adjusted so that it is perpendicular to the centre of the table top and the coronal plane parallel to it. The scan plane is perpendicular to the long axis of the body to enable transaxial imaging to be undertaken. The scanner table height is adjusted to ensure that the coronal plane alignment light is at the level of the mid-axillary line. The patient is now moved into the scanner until the scan reference point is at the level of the xiphisternum.

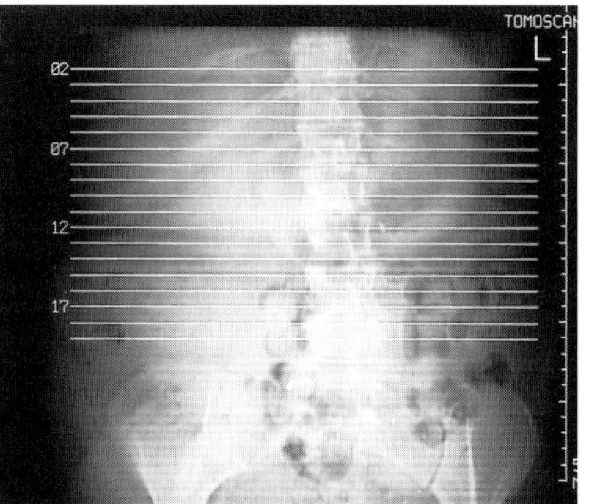


(b)

#### Imaging procedure

An anteroposterior scan projection radiograph is obtained, starting 5 cm above and ending 25 cm below the reference point. From this image, 10 mm contiguous sections are prescribed through the renal area. Scanning is performed on arrested respiration.

These pre-contrast images are reviewed and any area of abnormality is rescanned during the infusion of the contrast agent using the same imaging protocol. Scanning commences after 60 ml of the contrast agent has been administered.

If spiral scanning options are available, contrast-enhanced scans may also be acquired through the area of abnormality with a volume acquisition, using a 5 mm slice thickness and 5 mm table increments, but with a 3 mm reconstruction index to give overlapping sections.

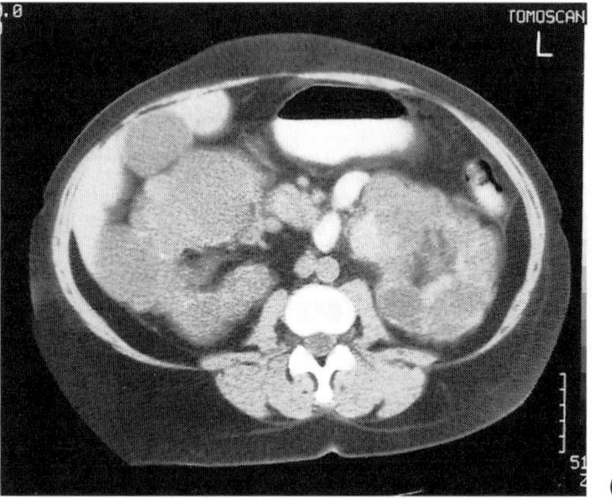


(c)

*Contrast media and injection data*

| *Volume* | *Concentration* | *Flow rate* |
|---|---|---|
| 100 ml | 300 mgI/ml | 2 ml/s |

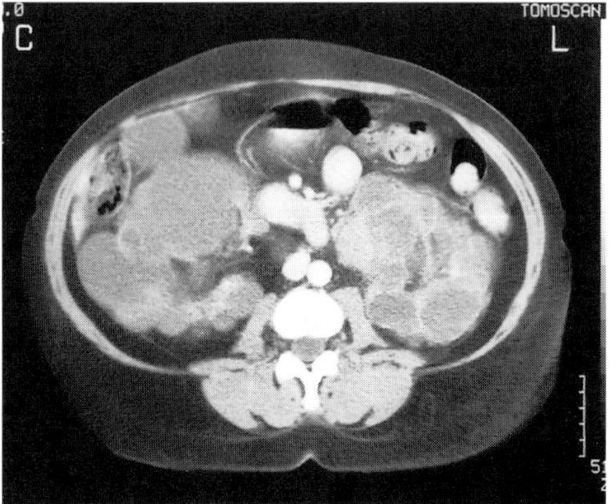


(d)

**Figure 6.18** (a) Patient in CT scanner; (b) scan projection radiograph showing prescribed scanning locations; (c,d) pre- and post-contrast enhancement scans, at the same level, demonstrating polycystic disease with haemorrhaging into the cysts

## Ureters and bladder

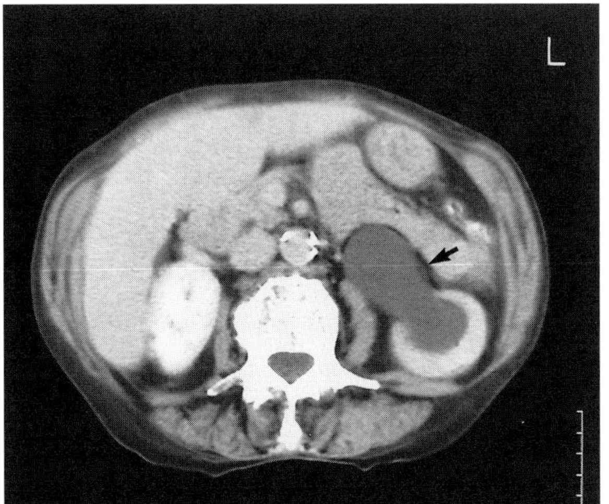


(a)

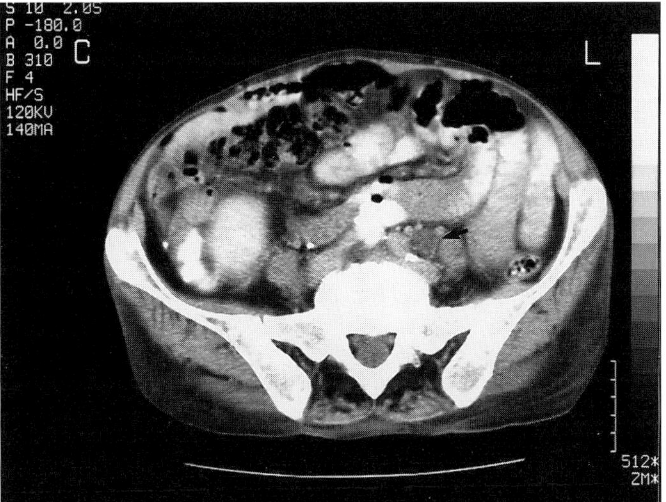


(b)

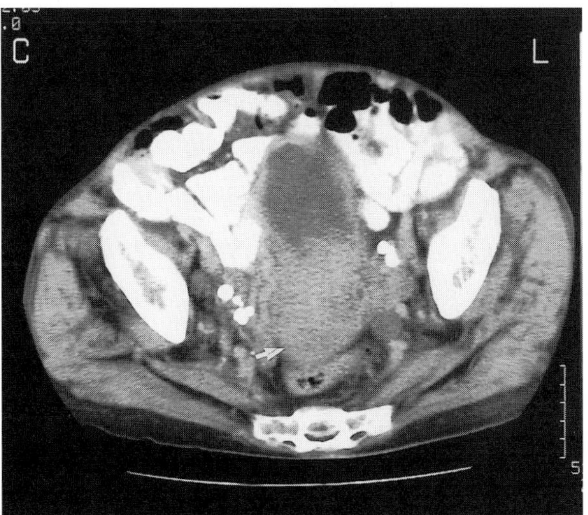


(c)

**Figure 6.19** Post-contrast enhancement CT series showing: (a) dilated left pelvi-ureteric system, (b) dilated left ureter at the level of the ASIS, and (c) section through a bladder mass compressing the left ureter

Transaxial images of the abdomen and pelvis may also be employed to demonstrate masses associated with the ureters and bladder. An oral contrast agent in the form of dilute Gastrografin or barium is also required to outline the alimentary tract. For female patients a tampon may be inserted in the vagina to act as a marker. Further images following injection of a non-ionic contrast agent to outline the ureters and to enhance suspected extrinsic lesions may form part of the imaging protocol.

### Indications

Retroperitoneal fibrosis and extrinsic tumours causing blockage of the ureters. External masses compressing the bladder and the staging of tumours of the bladder wall extending into the pelvis and malignant prostatic disease.

### Position of patient and imaging modality

The patient is positioned on the scanner table in a similar way to that described for the kidneys, with the scan reference point at the xiphisternum for examination of the ureters. For the bladder the reference point is at the level of the iliac crest.

### Imaging procedure – ureters

An anteroposterior scan projection radiograph is performed, starting 5 cm above and ending 40 cm below the xiphisternum to include the symphysis pubis. From this image, 10 mm sections at 20 mm table increments are prescribed through the abdomen, starting at the top of the kidneys to the symphysis pubis. These pre-contrast images are viewed, following which any abnormal area is rescanned during the infusion of a contrast agent using 10 mm sections and a table increment of 10 mm. Scanning commences after 60 ml of the contrast agent has been administered. All scans are acquired on suspended respiration.

### Imaging procedure – bladder

An anteroposterior scan projection radiograph is performed, starting 5 cm above and ending 20 cm below the iliac crests. The prescribed technique is 10 mm contiguous sections through the area of the bladder. These pre-contrast images are reviewed, following which the same area may be rescanned during the infusion of the contrast agent using the same imaging protocol. Scanning commences after 80 ml of the contrast agent has been administered.

When staging tumours, no I.V. contrast agent is used but the patient must have a full bladder.

*Contrast media and injection data*

| *Volume* | *Concentration* | *Flow rate* |
|---|---|---|
| 100 ml | 300 mgI/ml | 2 ml/s |

# 6 Urinary System

## Magnetic Resonance Imaging

The use of MRI within the urinary tract is, at the time of writing, mainly confined to imaging the bladder and has not been fully assessed for investigating disease of the renal areas. Multiplanar images not only provide information on the bladder but the spread of disease into the bony pelvis. Because of the relatively long scanning times there will be some image degradation due to motion artefacts. These may, however, be reduced by applying compression to the pelvis and using respiratory gating facilities. Peristalsis may be reduced by administering a suitable drug immediately prior to the examination if this is not clinically contraindicated.

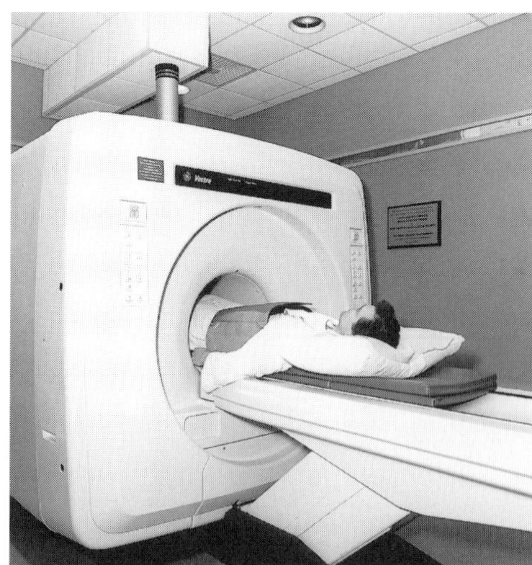

**Figure 6.20a** Patient in MRI scanner

### Indications

Tumours of the bladder wall and other pelvic structures, lymphadenopathy and assessment of renal involvement.

### Position of patient and imaging modality

The patient lies supine, feet first on the scanner table, with the median sagittal plane perpendicular to the centre of the table. Using the alignment lights the external reference point is obtained at the level of the anterior superior iliac spines. From this position the patient is moved the fixed distance to the iosocentre of the magnet which is also the centre of the radiofrequency transmitter/receiver coil.

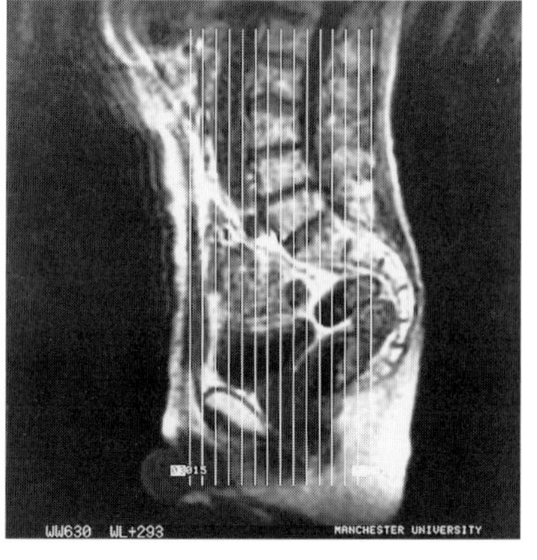


**Figure 6.20b** Sagittal localiser scan image showing the position of prescribed coronal sections

**Table 6.1 Tumour location and optimum scanning planes**

| *Bladder tumour location* | *Optimum scanning plane* |
|---|---|
| Dome or base only | Sagittal/coronal |
| Lateral wall only | Transaxial/coronal |
| Dome or base and the anterior and posterior walls | Sagittal/transaxial |
| Dome or base and the lateral walls | Coronal/transaxial |

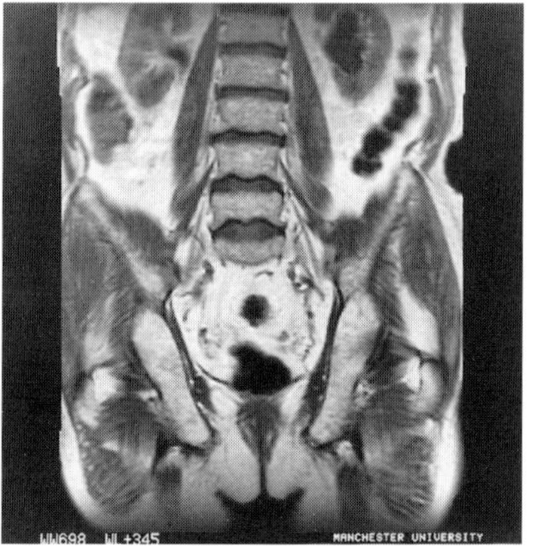


**Figure 6.20c** Coronal $T_1$ weighted image showing kidneys

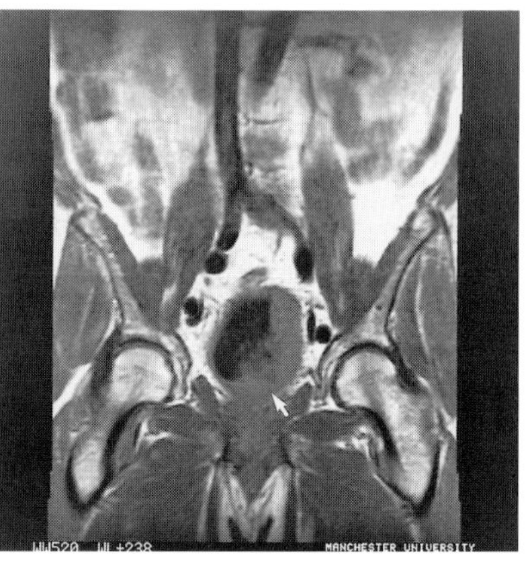


**Figure 6.20d** Coronal $T_1$ weighted image showing bladder tumour

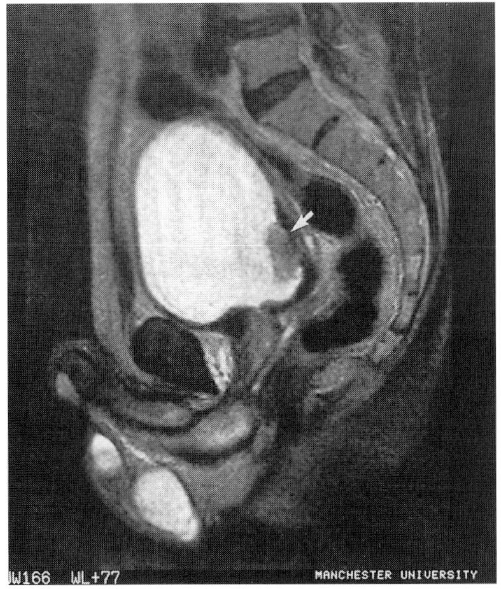


**Figure 6.21a** Sagittal $T_2$ weighted scan showing bladder wall tumour

## Imaging procedure

An initial midline sagittal localiser scan is performed to include the lower abdomen and pelvis. Using this image a series of coronal $T_1$ weighted scans are prescribed from the sacrum posteriorly to the symphysis pubis anteriorly. A large scan field of view is chosen, including the kidneys superiorly and the symphysis pubis inferiorly.

From the middle coronal section, a series of $T_2$ weighted images are prescribed in the optimum plane, depending on the anatomical location of the tumour (Table 6.1).

To assess pelvic and para-aortic lymphadenopathy, a final transaxial $T_1$ weighted series is acquired from the symphysis pubis inferiorly to the aortic bifurcation and, if clinically indicated, the renal hila superiorly.

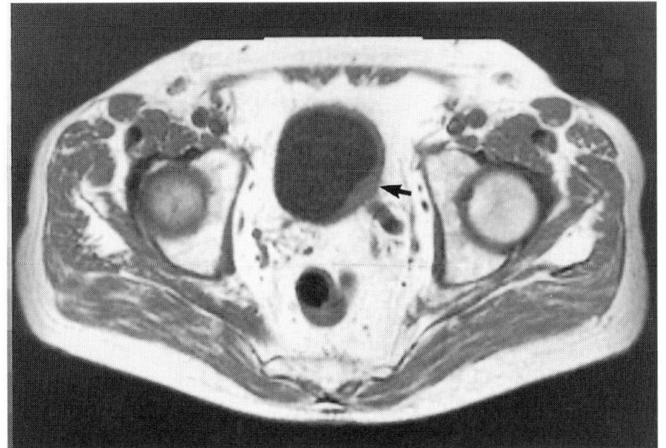

**Figure 6.21b** Transaxial $T_1$ weighted scan showing bladder wall tumour

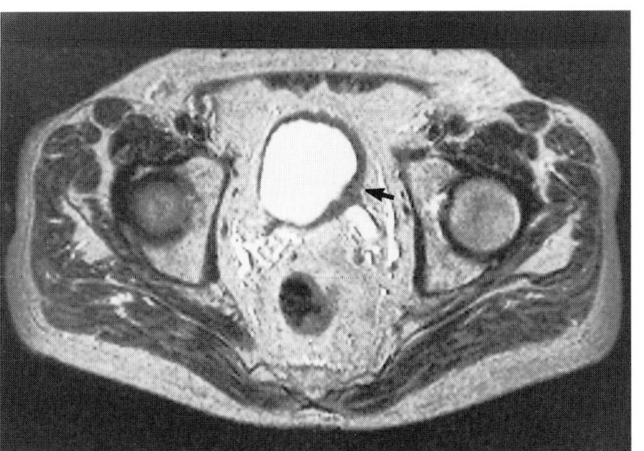

**Figure 6.21c** Transaxial $T_2$ weighted scan showing bladder wall tumour

**Table 6.2 Imaging parameters**

| *Imaging plane* | *Imaging sequence* | *TR* | *TE* | *Field of view* (cm) | *No. of NEX* | *Slice width/ gap* (mm) | *Matrix (horizontal–vertical)* |
|---|---|---|---|---|---|---|---|
| Coronal | Spin-echo $T_1$ weighted | 600 | 25 | 40 | 2 | 7/2 | 192 × 256 |
| Optimum | Fast spin-echo $T_2$ weighted | 3500 | 100 | 40 | 3 | 7/2 | 224× 128/160 |
| Transaxial | Spin-echo $T_1$ weighted | 500 | 25 | 30–40 | 2 | 7/2 | 256 × 192 |

# 6 Urinary System

## Angiography

The renal arteries and renal circulation are best examined using dedicated angiographic equipment combined with a digital imaging facility, enabling DSA or rapid serial radiography to be undertaken. This involves selective catheterisation of a renal artery using a preshaped catheter following femoral artery catheterisation and a hand injection of a non-ionic contrast agent. An aortogram similar to that described on page 294 enables both kidneys be examined simultaneously; in this case a pigtail catheter is sited in the aorta proximal to the renal arteries.

Intravenous DSA may be used when detailed anatomical information is not a priority and when femoral artery catheterisation is contraindicated.

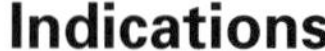

### Indications

Renal artery stenosis, diagnosis of difficult spaces-occupying lesions and renal artery embolisation.

### Position of patient and imaging modality

Postero-anterior projection images are taken of the affected renal area or of both kidneys. The patient lies supine in the middle of the imaging couch, with the head raised on a shallow pillow. The image intensifier/film changer is parallel to the imaging couch which is moved to align the renal area to the central X-ray beam.

Oblique projections may also be required to align the intensifier parallel to the renal artery to assess renal artery stenosis.

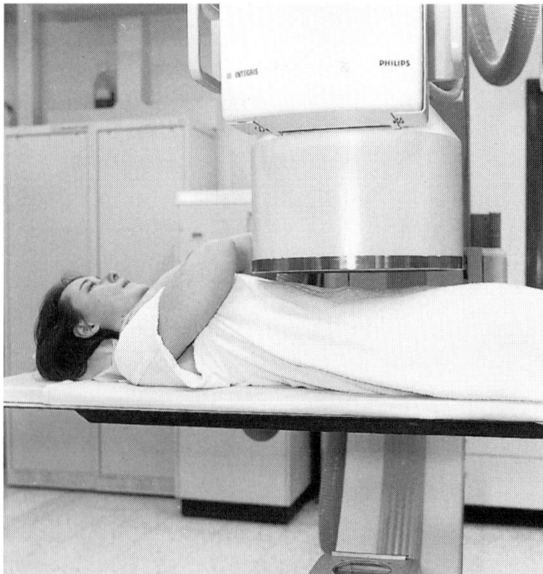


**Figure 6.22a** Patient and equipment

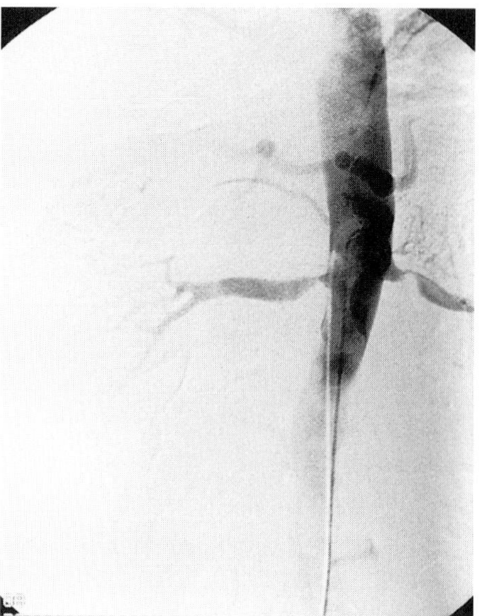

**Figure 6.22b** Early series aortogram image of the right kidney

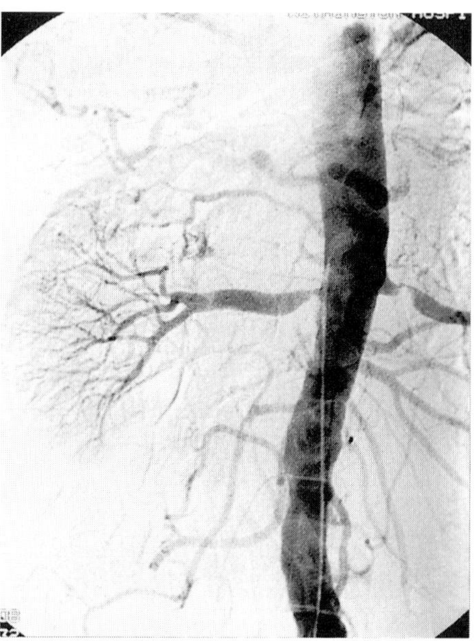

**Figure 6.22c** Mid-series aortogram image showing bilateral renal artery stenosis

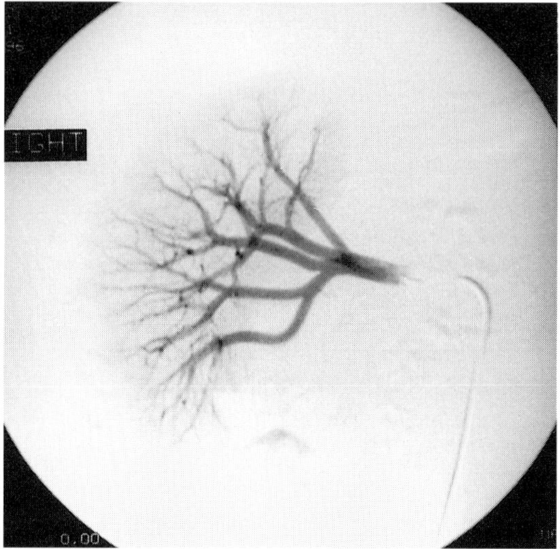

**Figure 6.22d** Arterial phase image following selective catheterisation of the right renal artery

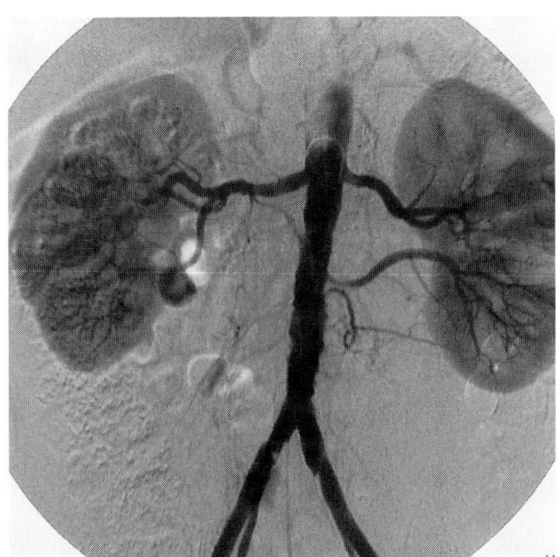

Figure 6.23a Mid-series aortogram image showing a second renal artery supplying the lower pole of the left kidney

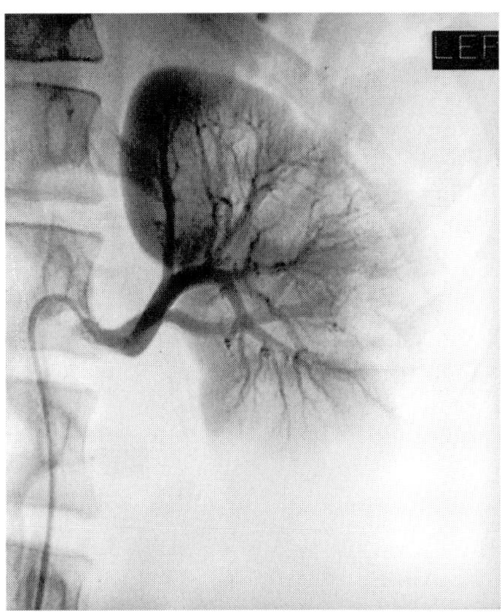


Figure 6.23b Arterial phase image following selective catheterisation of the left renal main artery showing the upper and mid-portions of the left kidney

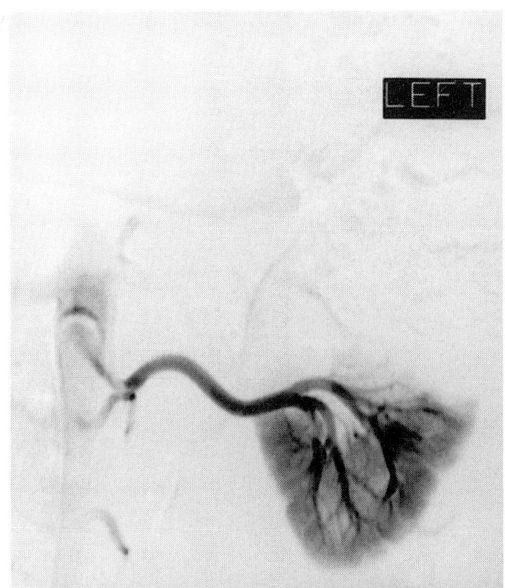


Figure 6.23c Arterial phase image following selective catheterisation of the second artery supplying the lower pole of the left kidney

## Imaging procedure

For selective angiography an aortogram may be performed initially to assess the renal arterial supply. Following catheterisation of the appropriate renal artery, a bolus of contrast is injected by hand, following which image acquisition commences immediately. When intravenous DSA is employed, an exposure delay of approximately 4 s is normally employed.

The imaging protocol is dependent on the individual radiologist and will normally be set to demonstrate arterial, venous and nephrogram phases, dependent on the patient's condition.

*Imaging parameters*

| *Selective angiography* | | *Aortography* | |
|---|---|---|---|
| *Images/s* | *Run time* | *Images/s* | *Run time* |
| 3 | 2 | 3 | 2 |
| 0.5 | 4 | 2 | 3 |

*Contrast medium and injector data*

| | *Selective* | *Aortography* |
|---|---|---|
| *Volume* | 8–10 ml | 40 ml |
| *Concentration* | 300 mgI/ml | 300 mgI/ml |
| *Flow rate* | Hand inj. | 15 ml/s |

In DSA, the concentration may be reduced.

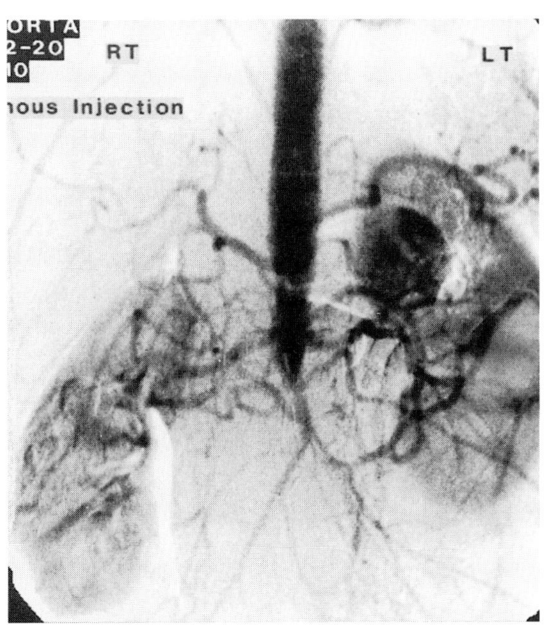


Figure 6.23d Intravenous DSA image showing obstruction in the aorta below the level of the renal arteries

# 6 Urinary System

## Retrograde Pyelography

Retrograde pyelography, also known as ascending pyelography, involves a mechanical filling procedure to demonstrate the renal calyces and pelvis with a suitable organic iodine contrast agent. Cystoscopy is first performed under general anaesthesia to locate a radio-opaque ureteric catheter in the affected kidney. The procedure may be carried out in theatre using a mobile image intensifier or after recovery in the imaging department using conventional fluoroscopic equipment.

### Indications

To demonstrate the anatomy of the calyces and pelvis of a non-functioning kidney or to examine strictures or space-occupying lesions within the collecting system.

### Patient preparation

For cystoscopy the patient is prepared for a general anaesthetic.

### Position of patient and imaging modality

Postero-anterior projection images of the renal areas and ureters are taken with the patient supine and the image intensifier/film changer parallel to the imaging couch.

### Imaging procedure

During fluoroscopy, between 5 and 20 ml of the contrast agent is introduced via the ureteric catheter into the affected renal pelvis. The injection is discontinued if the wakened patient complains of slight discomfort in the loin. Permanent images are acquired of the contrast-filled calyces and ureter. The catheter is withdrawn using fluoroscopy to observe emptying of the contrast into the bladder. Images are taken as and when required to record any abnormalities.

*Contrast medium and injection data*

| *Volume* | *Concentration* | *Flow rate* |
|---|---|---|
| 5–20 ml | 150 mgI/ml | Hand injection |

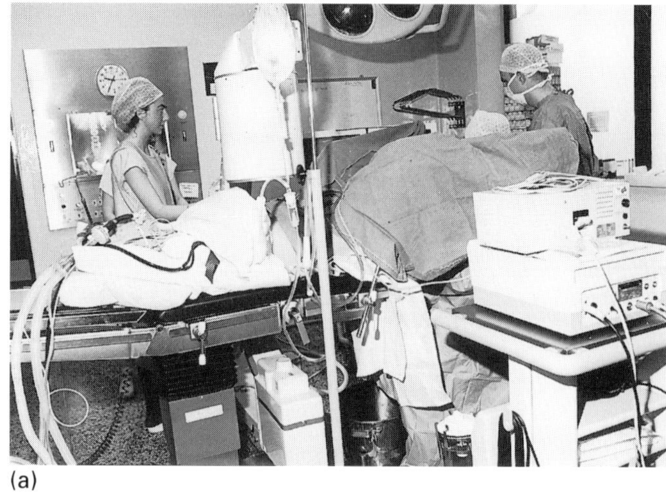

(a)

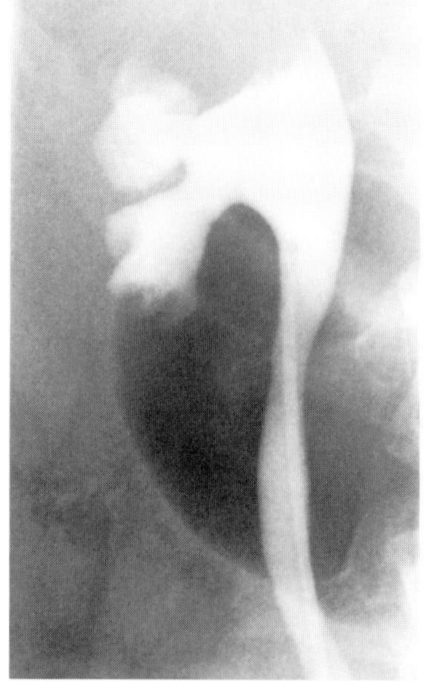

(b)

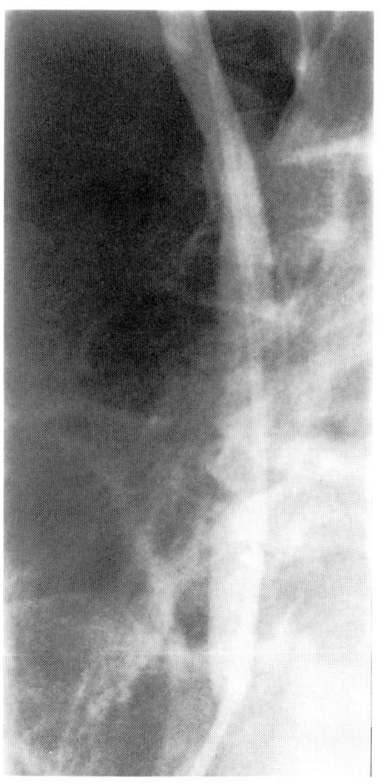

(c)

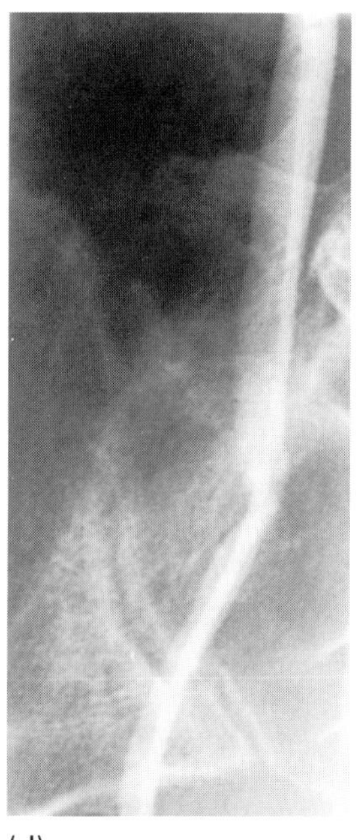

(d)

**Figure 6.24** (a) Theatre scene; (b–d) serial images from a retrograde pyelogram of the right kidney with a transitional cell tumour of the upper calyceal group

## Antegrade Pyelography

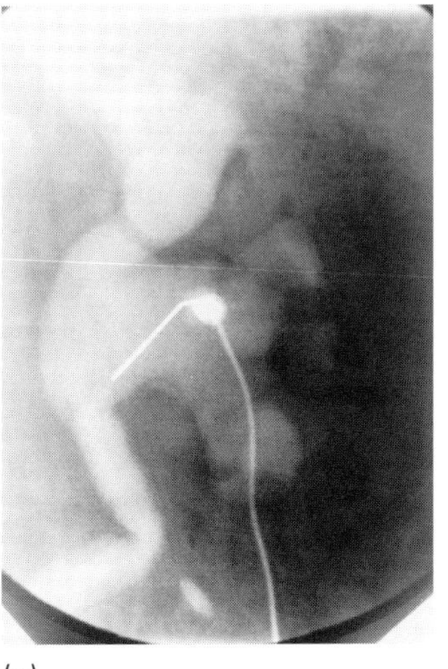

(a)

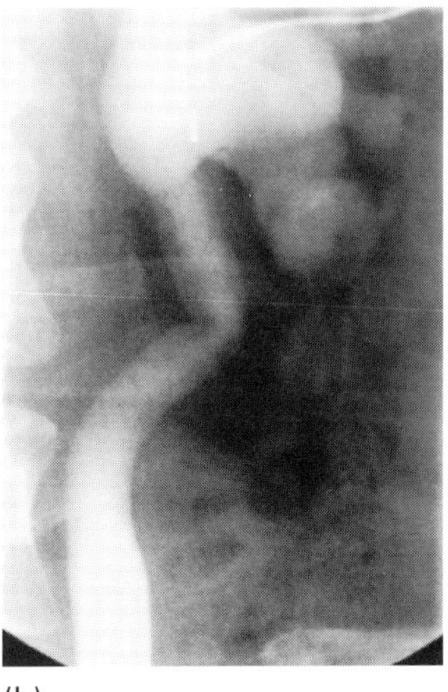

(b)

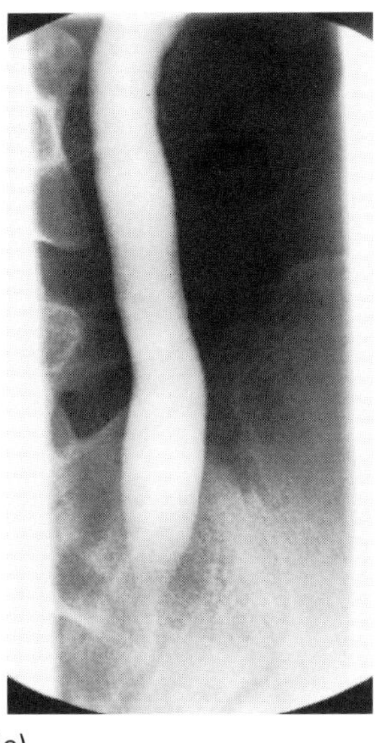

(c)

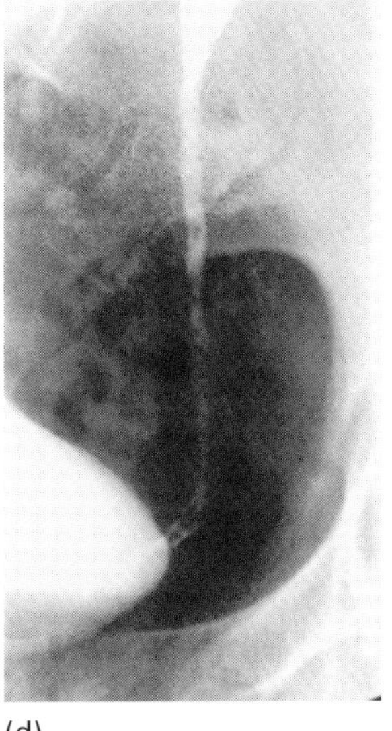

(d)

**Figure 6.25** (a–d) Serial images from an antegrade pyelogram of the left kidney and ureter demonstrating a stricture of the lower end of the ureter following radiotherapy treatment to the pelvis

Antegrade pyelography is used to demonstrate the renal calyces and pelves. This requires direct percutaneous puncture of the affected kidney with a thin-gauge needle, following which a suitable iodine contrast agent is injected into the pelvicalyceal system. The procedure is carried out using fluoroscopic equipment and ultrasound or fluoroscopy combined with intravenous urography to aid the percutaneous puncture. It is performed using local anaesthetic and it enables sampling of the pelvic contents.

### Indications

To demonstrate the anatomy of the calyces and pelvis of a non-functioning kidney when all other imaging modalities have been ineffective. Localisation of the cause of urinary tract dilatation.

### Contraindications

Uncorrected bleeding diathesis.

### Imaging procedure

The patient is positioned prone or prone oblique, with the affected side raised, to facilitate localisation and percutaneous puncture of the affected kidney. This, for a functioning kidney, can be accomplished using fluoroscopy and intravenous urography when the renal collecting system is visualised using contrast media. Real-time B-mode ultrasound can also be used and is useful for the non-functioning kidney. Once punctured, a flexible tube can be connected to the needle for withdrawal of a urine specimen.

During fluoroscopy between 5 and 20 ml of contrast is injected via the tubing into the renal pelvis to opacify the collecting system and ureter.

Permanent anteroposterior or anterior oblique projection images of the renal area and ureters are taken with the patient prone or oblique and the image intensifier/film changer parallel to the imaging couch. The patient may be tilted erect to assist in localising the site of an obstruction. Following the procedure, the contrast agent may be aspirated if obstruction is diagnosed.

*Contrast medium and injection data*

| *Volume* | *Concentration* | *Flow rate* |
|---|---|---|
| 5–20 ml | 150 mgI/ml | Hand injection |

## Cystography

Cystography is the radiographic examination of the urinary bladder following the introduction of a suitable contrast agent into the bladder. The procedure normally involves bladder catheterisation, withdrawal of any urine, and the removal of the catheter from the urethra after the bladder has been filled with contrast. Alternatively, suprapubic puncture may be required when catheterisation is impossible.

An organic iodine contrast medium with a low iodine concentration is selected to show detail both within and adjacent to the bladder. Too high a concentration may obscure defects within or adjacent to the bladder wall. The contrast is normally presented in a 250 ml sterile bottle which is warmed to body temperature.

The examination is performed using fluoroscopic equipment combined with digital imaging facilities or alternatively 100/105 mm camera film or conventional film/cassettes are used to record permanent images of the bladder.

The procedure described below assumes the use of a remote control imaging table with an overcouch X-ray tube. This has the advantage of allowing angulation of the central X-ray beam to better demonstrate the bladder.

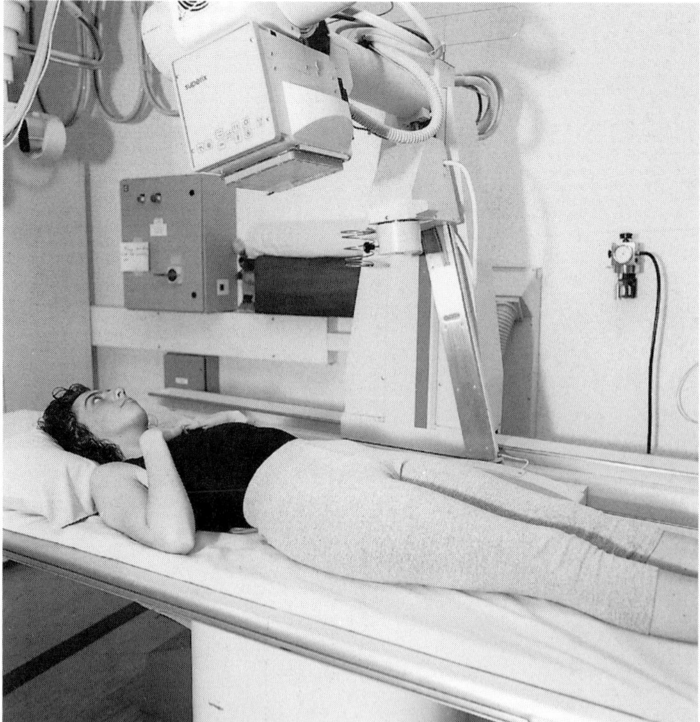

**Figure 6.26a** Cystography – patient in position for AP projection

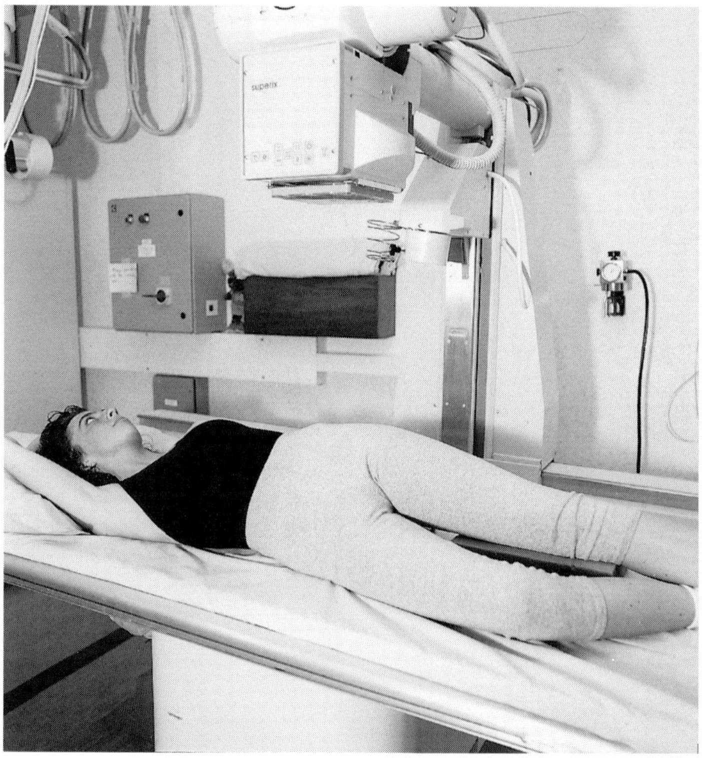

**Figure 6.26b** Cystography – patient in position for oblique projection

### Indications

Vesico-ureteral reflux, pathology such as diverticula and tumours, trauma and rectal or uterine fistulae. It is also employed prior to micturating and urethral studies.

### Contraindications

Care should be exercised with patients who may be sensitive to iodine contrast agents. Trauma to the urethra may prevent catheterisation.

### Patient preparation

Bladder catheterisation is performed prior to the procedure under strict aseptic conditions. Urethral anaesthesia is achieved using an appropriate anaesthetic jelly.

### Imaging procedure

Following catheterisation, the bladder is drained of urine, and with the patient supine an administration kit is connected to the catheter. A full bottle of contrast, followed by normal saline, is allowed to flow into the bladder under fluoroscopic control until the bladder is well filled. Once filled, the patient may be rolled through 180° to ensure that the bladder is evenly opacified.

A series of anteroposterior, right and left posterior oblique and lateral images are acquired to demonstrate the bladder outline and to demonstrate any filling defects. The optimum degree of patient obliquity is best determined by reference to the fluoroscopic image.

*Contrast medium and injection data*

| *Volume* | *Concentration* | *Flow rate* |
|---|---|---|
| 250–300 ml | 150 mgI/ml | Gravity |

## Cystography

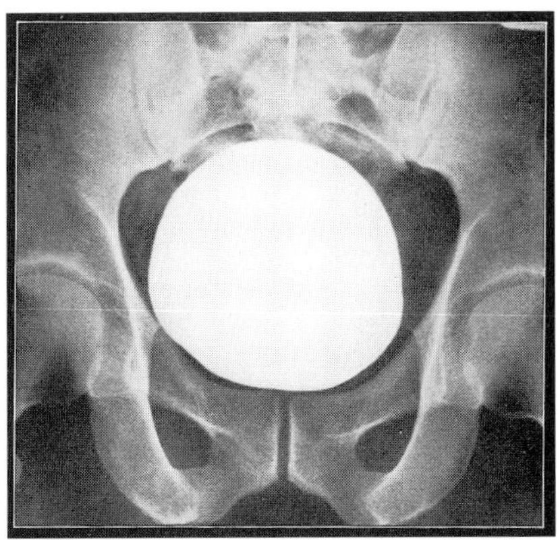

Figure 6.27a AP image of bladder

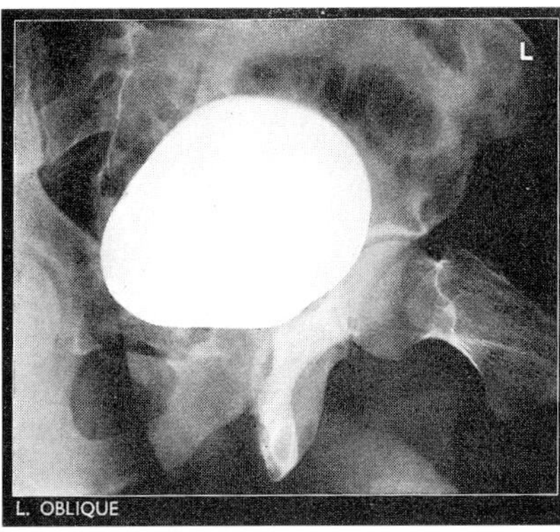


Figure 6.27b Left posterior oblique image of bladder

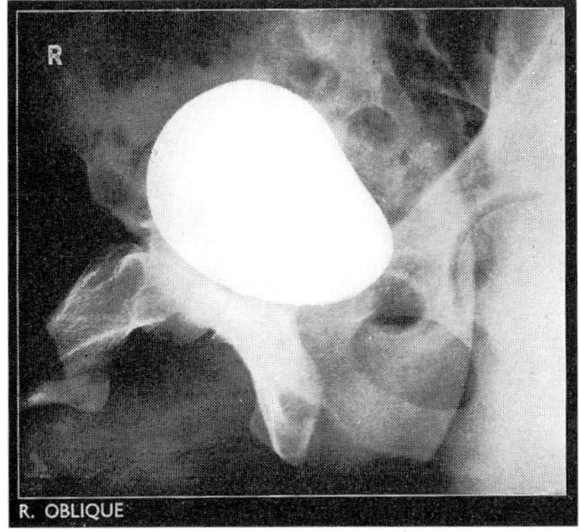


Figure 6.27c Right posterior oblique image of bladder

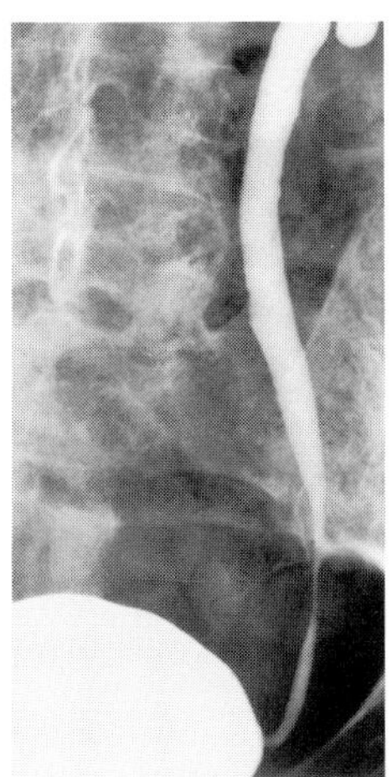

Figure 6.27d Reflux demonstrated in the left ureter

### Anteroposterior projection

This projection is used to demonstrate the rounded form of the bladder when slightly distended with contrast. The foot of the imaging couch may be raised 10° in order to fill the fundus of the bladder. It is important that the bladder is adequately filled with contrast otherwise, in the supine position, only the posterior proportion that is filled will be visualised.

*Position of patient and imaging modality*

The patient lies supine on the imaging couch, with the median sagittal plane at right angles to and coincident with the central long axis of the couch. The pelvis is adjusted so that the anterior superior iliac spines are equidistant from the couch top.

When selected, an 18 × 24 cm cassette is placed longitudinally in the cassette tray and displaced caudally so that the symphysis pubis is included on the lower part of the film.

*Direction and centring of the X-ray beam*

The central ray is directed 15° caudally and centred 5 cm above the upper border of the symphysis in the midline.

### Right and left posterior oblique projections

These projections demonstrate the lateral walls of the bladder and any vesico-ureteral reflux. The lower part of each ureter, as it passes from the lower lumbar region into the cavity of the pelvis, is also demonstrated by rotation of the pelvis. The ureter visualised corresponds to that of the raised side of the patient.

*Position of patient and imaging modality*

With the patient supine, the left and right sides are raised in turn through 30°. The actual degree of rotation is best determined with the aid of fluoroscopy. The hips and knees are flexed and the patient supported on non-opaque pads. A point mid-way between the anterior superior iliac spine, on the side nearest the couch, and the midline should be central to the couch.

When selected, an 18 × 24 cm cassette is placed longitudinally in the cassette tray.

*Direction and centring of the X-ray beam*

The perpendicular central ray is directed just below the anterior superior iliac spine on the raised side, examining each side in turn. The image must be clearly labelled as to the side in contact with the image couch.

# 6 Urinary System

## Micturition Cystography

Micturition cystography, known as cysto-urethrography, is primarily used in the female adult patient to demonstrate the angle between the bladder and urethra. The procedure can also be employed to demonstrate vesico-ureteric reflux during micturition, but has been largely replaced for this purpose in older children by the use of indirect radionuclide imaging micturition cystography, as described on page 212. The technique, however, is still used in examining infants and younger children who cannot co-operate with indirect micturition cystography, where in addition to demonstrating vesico-ureteric reflux it provides a means of imaging the bladder neck and urethra during voiding.

The procedure may be performed using fluoroscopic equipment as described for cystography, using a remote control imaging couch with an overcouch X-ray tube. However, conventional fluoroscopy with an undercouch X-ray tube and overcouch image intensifier may be preferred when examining young children and may be the system of choice during voiding, as the image intensifier housing offers a degree of privacy.

Due to the dynamic nature of the procedure, dynamic images are acquired using a video recorder, with static images recorded using digital imaging facilities or alternatively on 100/105 mm camera film or conventional film/cassettes. An organic iodine contrast agent is selected which will demonstrate both bladder and urethra.

### Indications

To investigate the presence and cause of stress incontinence in women, vesico-ureteric reflux in infants and young children and congenital urethral anomalies in boys (posterior urethral valves).

### Imaging procedure – stress incontinence

The patient is placed supine on the imaging couch and following catheterisation the bladder is filled with contrast in a similar way to that described for cystography. The catheter is clipped at the level of the termination of the urethra with a rubber-covered metal clip which will be visible in the recorded images. The free end of the catheter is strapped to the thigh. The imaging couch is tilted to the vertical and the patient, now standing, is turned into the lateral position with a plastic receptacle and collecting bag positioned between the legs to retain urine. Alternatively, the patient is seated on a non-opaque commode-type stool which is positioned between the couch top and image intensifier or X-ray tube. During fluoroscopy, images of the bladder and urethra are recorded with the patient in the lateral position relaxed and straining, the latter with the patient 'bearing down' very firmly without emptying the bladder. On removing the catheter, further static and dynamic images are acquired with the patient micturating.

*Contrast medium and injection data*

| *Volume* | *Concentration* | *Flow rate* |
|---|---|---|
| 250–300 ml | 150 mgI/ml | Gravity |



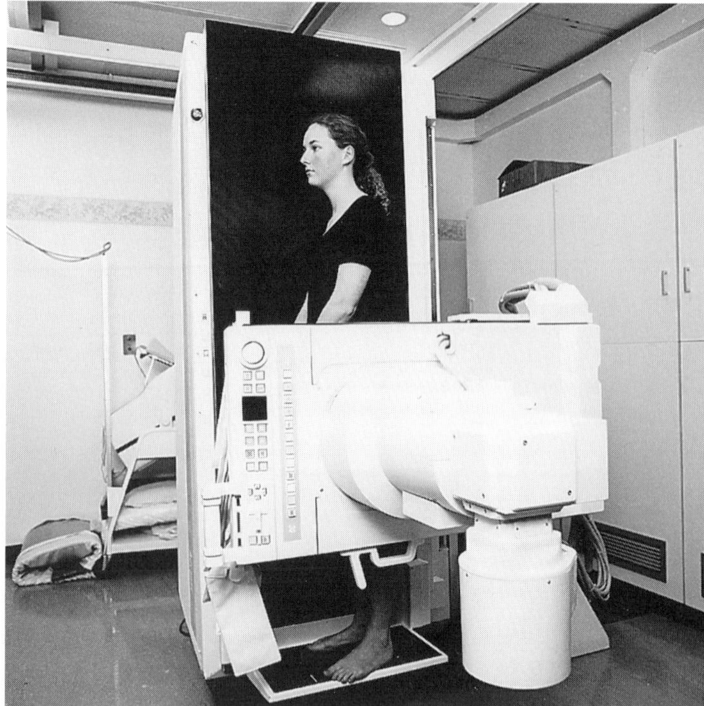

(a)

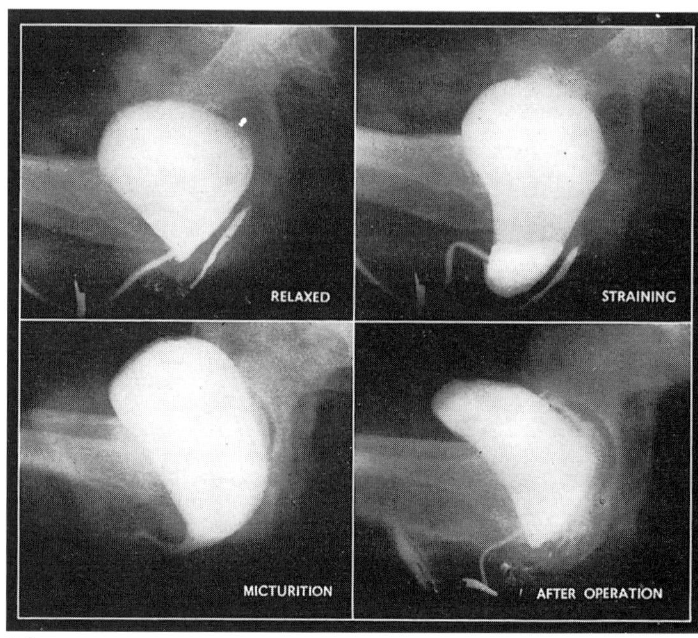


(b)

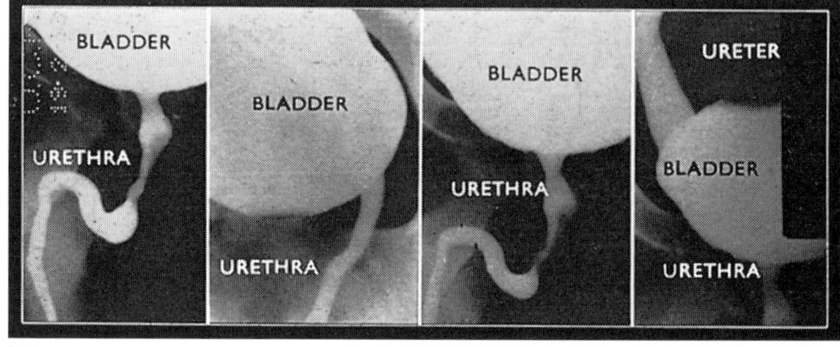


(c)

**Figure 6.28** (a) Patient in lateral position for micturition cystography; (b,c) composite images

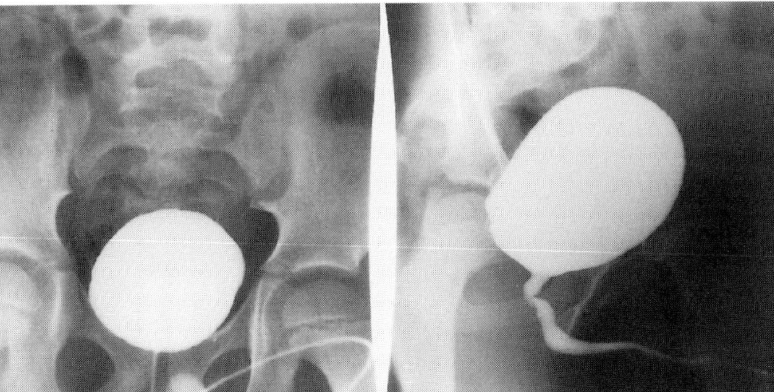

**Figure 6.29a** Postero-anterior and oblique images showing a full bladder with no reflux in the PA image. During bladder filling a trace of reflux was shown into the lower end of the right ureter

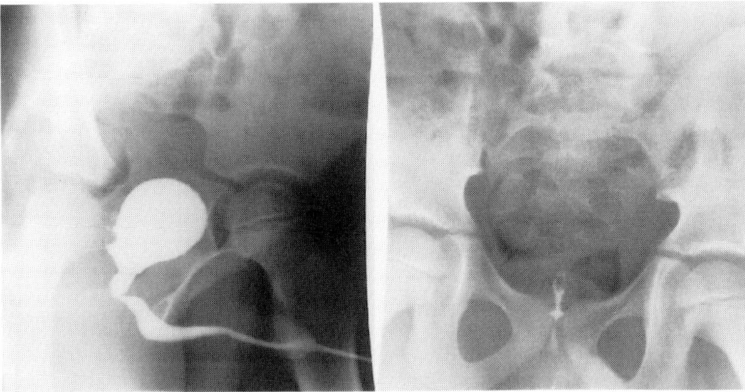

**Figure 6.29b** Oblique and postero-anterior images showing bladder emptying and normal urethra and an empty bladder

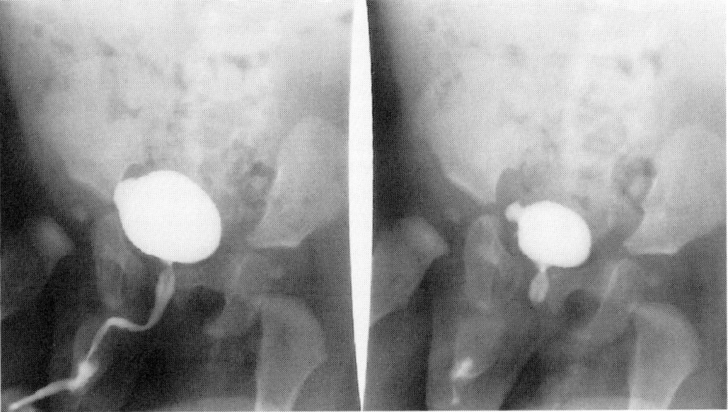

**Figure 6.29c** Postero-anterior images of a bladder during micturition showing a small right-sided diverticulum

## Imaging procedure – paediatric

Infants and young children are examined with the aid of fluoroscopy, preferably using a conventional imaging couch.

Catheterisation is performed under strict aseptic control either in the imaging department or on the paediatric ward, depending on the age of the child and departmental protocol. If catheterisation is performed on the ward it is important that the catheter, e.g. an infant nasogastric feeding tube, is secured to the child's leg to prevent the tube becoming dislodged from the bladder prior to the examination.

The bladder should be emptied prior to the procedure.

For infants, the bladder is filled under fluoroscopic control by gravity from a bottle until spontaneous micturation occurs.

For young children, the bladder is filled until the child complains of discomfort. Care should be taken not to overfill the bladder and as a rule of thumb the volume selected should be equal to 33 ml, multiplied by the age of the child in years, plus 50 ml, up to a maximum of 300 ml.

Encouraging young children to void may be difficult, owing to a child's embarrassment, and action such as running a cold-water tap may be employed to encourage the child to micturate. When possible the parents should accompany the child to encourage the child and relieve any distress.

During the procedure, with the aid of fluoroscopy anteroposterior images are acquired of the complete urinary tract to demonstrate any reflux as the patient voids. Additionally, oblique or lateral images are acquired during micturition to demonstrate the urethra and an empty bladder. In boys, it is important to demonstrate the posterior urethra to rule out the presence of congenital urethral valves.

# Urethrography – Male

Urethrography is the term applied to the radiographic examination of the male urethra using a water-soluble iodine contrast agent. Retrograde filling of the contrast agent into the urethra is described as ascending urethrography. This may be performed using a clamp-type device to seal off the tip of the penis and injection of contrast directly into the urethra. More commonly, contrast is injected via a rubber-nosed urethral syringe or a small Foley balloon catheter with its balloon inflated with 1 ml of water in the fossa navicularis just proximal to the urethra orifice. The disadvantage of this method is that it does not demonstrate the posterior (prostatic) urethra adequately. Alternatively, the urethra may be demonstrated during micturition having previously introduced contrast into the bladder following catheterisation. This method, described as descending urethrography, with antegrade filling of the urethra, may also be performed in certain circumstances following suprapubic puncture of the bladder.

The examination is performed using fluoroscopic equipment combined with digital imaging facilities, or alternatively 100/105 mm camera film or conventional film/cassettes are used to record permanent images of the urethra filled with contrast. The procedure described below assumes the use of a remote control imaging table with an overcouch X-ray tube.

Rarely, a urinary calculus becomes impacted in the urethra and can be demonstrated on plain films.

## Indications

Stricture and rupture of the urethra following trauma when retrograde filling is essential. Additionally, a retrograde approach is employed when investigating prostatic abnormalities, filling defects and indeterminate genital anatomy. It may also be necessary prior to catheterisation following major pelvic trauma to assess for any urethral damage. Descending urethrography is used to demonstrate obstruction and congenital urethral valves in young boys.

## Contraindications

Care should be exercised with patients who may be sensitive to iodine contrast agents. Trauma to the urethra may prevent catheterisation.

## Patient preparation

If a clamp device is used, anaesthetic jelly is applied to the urethra. Prior to urethral catheterisation anaesthetic jelly such as Instillagel or Xylocaine 1% jelly is applied to the entrance to the urethra, following which up to 11 ml, for adults, is instilled slowly into the urethra via syringe. A wait of 3–5 min is necessary while the anaesthetic takes effect.

## Imaging procedure

For ascending urethrography, the patient lies supine on the imaging couch and the urethral catheter or small Foley catheter is introduced into the meatus of the urethra.

Images are acquired with the patient in the oblique position, to outline the entire length of the urethra. Additionally, anteroposterior images of the penis may be acquired, although in this position there is foreshortening of the urethra.

Using a 20 ml syringe filled with contrast, image acquisition commences, under fluoroscopic control, immediately after 6–10 ml of contrast is injected. Further spot images may be acquired, if necessary, during the injection of further contrast to demonstrate the extent of any filling defect.

For descending urethrography, dilute contrast medium, as described for cystography on page 222, is introduced to outline the bladder. Images of the urethra are acquired, under fluoroscopic control, with the patient erect and in an oblique position as the patient voids.

*Contrast medium and injection data*

**Retrograde filling (ascending urethrography)**

| *Volume* | *Concentration* | *Flow rate* |
|---|---|---|
| 6–10 ml | 240 mgI/ml | Hand injection |

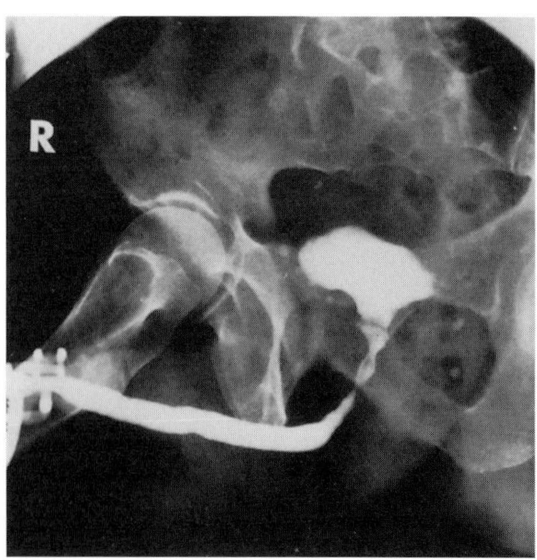


**Figure 6.30a** Ascending urethrogram – oblique position

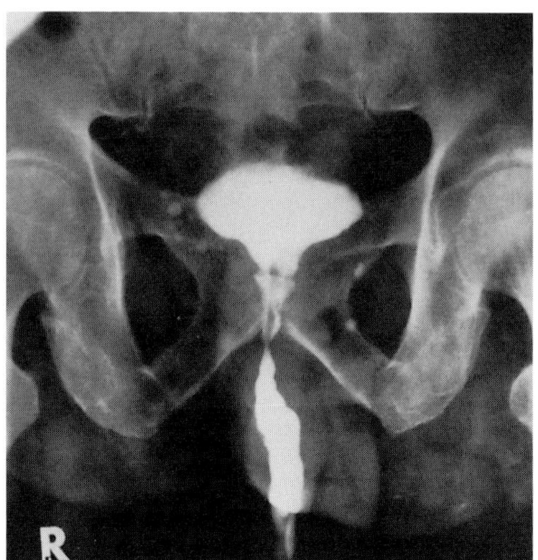


**Figure 6.30b** Ascending urethrogram – anteroposterior position

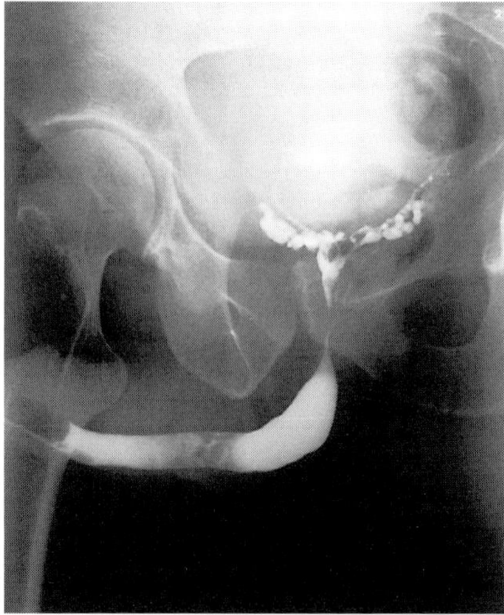

**Figure 6.30c** Ascending urethrogram showing a benign stricture and filling of the seminal vehicles and vas deferens

## Urethrography – Male

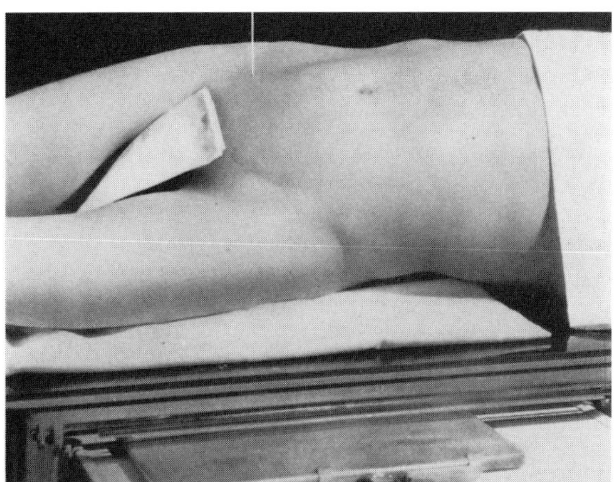
(a)

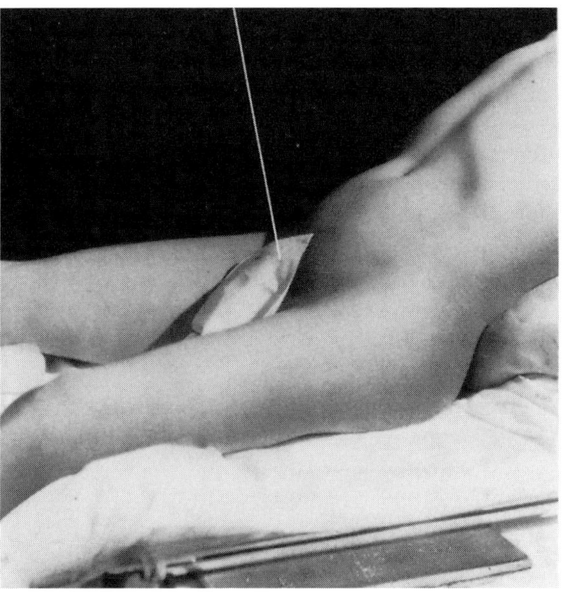
(b)

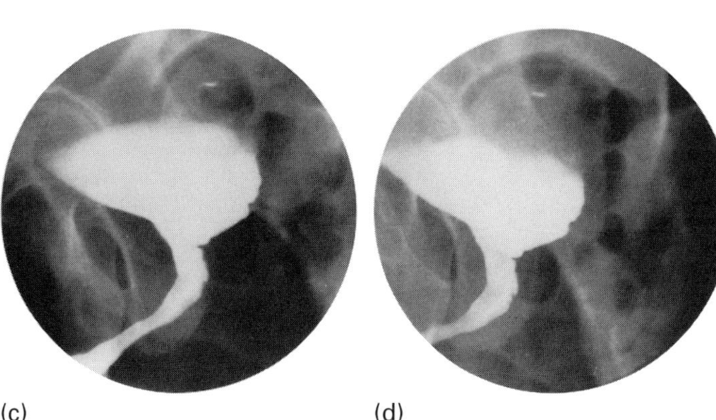
(c) (d)

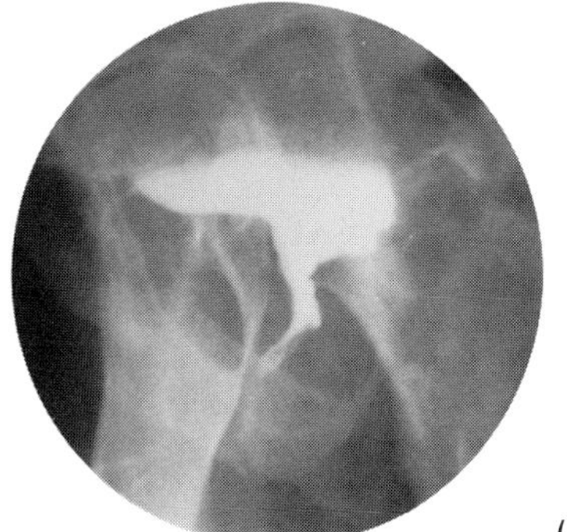
(e) **Figure 6.31** (a–b) patient in position; (c–e:) Images from a descending urethrogram

### Right and left posterior oblique projections

These projections, with the patient supine, are used in ascending urethrography to demonstrate the full length of the urethra and the bladder. For descending urethrography, the patient may be positioned erect to aid micturition.

*Position of patient and imaging modality*

With the patient supine, the left and right sides are raised in turn through 30°. The hip and knee joints are flexed and the raised side supported on non-opaque pads.

The penis is adjusted to overlay the soft tissues of the inner aspect of the thigh and the patient centred relative to the central longitudinal axis of the couch. Exact patient positioning is aided by fluoroscopy.

When selected, an 18 × 24 cm cassette is placed longitudinally in the cassette tray.

*Direction and centring of the X-ray beam*

The perpendicular central ray is directed just below the symphysis pubis. The image must be clearly labelled as to the side in contact with the image couch.

### Anteroposterior projection

This projection may be used to complement the oblique projections. However, with this projection there will be a degree of foreshortening of the urethra.

*Position of patient and imaging modality*

The patient is supported in a semi-recumbent position on the imaging couch, with a large triangular wedge pad or pillows supporting the back. The median sagittal plane is adjusted to coincide with the central longitudinal axis of the couch. The anterior superior iliac spines should be equidistant from the couch top.

The legs are separated and the penis adjusted to lie in a natural position between the legs.

When selected, an 18 × 24 cm cassette is placed longitudinally in the cassette tray.

*Direction and centring of the X-ray beam*

Centre over the symphysis pubis with the X-ray tube angled 10° towards the head.

# 6 Urinary System

## Percutaneous Nephrostomy

Percutaneous nephrostomy (PCN) is the term applied to the percutaneous catheterisation of the renal pelvis and ureter. The procedure is used for both diagnostic and therapeutic purposes and involves the use of both ultrasound and conventional fluoroscopy equipment. The procedure is similar to that described for antegrade pyelography on page 221, but instead of a thin-gauge needle a nephrostomy tract is created in the renal cortex to enable insertion of a retention drain or larger instruments associated with percutaneous nephrolithotomy (PCNL).

The technique is often carried out as an emergency procedure to relieve obstruction of the renal collecting system and is performed under aseptic conditions.

### Indications

Anatomical assessment of the renal pelvis and ureter and relief of obstruction to the renal collecting system. It may be employed following failed retrograde pyelography. Therapeutically, it is used to decompress the renal pelvis in cases of ureteric obstruction by facilitating drainage of the kidney. It is also used to bypass a benign or malignant structure.

### Patient preparation

A full blood count, coagulation profile, tests for serum creatinine, blood urea nitrogen (BUN) and serum electrolytes, and urine culture, are taken. All patients are given appropriate intravenous antibiotics, which should be administered immediately prior to the start of the procedure. Sedation should also be given just prior to and during the procedure. An ultrasound examination is performed initially to demonstrate the location and depth of the kidney as well as the degree of hydronephrosis. The outline of the affected kidney is marked on the patient's back in mid-inspiration. Location of a functioning kidney may also be aided using intravenous urography, during which the renal pelvis and collecting system is opacified.

### Imaging procedure

The patient is positioned prone or prone oblique on the fluoroscopy table, with the affected side uppermost. Initially, an antegrade pyelogram is performed, using a 22-gauge needle, to opacify the renal pelvis and thus assist in assessing the depth and angle for the oblique nephrostomy puncture. The selected puncture site is infiltrated with local anaesthetic. The preferred site is just medial to the posterior axillary line and immediately below the 12th rib. A fine-gauge needle attached to a flexible connecting tube is introduced and advanced, under fluoroscopy control, into the renal pelvis. When clear urine is aspirated, 3–5 ml of contrast is injected to check the needle position in relation to the collecting system. The sample of urine is sent for culture. A fine, torquable guide wire is then threaded through the fine-gauge needle toward the ureter and the needle then removed. A 6.3F guide wire converter, reinforced by a cannula, is then advanced over the fine guide wire which is then extracted from the kidney. A 0.038 in J guide wire is advanced along the cannula to exit through a side window, near its tip, and if possible is placed in the ureter. The guide wire converter is now removed, following which the nephrostomy tract is dilated, starting with a 6F dilator, following which a 6F or 8.3F loop nephrostomy drain, with its reinforcing cannula, is threaded over the guide wire into renal pelvis. Following removal of the cannula and guide wire the drain loop is re-formed by suture tension or clockwise rotation of the drain shaft. The drain is connected to a plastic bag, and to prevent accidental removal of the drain it is sutured to the patient's skin.

Alternatively, instead of the needle/guide wire converter, puncture of the renal pelvis is made under fluoroscopic control with an 18-gauge sheathed needle (Kellett). Following this the 0.038 in J guide wire is introduced to facilitate dilatation of the nephrostomy tract.

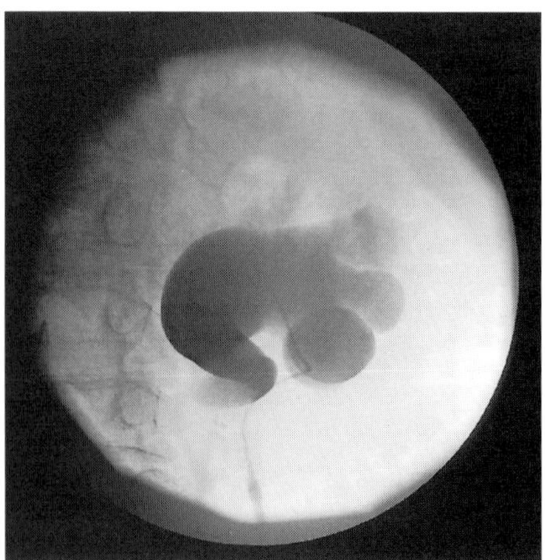

**Figure 6.32a** Opacified renal pelvis following antergrade pyelogram

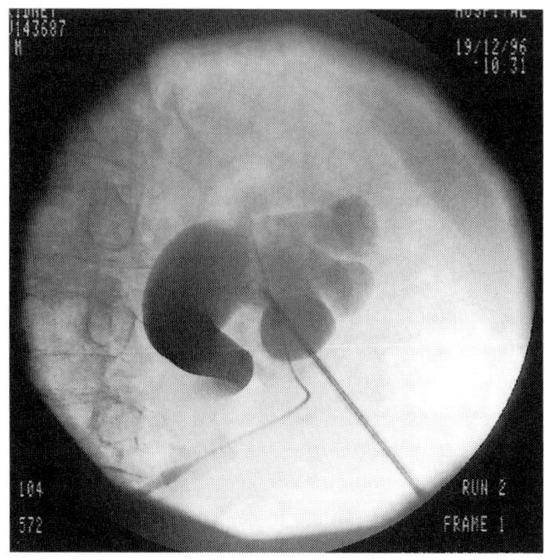


**Figure 6.32b** Tip of a Kellett needle lying within a selected calyx

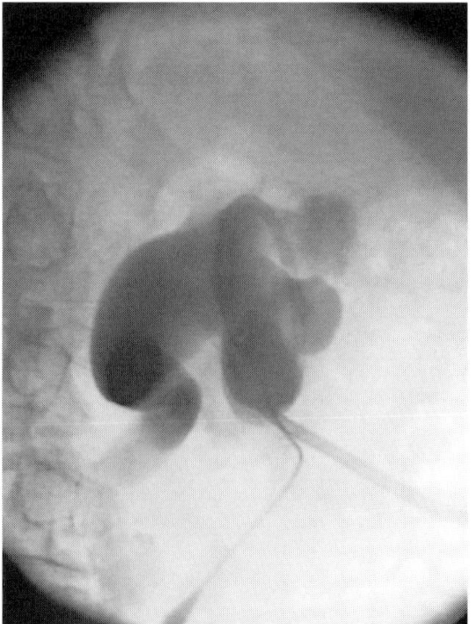

**Figure 6.32c** Nephrostomy tube within the renal pelvis

## Percutaneous Nephrolithotomy

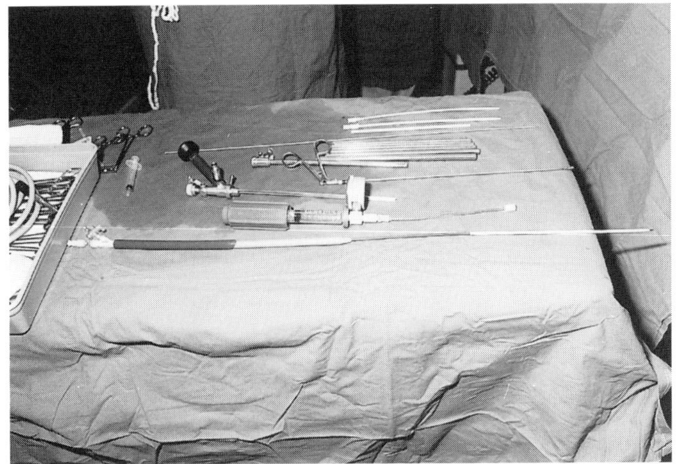

**Figure 6.33a** Dilators and nephroscope

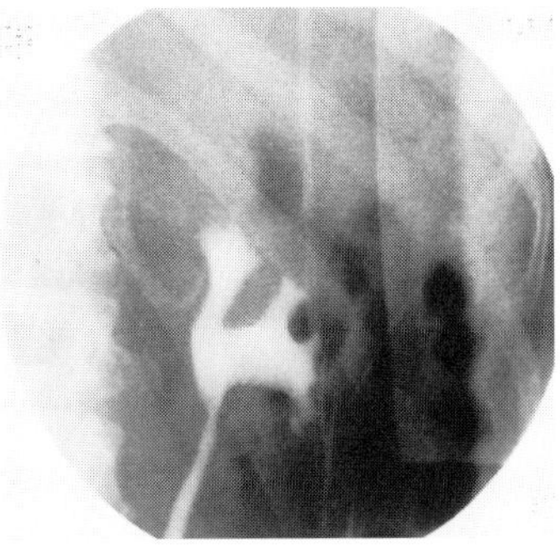

**Figure 6.33b** Retrograde filling of left kidney

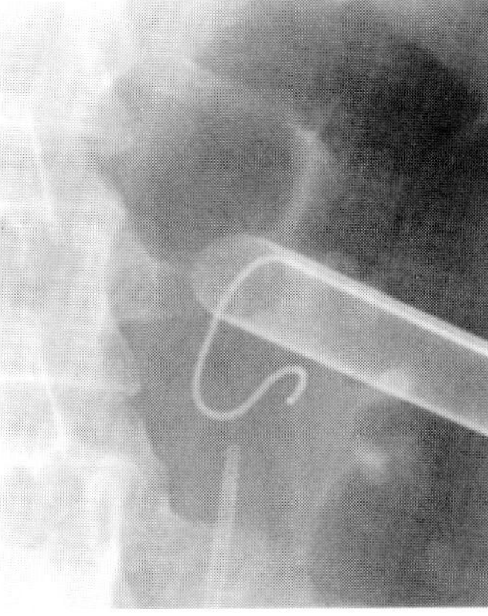

**Figure 6.33c** Sheath situated in the renal pelvis

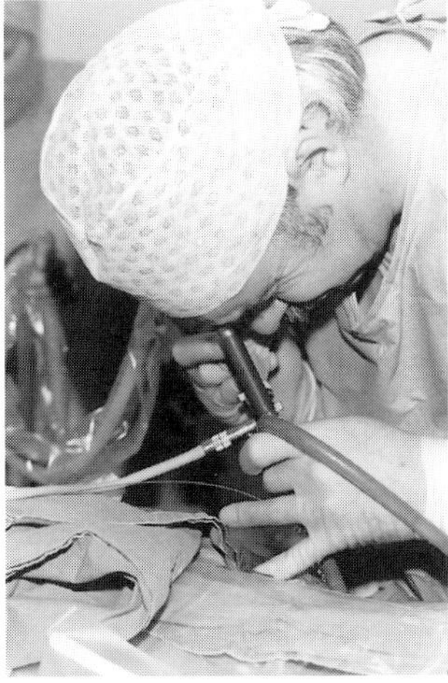

**Figure 6.33d** Nephroscope and irrigation tubing

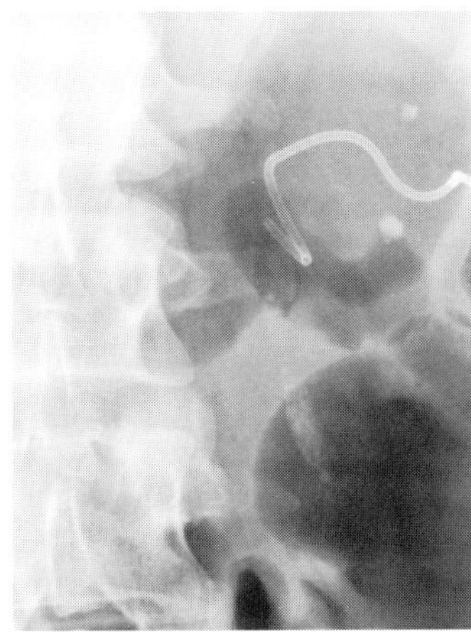

**Figure 6.33e** Pigtail catheter left in situ

Percutaneous nephrolithotomy (PCNL) is an interventional procedure used to remove renal stones directly via a nephrostomy tract. It is undertaken using a general anaesthetic or occasionally spinal anaesthesia.

The procedure requires the use of fluoroscopy and may be carried out in the imaging department using fluoroscopic equipment or in the operating theatre using a mobile image intensifier with a last image hold facility.

Small stones less than 1 cm which have proved unsuitable for treatment by lithotripsy are removed by special instruments in conjunction with endoscopy. Larger stones, e.g. staghorn calculus, require first to be disintegrated by electrohydraulic lithotripsy or ultrasound shock waves.

The procedure described assumes the use of a mobile image intensifier in a theatre environment.

### Imaging procedure

With the patient supine on the operating table for cystoscopy, a retrograde catheter is placed in the renal pelvis or upper ureter on the affected side. This facilitates contrast medium (150 mgI/ml) or methylene blue solution to be injected into the renal pelvis throughout the procedure. The patient is then carefully turned into the prone oblique position, with the affected side uppermost.

After opacification of the collecting system with contrast and methylene blue solution, the posterior calyx of the lower calyceal group is punctured using an 18-gauge needle cannua. Imaging is performed during this procedure with the C-arm vertical and angled obliquely across the long axis of the body to aid localisation of the kidney.

Following removal of the central needle and aspiration of the mixture of urine, contrast and methylene blue to ensure an accurate position within the collecting system, a soft J-wire and then a stiff wire are passed in an antegrade manner into the kidney. This tract is then dilated up to 30F size (1 cm) using either a series of plastic dilators or alternatively a combination of dilators and a dilatation balloon. A 1 cm sheath is then placed over the largest dilator or dilated balloon directly into the renal pelvis.

A nephroscope, with its light source, is passed through the sheath to visualise the collecting system and facilitate the passing of instruments required to disintegrate and remove the calculus. During the procedure an irrigation system, incorporated into the nephroscope, will wash clear any calculus fragments from the renal pelvis. Attention should be paid that any access water from this process does not come in contact with the image intensifier.

At the end of the procedure a 6F pigtail catheter is left in the pelvis to allow antegrade drainage of the kidney and to perform antegrade contrast studies if required to check for residual stone fragments.

Careful collimation of the X-ray beam should be employed during this long imaging procedure.

# 6 Urinary System

## Extracorporeal Shock-Wave Lithotripsy

Both large renal stones and impacted ureteral stones can be treated using extracorporeal shock-wave lithotripsy (ESWL). In this process, stones are shattered by a series of shock waves which are generated by the electromagnetic principle and focused by an acoustic lens system.

### Patient preparation

No solid food for 2 h prior to treatment. Blood pressure and urine are checked as a diastolic pressure exceeding 110 mmHg and urinary infections are contraindications. A full-length abdominal radiograph is normally taken immediately prior to treatment to assist in the treatment plan. A consent form should be signed and any premedication arranged prior to treatment.

The patient is prepared for ECG minitoring during the procedure, as one of the side-effects is bradycardia.

### Equipment

A variety of lithotripsy treatment units are available for this process which are multifunctional in nature, in that both the shock-wave head and imaging facilities are interlinked in order that a stone can be localised precisely in the isocentre of the pressure wave source prior to commencement of treatment. Imaging may be by means of a combination of fluoroscopy and ultrasound or alternatively by fluoroscopy or ultrasound only.

Treatment units, complete with full imaging and support facilities, may be housed in a purpose-built 'Portacabin-type' unit which can be transported from hospital to hospital. Other treatment units supplied with ultrasound only are portable in nature and can be transported by vehicle from hospital to hospital. At the hospital the unit is wheeled to a suitable treatment room where it may be used in conjunction with a mobile C-arm image intensifier, usually supplied by the hospital.

The ultrasound system usually consists of a 3.5 or 5 MHz high-resolution sector scanner transducer incorporated into the shock-wave source.

The built-in fluoroscopy unit described consists of a C-arm system with fixed +30° and –10° rotational movements, from the vertical, around the long axis of the treatment table to enable isocentric localisation of the stone. A 23 cm image intensifier, coupled with twin television monitors, one for last image hold, pulsed digital fluoroscopy and image recording facilities are desirable.

The shock-wave head operates on the electromagnetic principle and has motor-driven movements to facilitate precise coupling with the patient's body.

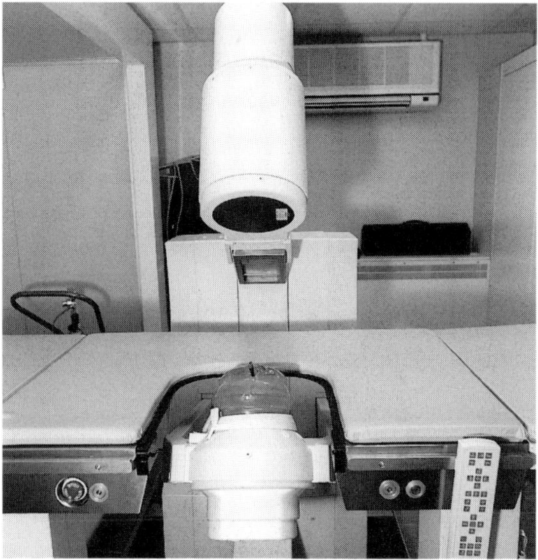

**Figure 6.34a** Lithotripsy treatment unit with image intensifier

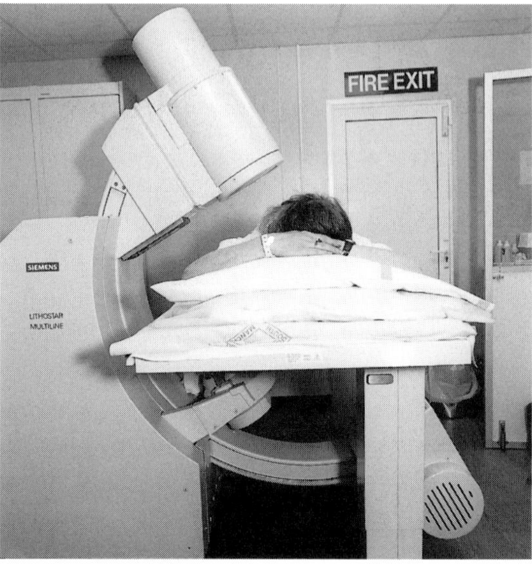


**Figure 6.34b** First localisation plane – C-arm at +30°

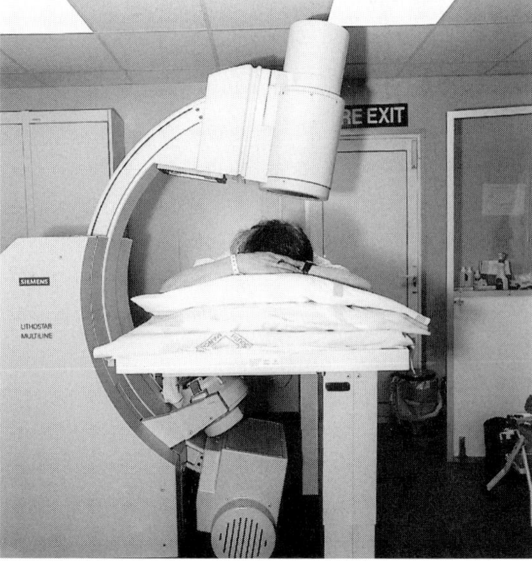


**Figure 6.34c** Second localisation plane – C-arm at –10°

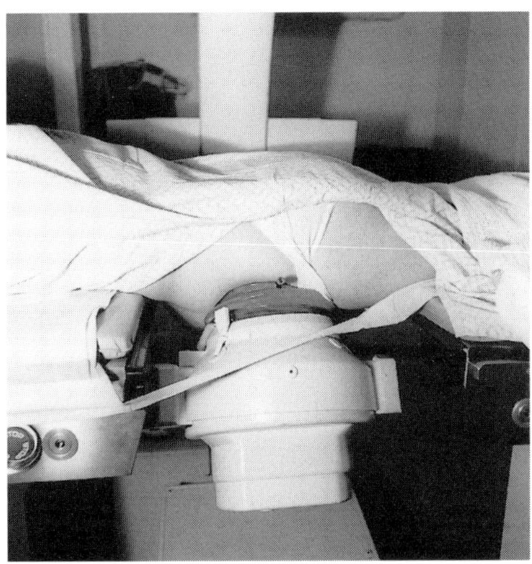

**Figure 6.35a** Patient prone with treatment head in position

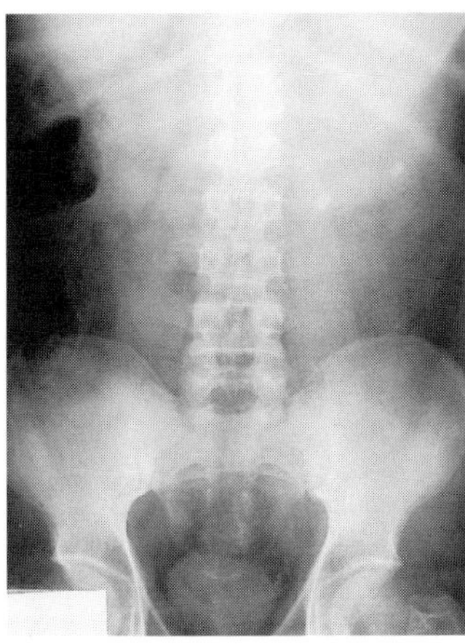

**Figure 6.35b** Left renal calculi prior to lithotripsy

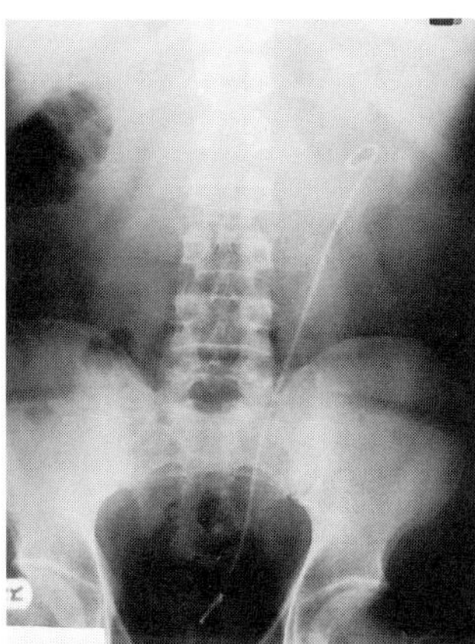

**Figure 6.35c** Fragmented calculi following lithotripsy

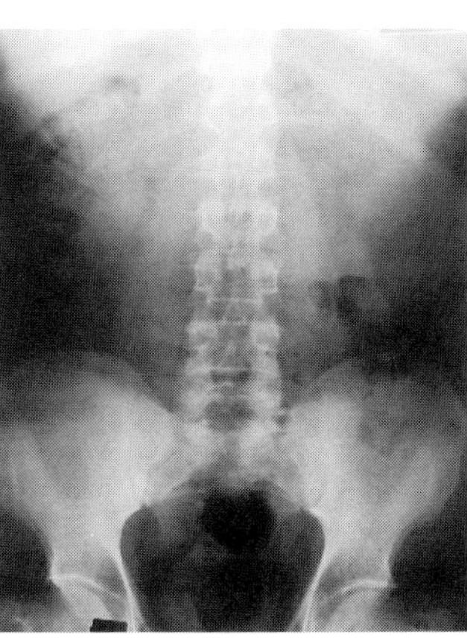

**Figure 6.35d** Follow-up radiograph 6 weeks later, following removal of stent, and showing no fragments

## Position of patient and imaging modality

The treatment table is initially lowered, with the shock-wave head in its parked position. The central removable section of the table is secured in position, together with the appropriate table top extensions.

The patient is assisted to lie either supine on the table for renal stones or prone for stones in the distal ureter. As the shock-wave head will be moved into the same fixed position for treatment, the patient will lie with the head either to the right or left of the table to position the correct anatomical part in line with the shock-wave head.

Once the patient is correctly positioned the table is raised to the treatment mode height, with the C-arm image intensifier in the vertical position.

With the aid of fluoroscopy the abdomen is screened until the stone is positioned in the centre of the beam, which is demonstrated on the television monitor when the stone is near the crosslines on the monitor.

For precise targeting of the stone, to bring it into the isocentre of the C-arm, the C-arm is moved first into the first localising plane (+30° position), following which using fluoroscopy the stone is brought to the point of intersection of the crosslines on the first television monitor. The C-arm is then move to the second localising plane (–10° position) when again using fluoroscopy the stone is brought to the point of intersection of the crosslines on the second television monitor. With this task completed, the central table top cover is removed and the shock-wave head moved into the coupling position when a suitable coupling gel is applied to the shock-wave head and skin surface, ensuring that there are no gas bubbles.

The shock-wave head is then coupled to the patient, following which using fluoroscopy as described above, first in the –10° position and then the +30° position, the stone is precisely located at the isocentre for treatment.

## Shock-wave treatment

During the treatment a series of up to 3000 shock-wave pulses are prescribed at an energy level, dependent on the size and type of stone. Digital fluoroscopy and/or ultrasound is employed at regular intervals to check the position and monitor for any effects. To ensure the stone is always in focus, despite organ movement due to respiration, respiratory triggering equipment can be employed to control the release of shock waves. This process, however, will greatly prolong the duration of the examination. ECG triggering is also a facility available on some equipment.

# 7

# Reproductive System

## CONTENTS

# 7 Female Reproductive System

## Introduction

For the purposes of this chapter, imaging of the female reproductive system will be divided into gynaecology and obstetric applications.

### Recommended imaging procedures

The placenta and fetus are now almost exclusively assessed using ultrasonography. There are no indications for radiography in early pregnancy and this is only performed in advanced pregnancy if ultrasound proves to be inconclusive.

Pelvimetry measurements can be obtained using a modified radiographic technique which minimises radiation dose. Low-dose CT can also be used and, where available, MRI.

Ultrasonography is used to demonstrate the contents of the female pelvis.

Hysterosalpingography is used to determine the patency of the fallopian tubes and to demonstrate uterine anomalies, but as ultrasound contrast medium becomes available this technique may gradually be replaced by ultrasonography.

As MRI becomes more widely available, applications can be found in both gynaecology and obstetrics. It presently plays an important role in the assessment and staging of endometrial cancer and has been used in the later stages of pregnancy to assess the degree of placenta praevia when ultrasound is inconclusive.

Computed tomography has a limited role and is mainly used to assess the extent of pelvic tumour masses and the spread of disease into the surrounding lymph nodes.

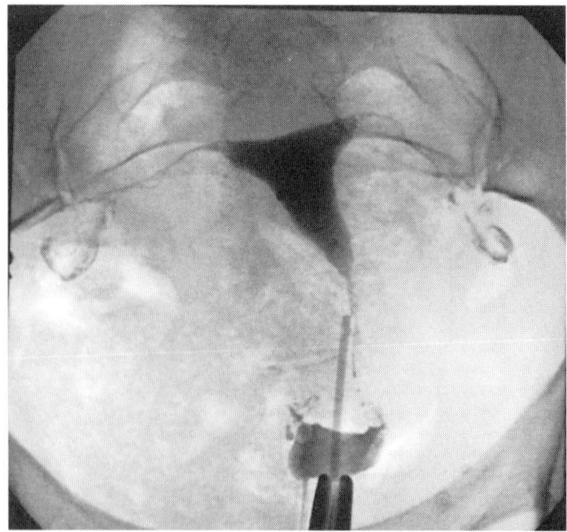

**Figure 7.1a** Hystersalpingogram image showing uterus and fallopian tubes filled with contrast

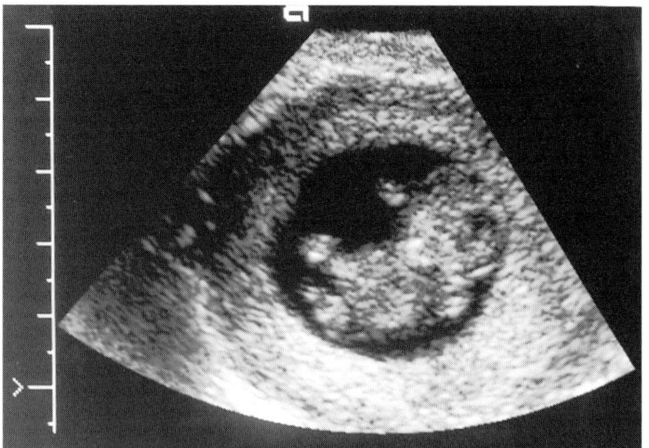

**Figure 7.1b** Ultrasound image showing 12-week-old fetus

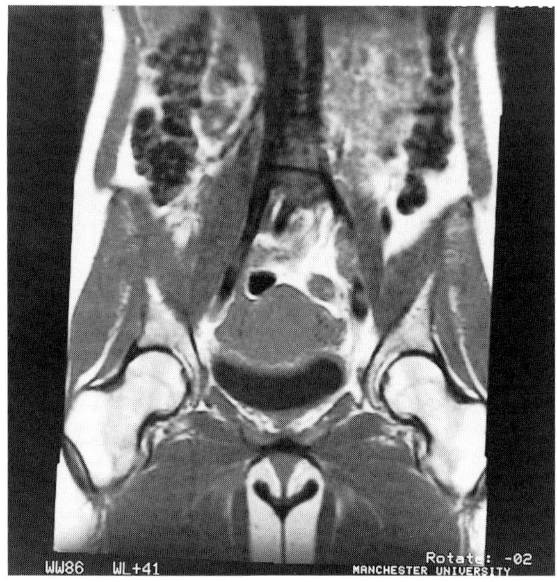


**Figure 7.1c** MR image showing a $T_1$ weighted coronal section through the female abdomen and pelvis

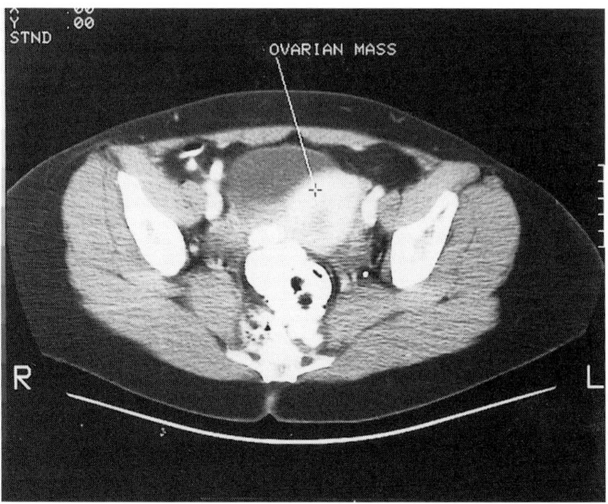


**Figure 7.1d** CT image showing a transaxial section through the female pelvis

# Female Reproductive System 7

## Ovaries, Uterus, Vagina (Gynaecology)

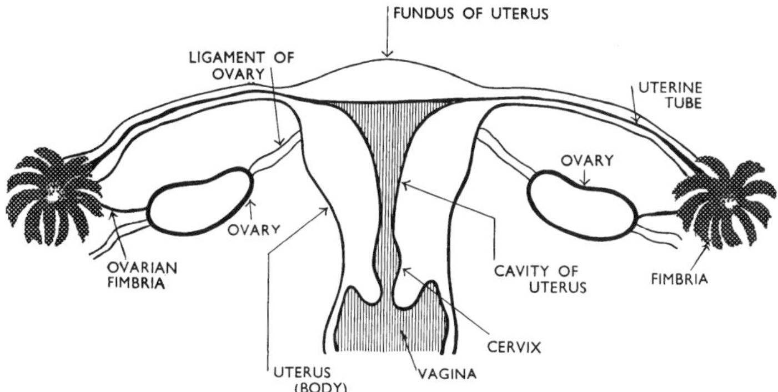


**Figure 7.2a** Female reproductive organs

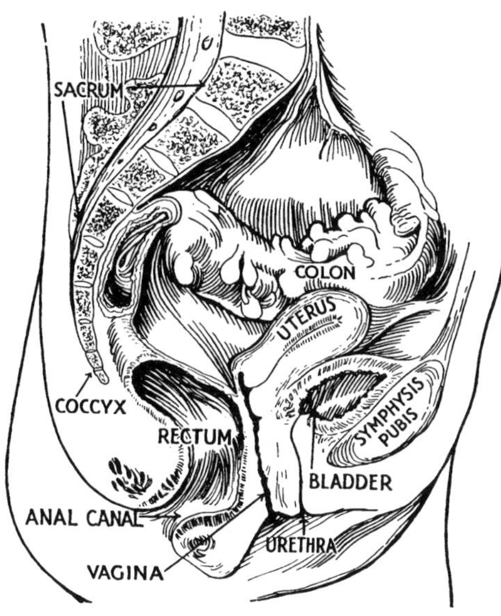


**Figure 7.2b** Median sagittal section through the female pelvis

The ovaries are paired organs which lie on either side of the uterus adjacent to the lateral pelvic wall. The paired uterine (fallopian) tubes measure approximately 10 cms in length and connect the lateral margin of the fundus of the uterus with the ovaries. The uterus is situated posterior to the bladder and anterior to the rectum. It is divided into three portions: the body, the cervix and the fundus. The body of the uterus is composed of three layers:

- perimetrium which is a covering of peritoneum
- myometrium which is a thick muscle layer
- endometrium which is the lining of the uterus

The uterine cervix is 2.5 cm in length and communicates at the internal os with the isthmus of the body and opens into the vagina at the external os.

The vagina lies between the bladder and urethra anteriorly and the rectum and anal canal posteriorly.

### Recommended imaging procedures

Ultrasound is the initial imaging examination of the female pelvis. It is widely available, giving excellent diagnostic capabilities at comparatively low cost with no known adverse effects at diagnostic levels. However in some instances, for example the staging of pelvic malignancies, it has proved to be inadequate. Computed tomography is widely used in staging pelvic tumours but has the associated disadvantages of using ionising radiation and iodinated contrast media.

Magnetic resonance imaging with non-ionising properties, multiplanar imaging and excellent inherent soft tissue contrast is now an accepted method to investigate pelvic disease, particularly if ultrasound proves inconclusive. General radiographic techniques are rarely undertaken, the exception being hysterosalpingography.

# 7 Ovaries, Uterus and Vagina (Gynaecology)

## Ultrasound

Transabdominal multiplanar images are initially obtained using a two-dimensional real-time ultrasound unit incorporating either a 3.5 or 5 MHz sector transducer. Following this examination, endovaginal ultrasound may be undertaken using dedicated equipment with a high-frequency transducer (6.5–7.5 MHz). For optimum image quality in both techniques, full use must be made of the equipment controls, i.e. focus, time/gain compensation, power and transducer size. Strict aseptic techniques must be followed when using endovaginal probes. Also, patient orientation must be correctly selected. In endovaginal ultrasound, coronal, sagittal and transverse planes are not anatomically correct, resulting in confusion in orientation. A solution commonly used is 'target organ scanning', whereby the operator searches for a specific organ as a main target without resorting to 'body planes'.

**Indications**

Incomplete/complete abortions, ectopic pregnancy, polycystic ovarian disease, to identify the nature of pelvic masses, pelvic inflammatory disease, endometriosis, post-partum haemorrhage, location of intrauterine contraceptive device, infertility procedures.

**Preparation of the patient**

A full explanation of the techniques involved must be given to the patient. This is of particular importance in endovaginal ultrasound, as most patients are unaware of the invasive nature of the examination. Patient consent is required, to avoid accusations of diagnostic rape. It is also the right of the patient and the sonographer to be chaperoned. For transabdominal scanning the patient must attend with a full bladder which provides a good acoustic window to aid visualisation of pelvic organs. The bladder, however, must be emptied prior to the endovaginal procedure.

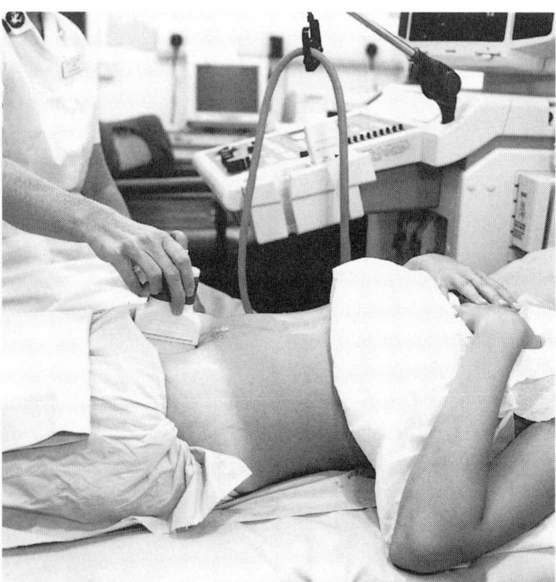

 **Figure 7.3a** Transducer positioned for midline sagittal image

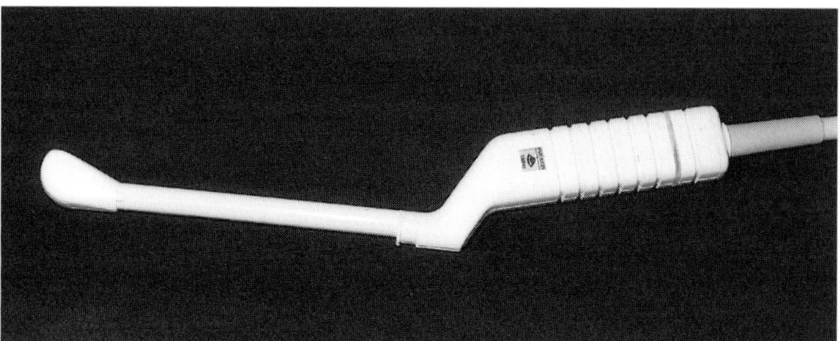

**Figure 7.3b** Transvaginal transducer

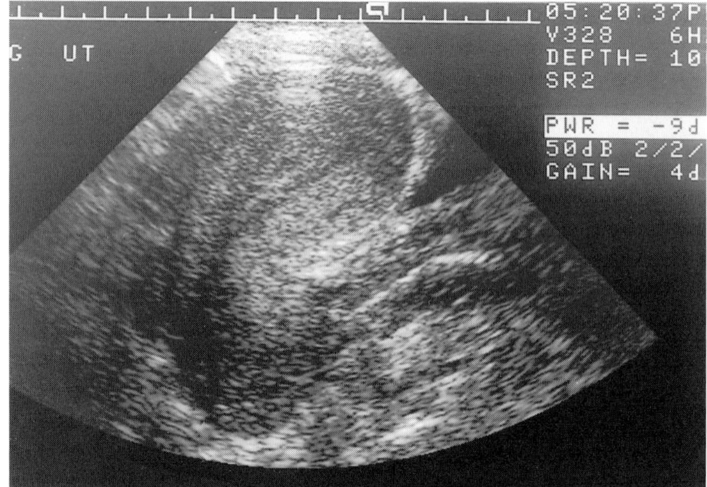


**Figure 7.3c** Pelvic area, with poor patient preparation, showing inadequately filled bladder for transabdominal ultrasound examination

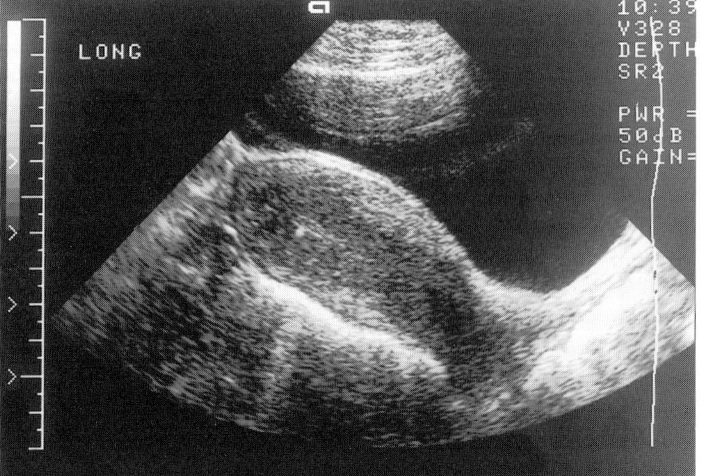


**Figure 7.3d** Pelvic area, with adequate preparation, showing full bladder used as an ultrasonic window to visualise pelvic anatomy

# Ovaries, Uterus and Vagina (Gynaecology) 7

## Ultrasound

### Imaging procedure (transabdominal)

The patient lies supine on the imaging table and ultrasound coupling gel is applied to the lower abdomen. The long axis of the transducer is placed vertically above the symphysis pubis in the midline, producing a midline sagittal image. The transducer is moved across the pelvis to each ovary in turn, thus examining the whole of the pelvis in the sagittal plane.

The transducer is then turned through 90° and, starting immediately above the symphysis pubis, transverse images are obtained moving cranially towards the umbilicus.

Oblique images may be required to demonstrate the ovaries adequately. Two images are obtained, one at right angles to the other.

### Imaging procedure (endovaginal)

Because of the nature of the examination, cross-contamination is relatively easy. To prevent this the transducer probe must be disinfected immediately prior to and after use. Before insertion into the vagina, ultrasound gel is applied to the probe which is then covered with a condom. Sterile gloves must be worn by the sonographer.

The patient lies supine in the lithotomy position, with the head slightly lowered and a pillow under the buttocks. The labia are separated and the probe guided posteriorly into the proximal vagina. From this position the probe is gently manoeuvred to visualise the anatomical structures. The probe is angled as anteriorly as possible and then rotated to provide a longitudinal image of the uterus. To view a retroverted uterus the probe is angled posteriorly before rotation. Lateral angulation, combined with push–pull and rotational manoeuvres, is required to visualise the ovaries.

### Image analysis

During both ultrasound procedures measurements are made of endometrial thickness, uterine and ovarian size (including any abnormal mass). Also, follicular measurements can be made.

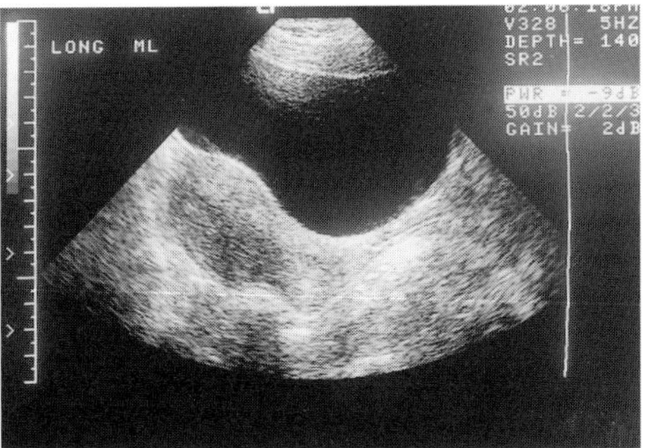


**Figure 7.4a** Transabdominal scan – midline long axis view of normal uterus

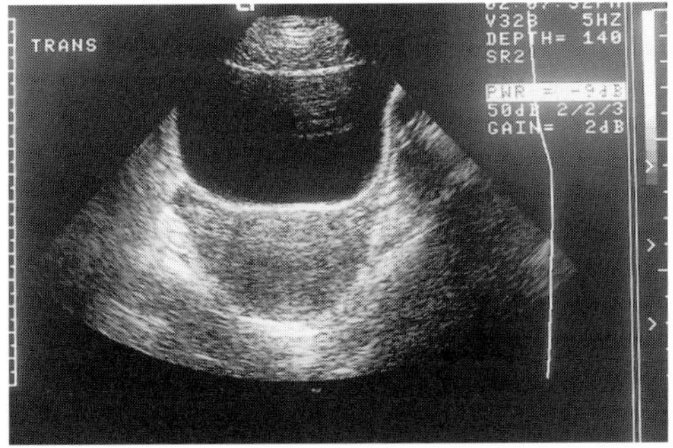


**Figure 7.4b** Transabdominal scan – transverse view of normal uterus

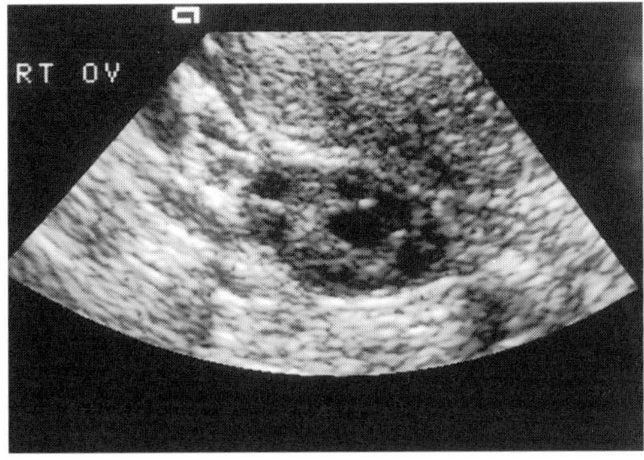


**Figure 7.4c** Endovaginal scan showing normal ovary demonstrating follicles

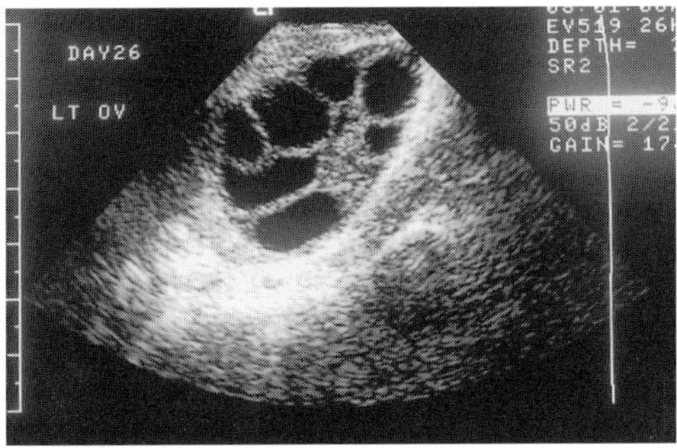


**Figure 7.4d** Endovaginal scan showing left ovary after sub-fertility treatment

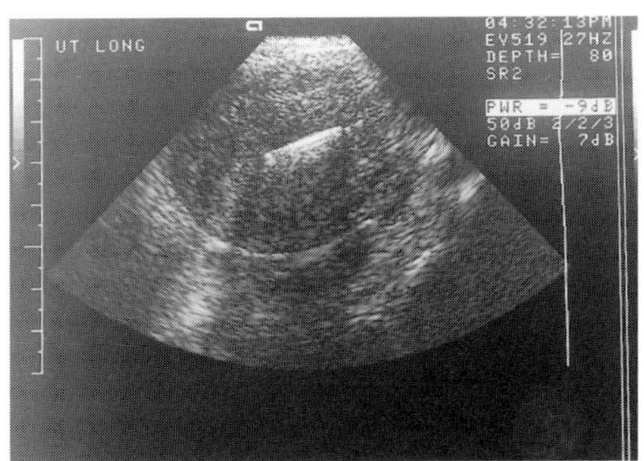


**Figure 7.4e** Endovaginal scan demonstrating intrauterine contraceptive device

# 7 Ovaries, Uterus and Vagina (Gynaecology)

## Hysterosalpingography

This examination is undertaken to determine the patency of the uterine tubes, demonstrating any cause of obstruction or abnormality of the uterine cavity. It involves injecting a contrast agent into the uterine cavity via the cervix. Fluoroscopic equipment is essential, with subsequent PA/AP radiographs taken using either a rare earth screen/film combination or digital imaging. Close beam collimation is essential to minimise radiation dose.

**Indications**

Primary and secondary infertility, recurrent abortions, the assessment of tubal surgery and prior to artificial insemination.

**Contraindications**

Pregnancy, purulent discharge (increased infection risk), recent abortion, dilatation and cauterisation, and unprotected intercourse.

**Preparation of patient**

The examination is undertaken during the 10th–14th day of the menstrual cycle, during which time the uterine mucosa is restored and the cavity is free from clots and debris.

The bladder and rectum must be evacuated and premedication administered if necessary.

Care must be taken at all times to reassure the nervous patient and to maintain privacy and dignity.

**Imaging procedure**

The patient is placed in the lithotomy position. Using an aseptic procedure a speculum is introduced to dilate the vagina and a cervix adaptor attached. Suction is now applied to seal the uterine cavity. A contrast agent is then administered under fluoroscopic control and a maximum of three radiographs taken. The first radiograph demonstrates the uterine cavity and tubal filling, the second shows tube spillage and the third, taken 20 min from commencement, shows peritoneal spillage.

*Contrast medium and injector data*

| *Volume* | *Concentration* | *Flow rate* |
|---|---|---|
| 10–20 ml | 300 mgI/ml | Hand injection |

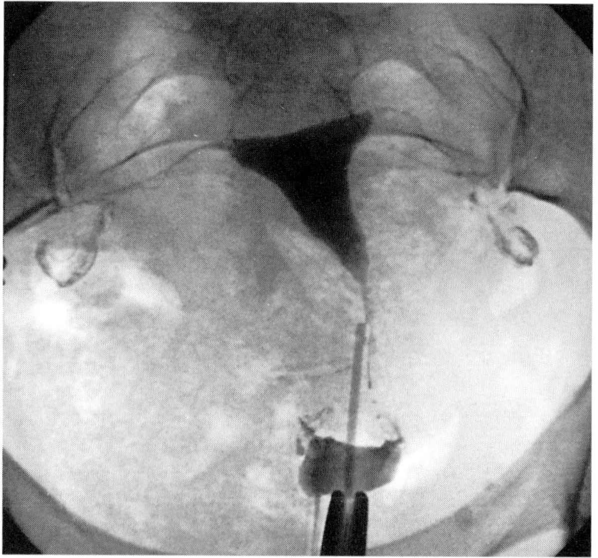

**Figure 7.5a** Initial image showing uterine cavity and tubal filling

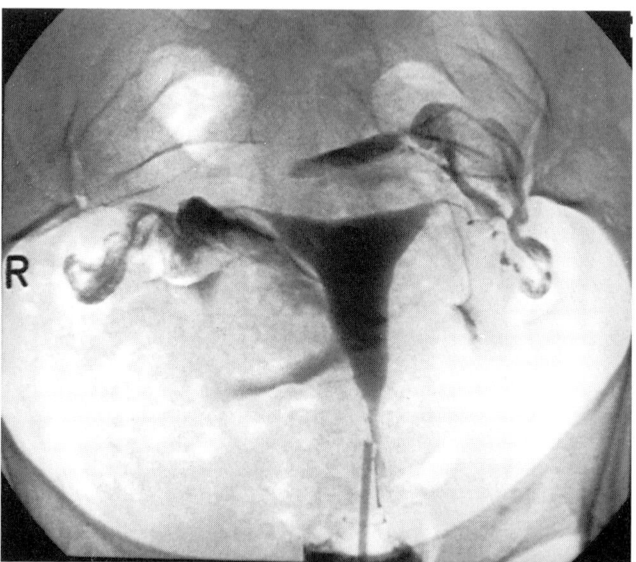


**Figure 7.5b** Second image in the series showing tube spillage

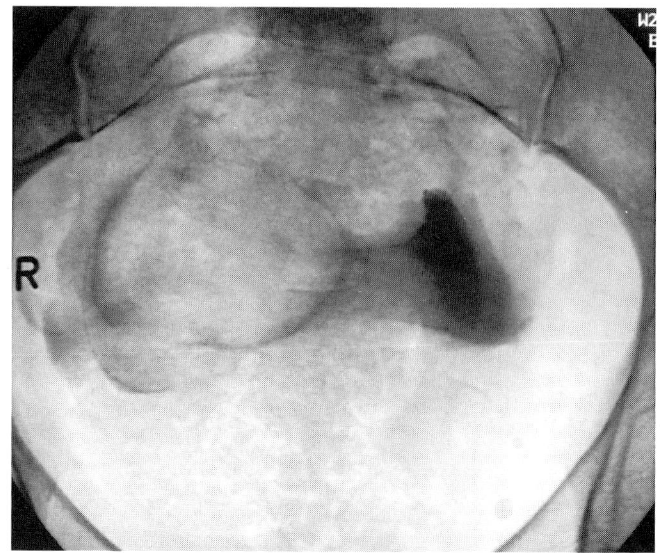


**Figure 7.5c** Delayed image showing peritoneal spillage

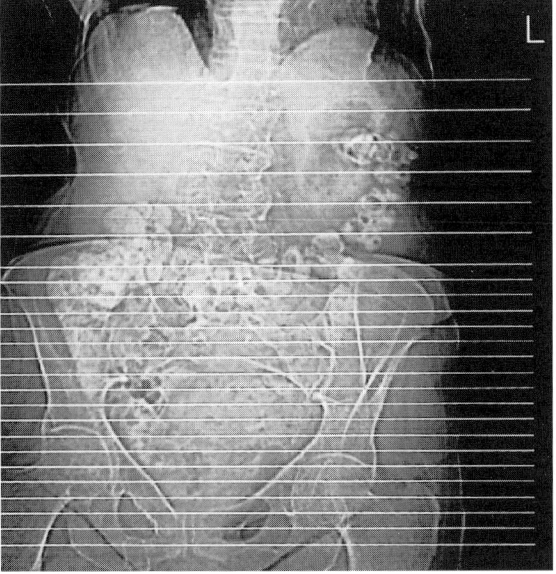


(a)

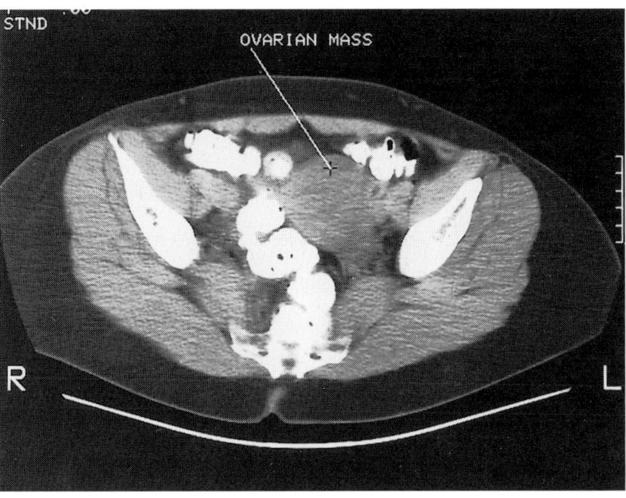


(b)

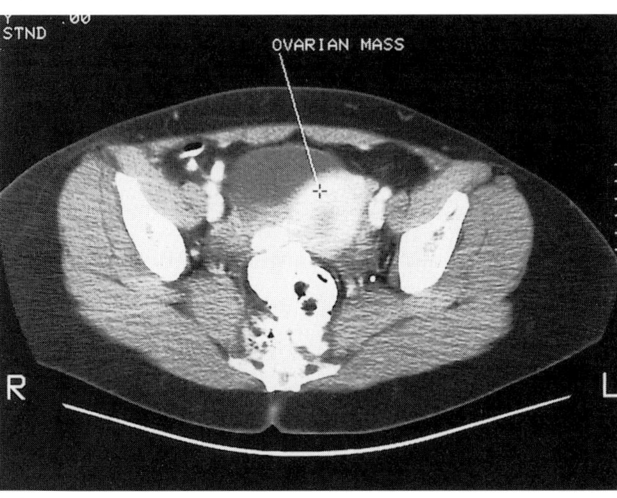


(c)

**Figure 7.6** (a) AP scan projection radiograph showing prescribed scanning sections. (b,c) Pre- and post-contrast enhancement transaxial images through the pelvis demonstrating an ovarian mass

# Ovaries, Uterus and Vagina (Gynaecology) 7

## Computed tomography

Transaxial images are obtained from the symphysis pubis to the renal hila. Contrast enhanced scans may be required to increase soft tissue contrast of tumour and surrounding anatomical structures.

### Indications

The staging of pelvic tumours.

### Patient preparation

It is necessary to opacify the bowel using dilute Gastrografin or barium sulphate solution, as described on page 36. A tampon may be inserted to outline the vagina. To outline the bladder it may be necessary to administer 20 ml of a non-ionc contrast agent intravenously.

### Position of patient and imaging modality

The patient lies supine, head first on the scanner table. Arms are raised and placed behind the patient's head, out of the scan plane. Positioning is aided by transaxial, coronal and sagittal alignment lights. The median sagittal plane is adjusted to be perpendicular to the centre of the table top and the coronal plane parallel to it. The scan plane is perpendicular to the long axis of the body to enable transaxial imaging to be undertaken. The scanner table height is adjusted to ensure that the coronal plane alignment light is at the level of the mid-axillary line. The patient is now moved into the scanner until the scan reference point is at the level of the symphysis pubis.

### Imaging procedure

An anteroposterior scan projection radiograph is obtained commencing 5 cm below the reference point and ending 30 cm above it to include the renal area. From this image, 10 mm sections at 10 mm table increments are prescribed from the symphysis pubis to the iliac crests. Scanning is performed on arrested respiration. After review, 10 mm contiguous sections are prescribed through any area of abnormality during the infusion of a contrast agent, using the same imaging protocol. Scanning then continues up to the level of the renal hila to demonstrate lymph node involvement, and 10 mm sections are prescribed at 20 mm table increments. Scanning commences after 80 ml of the contrast agent has been administered.

If spiral scanning options are available, post-contrast enhanced scans may be acquired through the area of abnormality with a volume acquisition, using a 10 mm slice thickness and 10 mm table increments, but with a 5 mm reconstruction index to give overlapping sections.

*Contrast media and injection data*

| *Volume* | *Concentration* | *Flow rate* |
|---|---|---|
| 100 ml | 240 mgI/ml | 2 ml/s |

# 7 Ovaries, Uterus and Vagina (Gynaecology)

## Magnetic resonance imaging

The high inherent contrast, the direct multiplanar imaging capability and the non-invasive nature of the modality all combine to make MRI an excellent tool for evaluating female pelvic disease, particularly if ultrasound is inconclusive.

Because of the relatively long scan times, however, there may be image degradation due to motion artefacts. These may be reduced by applying compression to the pelvis and using respiratory gating facilities. Peristalsis may be reduced by administering a smooth muscle relaxant drug immediately prior to the procedure if there is no clinical contraindication.

### Indications

Magnetic resonance imaging is used to determine the nature, origin and extension of pelvic tumours, preoperative staging and recurrent disease.

### Position of patient and imaging modality

The patient lies supine, feet first on the scanner table, with the median sagittal plane perpendicular to the centre of the table. Compression is applied. Using external alignment lights the external reference point is obtained at the level of the iliac crest. From this position the patient is moved the fixed distance to the isocentre of the magnet which is also the centre of the radiofrequency transmitter/receiver body coil.

### Imaging procedure

An initial midline sagittal localiser scan is performed to include the lower abdomen and pelvis. Using this image a series of coronal $T_1$ weighted scans are prescribed from the sacrum posteriorly to the symphysis pubis anteriorly. A large-scan field of view is chosen, including the kidneys superiorly and the symphysis pubis inferiorly, to assess renal impairment, lymphadenopathy and lateral tumour extension. Further $T_1$ and $T_2$ weighted transaxial images are acquired from the lower border of the symphysis pubis to the renal hila to assess tumour extension and its relationship to surrounding anatomical structures. To complete the examination, sagittal $T_2$ weighted scans are prescribed through the abnormality to assess tumour extension into adjacent anatomical structures.

Oblique images perpendicular to the line of the cervical canal may give information in carcinoma of the cervix.

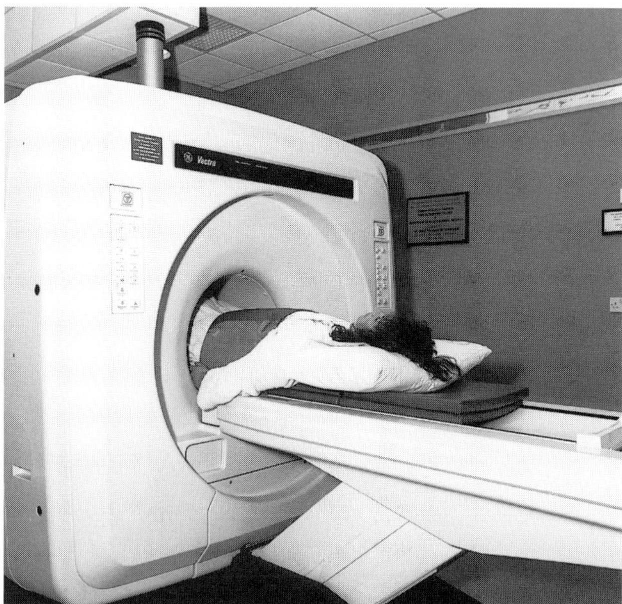

**Figure 7.7a** MRI scanner

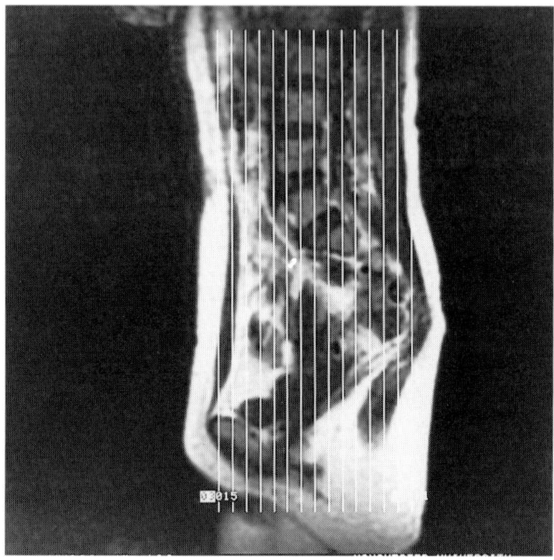

**Figure 7.7b** Midline sagittal localiser scan showing prescribed coronal sections

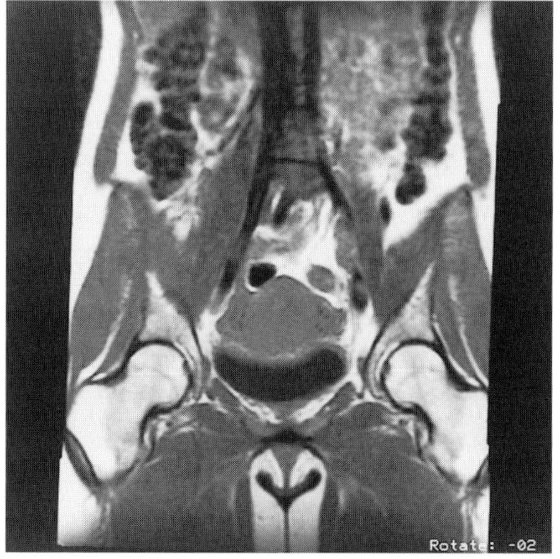

**Figure 7.7c** Coronal $T_1$ weighted image, using a large field of view, demonstrating the lower abdomen and pelvis

# 7 Ovaries, Uterus and Vagina (Gynaecology)

## Magnetic resonance imaging

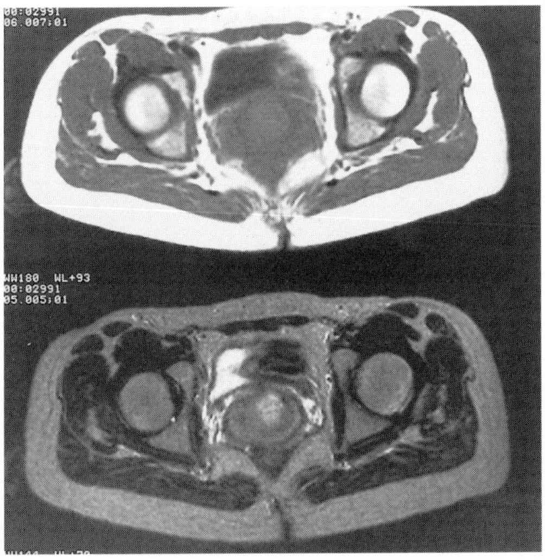

**Figure 7.8a** Transaxial $T_1$ (top) and $T_2$ (bottom) weighted images through the uterus

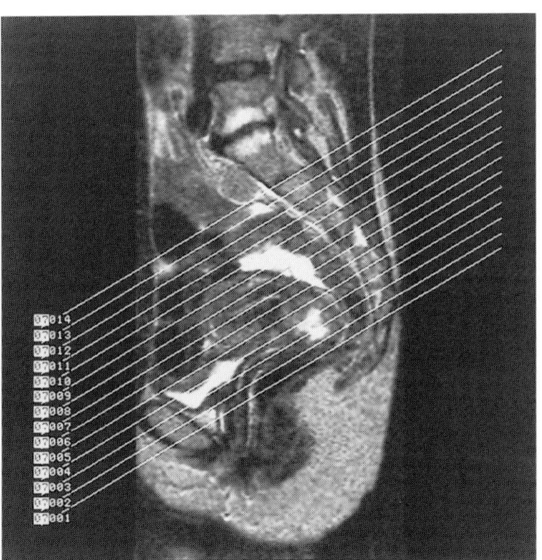

**Figure 7.8b** Sagittal localiser scan showing prescribed positions for oblique images perpendicular to the line of the cervical canal

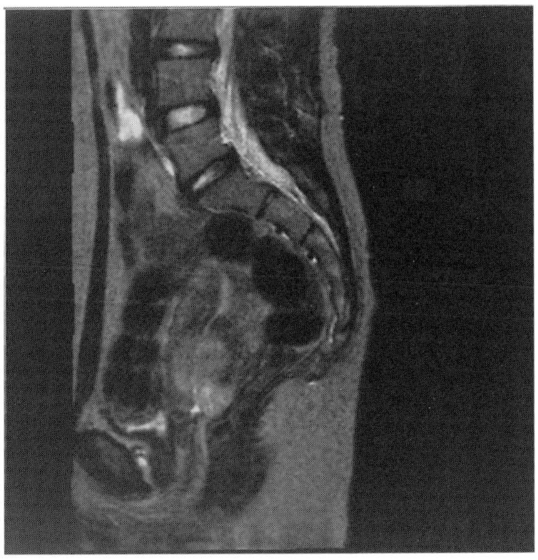

**Figure 7.8c** Sagittal $T_2$ weighted image showing uterus and vagina

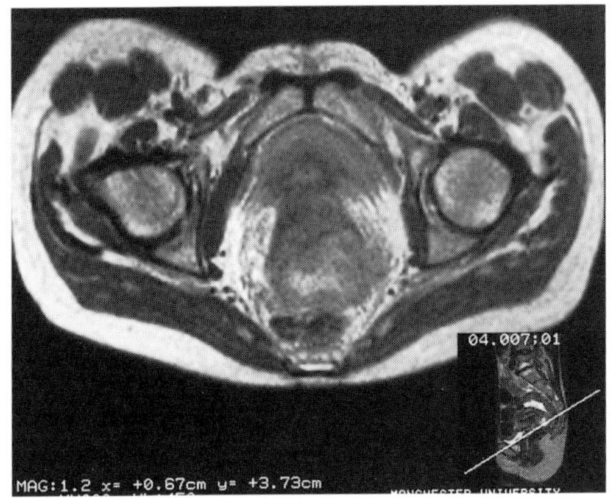


**Figure 7.8d** Oblique $T_2$ weighted image through the uterus and vagina. Note selection plane insert

**Table 7.1 Imaging parameters**

| *Imaging plane* | *Imaging sequence* | *TR* | *TE* | *Field of view* (mm) | *No. of NEX* | *Slice width/ gap* (mm) | *Matrix (horizontal–vertical)* |
|---|---|---|---|---|---|---|---|
| Coronal | Spin-echo $T_1$ weighted | 600 | 25 | 40 | 4 | 8/2 | 192 × 256 |
| Transaxial | Spin-echo $T_1$ weighted | 500 | 25 | 35–45 | 4 | 8/2 | 256 × 192 |
| Transaxial | Fast spin-echo $T_2$ weighted | 3500 | 100 | 35–45 | 3 | 5/2 | 256 × 192 |
| Sagittal | Fast spin-echo $T_2$ weighted | 3500 | 100 | 30 | 4 | 5/2 | 192 × 256 |
| Oblique | Fast spin-echo $T_2$ weighted | 3500 | 100 | 35–45 | 3 | 5/2 | 224 × 224 |

# 7 Female Reproductive System

## Obstetrics

### Ultrasound

Transabdominal two-dimensional real-time ultrasound incorporating a 3.5 or 5 MHz transducer is the imaging method used routinely to assess the pregnant abdomen. A large curvilinear array transducer is useful in the latter half of pregnancy. This gives a wedge-shaped image with a wider near field of view than a sector probe. Various measurements are made to assess fetal age and growth, including crown rump length, bi-parietal diameter, femur length, abdominal circumference and head circumference. In all instances the measurements are compared to standard gestational age by last menstrual period (LMP) and dating charts. Sequential measurements may be plotted to obtain the growth curve for any particular fetus.

Endovaginal ultrasound is also used in the first trimester to assess viability, exclude ectopic pregnancy or assessment of gynaecological related problems. In the second trimester this technique is used mainly to assess a low-lying fetus and in the third trimester to assess placenta praevia. This procedure is described on page 237.

Listed below are the indications for transabdominal ultrasound.

**Indications**

**1st trimester**

- Ectopic pregnancy.
- Viability of the fetus.
- Pregnancy dating.
- Multiple gestation.
- Related gynaecological problems.
- Location for chorionic villus sampling.

**2nd trimester**

- Fetal assessment.
- Placental site.
- Localisation for:
  - (a) amniocentesis
  - (b) fetal blood sampling
  - (c) placental biopsy.

**3rd trimester**

- Intrauterine growth retardation.
- Placenta praevia.
- Fetal well-being.
- Localisation for intrauterine transfusion.
- Certain fetal anomalies, e.g. some renal or intestinal anomalies.

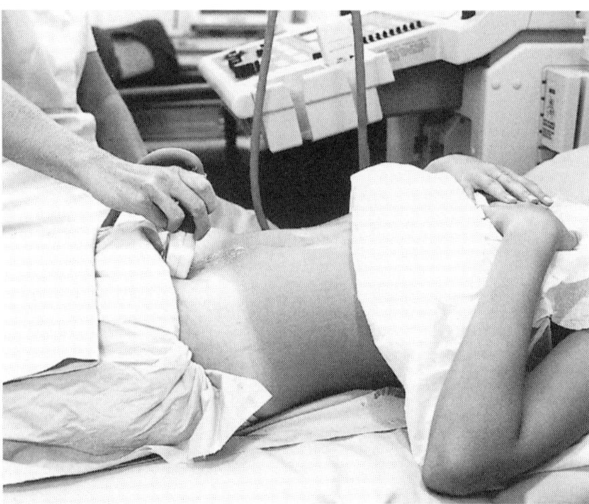

**Figure 7.9a** Transducer positioned for a transverse scan

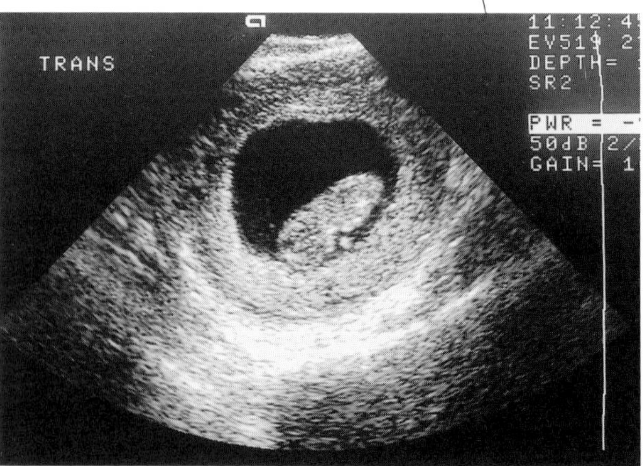


**Figure 7.9b** Transverse image of abdomen showing fetus in first trimester (8–9 weeks' gestation)

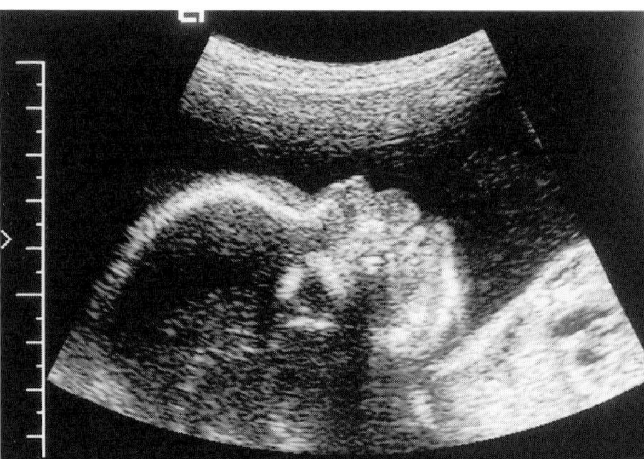

**Figure 7.9c** Parasagittal scan showing fetal profile in second trimester

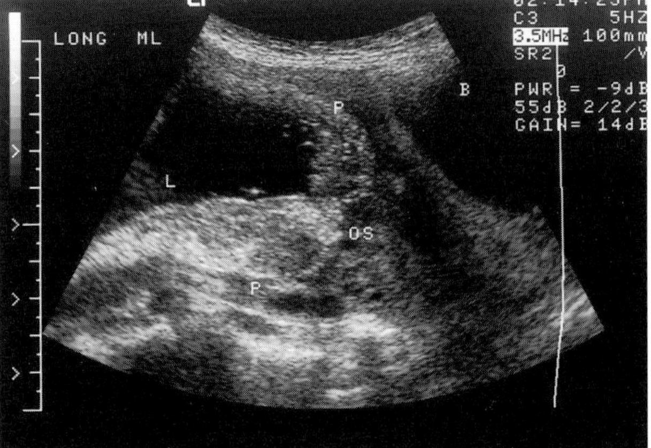


**Figure 7.9d** Midline sagittal image demonstrating placental position in third trimester (P, placenta; os, internal os; B, bladder; L, liquor)

## Transabdominal ultrasound

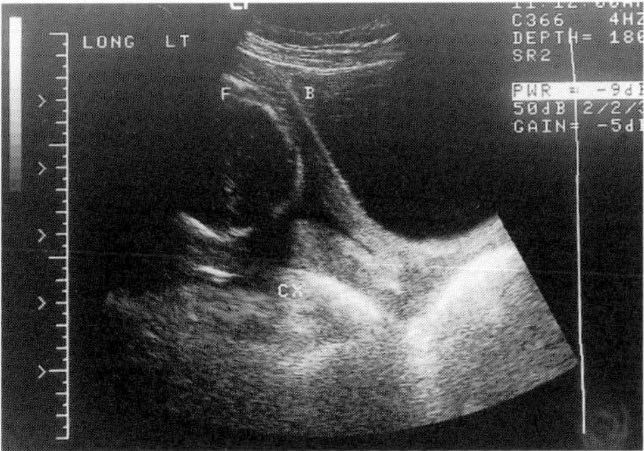


**Figure 7.10a** Long axis view of lower uterus, demonstrating the relationship between fetal parts and the internal os (B, bladder; F, fetus; cx, cervix)

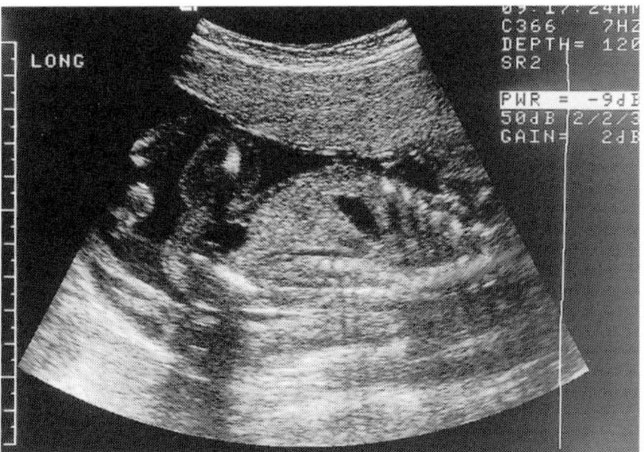


**Figure 7.10b** Long axis view of fetus demonstrating abdominal anatomy

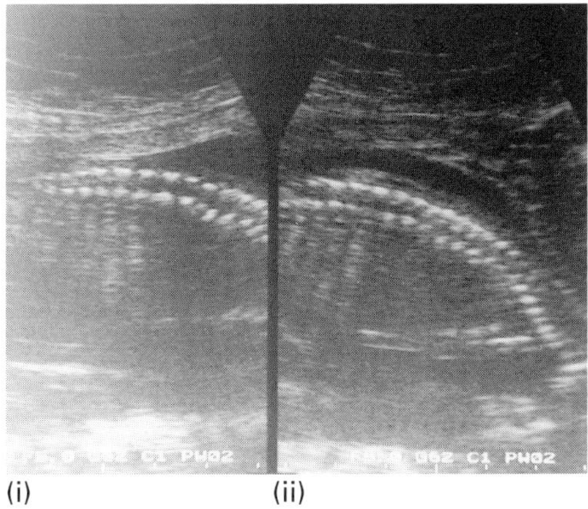

(i) (ii)

**Figure 7.10c** Long axis view of fetal spine showing: (i) sacrum, (ii) thoracic/lumbar spine

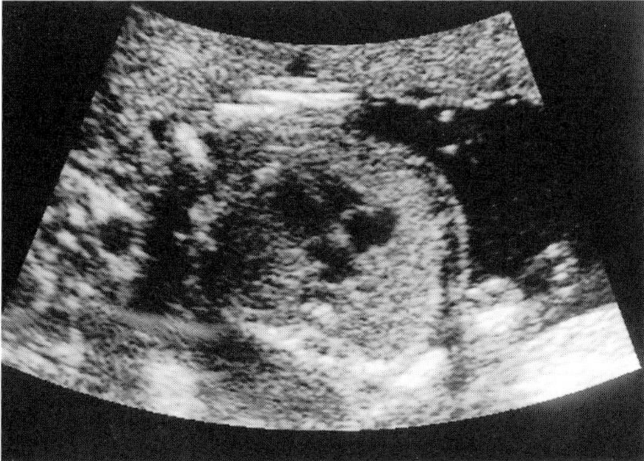

**Figure 7.10d** Transaxial view of fetal thorax showing normal cardiac anatomy (four-chamber view)

### Preparation of patient

For transabdominal ultrasound the patient must attend with a full bladder which provides an acoustic window to aid visualisation of pelvic structures and displaces bowel gas superiorly, preventing scattering of the ultrasound beam. An explanation of the procedure is given, the date of the patient's last menstrual period and any relevant medical history noted.

### Imaging procedure

The patient lies supine on the imaging table and ultrasound coupling gel applied to the lower abdomen. The long axis of the transducer is placed vertically above the symphysis pubis in the midline, producing a midline sagittal image (long axis view). From this position parasagittal scans are obtained by moving the transducer in a continuous scanning action to each side of the lower abdomen and pelvis.

The transducer is rotated through 90° and, starting immediately superior to the symphysis pubis, transverse images are obtained moving cranially towards the fundus of the uterus, again using a continuous scanning action.

Additional oblique projections are necessary to complete the examination.

### Image analysis

- Examination of the fetal head to exclude major spina bifida, anencephaly, ventriculomegaly, and sometimes to alert one to chromosomal problems, e.g. trisomy 18.
- Spinal examinations to exclude both spina bifida occulta and spina bifida aperta.
- Examination of the anterior abdominal wall to exclude omphalocele and gastroschisis.
- Examination of the limbs to exclude skeletal dysplasias.
- The four-chamber heart view to exclude major defects of ventricles and atria.
- Stomach visualisation to exclude oesophageal, duodenal and jejunal atresia.
- Visualisation of the bladder to exclude renal atresia.
- Visualisation of normal kidneys to exclude dysplastic kidneys and multicystic kidneys.
- Normal liquor to exclude polyhydramnios and oligohydramnios.

Polyhydramnios can indicate gestational diabetes, anterior wall defects and facial defects or heart defects. Oligohydramnios or reduced liquor can indicate renal problems, chromosal problems and intrauterine growth retardation (IUGR) in the third trimester.

# 7 Female Reproductive System (Obstetrics)

## Fetal measurement techniques

### Crown–rump length (CRL)

This is the longest demonstrable length of the fetus, from the crown to the rump, and is used to establish gestational age (GA) in the first trimester. There is a high correlation between fetal length and age, because it is a linear measurement. If done correctly it is the most accurate parameter for assessment of GA.

*Imaging procedure*
A long axis view of the fetus is obtained. Two calipers are placed on the freeze-frame image on the display screen, one on top of the head (crown) and one at the base of the spine (rump). The yoke sac and limbs must be excluded. Several images are obtained to ensure accuracy.

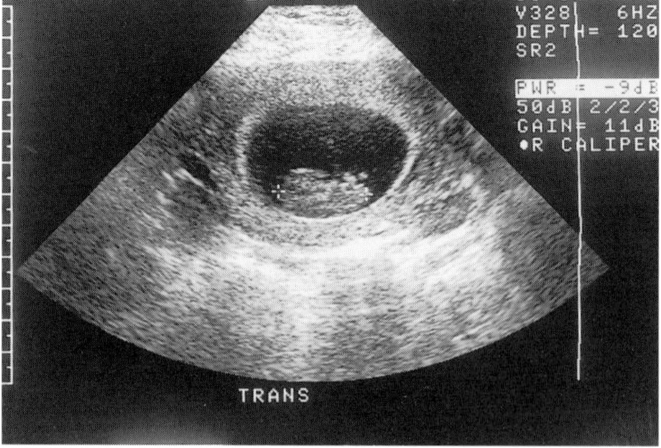


**Figure 7.11a** Transverse scan demonstrating first trimester fetus with crown–rump length 29.3 mm

### Bi-parietal diameter (BPD)

This is the greatest distance between the parietal bones and is measured in the transaxial plane at the level where the midline echo is broken by the cavum septum pellucidum. Measurements are taken from the outer to inner borders of the skull on the parietal eminences. This technique is a measurement of GA and is accurate to within ± 5 days prior to 20 weeks' gestation and to within ± 10 days between 20 and 28 weeks' gestation. Accuracy diminishes to within ± 2–4 weeks after the 24 th week of pregnancy.

*Imaging procedure*
A long axis view is obtained of the fetal cervical spine entering the base of the skull. The angle of the transducer to the maternal abdomen is noted (angle of asynclytism). A transaxial image of the fetal skull is obtained by rotating the transducer through 90° while maintaining the angle of asynclytism. Small adjustments of the transducer will produce the required image which should then be magnified and the measurements taken from this image.

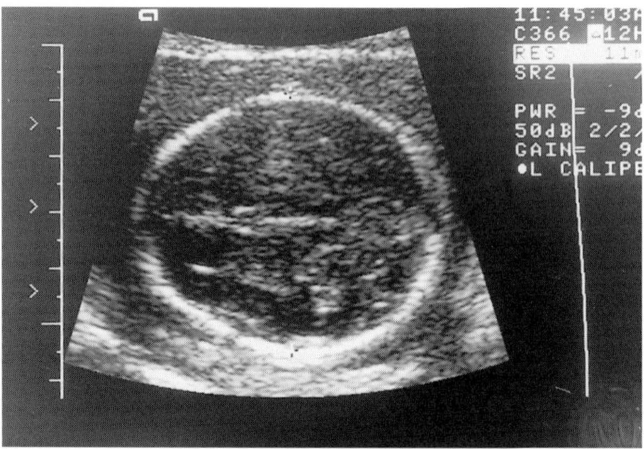


**Figure 7.11b** Image demonstrating position of calipers for bi-parietal diameter measurement in second trimester

### Femur length measurement (FLM)

This is used to confirm GA and can be measured from 14 to 15 weeks. Accuracy is similar to the bi-parietal diameter. It is also used to diagnose microcephaly if an accurate LMP is available.

*Imaging procedure*
A transaxial image is obtained of the fetal pelvis, identifying the bladder and iliac bones. The transducer is rotated until the long axis of the femur is parallel to the ultrasound beam. Acoustic shadowing must be apparent posterior to the femur to ensure a true longitudinal section. Measurements are taken of the femoral shaft. The neck of the femur and condyles are not included.

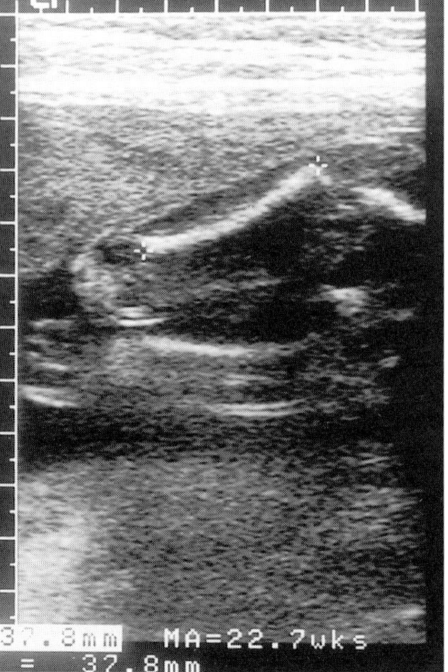


**Figure 7.11c** Image demonstrating femur length measurement of 37.8 mm

## Fetal measurement techniques

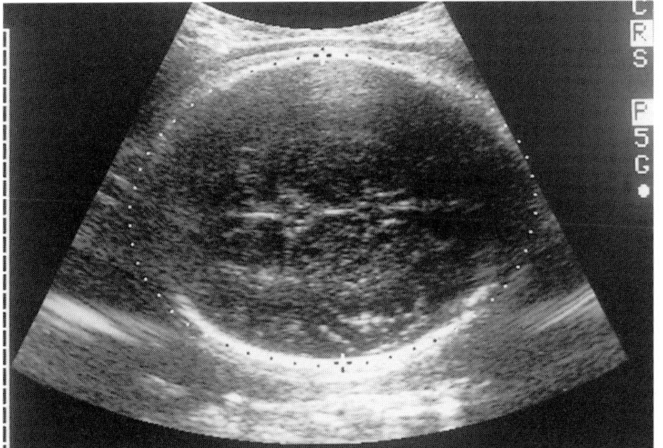

**Figure 7.12a** Image demonstrating caliper positioning for head circumference measurement in third trimester

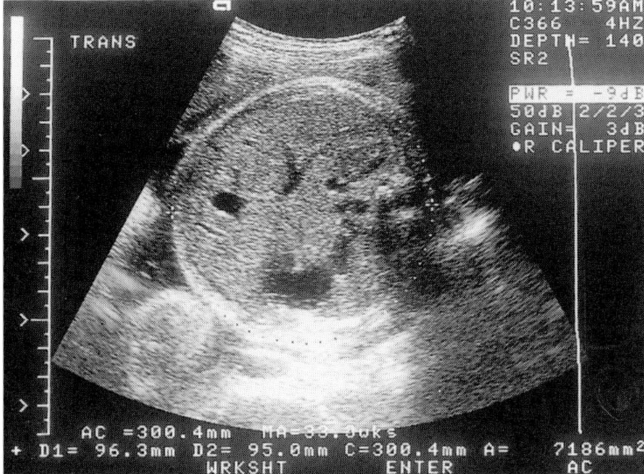


**Figure 7.12b** Transverse scan demonstrating position of calipers for abdominal circumference measurement

### Head circumference (HC)

This measurement is obtained from an identical image produced for the BPD. This measurement is more accurate than the BPD in later pregnancy as it is not affected by fetal position. When compared to the abdominal circumference measurement, it is used to assess symmetrical versus asymmetrical growth retardation.

*Imaging procedure*

From the freeze-frame image obtained the electronic calipers are adjusted and both are placed on the outer table of the fetal skull. The head circumference measurement is calculated by either using the automatic computer facility if available or by using the formula:

Occipitofrontal diameter + Bi-parietal diameter
× 1.62 (OFD + BPD × 1.62).

### Abdominal circumference (AC)

This is recorded to detect intrauterine growth, macrosomia and large fetus, and to confirm suspected microcephaly when compared with the head circumference measurement. Fetal weight can be estimated and fetal growth monitored. The measurement is usually taken in the third trimester, but in cases of suspected fetal anomaly or early growth retardation may be used as early as 24 weeks' gestation.

*Imaging procedure*

A long axis view is obtained of the fetal body to include aorta, stomach and bladder. The transducer is rotated through 90° to obtain a transaxial view and a measurement taken at the level of the bifurcation of the portal vein of the fetus. From this freeze-frame image, electronic calipers are placed on the skin line posterior to the lumbar vertebrae and the anterior abdominal wall. The abdominal circumference measurement is calculated by either using the automatic computer facility if available or the formula:

Transverse diameter + Anteroposterior diameter
× 1.57 (TD + AP × 1.57).

The AP diameter is measured from the tip of the spinous process of the lumbar vertebra to the skinline of the anterior abdominal wall and the TD is measured along a line perpendicular to the AP diameter.

### Head circumference/abdominal circumference ratio

The HC/AC ratio is used to distinguish between the different causes of abnormal fetal growth, e.g. to distinguish between macrosomia due to 'normal large baby' and macrosomia due to maternal diabetes mellitus (also called gestational diabetes). It also distinguishes between a normal small baby and IUGR due to placental insufficiency. The degree of disproportionality is evaluated by determining the HC/AC ratio.

# 7 Transabdominal Ultrasound (Obstetrics)

## Charts for dating

As discussed previously, estimation of gestational age is determined by reference to CRL, BPD and FLM charts. Fetal growth assessment is estimated by reference to AC, HC and the HC/AC ratio charts. Search of the literature reveals a variety of charts and those illustrated are typical of the ones available. The chart opposite illustrates the upper (95th centile) and lower limits (5th centile) of normality as well as the median (50th centile). The charts on the opposite page show the 3rd, 10th, 50th, 90th and 97th percentiles and relate to the exact length of gestation.

For each chart there is also a corresponding set of table values.

When assessing GA, e.g. in the CRL graph opposite, the measurement values (in millimetres) are located on the horizontal axis of the graph with the GA (in weeks) located on the vertical axis.

To estimate fetal age from a recorded measurement a vertical line is drawn up from that value on the horizontal axis to where it intersects the bold median curve (50th centile). From this point a horizontal line is drawn to where it intersects the vertical axis.

When assessing fetal growth, using the HC and AC graphs opposite, the GA is found on the horizontal axis, with the predicted growth measurement on the vertical axis.

In assessing growth it is normal to plot by LMP if the first scan and the LMP agree within 7 days. If not, growth is plotted by using the estimated GA as a baseline.

HC and AC may be measured serially every 4 weeks after 24 weeks' gestation, or every 2 weeks if growth deviates from expected lines.

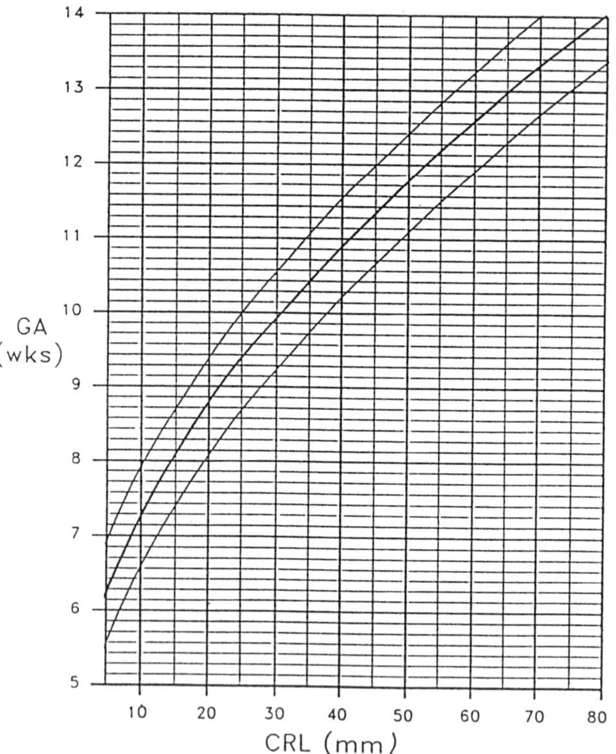


**Figure 7.13** Graph of gestational age vs. crown–rump length (After Robinson and Fleming, 1990)

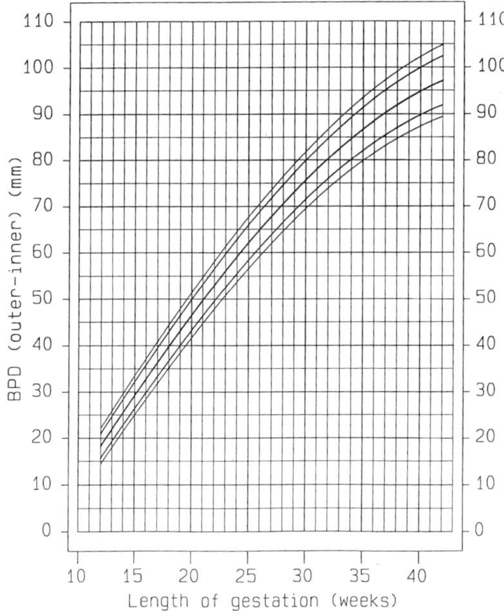


**Figure 7.14a** Biparietal diameter (outer–inner) – 3rd, 10th, 50th, 90th and 97th centiles (© Chitty and Altman, 1994; published in modified form with permission from the *British Journal of Obstetrics and Gynaecology*, **101**, 35–43)

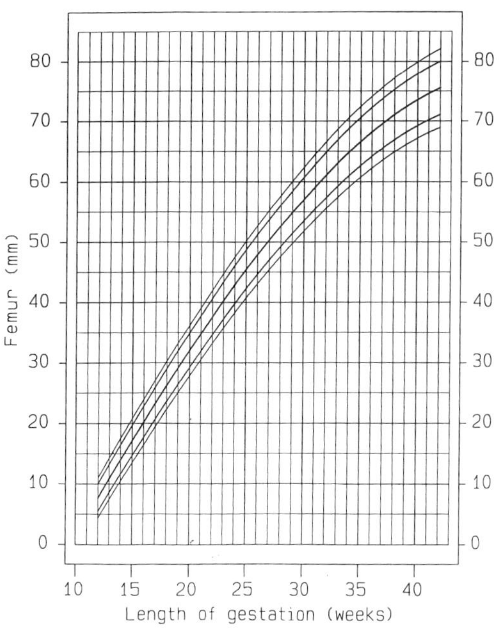


**Figure 7.14c** Femur – 3rd, 10th, 50th, 90th and 97th centiles (© Chitty and Altman, 1994; published in modified form with permission from the *British Journal of Obstetrics and Gynaecology*, **101**, 132–135)

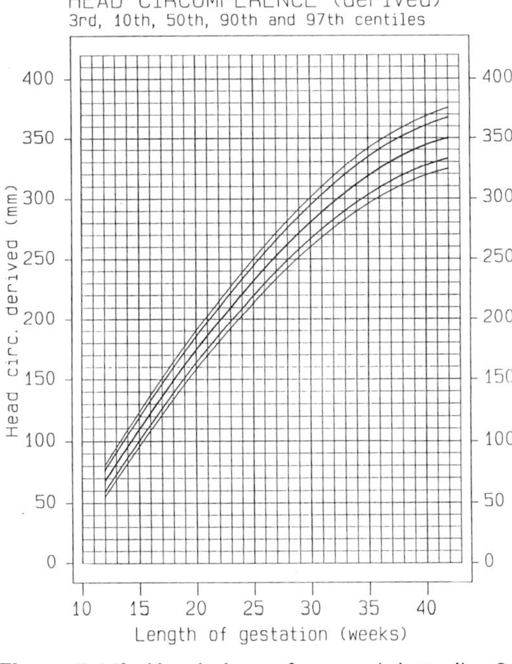


**Figure 7.14b** Head circumference (plotted) – 3rd, 10th, 50th, 90th and 97th centiles (© Chitty and Altman, 1994; published in modified form with permission from the *British Journal of Obstetrics and Gynaecology*, **101**, 35–43)

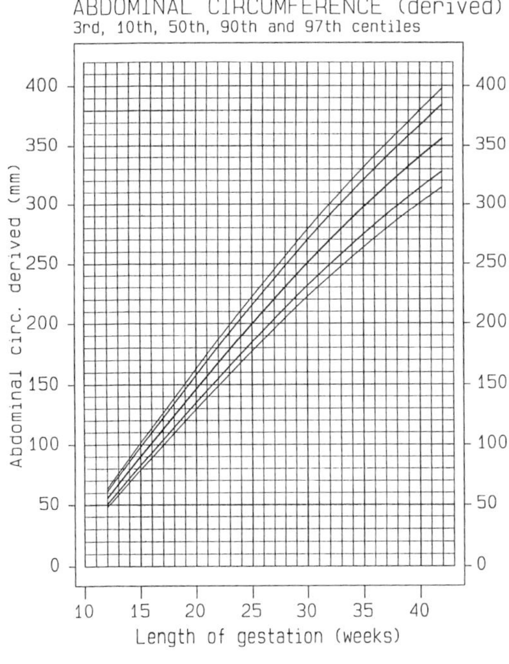


**Figure 7.14d** Abdominal circumference (plotted) – 3rd, 10th, 50th, 90th and 97th centiles (© Chitty and Altman, 1994; published in modified form with permission from the *British Journal of Obstetrics and Gynaecology*, **101**, 125–131)

# 7 Female Reproductive System (Obstetrics)

## Conventional Radiography

Conventional radiography is very rarely indicated and is only undertaken in the late stages of pregnancy, usually if the ultrasound examination proves inconclusive. The preferred technique to demonstrate the fetus more clearly is the postero-anterior oblique projection or alternatively the anteroposterior oblique projection. If clinically warranted further postero-anterior and anteroposterior projections may be necessary. All radiographs are taken on suspended respiration. In all cases compression is gradually applied to limit movement of the fetus and mother and to reduce the depth of tissue through which the radiation has to penetrate. This effectively reduces radiation dose and scattered radiation, thus maximising image definition. Further reductions in radiation dose are achieved by using a carbon fibre table top and a carbon fibre fronted cassette, also employing a fast film intensifying screen combination.

### Indications

To assess fetal abnormality and GA only if ultrasound proves inconclusive.

### Postero-anterior oblique projection

The postero-anterior oblique projection is used in preference to the anteroposterior oblique projection as the patient is more able to adopt this position and remain still during the procedure. The patient's abdomen is naturally compressed, with the benefit that scattered radiation is reduced to both the fetus and mother.

Either the right or left anterior oblique position is selected, depending on the lie of the fetal spine and limbs which should be demonstrated away from the maternal spine. The position of the fetal spine is determined by palpation or ultrasound.

**Position of patient and imaging modality**

The patient lies initially in the lateral position on the selected side. From this position the patient is gently rotated forwards until the median sagittal plane is approximately 45° to the table top.

The arm on the raised side is flexed so that the hand rests near the head, while the opposite arm lies alongside and behind the trunk.

Positioning aids are used for support. A 35 × 43 cm cassette is placed longitudinally in the Bucky tray and positioned to include the symphysis pubis on the lower border of the film.

A compression band is gently applied.

**Direction and centring of the X-ray beam**

The vertical central ray is directed to the raised side at the estimated midpoint of the fetal spine, ensuring that the whole fetus is included on the radiograph as well as the maternal abdominal wall to include the placental site.

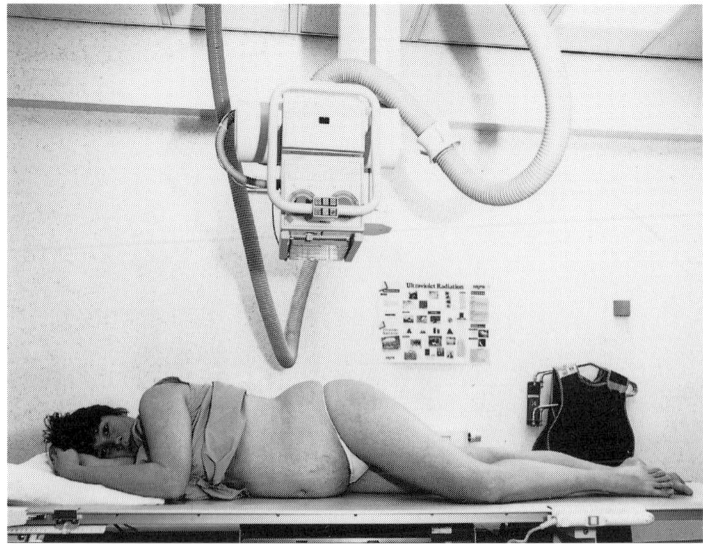

**Figure 7.15a** Conventional radiography in obstetrics – position of patient for PA oblique projection

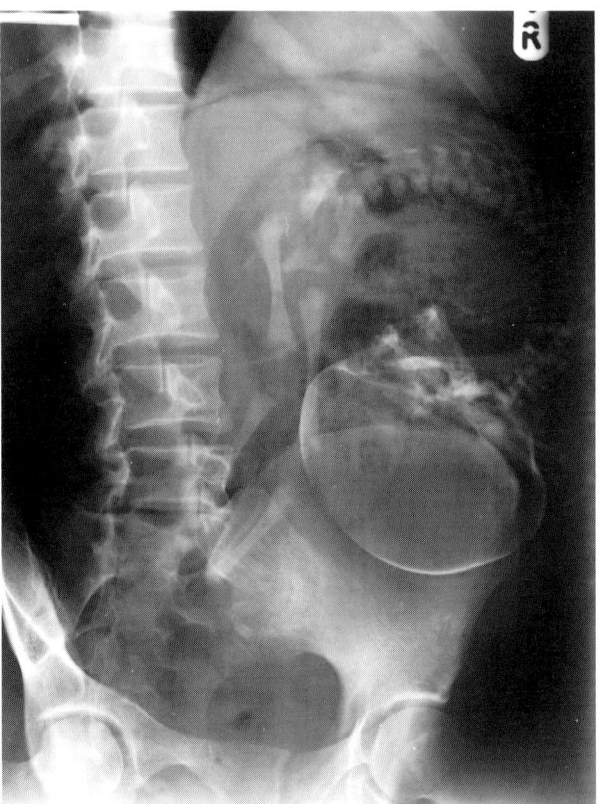


**Figure 7.15b** PAO radiograph of abdomen

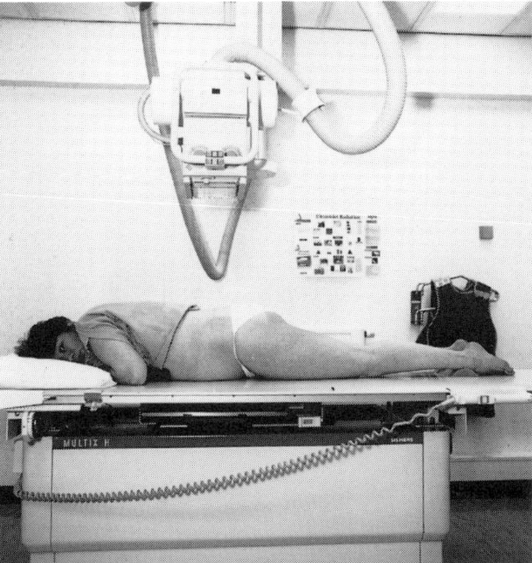

Figure 7.16a Patient in PA position

## Postero-anterior projection

**Position of the patient and imaging modality**

The patient lies prone on the imaging table, with the pelvis and thorax supported by radiolucent pads. The head is turned to one side and the arms raised and placed on the pillow. A sandbag is placed under the ankles for support. The patient's position is adjusted until the median sagittal plane is central and perpendicular to the imaging table. Gentle compression is applied.

A 35 × 43 cm cassette is placed longitudinally in the Bucky tray and positioned to include the symphysis pubis on the lower border of the film.

**Direction and centring of the X-ray beam**

The vertical central ray is directed towards the midline at the level of the fourth/fifth lumbar vertebrae.

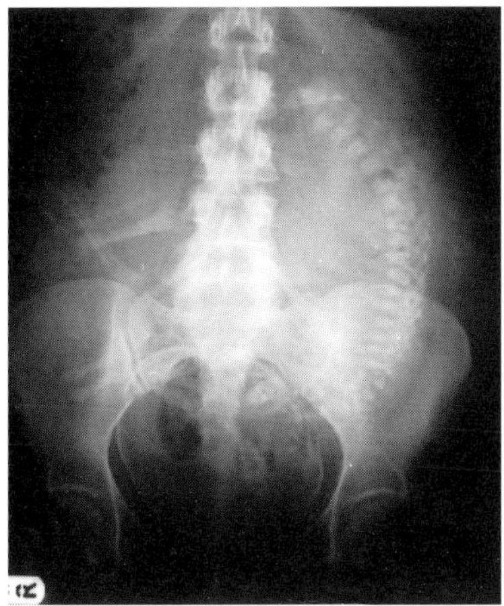

Figure 7.16b PA projection – vertex presentation

## Anteroposterior oblique projection

**Position of the patient and imaging modality**

The patient lies supine on the imaging table, hands resting on the chest, and a small pad is placed under the knees for comfort. The patient's position is adjusted until the median sagittal plane is central and perpendicular to the imaging table top. Compression is gently applied.

A 35 × 43 cm cassette is placed longitudinally in the Bucky tray and positioned to include the symphysis pubis on the lower border of the film.

**Direction and centring of the X-ray beam**

The vertical central ray is directed towards the midline at the level of the iliac crests.

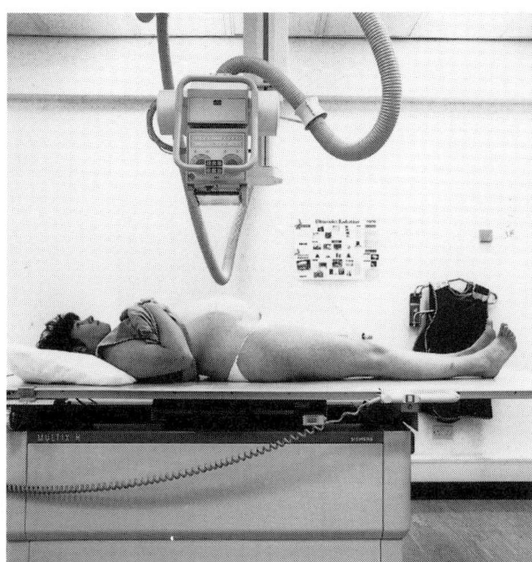

Figure 7.16c Patient in AP position

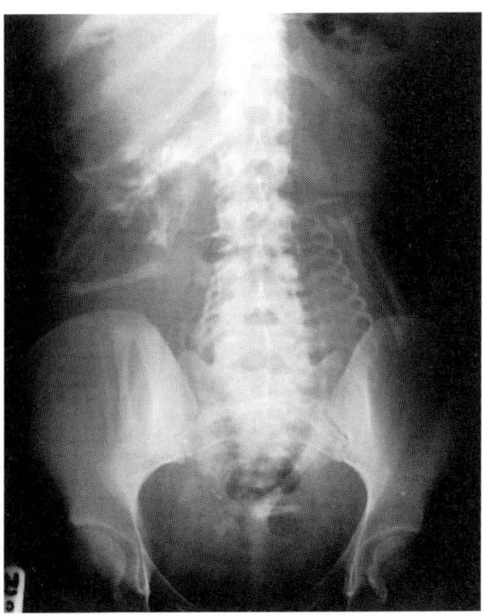

Figure 7.16d AP projection – breech position

# 7 Female Reproductive System (Obstetrics)

## Pelvimetry

### Internal diameters

Pelvimetry is the technique used to assess the internal diameters of the female pelvis. There are three imaging methods: conventional radiography, CT and MRI. The method of choice depends largely on the availability of equipment and local protocols.

As in all radiographic procedures, radiation dose must be kept to a minimum consistent with the diagnostic information required. Therefore the conventional radiographic method described is based on a low radiation dose technique devised in the Radiology Department, St. Mary's Hospital, Manchester, UK. More detailed information can be obtained by contacting the department directly.

The use of other conventional radiography techniques using higher radiation doses contributes greatly to the fetal dose and should be avoided.

For X-ray generated techniques, departments should evaluate patient and fetal doses for each modality and technique before establishing a standard imaging protocol.

From all three imaging methods, estimation can be made of:

- the *transverse inlet diameter* – the distance extending from side to side at the widest points of the pelvic brim
- the *bi-spinous diameter (interspinous)* – the distance extending between the ischial spines
- the *anteroposterior* inlet – the distance between the upper inner border of the symphysis pubis to the sacral promontory
- the *mid-plane*, anteroposterior, extending from the middle of the inner border of the symphysis pubis to the middle of the third sacral segment
- the *anteroposterior outlet* – the distance between the lower inner border of the symphysis pubis to the tip of the sacrum or, in the case of sacrococcygeal fusion, to the lower inner border of the first coccygeal segment
- the *oblique diameters*, if required, extending from the iliopubic eminence on the one side to the brim at the sacroiliac articulation on the other side.

### Indications

Cephalopelvic disproportion, breech presentation, previous caesarian section, small stature, pelvic injury and non-engagement of the fetal head in primigravida.

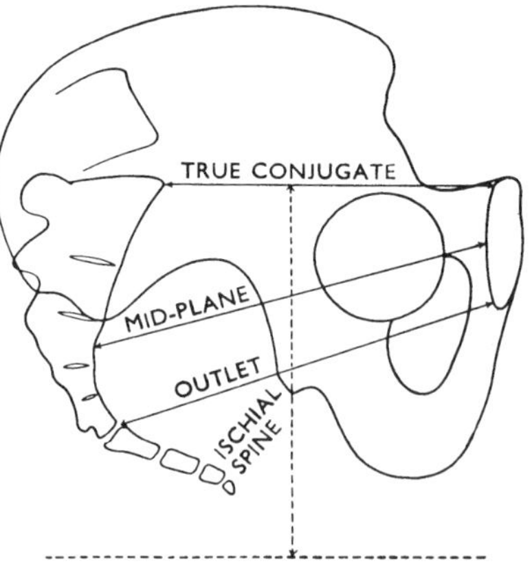


**Figure 7.17a** Diagram of lateral pelvis showing AP inlet, mid-plane and AP outlet dimensions

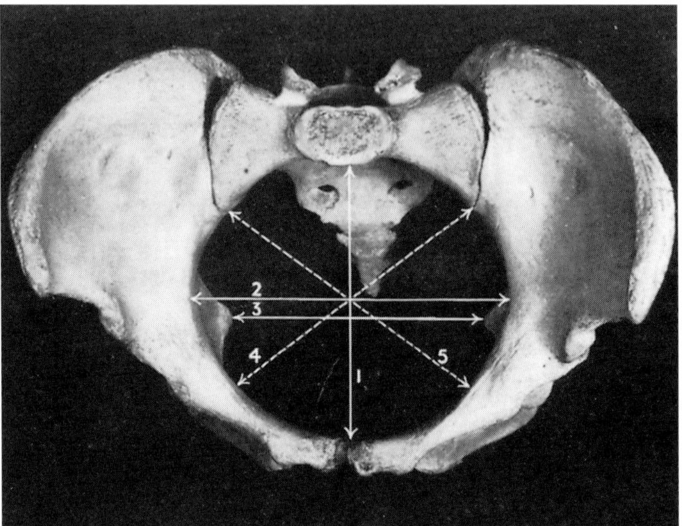


**Figure 7.17b** Photograph of pelvis demonstrating: 1, anteroposterior inlet; 2, transverse inlet diameter; 3, bi-spinous diameter; 4,5, oblique diameters

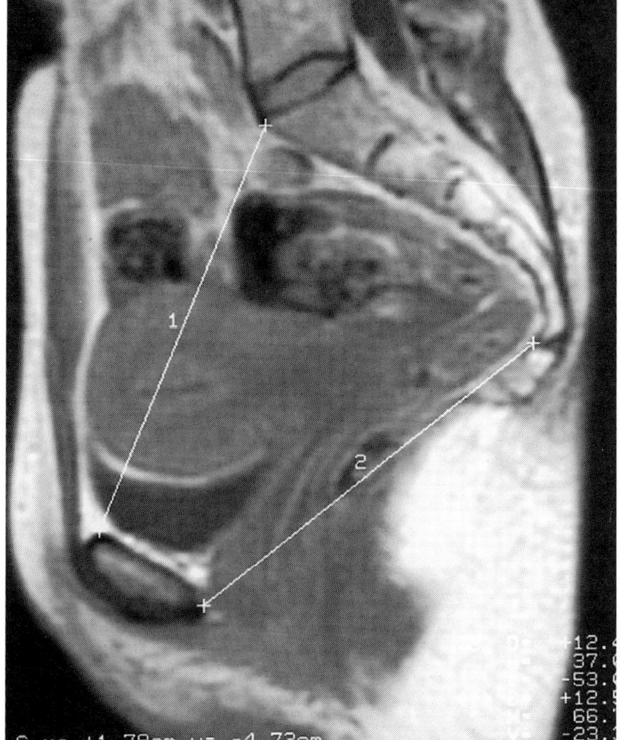


**Figure 7.18a** Spin-echo midline sagittal image showing (i) AP inlet measurement, and (ii) AP outlet measurement

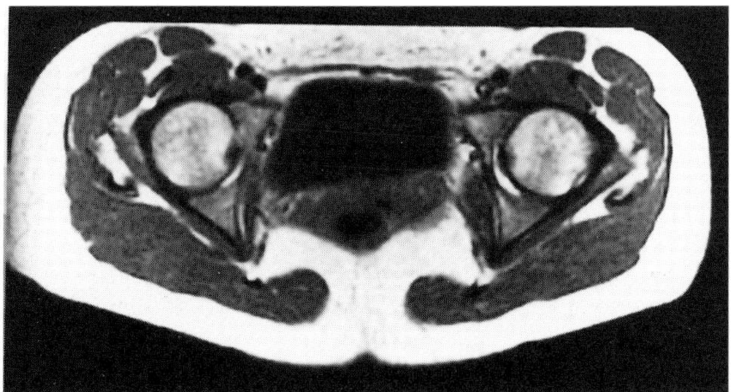

**Figure 7.18b** Transaxial spin-echo image at the level of the fovea

# Female Reproductive System (Obstetrics) 7

## Magnetic resonance pelvimetry

At the time of writing, MRI has a restricted role in obstetrics, only being used when ultrasound proves inconclusive and in preference to techniques involving the use of ionising radiation.

Magnetic resonance pelvimetry, however, is fast becoming a recognised technique to obtain traditional pelvis measurements.

### Position of patient and imaging modality

The patient lies supine, feet first on the scanner table, with the median sagittal plane perpendicular to the centre of the table.

Using the scanner alignment lights, the patient is moved until the sagittal alignment light is coincident with the median sagittal plane and the transverse alignment light is at the level of the anterior superior iliac spines. From this position the patient is moved the fixed distance to the iscocentre of the magnet which is also the centre of the radiofrequency transmitter/receiver body coil.

### Imaging procedure

A spin-echo midline sagittal scan is performed to include the lower abdomen and pelvis, to provide measurements of the available AP inlet and available AP outlet dimensions.

A spin-echo transaxial scan is obtained at the level of the fovea to obtain measurements of the transverse inlet and bi-spinous dimensions.

### Image analysis

By using the MR computer software facilities, direct measurement of selected distances can be made from the image on the image monitor. With this method, provided that the system is calibrated, there will be no magnification or diminution of the distances recorded.

Measurements should be taken twice and an average value used.

**Table 7.2 Imaging parameters**

| *Imaging plane* | *Imaging sequence* | *TR* | *TE* | *Field of view (cm)* | *No. of NEX* | *Slice width/gap (mm)* | *Matrix (horizontal–vertical)* |
|---|---|---|---|---|---|---|---|
| Sagittal | Spin-echo | 100 | 20 | 30 | 2 | 10 | 160 × 224 |
| Transaxial | Spin-echo | 100 | 20 | 35–40 | 2 | 10 | 224 × 160 |

# 7 Female Reproductive System (Obstetrics)

## Computed tomographic pelvimetry

Pelvimetry measurements can be obtained using the scan projection radiography facility available on CT systems, thus enabling scans to be obtained in the median sagittal and coronal planes. By optimising scanning technique factors and patient positioning, magnification errors can be eliminated and patient and fetal radiation dose minimised.

With some CT scanners, only postero-anterior scan projection radiographs are available, resulting in an additional transaxial section in some instances. In those patients who are restricted to being examined supine, the ischial spines are projected over the femoral heads and acetabulae, thus preventing a bi-spinous measurement from being made. To obtain this measurement, a transaxial section must be acquired at the level of the fovea.

To minimise operator error, it is recommended that a dedicated radiographic team perform and analyse this examination. The measurements should be taken twice and an average value used.

From the lateral scan projection radiograph, all measurements taken in line with the table movements are accurate irrespective of the table height.

In the anteroposterior or postero-anterior scan projection radiograph, the anatomical landmarks between which the measurements are made lie at 90° to the table movement.

To maintain accuracy these structures must be positioned at the centre of the gantry. In the supine position the transverse plane of the pelvic inlet lies at a level two-thirds of the distance between the anterior margin of the symphysis pubis and the table top. The ischial spines are located at one-third of this distance.

### Position of patient and imaging modality

The patient lies supine, head first on the scanner table, with the medial sagittal plane perpendicular to the scanner table and coincident with the central long axis of the table. The anterosuperior iliac spines should be equidistant from the table top. The arms are raised and placed behind the patient's head, out of the scan plane.

Positioning is aided by transaxial, coronal and sagittal alignment lights. The sagittal alignment light should coincide with the median sagittal plane and the scanner height is adjusted to ensure that the coronal plane alignment is at the level of the mid-axillary line. The patient is then moved into the scanner so that the scan reference point is at the level of the iliac crests.

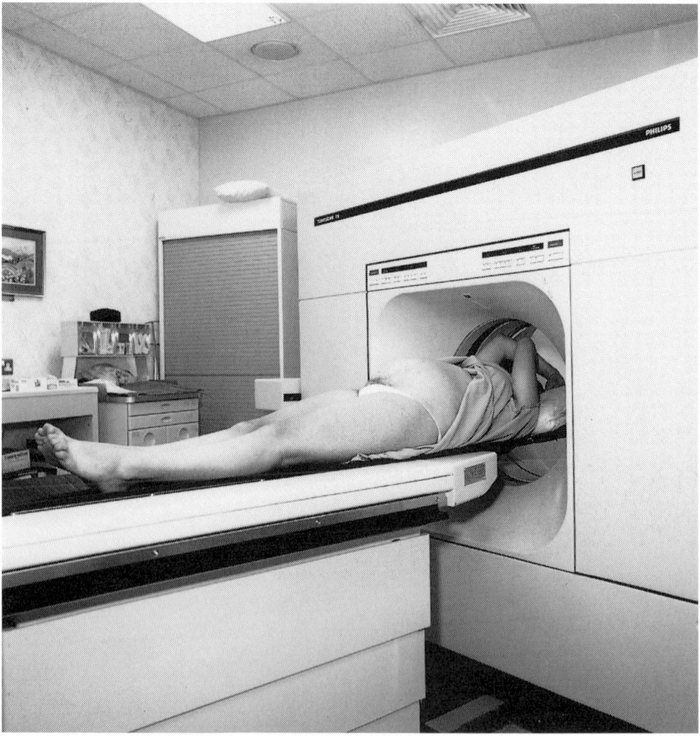

**Figure 7.19a** Patient on scanner table

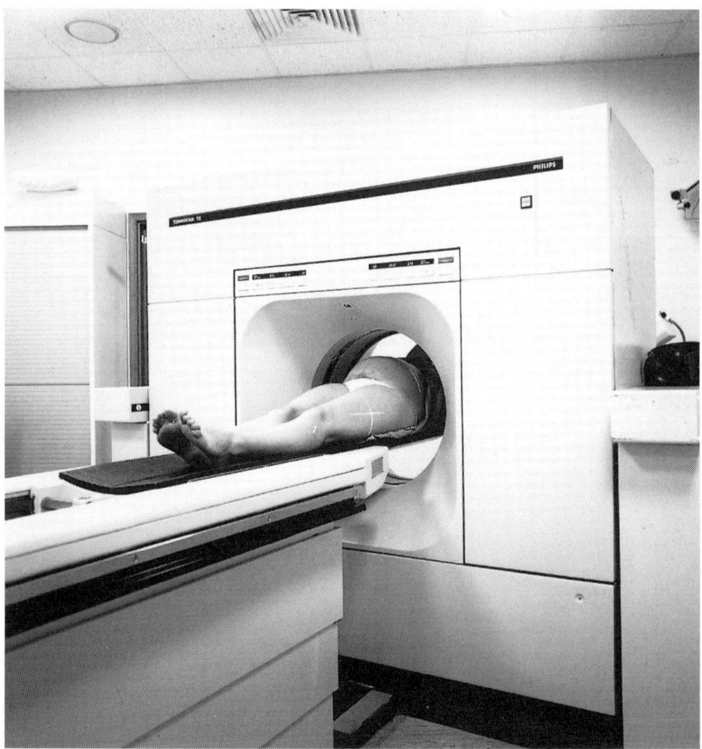

**Figure 7.19b** Patient in final position – table height adjustments made for AP/PA scan projection radiograph

## Computed tomographic pelvimetry

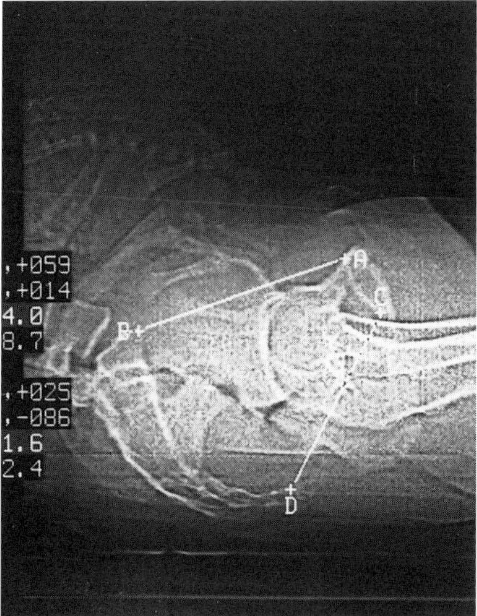


**Figure 7.20a** Lateral scan projection radiograph with markers and measurements

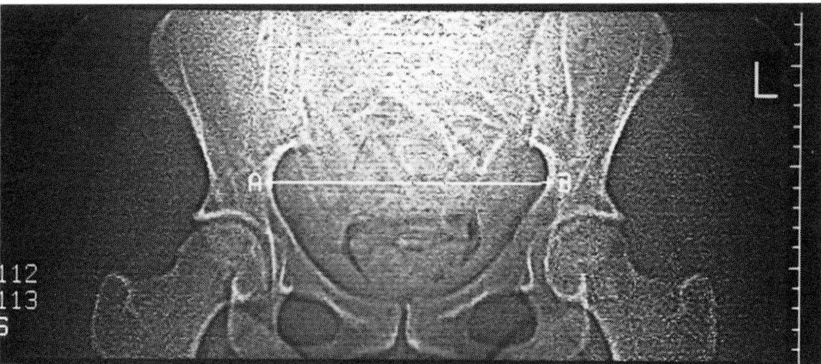


**Figure 7.20b** AP scan projection radiograph showing transverse diameter measurement

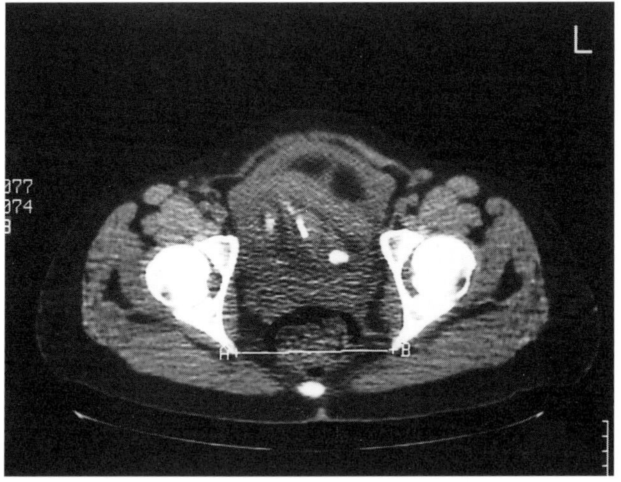


**Figure 7.20c** Transaxial image showing bi-spinous diameter

### Imaging procedure

*Lateral scan projection*

A lateral scan projection radiograph is taken, starting 3 cm above and ending 28 cm below the reference point, to include the lower border of the symphysis pubis.

During this procedure the patient is asked to remain still.

*Anteroposterior or postero-anterior scan projection*

From the lateral scan projection image the distance between the anterior margin of the symphysis pubis and the table top is measured to calculate the table height adjustments necessary to bring the pelvic inlet in the centre of the gantry.

A single scan projection radiograph is then taken, starting 3 cm above and ending 28 cm below the reference point, to include the relevant bony anatomy.

*Transaxial scan*

If necessary a single transaxial scan (section width 5 mm) is prescribed from a postero-anterior scan projection image at the level of the fovea to give the bi-spinous diameter.

To minimise radiation dose for the AP/PA scan projections and the transaxial scans the milliampere seconds (mAs) is reduced as much as possible. The resultant images will be degraded by 'noise', but the relevant bony landmarks will be visible and the appropriate measurements can be made.

### Image analysis

Using the distance cursor facility, the following measurements are made electronically:

(a) Lateral scan projection radiograph
- available anteroposterior inlet
- available anteroposterior outlet

(b) Anteroposterior scan projection radiograph
- transverse inlet
- bi-spinous diameter (assuming that any magnification is minimal)

(c) Postero-anterior scan projection radiograph
- transverse inlet

(d) Transaxial image
- bi-spinous diameter

# 7 Female Reproductive System (Obstetrics)

## Radiography method

**Recommended projections**

Routinely, an erect lateral projection, using an air-gap technique to reduce scatter without the dose penalty incurred by using a grid, and an orthodiagraphic projection are taken.

For the lateral projection the degree of magnification in the sagittal plane is constant for each examination as the anode to midline of the patient and the midline of patient to film distances are fixed. For the orthodiagraphic projection the degree of magnification or diminution is small.

Magnification correction scales are produced for both projections to correct for magnification of the anatomical structures.

### Erect lateral projection

Two measurements are recorded from this projection:

- the available anteroposterior inlet measurement
- the available anteroposterior outlet measurement and, if required, the mid-plane dimension

*Position of patient and imaging modality*

A metal positioning device with two horizontal markers is attached to the vertical cassette holder/chest stand. One marker is set at a fixed distance of 46 cm from the imaging cassette and is used to ensure that the midline structures, i.e. the maternal sacrum and symphysis pubis, are at a set distance. By maintaining the same object film distance (46 cm) a constant magnification factor is achieved for each patient irrespective of size. The second adjustable marker is used as a patient support and is positioned at the iliac crest.

The patient stands initially in the lateral position, with the spine parallel to the vertical imaging cassette (24 × 30 cm), the height of which is adjusted until the symphysis is at the level of the lower third of the cassette. The patient now stands aside and the horizontal central ray is directed to the centre of the imaging cassette, using a 230 cm focal film distance.

The X-ray beam is closely collimated to just within the dimensions of the cassette. A lead cut-out shield is then positioned between the X-ray tube and the imaging cassette to protect the fetus from primary radiation, allowing only the maternal sacrum and symphysis to be radiographed. The patient is now repositioned laterally with the vertebral column at the level of the horizontal marker (46 cm) from the imaging cassette, thus introducing the air gap. The patient stands with feet separated to preserve balance and arms folded across the chest. On viewing the patient from side, front and back, careful adjustment is made to avoid any tilting or rotation of the pelvis.

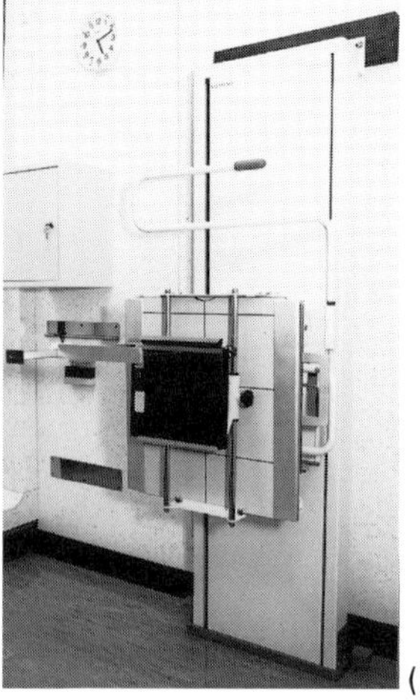
(i)

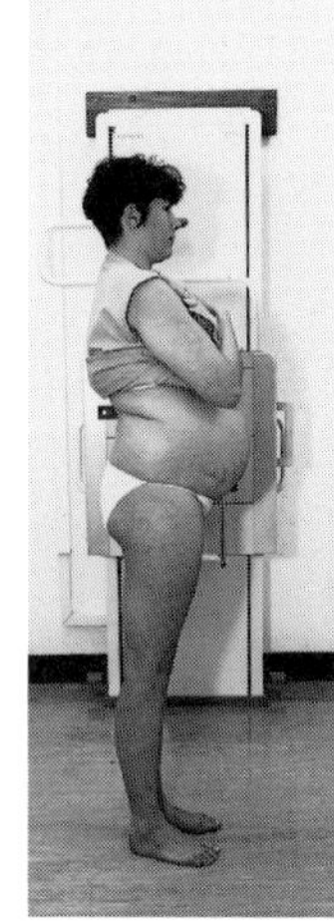
(ii)

**Figure 7.21a** Cassette/attachment and position of patient relevant to cassette

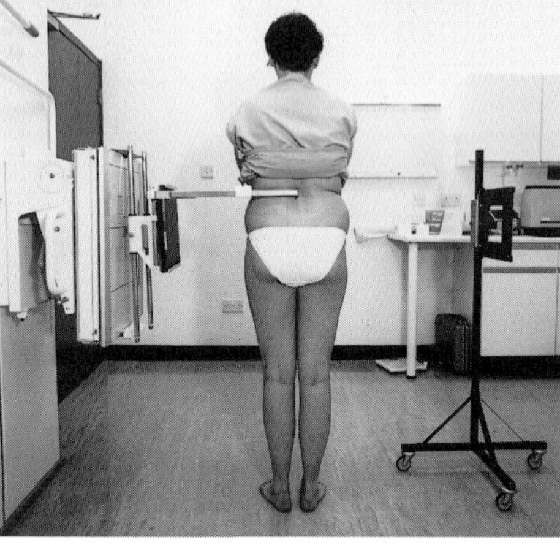

**Figure 7.21b** Patient in lateral position with vertebral column coincident at the level of the horizontal marker

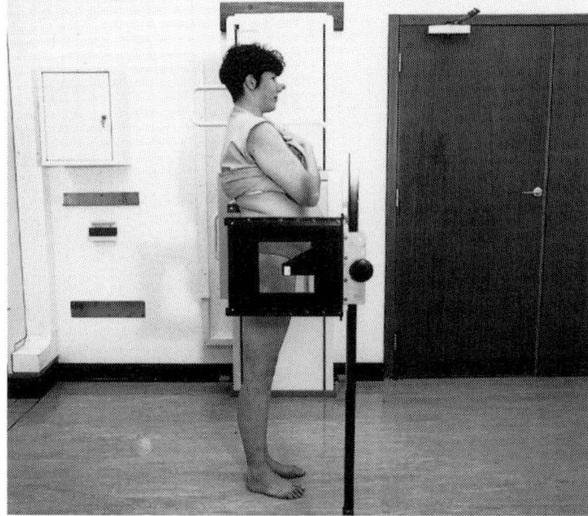

**Figure 7.21c** Lead cut-out shield in position

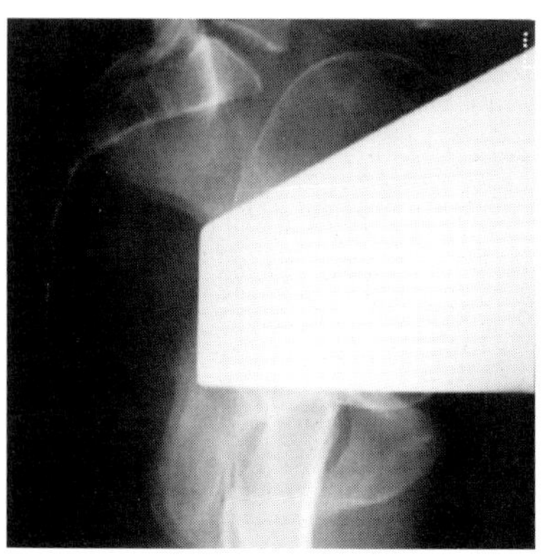

**Figure 7.21d** Lateral projection image

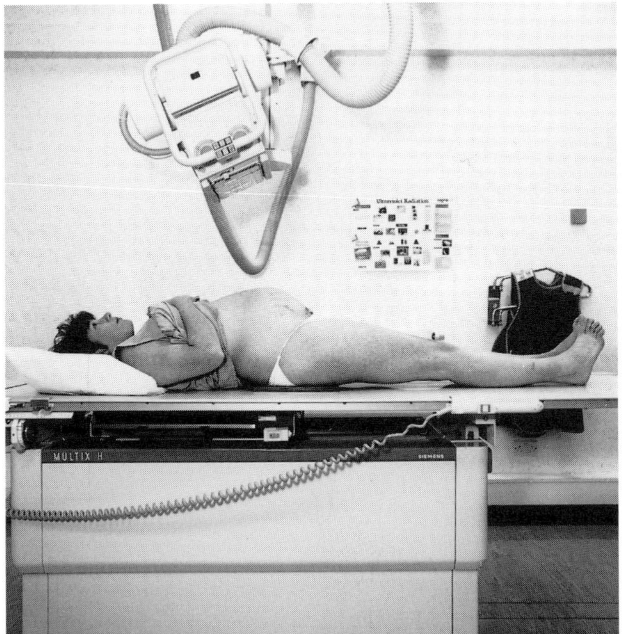


**Figure 7.22a** Patient positioned for orthodiagraphic projection

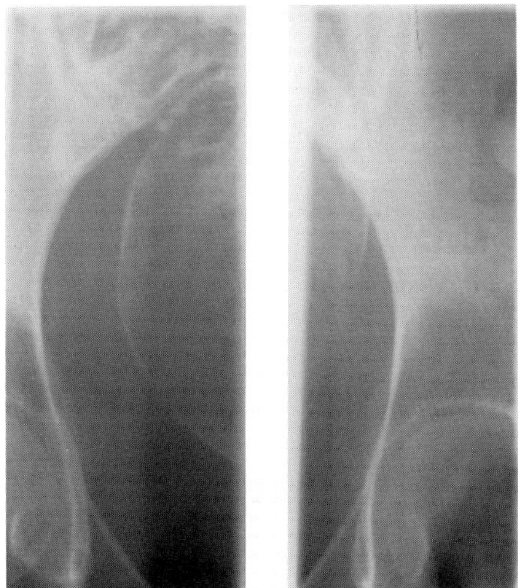

**Figure 7.22b** Orthodiagraphic projection

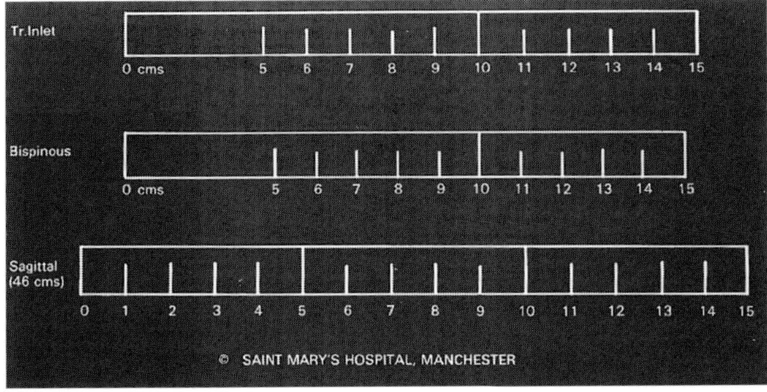


**Figure 7.22c** Magnification correction scales

## Orthodiagraphic projection

Two measurements are recorded from this projection:

- the transverse inlet measurement
- the bi-spinous measurement.

*Position of patient and imaging modality*
The patient lies supine on the imaging table, arms at the side and pelvis resting directly on the imaging cassette (24 × 30 cm), with the symphysis pubis 5 cm above the lower border of the cassette. Positional adjustments are made to bring the medium sagittal plane perpendicular to the centre of the cassette while ensuring the anterior iliac spines remain equidistant from the table top.

*Direction and centring of the X-ray beam*
The vertical central ray is angled 20° caudally and directed towards the midline 2.5 cm below the anterior superior iliac spines, with a focal film distance of 100 cm. Two separate exposures are made, each 5 cm lateral to the midline, with collimation set at 9 cm longitudinally by 3 cm transversely.

*Image analysis*
Measurements are made on the resultant radiographs using calipers or geometric dividers. This reading is then transferred to the appropriate magnification correction scale or alternatively the relevant scale is placed directly over an image for direct measurement.

### Magnification correction scales

A geometric correction scale is prepared for each projection type by radiographing a metallic ruler with notched markers at 1 cm intervals.

*(a) Transverse inlet correction scale*
The ruler is positioned 12 cm above, the assumed height of the pelvic inlet, and parallel to the cassette. With the focal film distance set at 100 cm, the X-ray beam is centred over the 0 point on the ruler and the beam is collimated to include only the 1 cm notch and exposure is made. The X-ray tube is then centred over the 10 cm notch and the beam collimated to include from 5 to 15 cm only. The previous exposed area is protected with lead rubber and another exposure made. The film is then developed.

*(b) Bi-spinous correction scale*
For the bi-spinous scale the film is exposed as previously described, but the ruler is positioned at 6 cm above the imaging cassette, the assumed height of ischial spines.

*(c) Lateral correction scale*
The scale is made by suspending the ruler at a distance of 46 cm from a cassette held vertically in the erect film holder/cassette stand. The horizontal X-ray tube is centred over the 10 cm notch using a FFD of 230 cm. The beam is collimated to the ruler and an exposure made.

# 7 Reproductive System

## Male Reproductive System

The male reproductive system consists of the following organs

- the two testes } within the scrotum
- the two epididymides } within the scrotum
- the two deferent ducts and spermatic cords
- the two seminimal vesicles
- the two ejaculatory ducts
- the prostate gland
- the penis.

The scrotum lies below the symphysis pubis, in front of the upper parts of the thighs and behind the penis. It contains the testes, the epididymides and the lower part of the two spermatic cords.

The testes are the reproductive glands of the male and are suspended in the scrotum by the spermatic cords which contain the testicular artery/vein, lymphatic vessels and the ductus deferens. Each testis consists of 200–300 lobules which form into tubules known as the seminiferous tubules, between which lie interstitial secretory cells. The tubules ascend in the upper pole of the testis, joining together to form the epididymis. The epididymis is a convoluted tubule which folds upon itself and descends to the lower border of the testis where it continues as the ductus deferens.

The ductus deferens passes upwards from the testis through the inguinal canal, ascending medially towards the posterior wall of the bladder to join the duct from the seminal vesicle to form the ejaculatory duct.

The seminal vesicles are two pouches which lie on the posterior aspect of the bladder. Their lower part narrows and opens onto two short ducts which join with the deferent ducts to form the ejaculatory ducts which pass forwards and downwards, to open into the prostate gland.

The prostate gland lies in the pelvic cavity immediately in front of the rectum and just behind the symphysis pubis and surrounds the commencement of the urethra. The male urethra forms a common pathway for the flow of urine and the flow of semen from the male reproductive organs and is approximately 20 cm long. It extends from the internal urethral sphincter of the urinary bladder to the extremity of the penis. It passes through the prostate gland and then turns at an angle of 90° through the perineum and then passes downwards, surrounded by the structures of the body of the penis. The penis is formed by three elongated masses of erectile tissue, fibrous tissue and involuntary muscle rich in blood supply. The two lateral columns are known as the corpora cavernosa which surrounds the middle column termed the corpus spongiosum. At the tip of the penis the corpus cavernosum is expanded into a triangular structure known as the glans penis, above which the skin is folded to form the foreskin and prepuce.

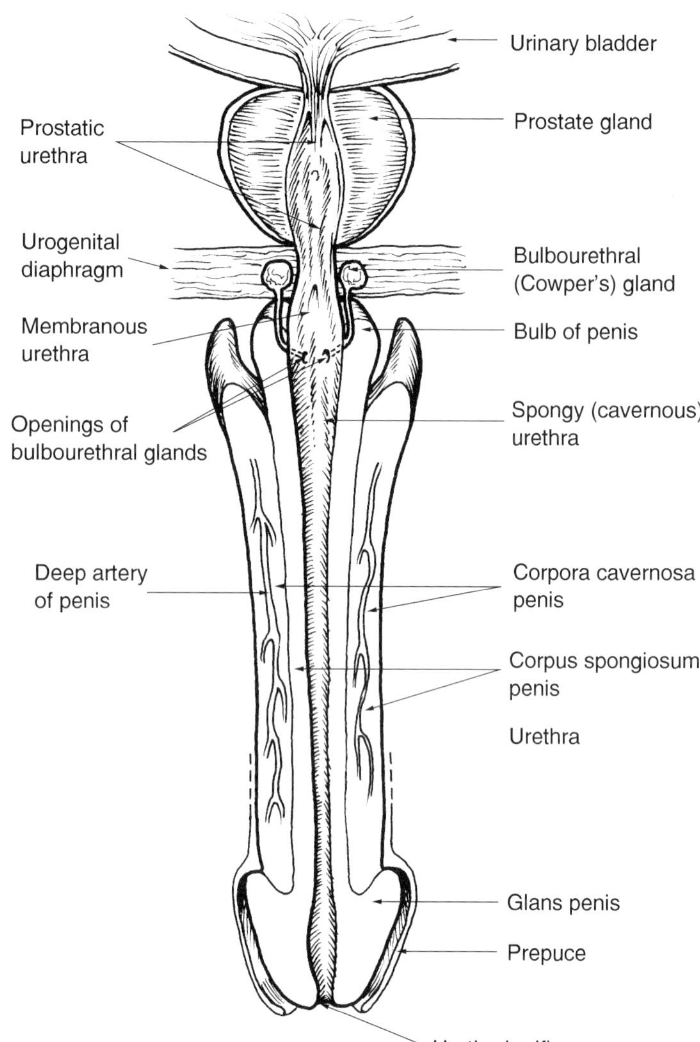


**Figure 7.23a** Internal structure of the penis

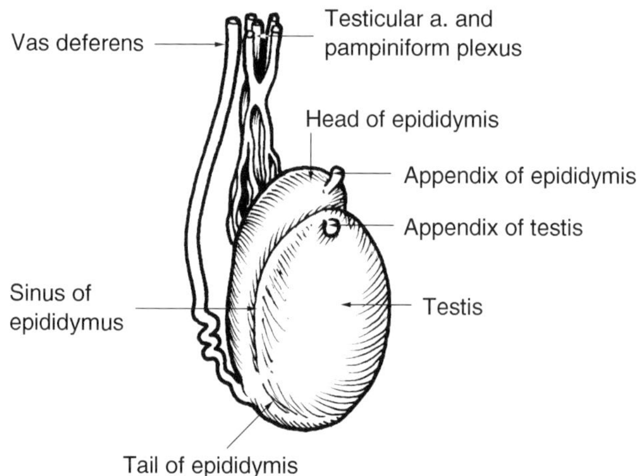


**Figure 7.23b** External aspect of the right testis and epididymis

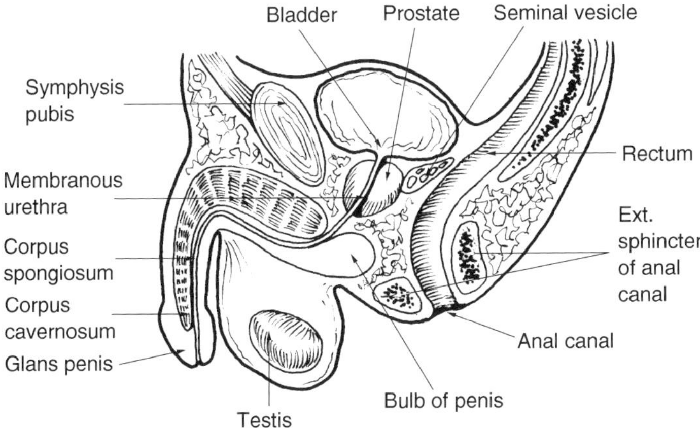


**Figure 7.24a** Sagittal section through male pelvis

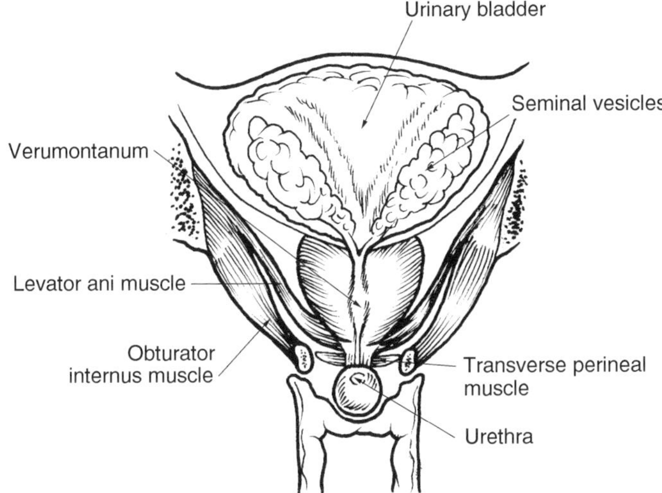


**Figure 7.24b** Coronal section through prostate gland

The prostate gland is situated between the neck of the bladder and the levater ani muscle. It is cone shaped, with the base uppermost. It is traversed vertically by prostatic urethra and, in the upper position, by paired ejaculatory ducts.

The gland is described as consisting of three glandular zones (central, transitional and peripheral) and one non-glandular zone which forms the anterior part of the prostate. The central zone is cone shaped, narrowing at its apex, the transitional zone lies around the proximal posterior urethra and the peripheral zone surrounds the others, forming the posterolateral and apical parts of the prostate.

## Indications

Pain, prostatism (poor urinary flow), urethral discharge and prostatitis are the most common reasons for radiological investigation. Also ultrasound may be used as a diagnostic screening tool for prostatic cancer.

## Recommended imaging procedures

Transrectal ultrasound (TRUS) is the imaging method of choice, clearly demonstrating zonal anatomy, gland symmetry, the prostatic urethra and the seminal vesicles. The high inherent soft tissue contrast in MR images enables this technique to be used in the staging of prostatic carcinoma and in assessing the spread of disease into adjacent pelvic structures. Endorectal surface coils at present under development should produce high-resolution images of the internal architecture of the gland itself and enable the full potential of MR imaging of the prostate gland to be assessed.

The inability of CT scanning to detect intracapsular malignancy severely limits the application of this technique in prostate imaging. Computed tomography is mainly used to demonstrate associated pelvic and abdominal lymphadenopathy.

The role of intravenous urography (IVU) in demonstrating prostatic disease has greatly diminished and is usually only undertaken in patients who have general urological symptoms.

# 7 Prostate Gland

## Transrectal ultrasound

Transrectal ultrasound allows multiplanar imaging of the prostate gland to be undertaken. Although uncomfortable, it is a relatively painless procedure carried out after an initial clinical digital rectal examination. No patient preparation is routinely required, although a cleansing enema may be necessary if there is a great deal of faecal material in the rectum. A slightly distended urinary bladder is also useful in imaging the base of the prostate.

Recent technological advances have produced a variety of handheld transducers, with frequencies ranging from 6 to 7.5 MHz. These can image in single or multiple planes (transverse, longitudinal or oblique). Some probes also permit colour Doppler imaging.

### Indications

This is used to detect prostatic carcinoma and it has been advocated in several countries as a screening tool for early detection of cancer. Prostatic biopsy is possible using this modality.

### Position of patient and imaging modality

Because of the nature of the examination, cross-contamination is relatively easy. To prevent this the transducer probe must be disinfected immediately before and after use. Gloves must be worn by the sonographer. To ensure good image quality, all air must be removed from the transducer assembly. To achieve this, a 50–60 ml syringe of distilled water is attached via a one-way valve to a piece of intravenous connecting tubing, the other end of which is connected to the transducer handle filling port. The water is then slowly injected until it emerges through the water exit port at the transducer tip. The transducer cover is then slipped over the transducer and held in place by an O-ring. Water is then injected into the cover and any air present allowed to gather around the exit port. By withdrawing the barrel of the syringe, the air is drawn back into the syringe.

This procedure is repeated several times to ensure that all air has been removed. Transducer coupling gel is then applied to the tip of the transducer which is covered with a condom.

The patient lies on the left side, arms resting on the pillow and knees flexed. After reassurance of the patient, the transducer is introduced into the rectum and 20–30 ml of water injected into the tip of the cover.

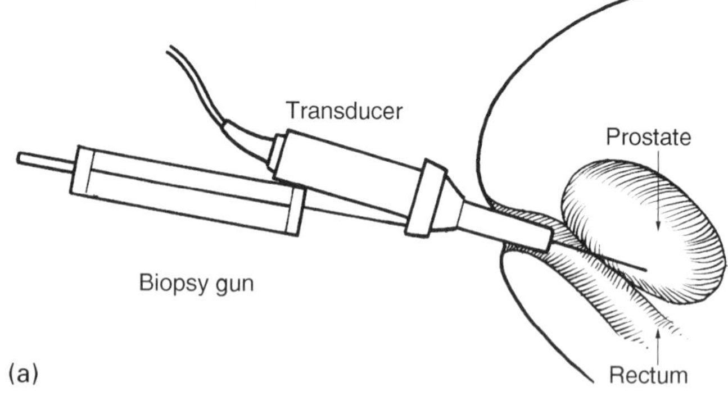


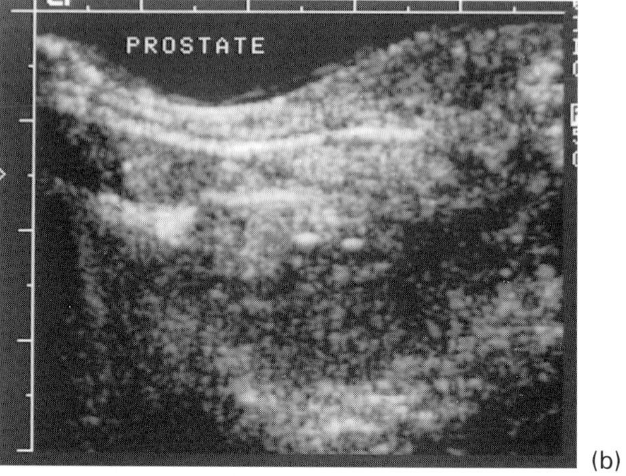


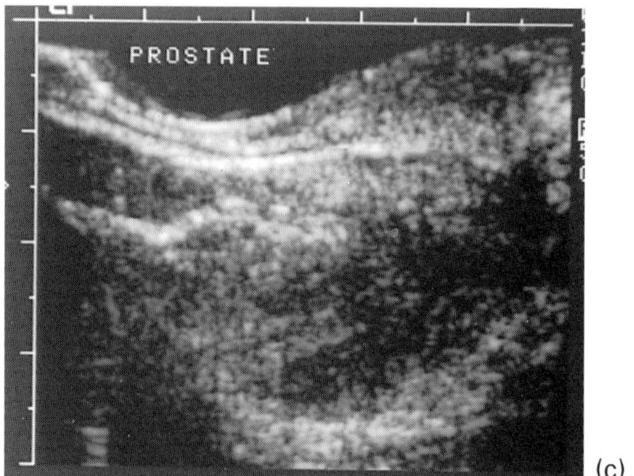


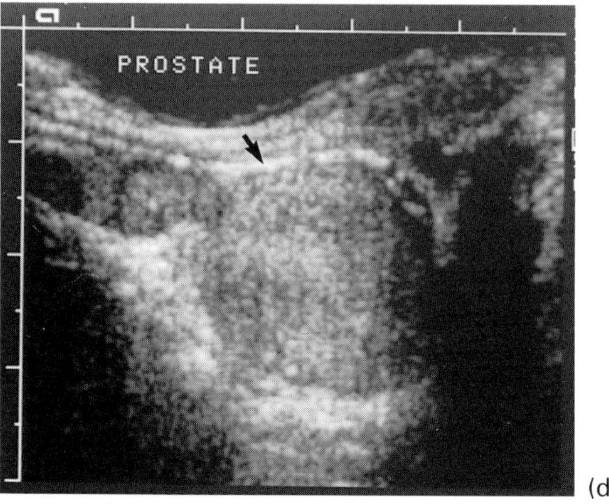


**Figure 7.25** (a) Diagram showing position of transducer, biopsy gun and needle attachment for transrectal biopsy; (b–d) series of longitudinal images through a normal prostate gland

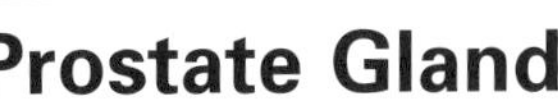



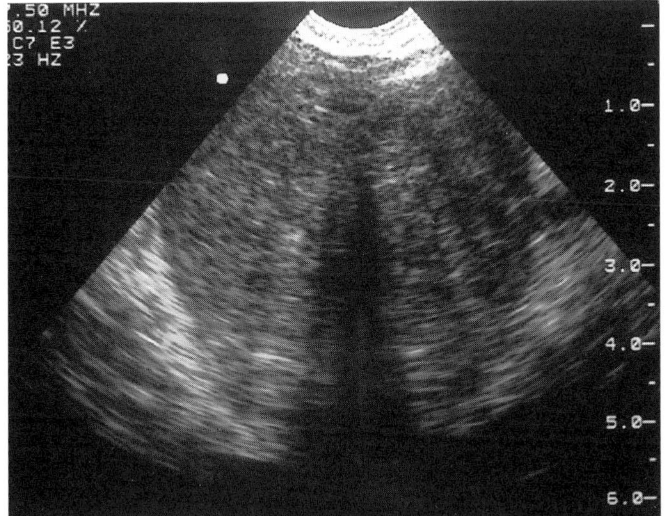


**Figure 7.26a** Transverse image showing prostate gland and echo from urethra

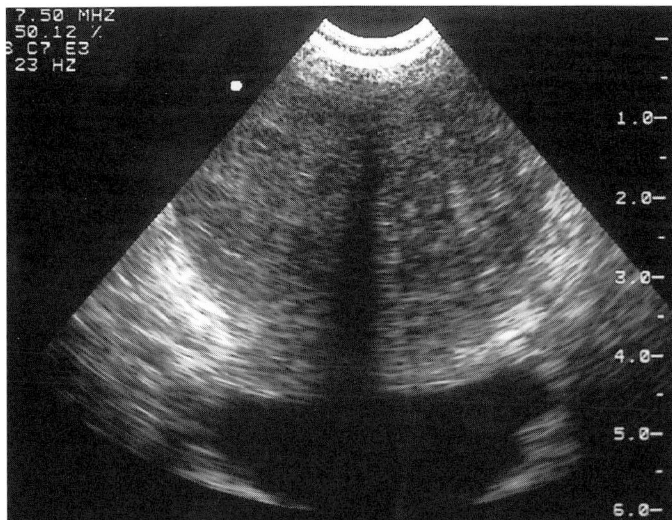


**Figure 7.26b** Transverse image showing prostate gland, urethra and bladder

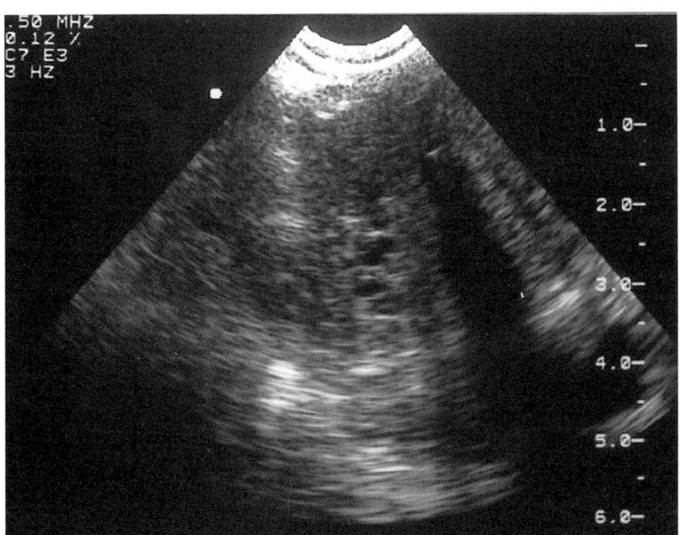


**Figure 7.26c** Transverse image showing biopsy needle in position

### Imaging procedure

To examine the prostate from apex to base, a multiplanar technique is required. Transaxial images starting at the level of the seminal vesicles and withdrawing the transducer in a caudad direction will demonstrate the seminal vesicles, central gland, peripheral zones and evaluate symmetry, size and shape of the gland. Sagittal imaging permits assessment of the seminal vesicles, the base, apex and lateral margin of the gland. The prostatic urethra is visible on a midline sagittal image.

If clarification of information gained from the transverse axial and sagittal views is required, the transducer may be rotated to produce an oblique coronal view which elongates the gland, demonstrating the periphery of the prostate.

### Biopsy

There are two biopsy methods – transrectal biopsy and transperineal biopsy. Using the former approach, bleeding can occur which may lead to sepsis. To overcome this, a course of broad-band antibiotics is prescribed for 1 week prior to biopsy.

In the latter, local anaesthetic is needed but the risk of infection is greatly reduced.

In both approaches, cores of tissue are obtained through an 18-gauge biopsy needle attached to an automatic trigger device. For transperineal biopsy the needle is placed through a special guiding device attached to the transducer. For transrectal biopsy the needle is directed mounted on the probe.

# 7 Prostate Gland

## Magnetic resonance imaging

Magnetic resonance is an excellent imaging tool in the evaluation of the male pelvis. Multiplanar images not only provide information on the prostate gland and the seminal vesicles, but the spread of disease into the surrounding lymph nodes and bony pelvis can also be assessed.

$T_2$ weighted sequences demonstrate intraprostatic disease. $T_1$ weighted sequences demonstrate periprostatic tumour extension.

Because of relatively long scanning times there will be image degradation due to motion artefacts. These may be reduced by applying compression to the pelvis. Prone imaging has been advocated, but this is often impossible for the patient to maintain. Peristalsis may be reduced by administering a smooth muscle relaxant drug immediately prior to the examination if not clinically contraindicated.

At the present time, endorectal coils which improve resolution are still being assessed. Therefore this technique is not described in this chapter.

### Position of patient and imaging modality

The patient lies supine, feet first on the scanner table, with the median sagittal plane perpendicular to the midline of the table. Compression may be applied. Using external alignment lights, the external reference point is obtained at the level of the anterior superior iliac spines.

From this position the patient is moved the fixed distance to the isocentre of the magnet/receiver body coil.

### Imaging procedure

An initial midline sagittal localiser scan is performed to include the lower abdomen and pelvis. Using this image, transaxial $T_1$ and $T_2$ weighted sequences are prescribed to cover the entire prostate gland and seminal vesicles.

Coronal $T_1$ weighted images are acquired from the sacrum posteriorly to the symphysis pubis anteriorly, to assess lymphadenopathy. A variable echo sequence, producing proton density and $T_2$ weighted scans in the sagittal plane, is performed to assess the relationships between the prostate, bladder, bladder base seminal vesicles and rectum.

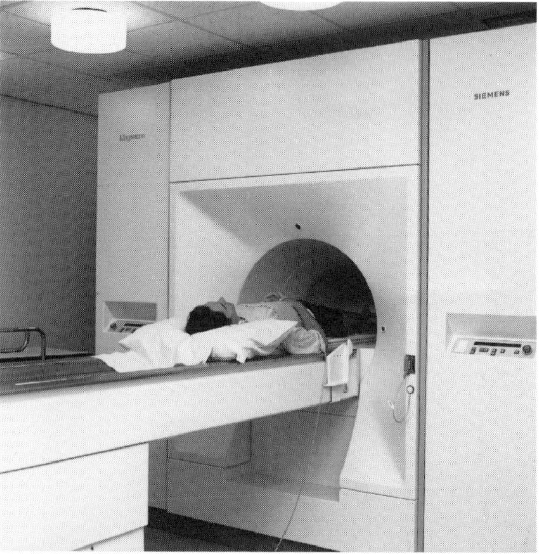


**Figure 7.27a** Patient positioned for MRI of prostate gland

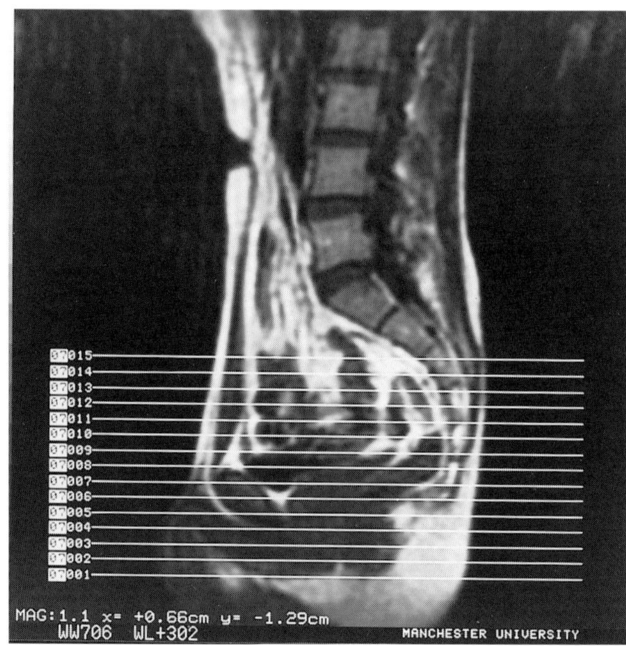


**Figure 7.27b** Localiser scan showing prescribed transaxial sections

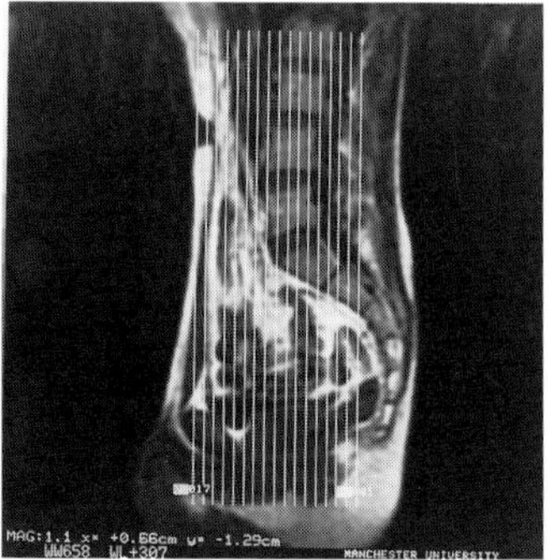

**Figure 7.27c** Localiser scan showing prescribed coronal sections

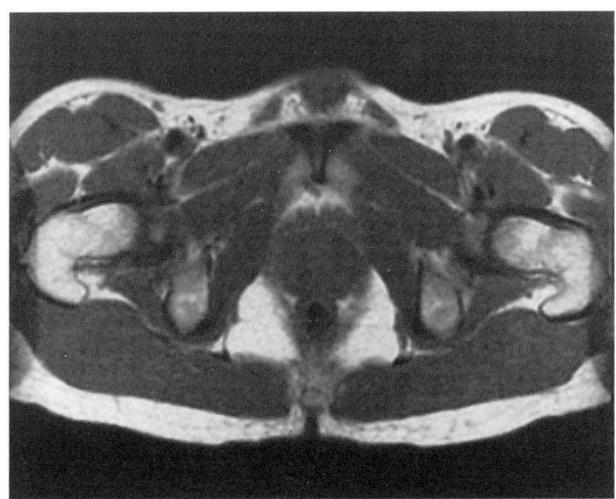

**Figure 7.28a** Transaxial $T_1$ weighted image

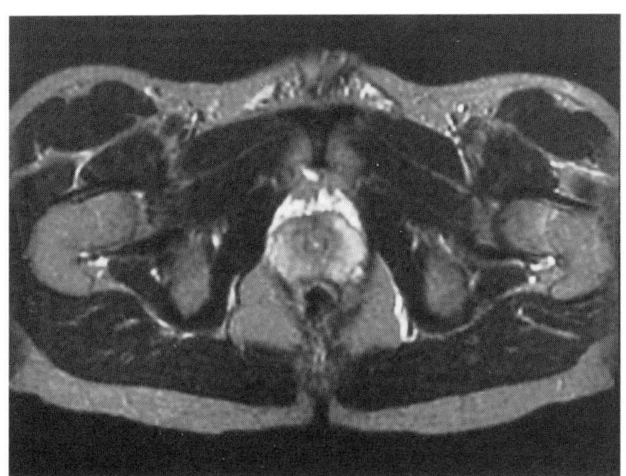

**Figure 7.28c** Transaxial $T_2$ weighted image

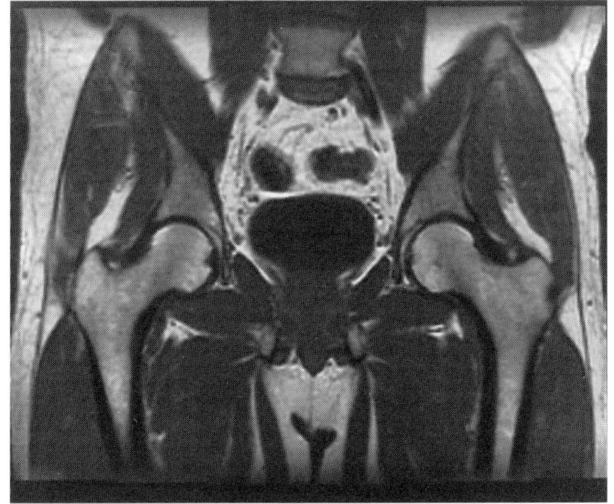

**Figure 7.28b** Coronal $T_1$ weighted image

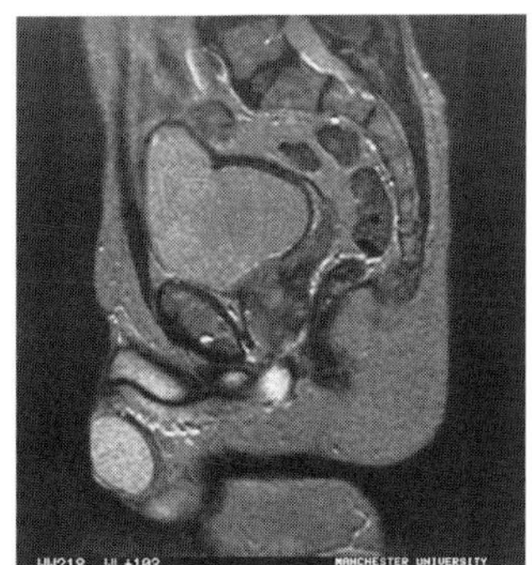

**Figure 7.28d** Sagittal $T_2$ weighted image

**Table 7.3 Imaging parameters**

| *Imaging plane* | *Imaging sequence* | *TR* | *TE* | *Field of view* (cm) | *No. of NEX* | *Slice width/ gap* (mm) | *Matrix (horizontal–vertical)* |
|---|---|---|---|---|---|---|---|
| Transaxial | Spin-echo $T_1$ weighted | 500 | 25 | 30–40 | 2 | 7/2 | 256 × 192 |
| Transaxial | Fast spin-echo $T_2$ weighted | 3500 | 100 | 35–40 | 3 | 5/2 | 256 × 192 |
| Coronal | Spin-echo $T_1$ weighted | 600 | 25 | 40 | 2 | 7/2 | 192 × 256 |
| Sagittal | Variable echo | 2000 | 35/90 | 30–40 | 2 | 5/2 | 192 × 256 |

# 7 Male Reproductive System

## Scrotum

The scrotum lies below the symphysis pubis, in front of the upper parts of the thighs and behind the penis. It contains the testes, the epididymides and lower spermatic cords.

### Indications

Pain, scrotal swelling, trauma, hydroceles and testicular torsion are the most common reasons for radiological investigation.

### Recommended imaging procedures

Ultrasound is the preferred imaging method. Computed tomography is used only to localise undescended testes.

### Ultrasound

A two-dimensional real-time ultrasound system using a 7.5–10 MHz linear array probe is selected.

**Position of patient and imaging modality**

The patient lies supine on the scanner table. The scrotum is elevated with a towel and the penis resting on the lower anterior abdominal wall. As much of the lower abdomen as possible is covered with a towel to preserve patient dignity. The presence of a chaperone is usually advised.

**Imaging procedure**

Direct contact imaging is the method usually undertaken. However, a 'stand-off' block can be used to reduce any near-field artefact which may be detrimental to image quality in units with older transducer technology.

Images are obtained in the transaxial and parasagittal planes, and the texture and size of each testis is compared, one with the other.

Colour Doppler ultrasound may be used to look at the arterial supply of the testes in cases of testicular torsion, tumours and varices (see Plate 3).

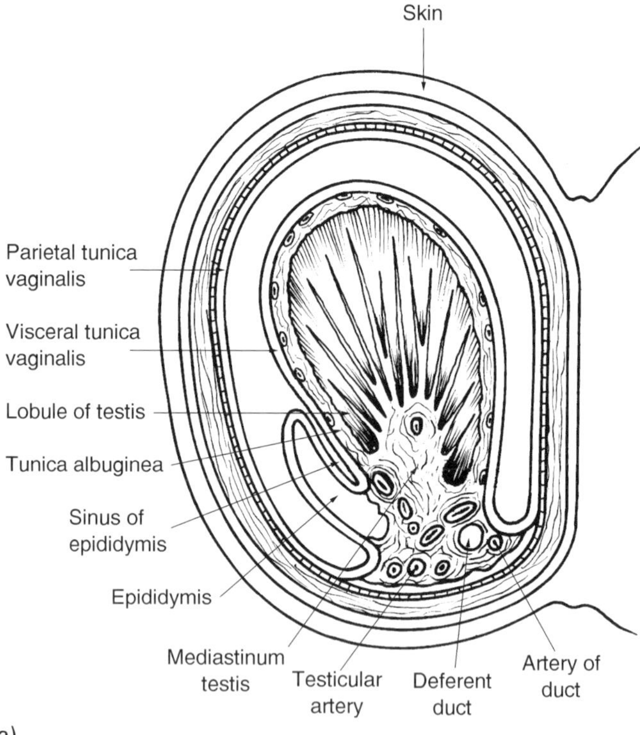


(a)

(b)

(c)

**Figure 7.29** (a) Transverse section through the left scrotum; (b,c) longitudinal sections through a testis showing focal abnormalities

## Computed tomography

Computed tomographic scanning is used to aid the localisation of undescended testes. Oral contrast medium in the form of either dilute Gastrografin or barium, as described in Chapter 1, is required to outline the small bowel.

**Position of patient and imaging modality**

The patient lies supine, feet first on the scanner table, with the median sagittal plane coincident with the centre of the table. Arms are raised and placed behind the patient's head, out of the scan plane. Positioning is aided by transaxial, coronal and sagittal alignment lights. The median sagittal plane is perpendicular and the coronal plane is parallel to the scanner table. The scan plane is perpendicular to the long axis of the body to enable transaxial cross-sectional imaging to be undertaken. The scanner table height is adjusted to ensure that the coronal plane alignment light is at the level of the mid-axillary line. The patient is then moved into the scanner until the scan reference point is at the level of the xiphisternum.

**Imaging procedure**

An anteroposterior scan projection radiograph is performed, starting at the level of the xiphisternum and ending just below the level of the symphysis pubis (table travel approximately 35 cm).

From this image, 10 mm contiguous sections are prescribed, starting at the symphysis pubis and ending at the anterior superior iliac spines. If no abnormality is detected on these images, further 10 mm sections are obtained at 20 mm intervals as far as the renal hilum.

If any abnormal mass is detected, contrast enhanced 10 mm contiguous sections are acquired through the area of abnormality.

If spiral scanning options are available, these images may be acquired with a volume acquisition, using a 10 mm slice thickness and 10 mm table increments, but with a 5 mm reconstruction index to give overlapping sections.

*Contrast medium and injector data*

| *Volume* | *Concentration* | *Flow rate* |
|---|---|---|
| 100 ml | 300 mgI/ml | 2 ml/s |

Scanning commences after 60 ml of contrast has been administered.

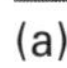

(a)

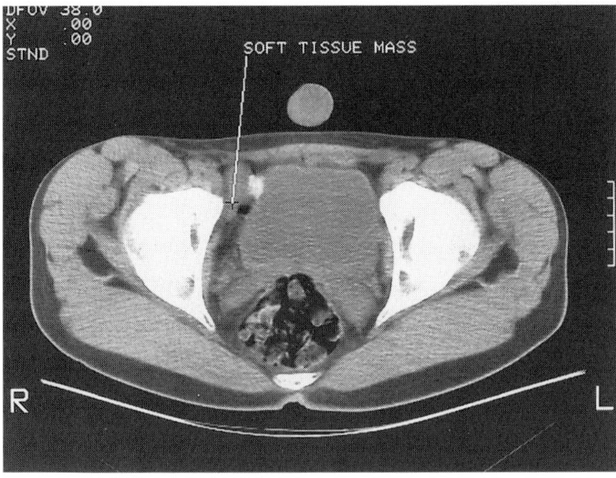

(b)

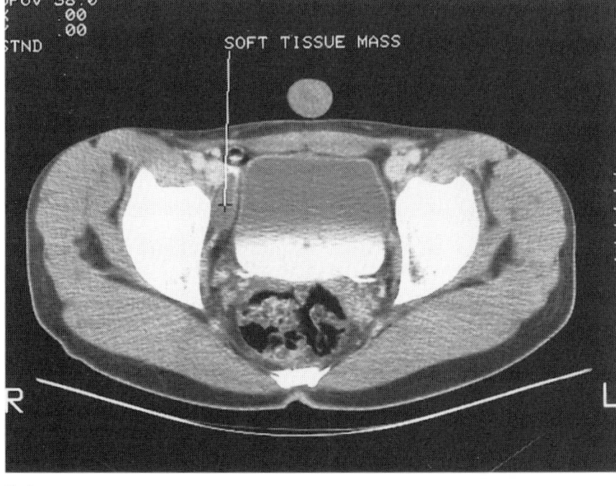


(c)

**Figure 7.30** (a) AP scan projection radiograph showing prescribed sections; (b,c) pre- and post-contrast enhancement scans at the level of the femoral heads showing a soft tissue mass between the right femoral head and bladder suggestive of an undescended testicle

# 7 Male Reproductive System

## Penis

The penis is formed by three elongated masses of erectile tissue, fibrous tissue and involuntary muscle rich in blood supply. The two lateral columns are known as the corpora cavernosa, surrounding the middle column – the corpus spongiosum. At the tip of the penis, the corpus cavernosum is expanded into a triangular structure known as the glans penis (see page 256 for diagram).

Arterial blood is supplied by the superficial and deep penile arteries and venous drainage by the superficial and deep dorsal veins and the cavernosal veins. During erection, the smooth muscles of the cavernosal walls relax and the veins are compressed, producing a rise in intracorporeal pressure.

### Indications

Erectile impotence is the main reason for radiological investigation which can be the result of arterial insufficiency or venous incompetence.

### Recommended imaging procedures

Doppler ultrasound is used to assess the arterial blood supply, with papaverine injected during the procedure to assess tumescence. If this appears normal, either cavernosography or pharmacocavernosography using conventional fluoroscopy is necessary to evaluate venous drainage. In the former, an erection is achieved by infusion of saline into the corpora cavernosa at the rate of up to 300 ml/min; in the latter, the smooth muscle relaxant papaverine is used in addition to saline.

### Cavernosography

**Imaging procedure**

The procedure assumes the use of a remote fluoroscopic unit with overcouch X-ray tube. The patient lies supine on the imaging couch and, under sterile conditions, a 19-gauge butterfly needle is inserted into each corpora approximately 2.5 cm proximal to the glans. One needle is connected to the infusion pump, while the other is used to record pressure measurements during the infusion. The rate of infusion varies depending upon the degree of tumescence and the pressure rise in the penis. The X-ray tube is adjusted to ensure that the exit of the central ray is 2.5 cm above the symphysis pubis in the midline. Under fluoroscopic control, anteroposterior and posterior oblique projections (with the patient rotated 45° to the right or left) are obtained before and after the infusion of 20 ml of a suitable contrast agent, demonstrating the draining veins in the flaccid state.

An erection is now induced by infusion of either saline alone or saline plus papaverine. The addition of a water-soluble contrast agent to the saline allows demonstration of venous leakage at the same time as pressure measurements are made.

*Contrast medium and injection data*

| *Volume* | *Concentration* | *Flow rate* |
|---|---|---|
| 20 ml | 180 mgI/ml | Slow infusion |

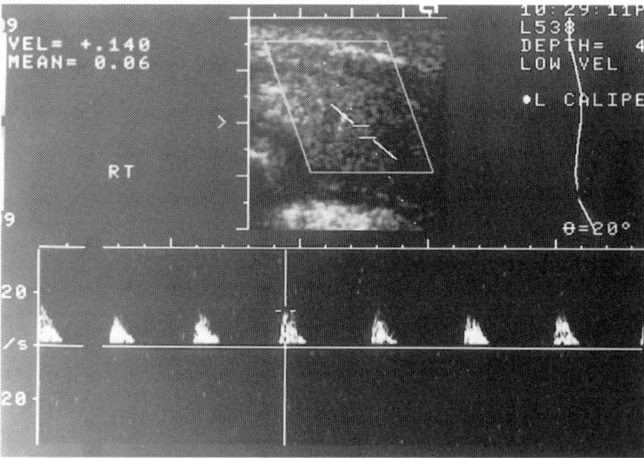


**Figure 7.31a** Doppler ultrasound study from cavernosal artery of flaccid penis

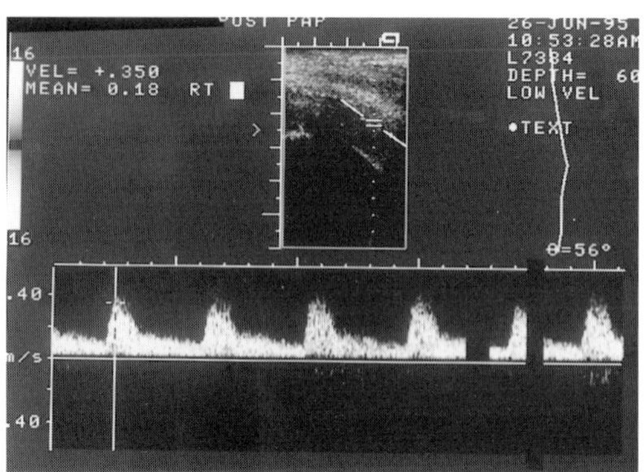


**Figure 7.31b** Doppler ultrasound study from the cavernosal artery of penis after injection of 60 mg of papaverine

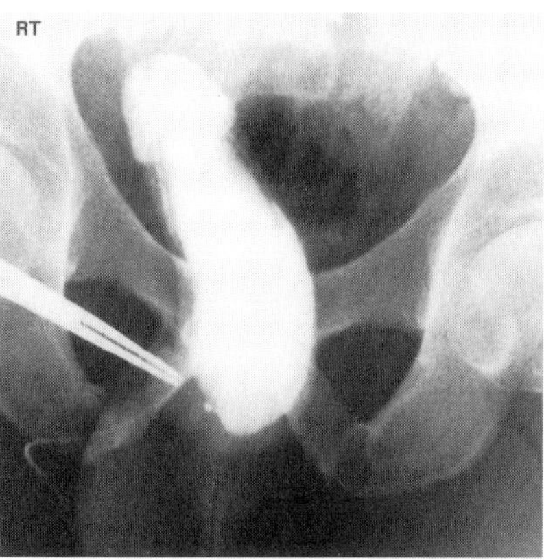


**Figure 7.31c** Early cavernosogram image during the infusion of contrast

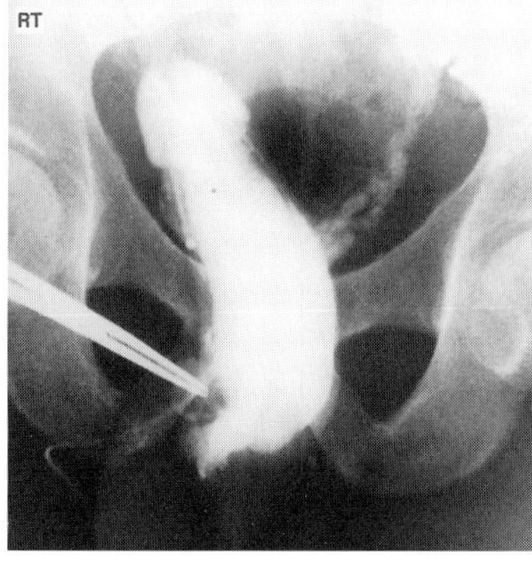


**Figure 7.31d** Late cavernosogram image demonstrating venous leakage consistent with impotence

# 8

# CARDIOVASCULAR SYSTEM

## CONTENTS

# 8 Cardiovascular System

## Introduction

This chapter deals with diagnostic investigations and interventional procedures of the heart, aorta, blood vessels of the neck, upper and lower limbs and the inferior vena cava.

Vascular investigations associated with other anatomical systems will be covered in the relevant chapter.

The nature of patient preparation and after-care will depend on the type of imaging procedure selected, and is fully discussed in Chapter 1.

### Recommended imaging procedures

Investigations of the cardiovascular system may be by means of angiography, ultrasound, RNI, MRI and CT.

The basis of selection should be related to the sensitivity of the equipment and the procedure in detecting the disease process under investigation.

Other factors such as the invasive nature of the investigation, possible reactions to contrast media and the adverse effects of ionising radiation may also be taken into consideration.

## Angiography

For a long time, angiography was the only imaging procedure available for detailed investigations of the heart and blood vessels. Today, although not always the first procedure of choice, it still plays an important role in the assessment of vascular and heart disease.

Using this procedure the heart (angiocardiography), arteries (aortography and arteriography) and veins (venography or phlebography) may be examined by means of contrast media and digital imaging equipment or rapid serial radiography.

Digital imaging offers many advantages compared with rapid serial radiography and enables smaller volumes and less concentrated contrast media to be used. It also facilitates 'real-time' digital image subtraction angiography (DSA) and provides sophisticated image processing functions to provide better qualitative and quantative diagnostic information.

A venous approach (IV.DSA) can in some circumstances replace arterial catheterisation (IA.DSA), thus reducing the invasive nature of the procedure.

When digital subtraction is unavailable, standard subtraction radiography techniques should be used to show vessels obscured by overlying bony structures.

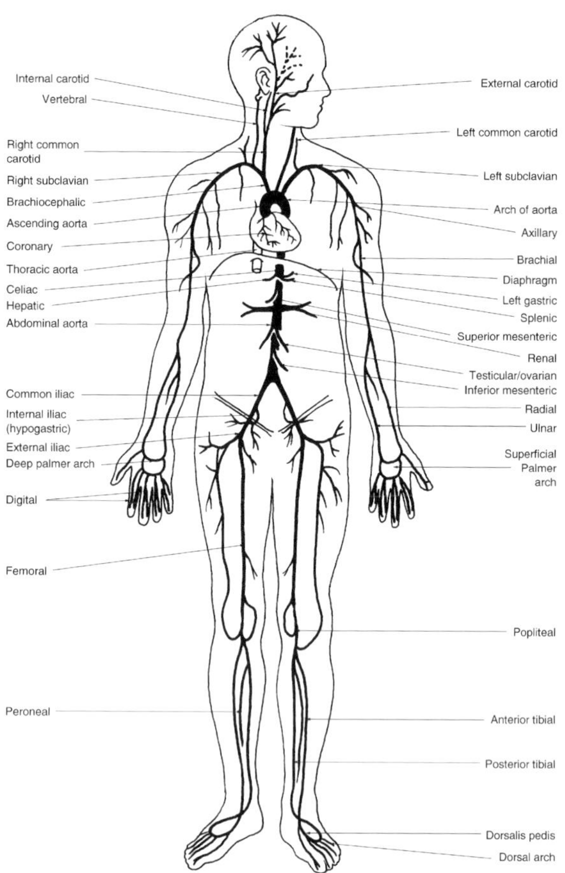


**Figure 8.1a** Arterial system – main vessels (anterior view)

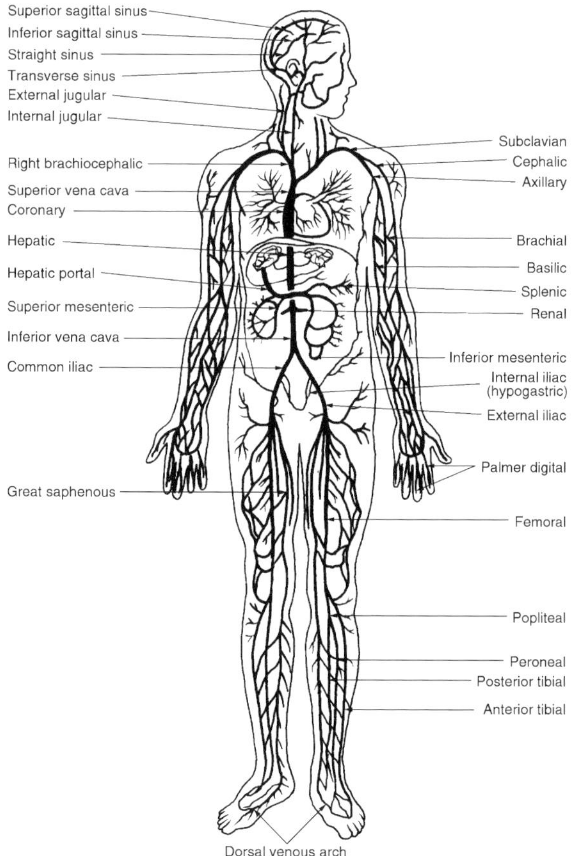


**Figure 8.1b** Venous system – main vessels (anterior view)

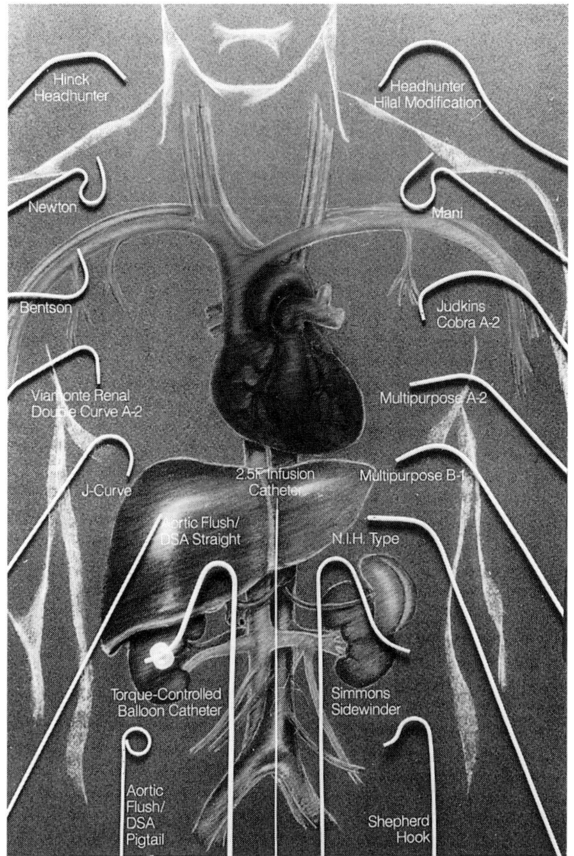


**Figure 8.2a** Typical types of angiography catheter (Courtesy of Cordis)

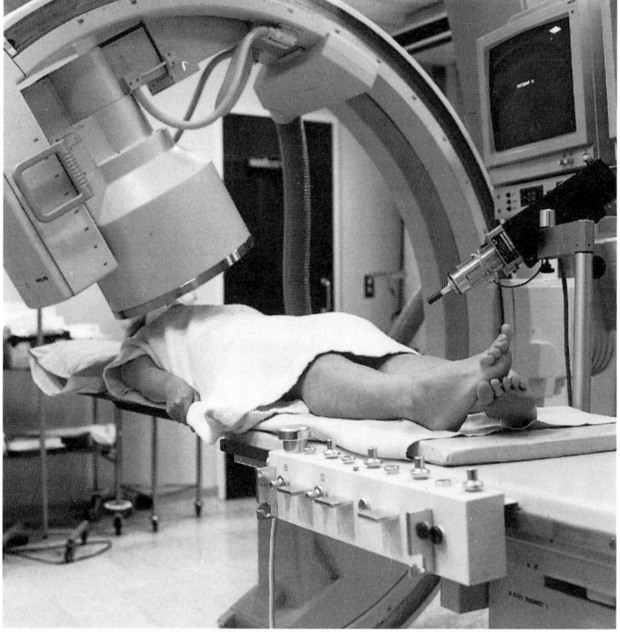

**Figure 8.2b** C-arm angiographic equipment with contrast pressure injector

## Contrast administration

Opacification of the cardiovascular system by means of arterial catheterisation is commonly performed following puncture of a common femoral artery. In this procedure, the catheter is passed in a retrograde fashion along the length of the iliac artery, aorta or aortic arch to the required anatomical location. A catheter may also be passed in an antegrade fashion down the length of an artery and its branches, such as employed in investigations and interventional procedures associated with the lower limbs. Access to the arterial system may also be by means of puncture of the brachial artery, with access to the descending aorta usually made from the left side. In this situation a catheter is directed in an antegrade manner as the catheter is advanced towards the abdominal aorta.

Occasionally, access is made by direct puncture of an artery such as the carotid artery or translumbar puncture of the abdominal aorta, although nowadays these procedures are rarely performed.

Arterial access may be by means of the Seldinger technique or alternatively a single-part needle technique through which a J-tip guide wire is inserted to facilitate introduction of the selected catheter (see page 38).

A sheath introducer system is adopted if more than one catheter is to be used during the procedure, thus reducing damage to the arterial wall. This also facilitates the artery being flushed with heparinised saline through a side line.

For many investigations, intra-arterial pressure monitoring may be required.

For IV.DSA, a bolus injection of contrast is injected into the superior vena cava or a suitable antecubital vein.

## Contrast pressure injector

A contrast pressure injector (see page 40) is required for most angiographic procedures. Using this equipment, a bolus of contrast, maintained at body temperature, is injected into a vessel or heart chamber under controlled conditions, e.g. defined volume and flow rate. A delay factor can also be selected to postpone the commencement of either contrast injection or X-ray exposure. Maximum injection pressure is adjusted to match the type of catheter selected for the procedure.

## Catheters

A variety of catheters are required to enable different arteries and veins to be accessed. These are distinguished by the shape of the end portion and side holes. Catheters are available in different lengths and diameters (French gauge size). Use of a guidewire is necessary as part of the catheterisation procedure. For IA.DSA, smaller French gauge catheters are used, which reduces trauma to the arterial wall and shortens patient after-care.

# 8 Cardiovascular System

## Neck Vessels

This section deals with the examination of neck vessels. Detailed examination of the intracranial vessels is described in Chapter 10.

### Indications

These include transient ischaemic attacks associated with impaired cerebral blood supply, aneurysms of the neck vessels and subclavian steals.

### Recommended imaging procedures

Imaging of the arterial vessels of the neck falls into two categories: screening procedures for the detection of significant arteriosclerosis and as a roadmap for surgical planning. The techniques used for screening procedures include ultrasound, MRI and IV.DSA. Both ultrasound and MRI are non-invasive, presenting no risk to the patient, but do require a high level of expertise. For surgical planning, conventional angiography using digital imaging subtraction is routinely undertaken. Assessment of the carotid arteries may also be made by the use of spiral CT, but at the time of writing this is not in widespread use.

### Angiography

The procedure is best performed using dedicated angiographic equipment with an image intensifier and digital imaging facilities, allowing image subtraction and blood flow analysis. Images can also be acquired using a rapid serial film changer. The vessels are demonstrated using a non-ionic contrast agent and pressure injector.

For intravenous angiography, digital imaging facilities are essential. During the procedure both postero-anterior and right or left anterior oblique projections are acquired.

#### Imaging procedure

The procedure usually involves demonstration of the great vessels prior to selective catheterisation of a specific carotid or vertebral vessel. This is necessary to determine the exact relationships of the different artery origins and to determine if any of the vessels are stenosed. It is most commonly performed by a Seldinger technique, with retrograde catheterisation of a femoral artery, and the tip of a small straight or pigtail catheter (4–5 F) positioned in the arch of the aorta proximal to the right brachiocephalic artery. Images are acquired of the great vessels following a bolus injection of contrast medium using the pressure injector. Selective catheterisation of specific vessels is performed with the aid of fluoroscopy and images acquired following hand injection of contrast medium.

*Contrast medium and injector data*

| | *Volume* | *Concentration* | *Flow rate* |
|---|---|---|---|
| Selective | 10 ml | 300 mgI/ml | Hand injection |
| IV.DSA | 25 ml | 370 mgI/ml | 10–12 ml/s |

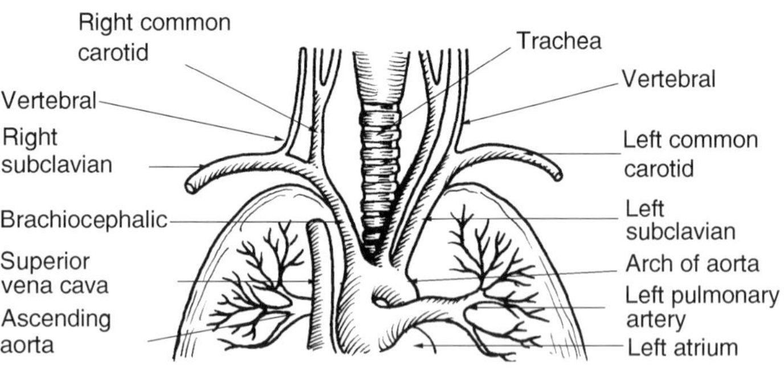


**Figure 8.3a** Aortic arch and neck vessels (anterior aspect)

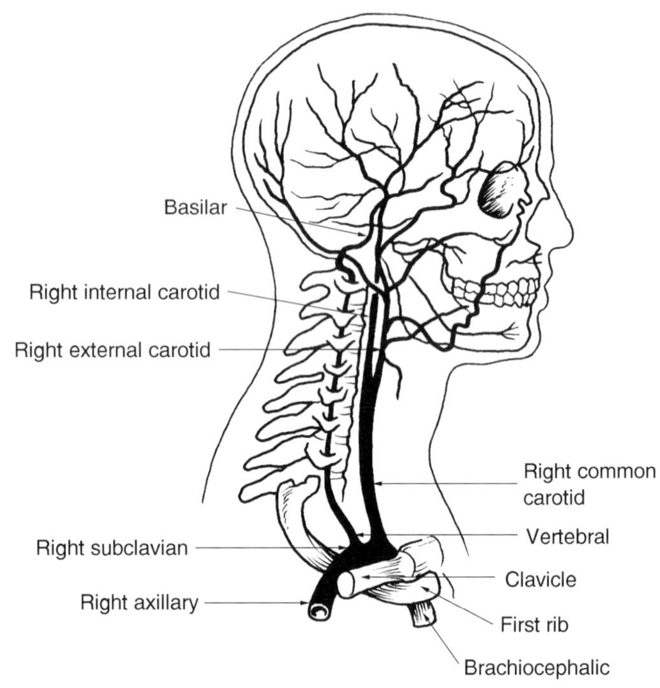


**Figure 8.3b** Arteries of the head and neck (right side)

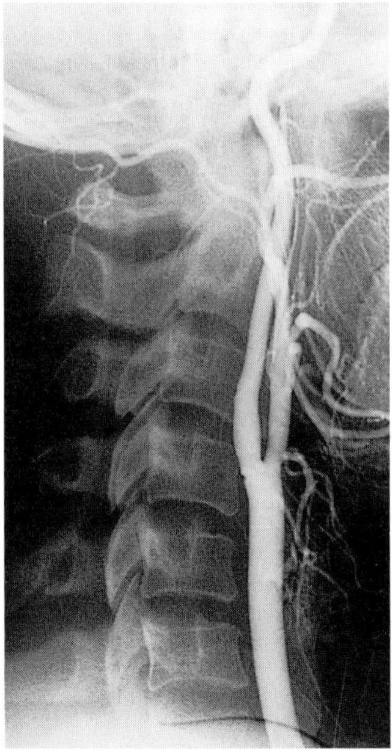

**Figure 8.3c** Lateral image of neck showing common carotid artery, internal and external carotid arteries and bifurcation

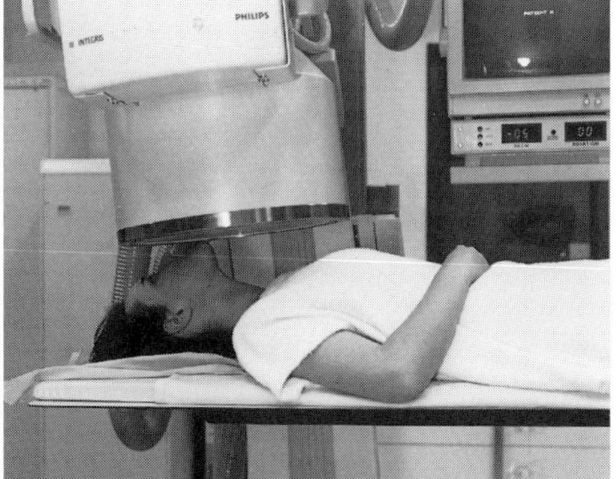

(a)

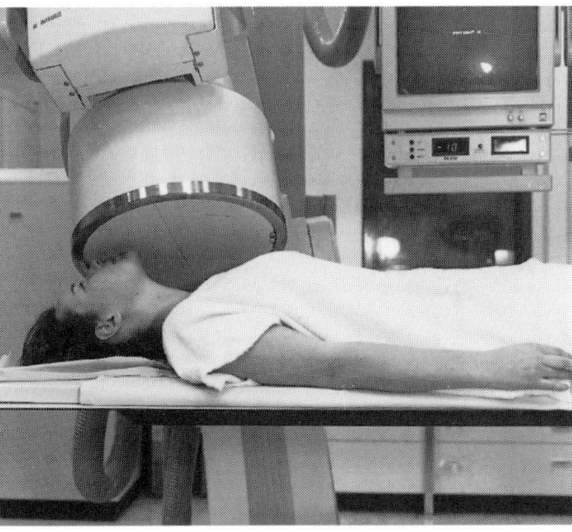

(b)

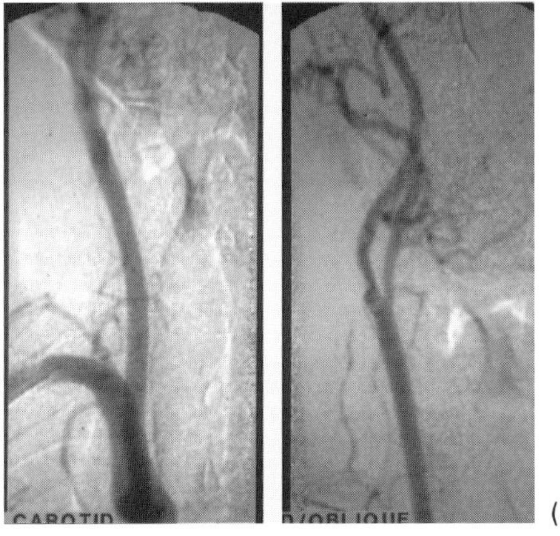

(c)

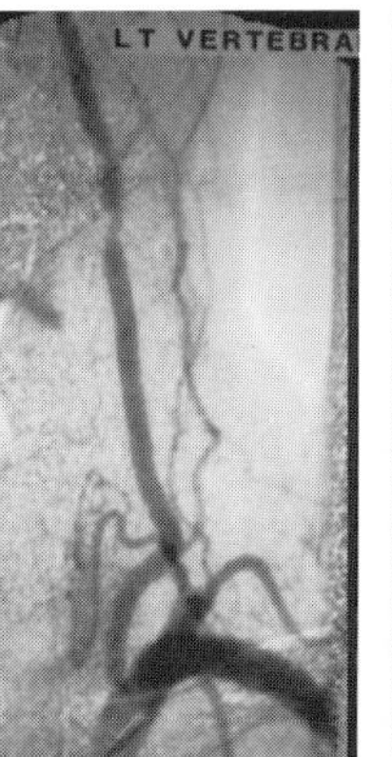


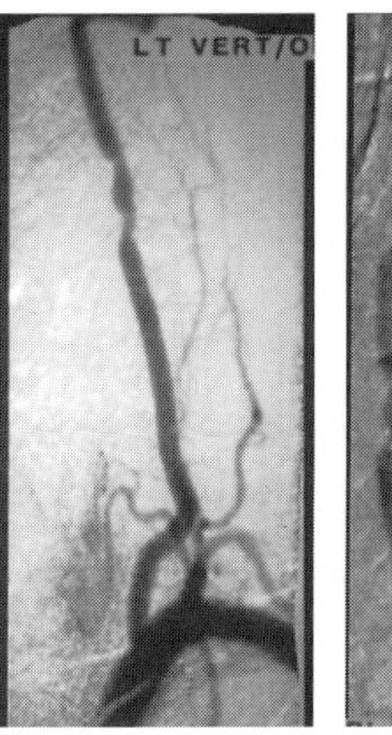


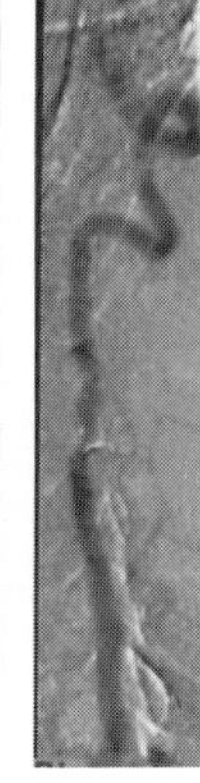

(d)

**Figure 8.4a** (a,b) Patient and equipment; (c) postero-anterior and oblique images of the right common carotid artery with some stenotic disease just distal to the bifurcation; (d) series of oblique images of the left vertebral artery showing two areas of stenotic disease

Prior to image acquisition the patient is advised to swallow and then arrest respiration. This reduces movement artefact which would otherwise lead to misregistration on subsequent subtracted images.

In digital subtraction angiography, a mask image is usually taken immediately preceding the contrast injection.

In IV.DSA, a contrast agent is introduced via a peripheral or a central vein.

## Postero-anterior

This projection is used to demonstrate carotid or vertebral vessels in the neck.

*Position of patient and imaging modality*

The patient is laid supine on the imaging couch, with the head adjusted to bring the median sagittal plane at right angles to the couch top. The neck is extended as far as can be comfortably maintained by the patient and centred in respect to the image intensifier which is positioned above the neck and parallel to the couch top.

*Direction and centring of the X-ray beam*

The central ray of the C-arm equipment is angled 5–10° caudally, to ensure that the lower border of the mandible and the occipital bone are superimposed, which will show the full extent of the vessels unobscured by bone.

## Anterior oblique

Both right and left anterior oblique projections are employed to enable the bifurcation of either carotid artery to be visualised adequately. The actual degree of C-arm angulation is best determined with the aid of fluoroscopy as the vessel anatomy will vary between patients.

*Position of patient and imaging modality*

The patient adopts a similar position to that described for the postero-anterior projection.

*Direction and centring of the X-ray beam*

With the central ray angled 10° caudally, the X-ray tube is angled 15–35° away from the side being examined. The image intensifier is then brought close to the side being examined.

**Table 8.1 Imaging parameters**

| *Images/s* | *Run time* | *Total images* |
|---|---|---|
| 2 | 2 s | 4 |
| 1 | 6 s | 6 |

A 0.5 s injector delay allows a mask image to be acquired.

# 8 Neck Vessels

## Magnetic resonance imaging

Magnetic resonance angiography plays an important role in the investigation of carotid artery disease and is used mainly as a second-line investigation following ultrasound when this is equivocal. Both two- and three-dimensional time of flight (TOF) imaging protocols, described in Chapter 1, may be used. The former allows a shorter acquisition time and greater sensitivity to slow flow within the vessels, while the latter gives better signal to noise with the advantages of higher spatial resolution and better signal from tortuous vessels.

In the following text a 2D TOF protocol is described. During this procedure a series of thin axial slices are acquired of the neck region to create a stack or volume containing the vascular structures. For optimum demonstration of the vessels it is important that blood flow is perpendicular to each slice. To complete this investigation, examination of the circle of Willis may be performed.

**Position of patient and imaging modality**

The patient lies supine on the imaging couch and a receive coil is placed in position around the neck region. The head is adjusted with the anthropological baseline positioned parallel to the transaxial alignment light and the sagittal alignment light in line with the median sagittal plane. The table is then moved until the external reference point is at the centre of the coil. From this position the patient and coil is driven into the centre of the magnet.

**Imaging procedure**

A sagittal pilot scan is performed to obtain reference points for image acquisition in the transaxial plane. For the carotid bifurcation, a TOF pulse sequence with a flip angle of 60° is employed with 50–70 contiguous 1 mm axial slices acquired using flow compensation to correct flow-related phase errors. A presaturation pulse, 3 cm wide and 0.5 cm superior to the slice, is applied above each slice to eliminate signal from overlapping venous structures. The saturation pulse moves superiorly with each successive slice.

The saturation pulse is applied below the imaging volume to eliminate arterial signal if venous images are acquired.

Following image data acquisition, the image volume is subjected to a maximum intensity pixel (MIP) tracing technique to produce multiple projection images of the vascular structures about the longitudinal axis of the slices.

When the velocity of blood is slow and saturation of blood causes loss of signal from a vessel, MR contrast agents that shorten the $T_1$ of blood can be used to improve signal.

**Table 8.2 Imaging parameters – 2D time of flight**

| *TR* | *TE* | *Field of view (cm)* | *No of scans* | *No. of NEX* | *Slice width/gap (mm)* | *Matrix (h–v)* |
|---|---|---|---|---|---|---|
| 45 | 10 | 16–20 | 64 | 1 | 1 mm (no gap) | 128 × 256 |

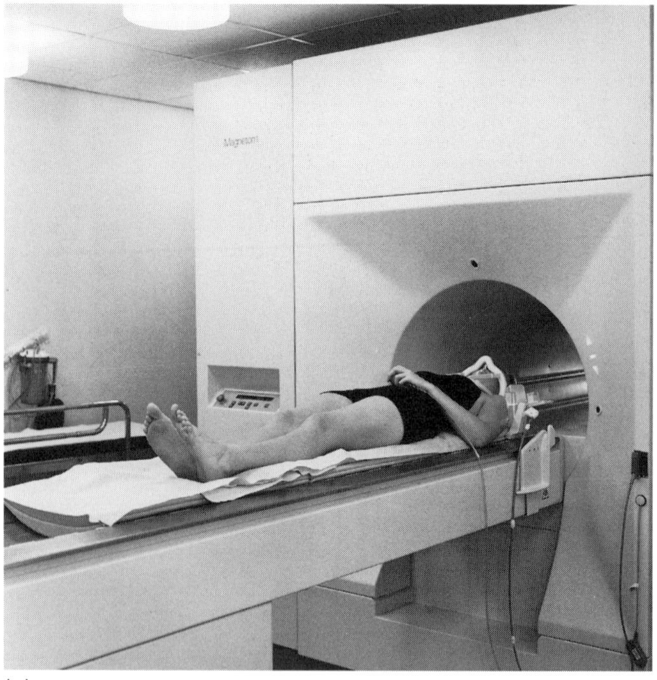

(a)

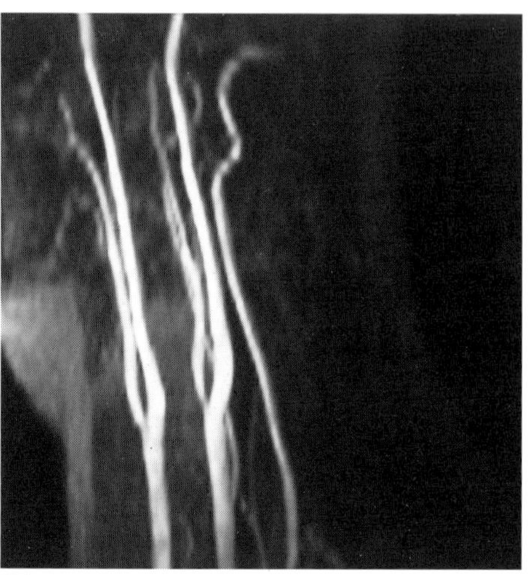

(b)

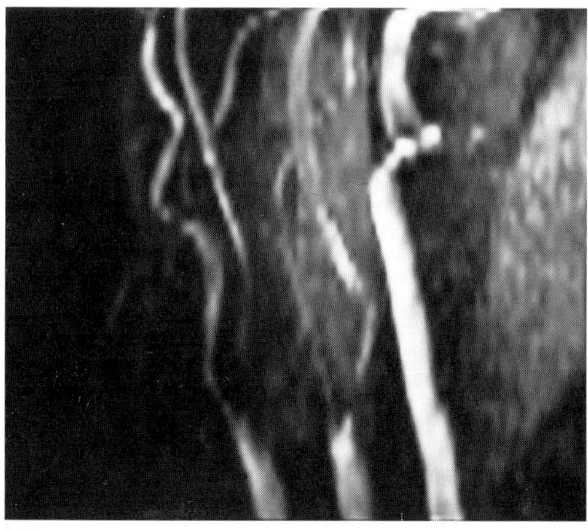

(c)

**Figure 8.5** (a) Patient and neck coil; (b) 2D TOF image showing normal carotid and vertebral arteries; (c) 2D TOF image showing abnormal carotid and vertebral arteries

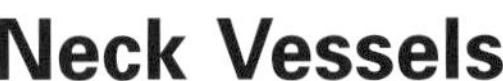

# Neck Vessels 8

## Ultrasound

(a)

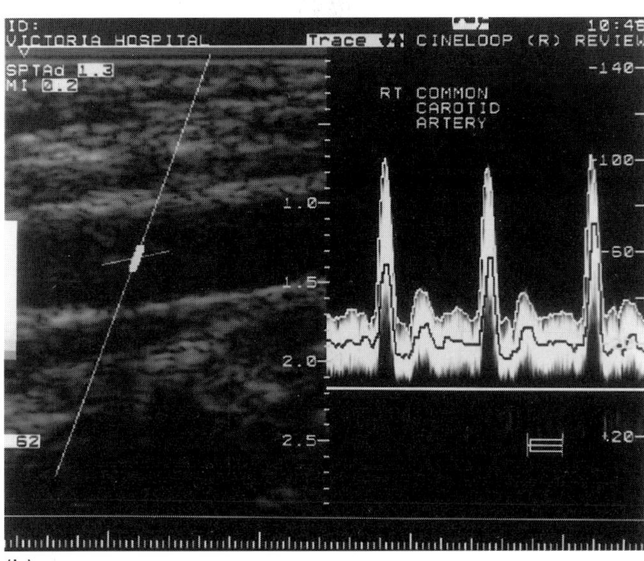


(b)

**Figure 8.6a** (a) Patient and transducer; (b) pulsed Doppler waveform from right common carotid artery

The neck vessels can be examined by means of ultrasound equipment which combines real-time B-mode imaging, pulsed Doppler and colour Doppler. Using this combination, vessel anatomy is demonstrated and blood flow quantified using spectral analysis.

### Indications

Suspected vascular disease at the carotid bifurcation, which is a common site of atherosclerotic lesions associated with transient ischaemic attacks.

### Position of patient and imaging modality

The patient normally is investigated supine. The neck is extended, with the head rotated away from the side being examined.

### Imaging procedure

A transverse scan is performed to locate the position of the carotid bifurcation and to orientate the vessels. The carotid arteries may then be imaged in the longitudinal plane by either an anterior or posterior oblique approach which will be decided on the basis of the transverse scan. Spectral analysis of the pulsed Doppler signal may be obtained by placing the sample volume at any point within the demonstrated vessel. A stenotic lesion is characterised by an increase in blood velocity, seen as an increase in frequency shift and spectral broadening. Beyond the site of the stenosis, marked changes in the flow waveform are seen due to flow turbulence a short way downstream from the lesion.

The dynamics of blood flow can also be demonstrated using colour flow mapping (see Plate 4). Blood flowing towards the transducer is seen by convention as shades of red and that flowing away as shades of blue. A colour bar scale on the screen will indicate the colour/velocity relationships. Abnormal turbulent blood flow at a site will be demonstrated on the image as a mosaic of colours.

**Table 8.3 Imaging modality parameters**

| | *Probe frequency* |
|---|---|
| B-mode | 7.5–10 MHz |
| Doppler | 4–5 MHz |

# 8 Cardiovascular System

## Heart

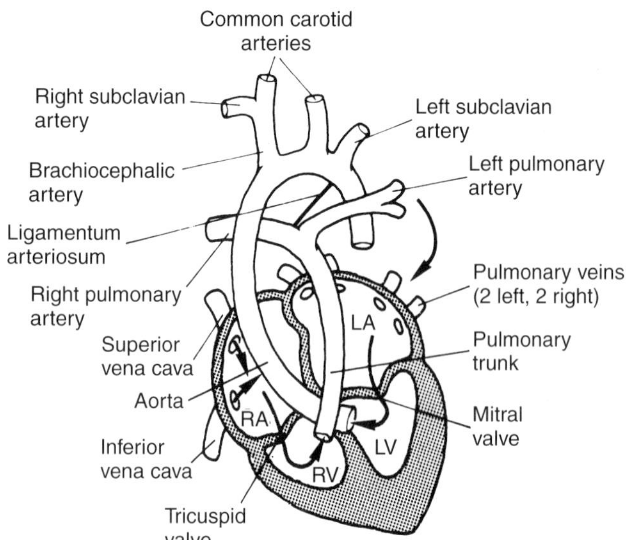


**Figure 8.7** Diagrammatic representation of blood flow through heart

The heart is a hollow muscular organ which, with the roots of the great vessels, is enclosed in a fibroserous sac, the pericardium. It is situated mainly to the left of the midline in the middle mediastinum attached to the central tendon of the diaphragm. The heart has four chambers: the right and left atria and the right and left ventricles. The atria are separated by the interatrial septum and the ventricles by the interventricular septum.

Blood circulates through the normal heart from the inferior vena cava and superior vena cava into the right atrium and through the tricuspid valve into the right ventricle. It then passes via the pulmonary valve into the pulmonary artery and on to the lungs. Blood returns to the heart via the pulmonary veins into the left atrium and then through the mitral valve into the left ventricle, where it passes through the aortic valve into the aorta. The blood supply to the cardiac muscle (myocardium) is by the coronary arteries which arise from the root of the aorta just above the aortic valve.

### Recommended imaging procedures

A postero-anterior radiograph is routinely performed to assess the shape and size of the heart. This may be supplemented with a lateral radiograph and occasionally a barium swallow is undertaken to identify abnormal impressions on the oesophagus as a result of enlargement of the heart and aorta.

Specialised investigations of the heart include the use of angiography, ultrasound using two-dimensional real-time scanning, M-mode, Doppler studies and intravascular techniques, RNI, MRI and CT. There are several RNI methods to evaluate cardiac disease and function. These include first pass studies (not described here – see reading list), perfusion and multi-gated acquisition (MUGA) scanning. These modalities are selected to demonstrate anatomy and to assess heart function which includes ventricular wall motion studies, measurement of ventricular volume and ejection fraction.

Where appropriate, a non-invasive modality such as ultrasound is selected as a preliminary investigation. This avoids the use of angiography which carries risks associated with ionising radiation, contrast agents and of the procedure itself.

### Indications

Included are ischaemic heart disease, valve disease, congenital defects, ventricular hypertrophy, arterial disease, tumours, thrombi, cardiomyopathy, and the detection of an aneurysm.

## Angiocardiography

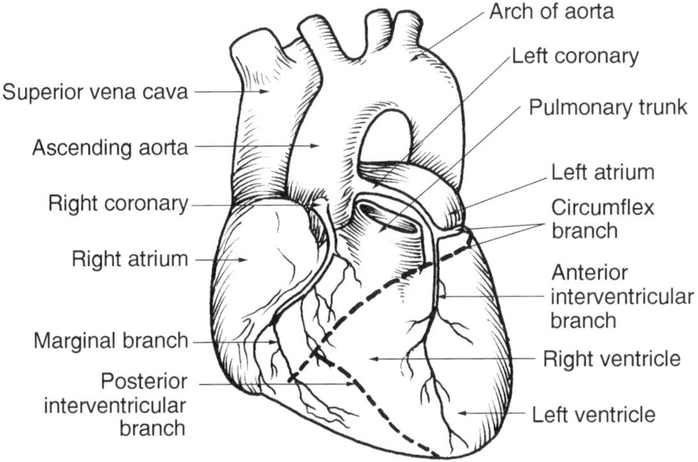


**Figure 8.8a** Coronary circulation – arterial

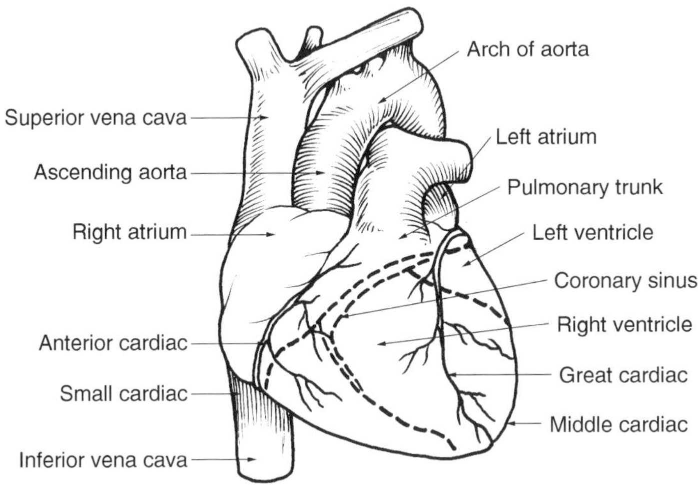


**Figure 8.8b** Coronary circulation – venous

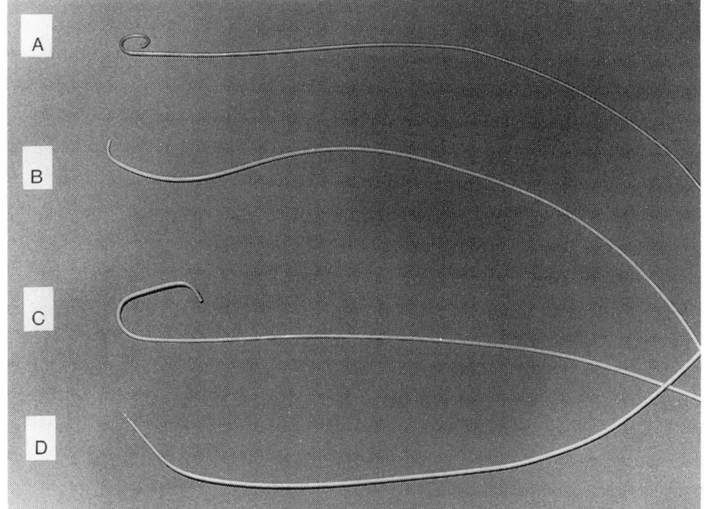


**Figure 8.8c** Typical catheters used in cardiac procedures: (A) 6F 'pigtail' for left ventricular angiogram and arch aortogram (high-pressure injection 900 psi); (B) 7F 'right coronary' catheter – hand injection; (C) 7F 'left coronary' catheter – hand injection; (D) 7F 'brachial' catheter for left ventricular angiogram and cannulation of the left coronary artery

Angiocardiography is the demonstration of the cardiac chambers and major vessels of the heart using a non-ionic contrast agent following cardiac catheterisation. In this section, left ventricular angiography (LVA) is described. Right ventricular angiography is not described but is similar to LVA and may be employed when investigating ventricular anatomy and dysplasia. A contrast pressure injector is employed for studies of the heart chambers, aorta ventricular and the pulmonary artery using catheter pressures up to 900 psi. Coronary arteriography is performed following selective coronary artery catheterisation with the contrast medium injected by hand.

Dedicated isocentric angiographic equipment, with single or preferably using bi-plane imaging, is necessary for the series of complex projections of the heart required for each study. Dynamic image acquisition is by means of digital imaging with the quantitative analysis facilities necessary for assessment of heart function and for quantifying the degree of coronary artery disease. Optimum image definition is provided using 23 cm image intensifiers. A number of centres may acquire dynamic studies using conventional 35 mm cine fluorography.

Access to the left side of the heart is commonly performed following retrograde catheterisation of a femoral artery or alternatively using a brachial approach. The right side of the heart is by means of a femoral vein or brachial vein approach. During all investigations the patient's ECG and blood pressure is continuously monitored. In a number of investigations blood samples are taken for evaluation of oxygen content together with recordings of intracardiac pressures.

A variety of catheters with special preformed shapes are available for these investigations to maximise optimum distribution of contrast within the heart chambers and to facilitate selective coronary artery cannulation.

### Indications

Congenital heart defects, ischaemic heart disease, ventricular dysfunction, cardiac aneurysms and valvular disease. Selective coronary angiography for mapping the position and extent of atheromatous plaques and arterial occlusions and during interventional procedures to monitor and assess the effect of treatment.

### Contraindications

In cases of gross heart failure, procedures may be postponed until the patient's condition has stabilised. Risks associated with known contrast allergies, hypertension, recent myocardial infarction and ventricular irritability will be assessed by the clinician, with appropriate care given to the patient prior to the procedure. There are no absolute contraindications. In serious cases, the benefits far outweigh the risks.

# 8 Heart

## Left ventricular angiography

This procedure is used to assess the function and regional wall motion of the left ventricle as well as demonstrating movement of the mitral and aortic valves. The right anterior oblique projection is usually selected and is supplemented by the left anterior oblique when more detail of the ventricle is required. A typical technique using a single plane unit is described.

**Position of patient and imaging modality**

The patient is supine in the middle of the imaging couch, with the arms raised above the head which rests on a shallow pillow. The image intensifier is first positioned above the anterior chest wall and parallel to the imaging couch. A 7F or 8F pigtail catheter is then positioned in the left ventricle under fluoroscopic control.

**Direction and centring of the X-ray beam**

*Right anterior oblique*: The X-ray tube is rotated towards the left side of the patient so that it is angled at 30° to the median sagittal plane. The image intensifier input field is positioned adjacent to the right anterior chest wall.

In this projection the anterior and inferior walls of the left ventricle and mitral valve are demonstrated.

*Left anterior oblique*: The X-ray tube is rotated towards the right side of the patient until it is angled at 40–60° to the median sagittal plane. The image intensifier is positioned adjacent to the left anterior chest wall.

In this projection the posterior wall of the ventricle, the interventricular septum and the aortic outflow tract are demonstrated.

**Imaging parameters:**

*Digital imaging*: Imaging lasts approximately 5–7 s using image acquisition speeds of 50 images/s for children and 25 images/s for adults.

*Cine fluorography*: 25 or 50 frames/s for approximately 5–7 s.

*Contrast medium and injector data*

| *Volume* | *Concentration* | *Flow rate* |
|---|---|---|
| 30–50 ml | 340–370 mgI/ml | 10–20 ml/s |

Using digital imaging the concentration may be reduced.

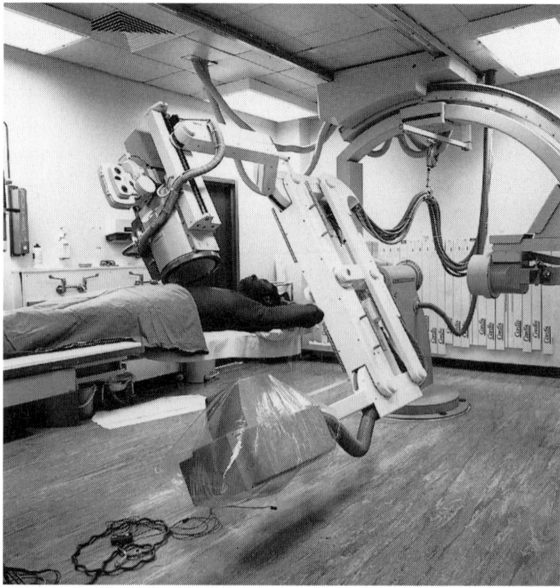

**Figure 8.9a** Positioning for RAO 30° projection

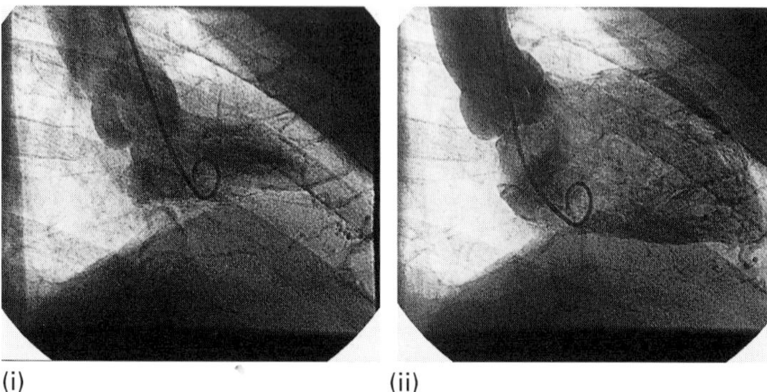

(i) (ii)

**Figure 8.9b** RAO 30° images in (i) end-systole, and (ii) end-diastole

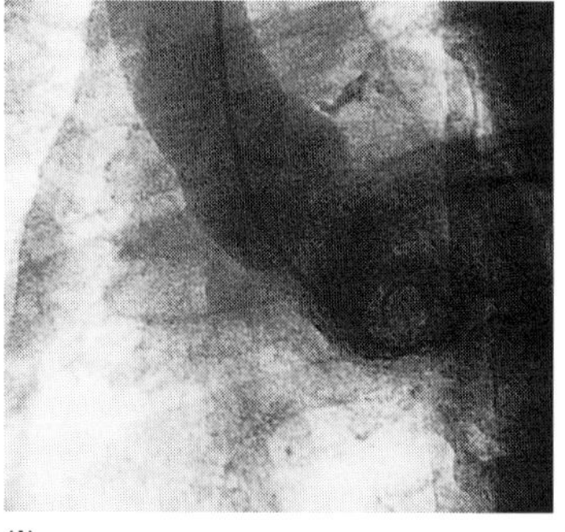

(i)

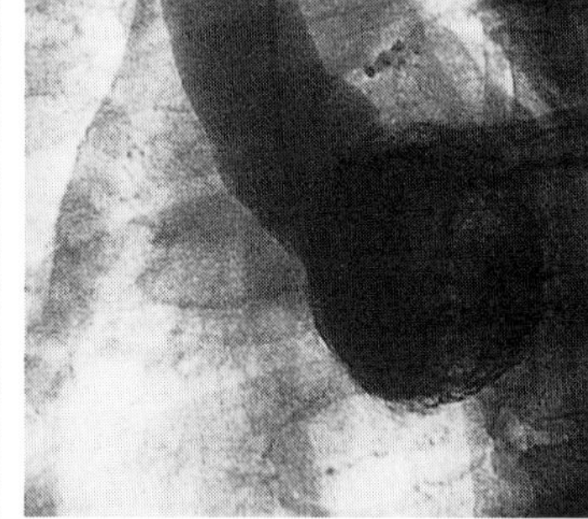

(ii)

**Figure 8.9c** LAO 45° images in (i) end-systole, and (ii) end-diastole

## Left ventricular angiography

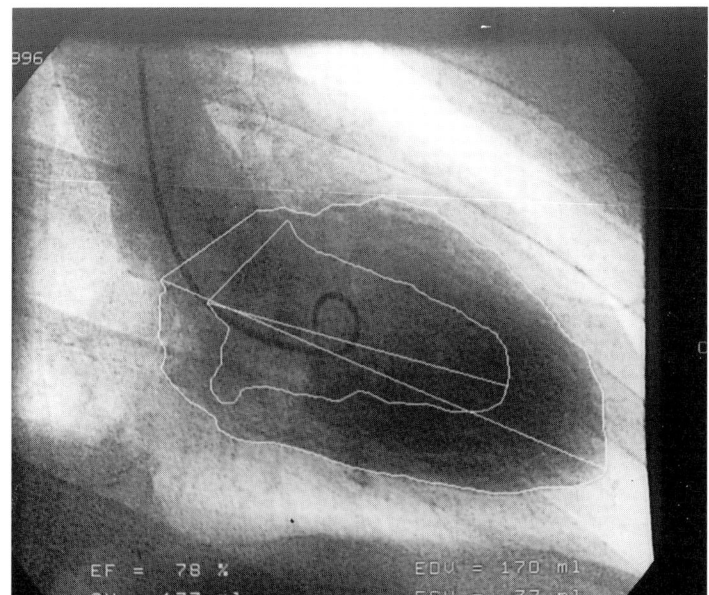


**Figure 8.10a** LVA image showing calculation of: ejection fraction, 78%; stroke volume, 133 ml; end-diastole volume, 170 ml; end-systole volume, 37 ml

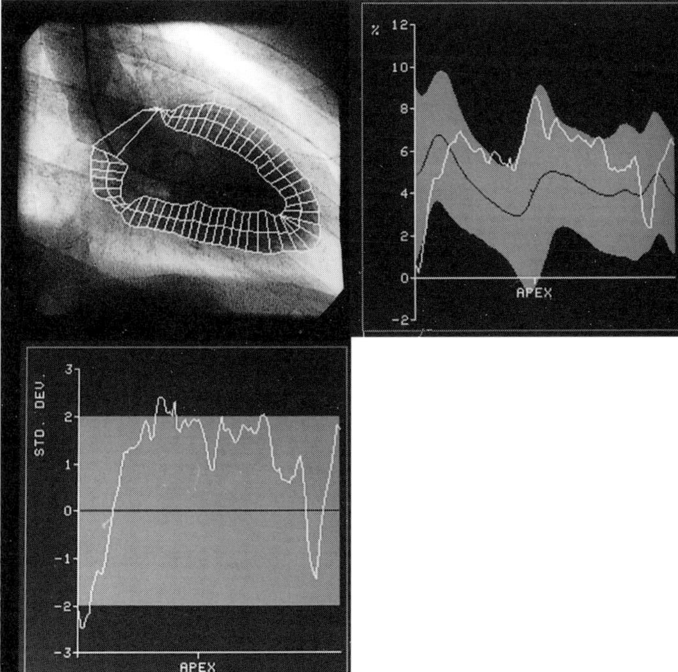


**Figure 8.10b** Composite image showing evaluation of left ventricular contraction using a centre-line wall motion program

### Analysis of LVA

Digital imaging review techniques or specialised cine projectors enable the dynamic function of blood flow through the heart chambers and valves to be assessed.

This is particularly relevant in the investigation of stenotic and incompetent valves and the abnormal blood flow patterns associated with congenital and acquired defects. Ventricular wall motion can also be determined when evaluating the effects of compromised myocardium due to aneurysms or ischaemia.

With the application of computer analysis techniques associated with digital imaging or specialised 35 mm cine projection systems, evaluation of cardiac ejection fraction is possible from images acquired in the RAO 30° projection.

In digital imaging a calibration routine is normally required, using a centimetre grid or sphere with a size of at least 3 cm to ensure accurate calibration. This is normally performed after the procedure, with the test object in the same position as the heart during the LV image acquisition. Images of the left ventricle at end-systole and end-diastole during the same image sequence, with the same imaging geometry, are selected. Contours of the ventricle in these phases are drawn either manually or automatically using edge detection techniques. The computer will then calculate the area and length of the ventricle and indicate the end-systolic and end-diastolic volumes together with the stroke volume and the ejection fraction.

Assessment of cardiac wall motion, in relative terms, is also possible with digital imaging using a variety of software applications, e.g. regional wall motion, centre-line wall motion and Slager wall motion which assesses regional left ventricular motion using endocardial landmarks. The centre-line wall motion program, seen opposite, is used to calculate and demonstrate the extent of contraction of the wall of the left ventricle between the ends of the diastolic and systolic phases of the heart cycle. Prior to running this program, an ejection fraction program is run to obtain the required data. As a result, there is available a selected image of the heart in the end-diastolic phase with superimposed outlines of the left ventricle in the end-systolic phase. Following selection of the wall motion function, a line is plotted on the monitor mid-way between the outlines of the left ventricle in its end-diastole and end-systole locations. Subsequently, 100 perpendicular chords are constructed across the line to meet the end-diastole and end-systole outlines, with every other one of these shown superimposed on the display image. The algorithm used assumes that each chord represents the line of direction of wall contraction in its area and the length of the chord is expressed as percentages of the end-diastole circumferences in their regions and is plotted graphically along with the expected normal range. An additional graph comparing the results with statistical data is also provided.

# 8 Heart

## Coronary arteriography

Selective coronary arteriography enables assessment of vessel anatomy and pathology and is performed in conjunction with interventional procedures such as angioplasty and stent insertion.

**Position of patient and imaging modality**

The patient is supine, the head rests on a shallow pillow and the arms raised above the head. The image intensifier is first positioned over the anterior chest wall and parallel to the imaging couch. In this position a suitable catheter is directed into either the right or left coronary artery under fluoroscopic control.

Investigations of the left and right coronary arteries and their respective branches involve the use of simple and compound projections to demonstrate vessels free of superimposition of other vessels. Each vessel requires multiple projections, often taken at right angles to each other, and the X-ray tube/image intensifier C-arm gantry is rotated into one of the standard preset positions ready for image acquisition. Adjustment to these angles may be required according to variations in individual anatomy. In all cases the image intensifier will be positioned as close as practicable to the patient's chest wall with the X-ray tube angled beneath the patient relative to the median sagittal plane. A selection of standard X-ray tube angulations which may be employed is seen in Table 8.4.

**Imaging procedure**

Image acquisition takes place during the hand injection of contrast medium, with the imaging couch top normally moved during the acquisition to ensure that the full extent of the arterial branches is demonstrated. Imaging lasts approximately 5–7 s, using digital acquisition rates of 12.5 or 25 images/s or with cine 25 or 50 frames/s.

*Contrast medium and injector data*

| *Volume* | *Concentration* | *Flow rate* |
|---|---|---|
| 3–10 ml | 340–370 mgI/ml | Hand injection |

Using digital imaging, the concentration may be reduced.

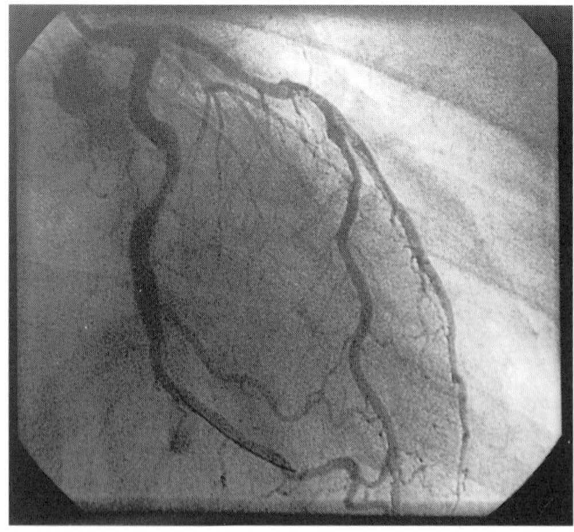

**Figure 8.11a** Routine RAO 30° image of left coronary artery

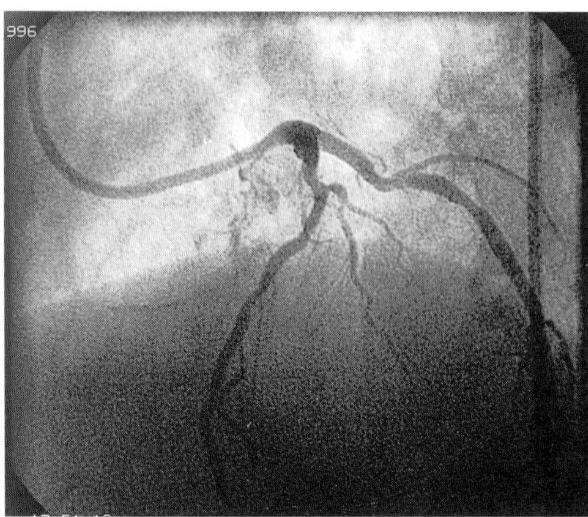

**Figure 8.11b** LAO 43° image with 30° cranial angulation of left coronary artery

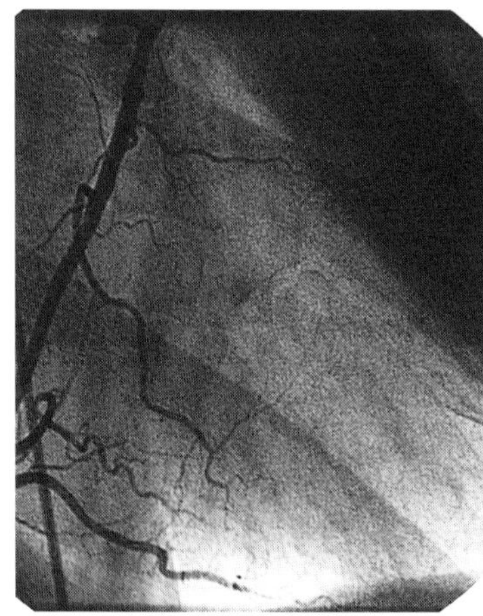

**Figure 8.11c** Routine LAO 50° image

**Table 8.4 Some X-ray tube angulations**

| *Artery* | *X-ray tube angulation* | *Vessels demonstrated* |
|---|---|---|
| Left | Right anterior oblique (RAO) 30° | Routine – view of main stem, circumflex system and left anterior descending (LAD) |
| Left | RAO 30° and 20° caudal | Separates LAD and diagonal arteries |
| Left | RAO 5° and 35° cranial | Profiles LAD |
| Left | LAO 50° and 25° cranial | Routine overall view |
| Left | Left lateral | Routine – good separation of LAD and circumflex |
| Left | Postero-anterior | Opens up left main coronary artery and LAD |
| Right | LAO 50° and 15° caudal | Routine – good visualisation of proximal and middle arteries |
| Right | RAO 5° and 35° cranial | Distal vessels, posterior descending and posterolateral vessels |
| Right | RAO 40° | Proximal and mid, posterior interventricular and collateral branches |

## Coronary arteriography

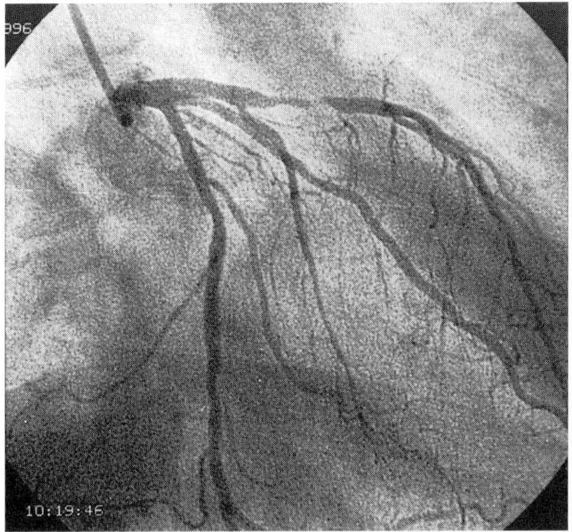


**Figure 8.12a** RAO 30° image with 23° caudal angulation showing a stenotic lesion in the left anterior descending artery

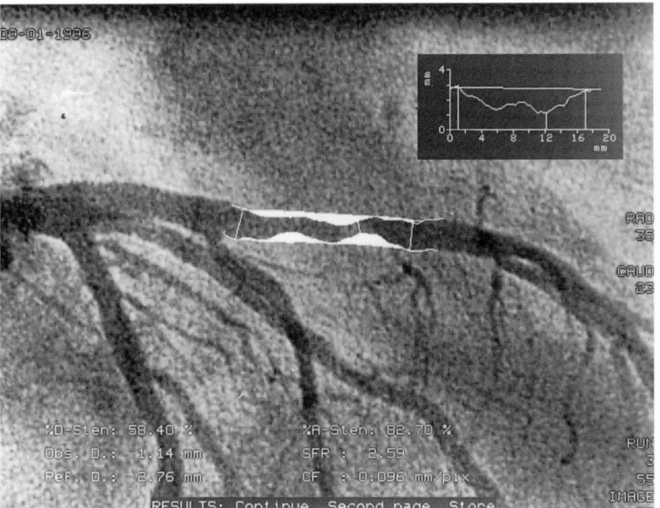


**Figure 8.12b** Digital image showing assessment of vessel diameter along the length of the stenotic lesion

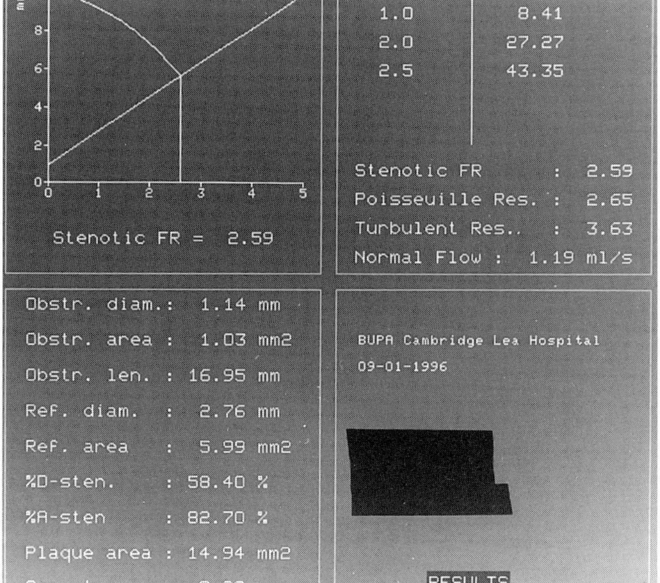


**Figure 8.12c** Typical printout of results following assessment of diseased vessel

**Image analysis**

Evaluation of blood flow through the coronary arteries and detailed study of vessel anatomy is accomplished by the use of either 35 mm cine projection or computer playback and analysis of digital images. For long-term viewing the digital data can be stored on various recording media, including optical disc, compact disc and video tape. Using digital imaging, quantitative assessment of vessel diameter and the severity of coronary artery narrowing can be accomplished. Other digital software features include roadmapping, contrast and edge enhancement, window width and window level adjustments, image inversion and zoom functions. Images of vessels from a 35 mm cine film frame or the digital imaging playback monitor can be recorded on single emulsion film.

The measurement of vessel diameter and assessment of the severity of vessel narrowing is performed using a software package supplied with the digital imaging equipment. Initially, a calibration routine is performed from an image of a catheter of a known size positioned in a coronary vessel. This determines the magnification factor which enables the computer to calculate actual vessel dimensions. Margins of a narrowed segment of artery are defined using automatic edge detection techniques, after which the computer presents a detailed set of geometric calculations relating to the length, diameter and cross-sectional area of the stenotic lesion. These results may be stored along with the accompanying image and kept to compare with the results of findings following angioplasty.

*Roadmapping*

Dynamic roadmapping of the coronary vessels during procedures such as angioplasty presents a challenge due to the fast action of the heart. Conventional roadmapping, however, as used with the peripheral vessels, is not suitable due to the misregistration of mask and 'real-time' images produced as a result of cardiac movement. To overcome this problem, acquisition of the live fluoroscopy image and the acquired image are synchronised to the patient's ECG.

In this way the dynamic roadmap follows the motion of the heart to allow precise placement of guide wires and balloon catheters. It is essential that neither the imaging equipment nor the patient moves during this procedure.

# 8 Heart

## Ultrasound (echocardiography)

Cardiac ultrasound, otherwise known as echocardiography, using two-dimensional real-time scanning, M-mode and Doppler, offers a non-invasive method of examining the heart. Both qualitative and quantitative information relating to heart disease and function is readily obtainable. In many cases echocardiography is the only imaging modality selected. The investigation is accomplished with specialised ultrasound equipment using a hand-held phased array electronic sector scanning probe. Two-dimensional imaging is employed initially and then used to direct M-mode and Doppler studies. Information from the different studies can be displayed on the same viewing monitor either in dynamic or still mode, with a record of an ECG tracing taken during the examination. Using a built-in microprocessor, various features can be measured and calculated. The equipment comes with a number of special features such as a zoom facility to magnify parts of the image and a speaker system to enable audible tones of Doppler blood flow to be heard. Video recordings of the examination gives a permanent record of the procedure which can be reviewed and used to assess changes in the patient's condition.

Echocardiography can also be performed using a 5 MHz transoesophageal probe. This gives better image detail, particularly of the atria and the valves.

Intravascular ultrasound, using an ultrasound imaging catheter, enables real-time cross-sectional imaging of the coronary arteries. This plays an important role before and during interventional procedures in providing information on plaque distribution and composition as well as enabling measurement of vessel size and plaque thickness. Accurate assessment of the type and extent of disease will enable the clinician to select the most appropriate interventional procedure.

### Indications

Congenital heart disease, myocardial abnormalities, tumours, valve disease, pericardial effusion and ischaemic heart disease.

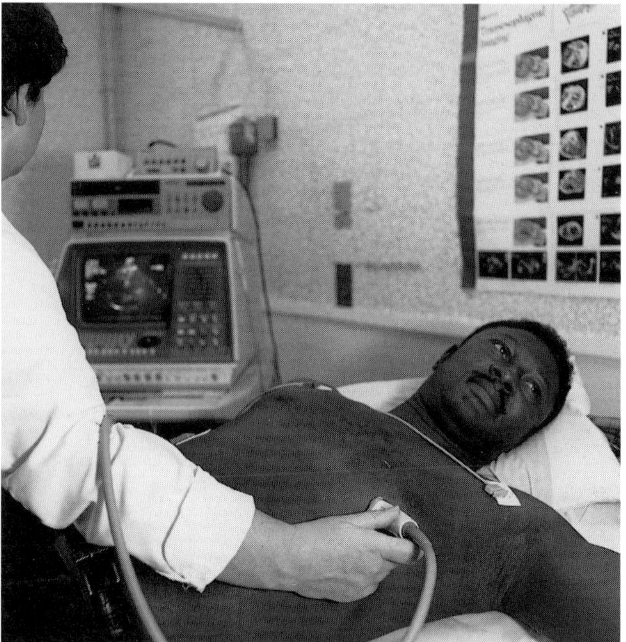

**Figure 8.13a** The transducer

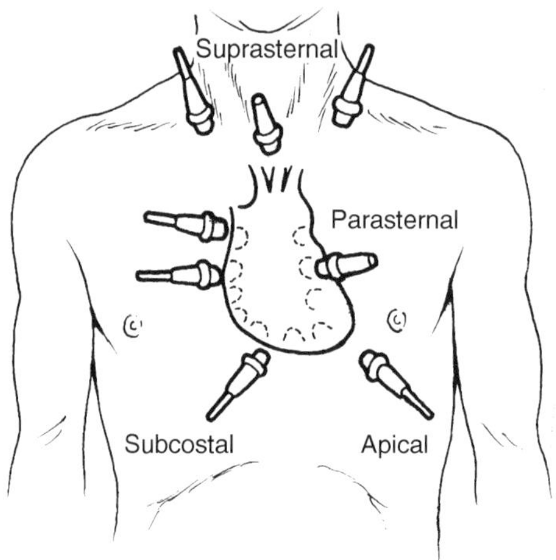


**Figure 8.13b** Typical scanning locations

### Two-dimensional imaging

The heart is examined in the long and short axes in order to assess its anatomy and function.

*Position of patient and imaging modality*

For the long axis, short axis, apical four-chamber and apical five-chamber views the patient is rotated from the supine position approximately 50° onto the left side. This allows the heart to assume a position closer to the chest wall to enable better imaging. For the subcostal and suprasternal views the patient lies supine on the examination couch.

**Table 8.5 Summary of views and scanning locations**

| *View* | *Location* |
|---|---|
| Long axis parasternal | Left parasternal 4th intercostal notch |
| Short axis parasternal | Left parasternal 4th intercostal notch |
| Apical four-chamber | Cardiac apex |
| Apical five-chamber | Cardiac apex |
| Suprasternal | Suprasternal notch |
| Subcostal | Sub-xiphoid |

## Ultrasound (echocardiography)

Figure 8.14a Long axis view showing aortic valve closed

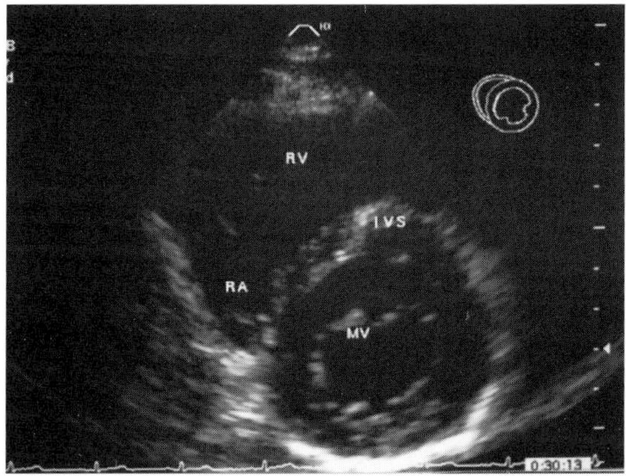


**Figure 8.14b** Short axis view at the level of the mitral valve

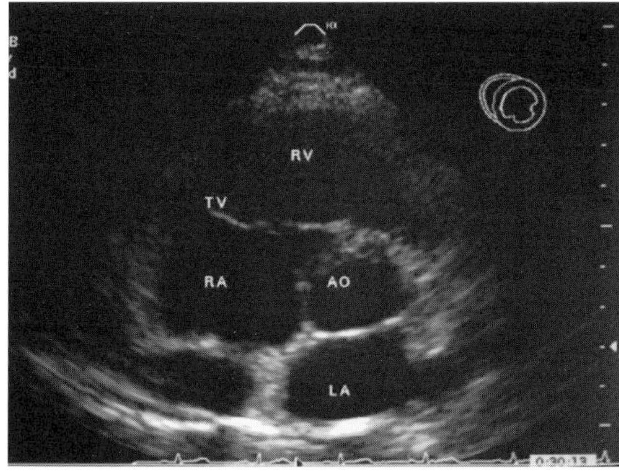


**Figure 8.14c** Short axis view at the level of the aortic root

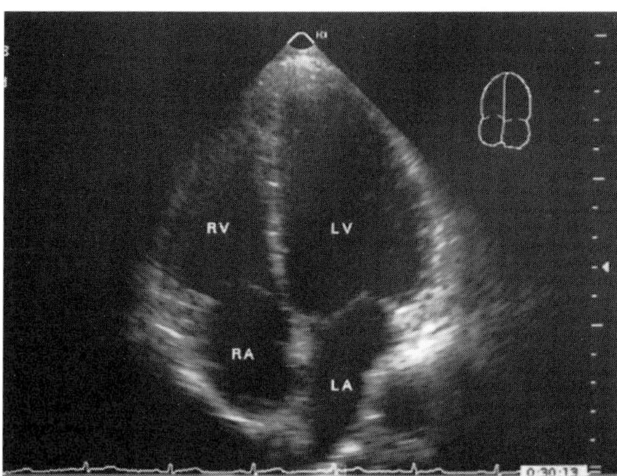


**Figure 8.14d** Four-chamber apical view

*Imaging procedure*

A typical imaging protocol comprises five views of the heart, starting with the parasternal long axis view, and continues with the short axis, apical four-chamber, five-chamber and subcostal views. The imaging transducer is positioned at selected locations for each view (Table 8.5). These locations represent acoustic windows, avoiding bony structures such as the ribs and sternum and air in the lungs. Careful angulation of the transducer at these locations will enable visualisation of different anatomical details at oblique angles from the planes selected.

Real-time scanning enables observation of cardiac wall motion and valve function.

Cardiac dimensions can also be measured from static images which make it possible to calculate valve area cross-sections and ventricular size.

Table 8.6 indicates the anatomical features demonstrated.

**Table 8.6 Summary of views with associated anatomical features**

| *View* | *Anatomy* |
|---|---|
| Long axis | Left ventricle (LV) and left atrium (LA)<br>Mitral valve (MV) and aortic valve (AV)<br>Right ventricle (RV)<br>Interventricular septum (IVS) |
| Short axis | LV and LA<br>RV and right atrium (RA) |
| Apical four-chamber | Both ventricles and both atria<br>Mitral and tricuspid valves (TV)<br>Interatrial septum<br>Interventricular septum |
| Apical five-chamber | As four-chamber view plus aortic valve |
| Suprasternal | Aortic arch<br>Great vessels |
| Subcostal | As four-chamber view plus interatrial septum and interventricular septum |

*Transducer parameters*

| *Type* | *Probe frequency* | |
|---|---|---|
| 80° phased array sector transducer | Adult | 2.5–5.0 MHz |
| | Child | 5.0–10.0 MHz |

# 8 Heart

## Ultrasound (echocardiography)

### M-mode studies

M-mode studies are performed in conjunction with two-dimensional echocardiography to assess function of the left ventricle, aortic valve and mitral valve. During acquisition, ECG tracings are recorded simultaneously to enable accurate timing of events in the cardiac cycle.

M-mode is best selected in the long and short axis views to produce tracings of the movement of cardiac anatomy perpendicular to the ultrasonic beam. From these tracings various parameters are measured: ventricular wall thickness, chamber size, contractility and ejection fraction. Valve thickness is determined and the degree of valve movement assessed. Slope characteristics of the rate of valve opening and closing may be measured and the information used to calculate the surface size of the valve orifice. The accompanying tracings are typical of a standard investigation, with Figure 8.15b indicating the relative positioning of the transducer.

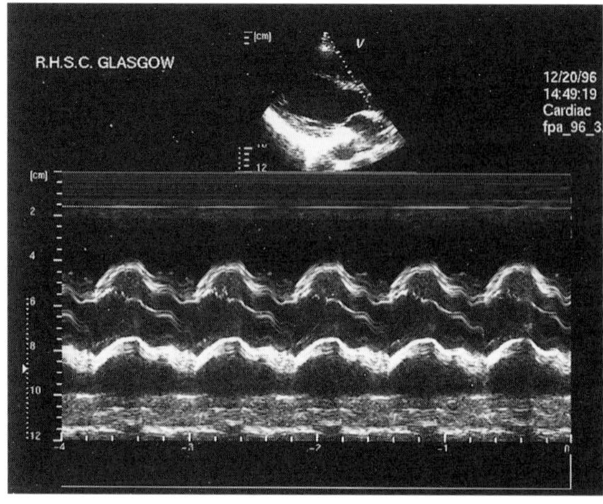


**Figure 8.15a** Tracing demonstrating aortic route diameter, aortic valve excursion, left atrium dimension, aortic route and left atrium cavity

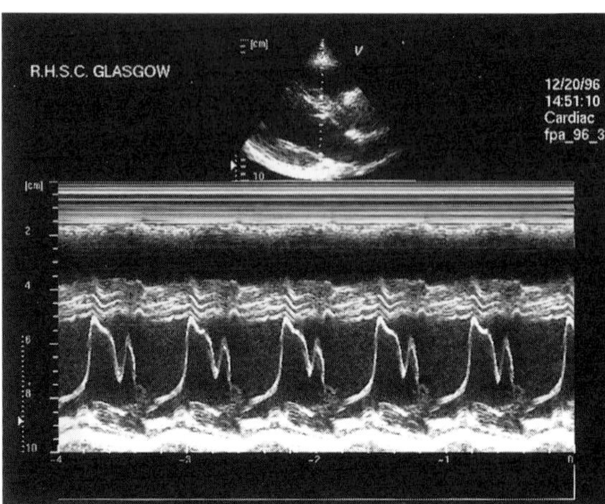


**Figure 8.15c** Tracing demonstrating right ventricle cavity and excursion of the anterior and posterior mitral valve leaflets

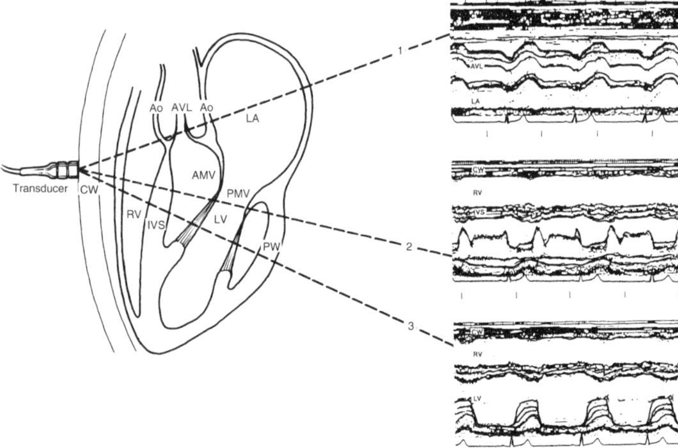


**Figure 8.15b** CW, chest wall; RV, right ventricle; IVS, interventricular septum; Ao, aorta; AVL, aortic valve leaflets; AMV, anterior mitral valve leaflets; PMV, posterior mitral valve leaflet; LA, left atrium; LV, left ventricle; PW, posterior LV wall

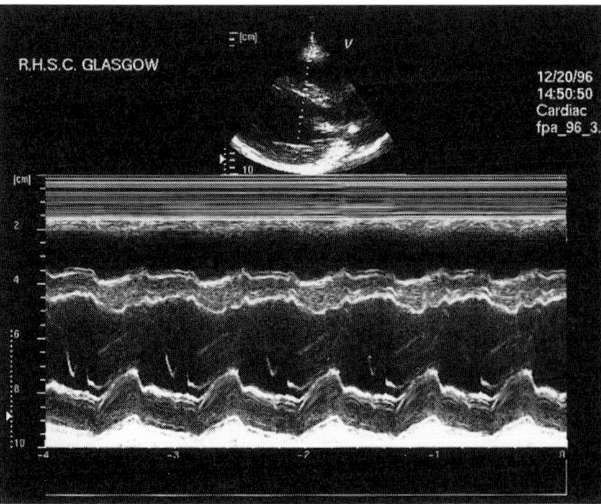


**Figure 8.15d** Tracing demonstrating right and left ventricular cavities, interventricular septum and posterior wall

### Doppler studies

Doppler studies are performed by means of pulsed wave Doppler (PWD), continuous wave Doppler (CWD) or colour flow (see Plates 5–8). These applications enable blood flow patterns and velocities through the heart chambers and valves to be studied. To ensure accurate velocity measurements, the transducer beam is positioned parallel to the direction of blood flow.

An assessment of the effect of valve disease can be made by positioning the sample volume cursor at the site of the valve and studying the velocity, direction of flow, timing and intensity of the spectral information obtained. Jets of blood associated with stenotic valves can be observed, as well as the regurgitation of blood associated with incompetent valves. By convention, blood flowing toward it will appear above the zero line and that flowing away from it below the line. PWD is only able to detect a limited range of flow velocities. If the peak velocity exceeds this range, an artefact known as aliasing occurs which renders measurements inaccurate. Continuous wave Doppler overcomes the problem, as it measures a greater range of velocities, but it has the disadvantage that the location of the sample within the patient is less well defined.

Pressure gradients within the heart can also be calculated from the peak velocity of flow by application of the modified Bernoulli equation, $P = 4V^2$, where $P$ = pressure gradient in mmHg, and $V$ = peak velocity of flow in m/s. Estimation of the severity of valve stenosis as a valve area, as in mitral stenosis, is also possible using Doppler. By calculating the pressure 'half-time', it is possible to estimate the valve area.

The dynamics of blood flow can be highlighted using colour flow mapping. Blood flowing towards the transducer is seen by convention as shades of red and that flowing away as shades of blue. A colour bar scale on the screen will indicate the colour/velocity relationships. Turbulent blood at a specific site is demonstrated on the image as a mosaic of colours. This procedure is useful in cases of congenital and septal defects. While colour Doppler is useful in many areas of heart disease, it is particularly helpful in congenital problems.

### Intravascular ultrasound (IVUS)

Real-time cross-sectional images of the endoluminal structures are produced using a special 10–30 MHz imaging catheter which is positioned in the selected coronary vessel using the conventional over-the-guidewire technique. During angioplasty it is used to measure luminal diameter and to calculate percentage stenosis, characterise tissue pathology and assist in the selection of the optimal balloon size. It is used to evaluate the lumen after intervention and is also used in the management of stenting and atherectomy.

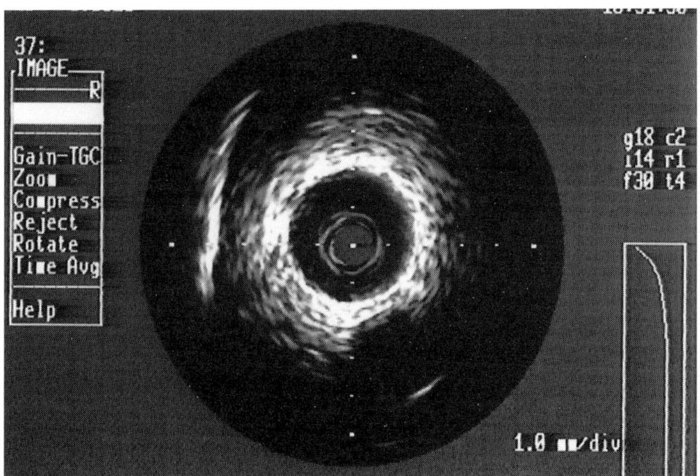


**Figure 8.16** Typical intravascular ultrasound image

# 8 Heart

## Radionuclide imaging – perfusion studies

Perfusion myocardial scanning is performed using either $^{201}$Tl, $^{99}$Tc MIBI (Cardiolite) or $^{99}$Tc tetrofosmin (Myoview) to assess myocardial blood flow.

Static imaging or single photon emission computed tomography (SPECT) is employed using a gamma camera linked to a computer for image analysis. Imaging is normally associated with some form of stress induction and a period of rest. Images acquired immediately post-exercise may show perfusion defects related to either ischaemia or necrosis. If repeat scans after a period of rest show reperfusion, ischaemia rather than infarction will be diagnosed. The procedure is supervised by a clinician with continual ECG monitoring of the patient.

### Indications

Atypical chest pain, suspected ischaemia and to assess improvement following coronary artery bypass grafting or angioplasty.

### Position of patient and imaging modality

*Static imaging*

Static imaging consists of four views: anterior, 45°, 55° or 70° left anterior oblique and left lateral. For the anterior view the patient is supine on the imaging couch, with both arms by the side of the body. The gamma camera head is positioned parallel to the imaging couch over the anterior chest wall, ensuring that the cardiac region is in the centre of the imaging field. From this position the camera head is rotated through the appropriate angle and placed against the left chest wall for the other views, with the left arm is raised above the head.

*SPECT*

SPECT is employed using a circular or elliptical tomograph with a 180° arc for $^{201}$Tl and a 360° or 180° elliptical arc for $^{99}$Tc MIBI or $^{99}$Tc tetrofosmin.

The patient lies supine on the imaging couch, with arms raised and held together above the head. The patient and camera head are centralised relative to the heart to ensure a safe sweep of the camera.

The camera starts in the 45° right anterior oblique position and terminates its movement in the 45° left posterior oblique position when employing the 180° arc.

*Imaging and radiopharmaceutical parameters*

| *Type* | *Administered activity* | *Principal energy* |
|---|---|---|
| $^{201}$Tl | 75 MBq | 65–82 keV |
| $^{99}$Tc MIBI | 300–400 MBq | 140 keV |
| $^{99}$Tc tetrofosmin | 300–400 MBq | 140 keV |

| *Window width* | | *Acquisition counts/time* |
|---|---|---|
| $^{201}$Tl | 20% | Static 300 000 counts |
| $^{99}$Tc MIBI | 20% | 360° SPECT – 64 views at 20–30 s per view |
| $^{99}$Tc tetrofosmin | 20% | 180° SPECT – 32 views at 25–30 s per view |

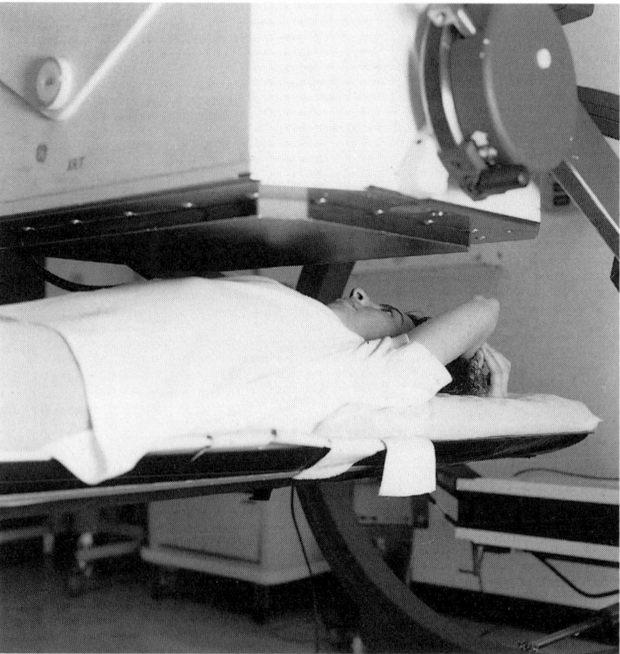

**Figure 8.17a** Gamma camera positioned for SPECT

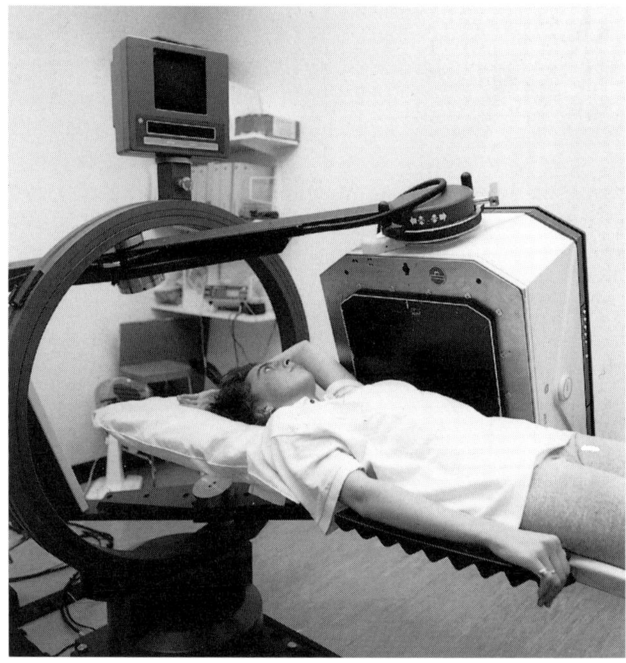

**Figure 8.17b** Gamma camera positioned for 70° left anterior oblique

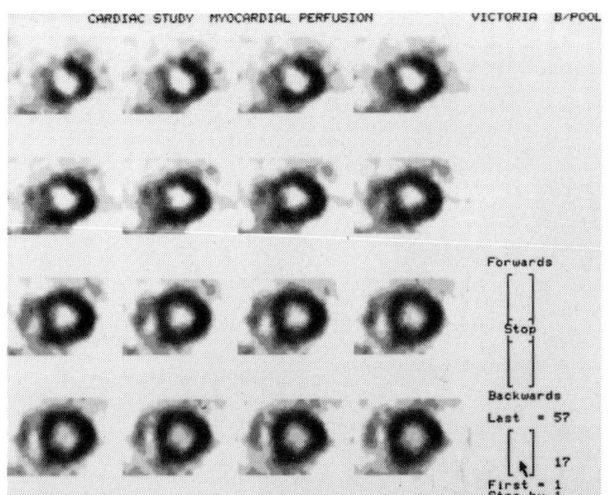

Figure 8.18a Series of 'stress' short-axis SPECT images

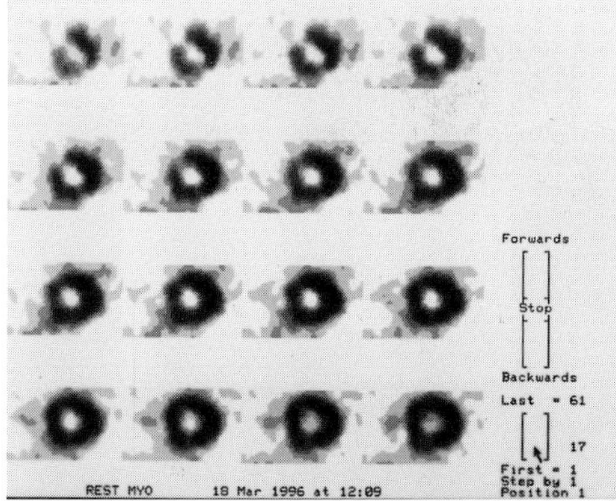

**Figure 8.18b** Series of 'rest' short-axis SPECT images

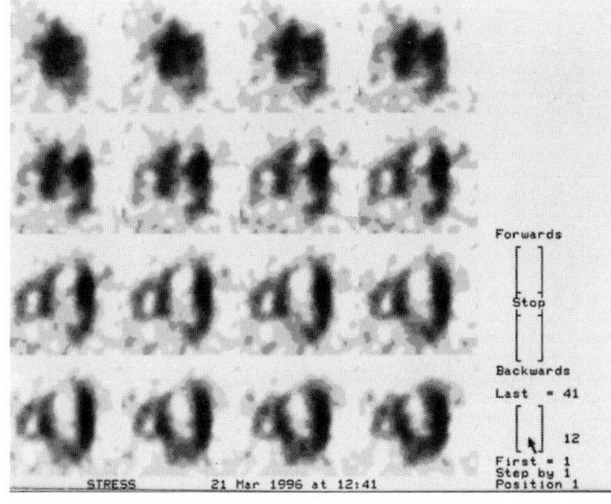

**Figure 8.18c** Series of 'stress' horizontal long-axis SPECT images showing decreased perfusion in the apical region

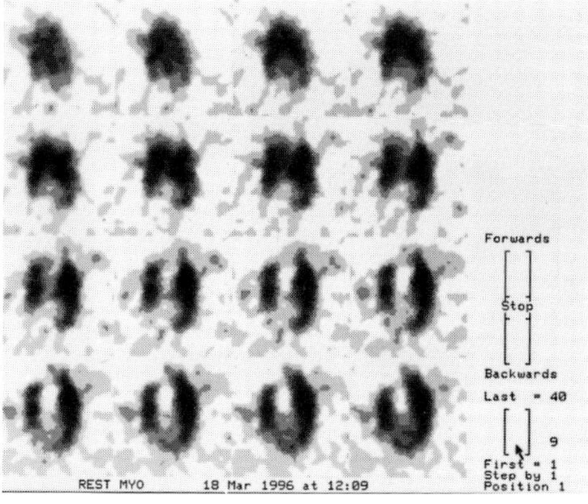

**Figure 8.18d** Series of 'rest' horizontal long-axis SPECT images



## Radionuclide imaging – perfusion studies

### Imaging procedure

A high-resolution collimator and an image magnification technique are selected. Unless clinically contraindicated, cardiac stress is induced using a treadmill or exercise bicycle. If the patient is unable to exercise, stress can be induced using a coronary vasodilator (e.g. dipyridamole). When the patient's heart rate reaches a rate of 225 minus age, the radionuclide is given i.v. and exercise continued for a further 1–2 min to maximise its distribution in the cardiac muscle. Constant ECG monitoring will indicate how long it takes for the heart rate to normalise. If thallium is injected, imaging commences immediately, with further rest images taken after a period of 2 h. When Cardiolite or Myoview is used, imaging may be delayed for 1/2–1½ h following exercise to allow the patient to recover and to have a fatty meal. The meal improves imaging by separating the stomach from the cardiac region and encourages hepatobiliary clearance of the radiopharmaceutical. As Cardiolite and Myoview do not redistribute the way thallium does, a further investigation on another day is required to demonstrate the cardiac muscle at rest.

### Image analysis

Following the acquisition of data and computer image enhancement techniques, subjective assessment of the static images is made by the clinician on the colour display monitor. If SPECT is employed, correction for the normal oblique position of the heart is made prior to the production of reconstructed segmented images taken in the vertical long, horizontal long and short axes of the heart. The resulting tomograms allow a qualitative assessment of perfusion.

The isotope images provided by both procedures can be used to differentiate regions of the myocardium supplied by specific coronary vessels. Perfusion defects in any region will be directly related to an occlusion or stenotic lesion associated with the vessel supplying it.

Hard copies of these images and quantitative information of isotope uptake are kept for further comparison at a later date.

Quantitative analysis and bull's-eye images can be produced with additional software.

# 8 Heart

## Radionuclide imaging – MUGA

Cardiac imaging using a multi-gated acquisition (MUGA) protocol assesses global myocardial wall motion and ventricular function. During this procedure a series of 16–32 gated images are taken of the cardiac blood pool for the duration of the cardiac cycle using $^{99m}$Tc labelled red blood cells. This is achieved by initially injecting a stannous red cell agent into the blood pool to coat the erythrocytes and act as a labelling mechanism for $^{99m}$Tc. Twenty minutes later the $^{99m}$Tc is now injected into the blood pool where it loads onto the stannous coated cells. Plate 9 shows MUGA cardiac review summary images.

### Indications

Assessment of ejection fraction, wall motion analysis, detection of an aneurysm and monitoring the effects on left ventricular function of stress and the use of cytotoxic drugs.

### Position of patient and imaging modality

The 45° left anterior oblique view which demonstrates both ventricles and the interventricular septum is normally selected. The procedure starts with the patient lying supine on the imaging couch, with head resting on a pillow. Using the persistence scope, the gamma camera head is positioned parallel to the imaging couch and over the anterior chest wall, ensuring that the cardiac region is in the centre of the imaging field. From this position the camera head is rotated 45° and placed against the left chest wall. A 5–10° caudal angulation of the camera head may be required to enable the ventricular septum to be seen clearly. An anterior, 70° left anterior oblique or right anterior oblique view may be required.

*Imaging and radiopharmaceutical parameters*

| *Type* | *Administered activity* | *Principal energy* |
|---|---|---|
| $^{99m}$Tc pertechnetate and stannous red cell agent. | 550–750 MBq | 140 keV |

| *Window width* | *Acquisition counts/time* |
|---|---|
| 20% | 4800 K counts for 24 frames |

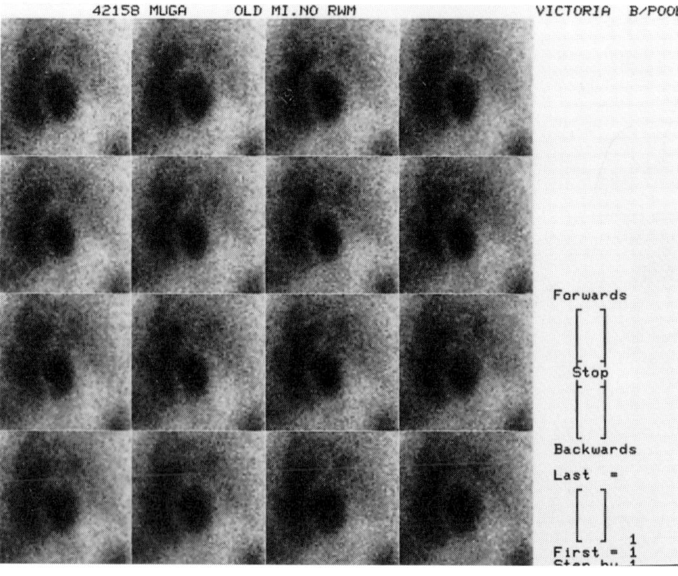


**Figure 8.19a** Series of MUGA static images acquired of the cardiac blood pool in a cardiac cycle

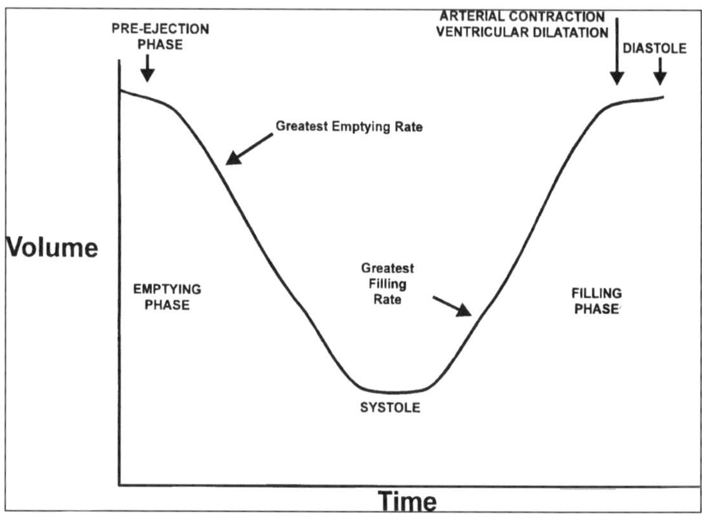


**Figure 8.19b** Cardiac analysis curve demonstrating the emptying and filling phases of the heart, with ventricular volume plotted against time, and produced to determine left ventricular ejection fraction

## Radionuclide imaging – MUGA

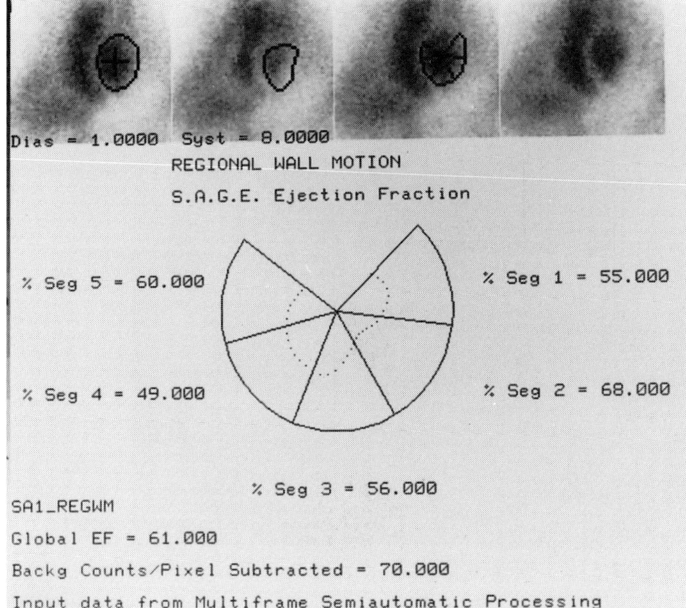


**Figure 8.20** Regional wall motion analysis demonstrating contractility of the left ventricle which is divided into five segments excluding the valve plane. This assists in the diagnosis of infarcted tissues and aneurysms

### Imaging procedure

A low-energy general-purpose collimator adopting a magnification technique is used for this procedure. Prior to the procedure the patient's ECG is checked for signs of atrial fibrillation as this will negate the study. The stannous red cell agent is injected i.v. via a butterfly needle and flushed through with saline. After a delay of 20 min the patient is positioned on the imaging couch with electrodes attached to the chest area and connected to the ECG monitor. The ECG leads and monitor controls are adjusted to provide an R-wave with a clear peak that will act as a trigger for the image acquisition program. The heart rate is monitored until the rate has stabilised and the equipment is adjusted to allow for a 10–20% change in this rate. The radiopharmaceutical is administered via the butterfly needle. As soon as a good heart rate average has been achieved and the equipment is detecting gamma emission, the acquisition protocol is started. The image acquisition parameters are set to acquire 16–32 individual gated frames for the duration of the cardiac cycle.

### Image analysis

Following data acquisition, computer image enhancement techniques such as filtering, background subtraction and edge enhancement are applied to enhance image visualisation. A subjective assessment of heart wall movement is made on a colour monitor by playing back the frames in each view in cine mode. This enables cardiac defects such as areas of akinesis associated with necrotic myocardium and aneurysms (which move paradoxically in respect to normal contraction) to be diagnosed. These conditions can be assessed objectively by the application of software programs which include the production of phase maps. These images allow the separation of normal from abnormal functioning myocardium by differences in phase during contraction. A phase histogram (see Plate 10) also gives an indication of the proportion of heart muscle which is moving in phase. An amplitude image (see Plate 10) gives a measure of the extent of cardiac muscle contraction during the cardiac cycle. The ejection fraction is calculated as the change in number of counts within a region of interest that includes the left ventricle during systole.

# 8 Heart

## Magnetic resonance imaging

Magnetic resonance imaging offers a non-invasive means of demonstrating the heart.

Cardiac and respiratory gating is an essential feature of this imaging procedure to ensure the production of motion-free images. There is no special patient preparation.

Using a spin-echo sequence, the cardiac chambers and major vessels are seen as areas of signal void due to the fact that blood flowing into or out of the image slice will have no signal. The chambers are seen in contrast to the higher signal received from the heart muscle and vessel walls. These images are best for demonstrating cardiac and mediastinal anatomy.

Using a gradient-echo pulse sequence, flowing blood has a high signal intensity. In this procedure, which can also be used for magnetic resonance angiography (MRA), rapid pulse repetition rates gives rise to partial saturation of static tissue which reduces signal intensity while flowing blood appears bright due to a refreshment effect. This sequence allows a rapid series of motion-free images to be acquired throughout the cardiac cycle in a relatively short period of time. Multi-phase images acquired in a cine acquisition can be played back in a cine loop to assess left ventricular wall motion. With the appropriate software, cine loops from contiguous slices can be combined to calculated ejection fraction and stroke volume. Other sophisticated pulse sequences enable techniques such as myocardial tagging, velocity mapping and breath-hold cine to be performed.

Coronary artery disease can be investigated by measuring blood flow in a vessel as an indication of narrowing. Using a high magnetic field system, chemical shift imaging and spectroscopy allow analysis of the chemical content of pathological lesions.

### Indications

Congenital heart disease, cardiac masses, thoracic aorta and pericardial disease. It also plays a role as a follow-up procedure after surgery to determine the patency of the coronary vessels.

### Contraindication

Patients with cardiac pacemakers are absolutely contraindicated. See Chapter 1 for other contraindications.

*Contrast medium and injection data*

MR contrast agents are not used routinely in cardiac imaging. It is hoped that, in the future, agents will be available to differentiate areas of normal myocardium, ischaemia and infarction.

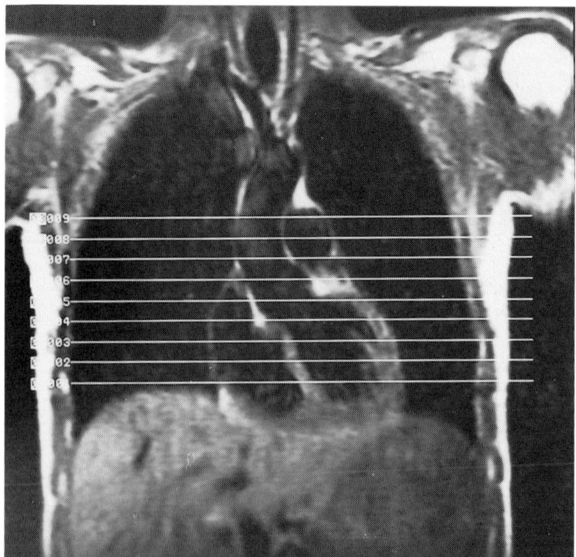

**Figure 8.21a** Coronal localiser for planning series of transaxial scans

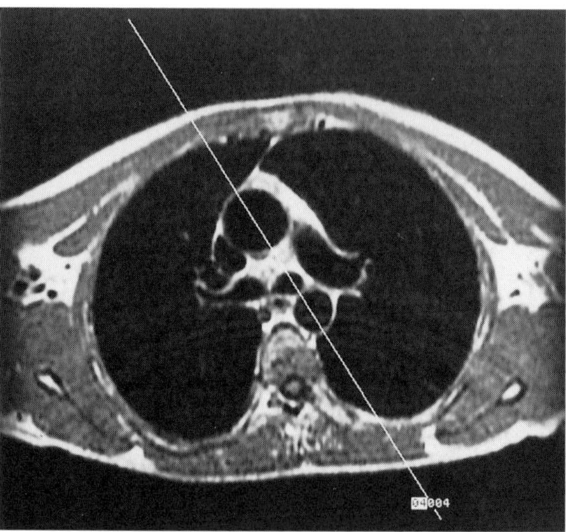

**Figure 8.21b** Transaxial section of thorax showing heart at the level of the ascending and descending aorta

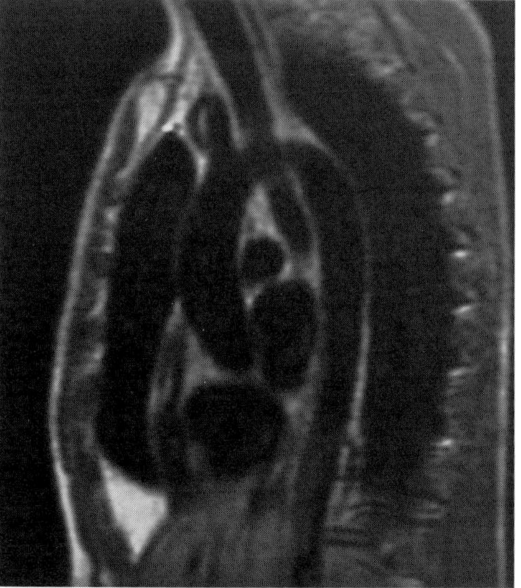

**Figure 8.21c** Sagittal oblique of thorax showing arch of aorta and descending aorta

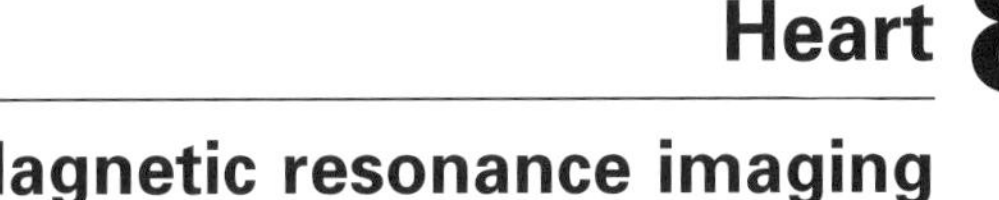



## Magnetic resonance imaging

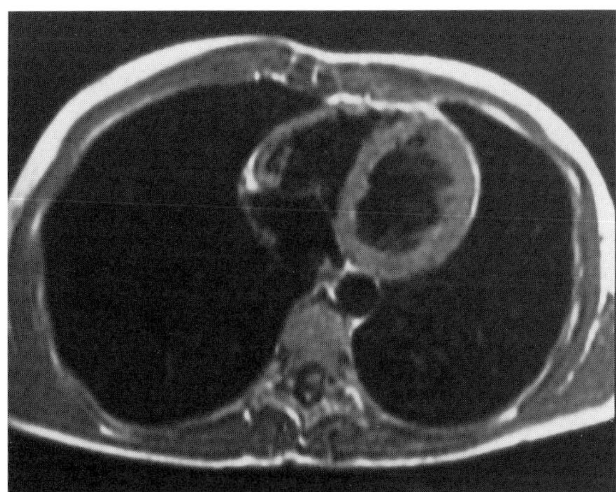

**Figure 8.22a** Transaxial image of the thorax at the level of the left ventricle

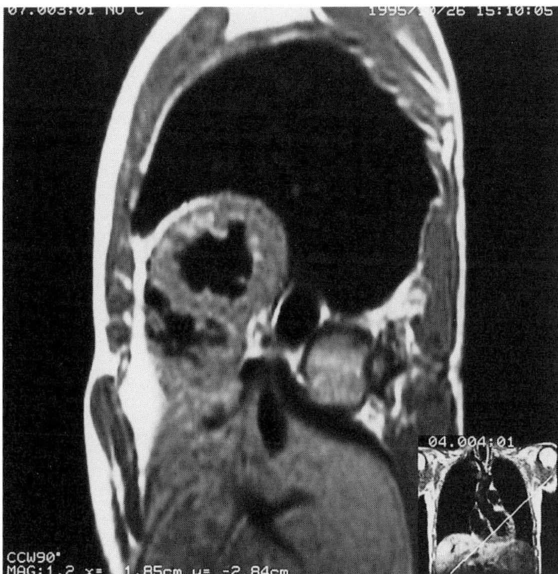


**Figure 8.22b** Short-axis image of the left ventricle

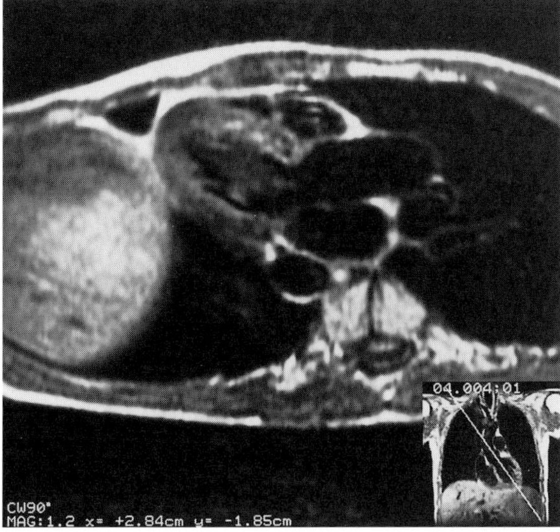


**Figure 8.22c** Long-axis (verticle) image of the heart

**Position of patient and imaging modality**

The cardiac gating facility is applied following the manufacturer's guidance to ensure patient safety and to give a well defined R peak to generate a reliabile triggering pulse. Three ECG leads are connected either to the back or front of the patient's thorax, ensuring that the leads are not directly in contact with the patient's skin or curled in a loop, as this may induce an unwanted current in the lead. The patient then lies supine, head first on the scanner couch, with the median sagittal plane perpendicular to the middle of the table and coincident with the sagittal alignment light and the transverse alignment light at the level of the manubrium. From this position the patient is moved the fixed distance to the isocentre of the radiofrequency receiver/transmitter coil.

**Imaging procedure**

*General overview*

A general examination of the heart, including the aorta, may consist of the following scans of the thorax:

- coronal localiser
- transaxial scans
- sagittal or sagittal oblique scans.

Initially a series of coronal spin-echo $T_1$ scans 3–8 mm thick, depending on patient size, with a small slice gap are prescribed through the thorax from the sternum anteriorly to the thoracic spine posteriorly. One of these images is selected as a localiser to plan a series of transaxial spin-echo $T_1$ scans, 3–8 mm thick, with a small slice gap from the inferior border of the heart to the superior aspect of the arch of the aorta. The subsequent images are reviewed for any pathology, following which an image showing the ascending and descending aorta is selected to plan a series of spin-echo $T_1$ sagittal oblique scans through the aorta. These scans are 3–4 mm thick, with a small slice gap, and extend from one lateral edge of the aorta wall to the other.

*Cardiac chambers*

The cardiac chambers may be further demonstrated by obtaining a series of scans parallel to the horizontal long-axis plane and short-axis plane of the heart.

For horizontal long-axis scans a transaxial image is acquired at the level of the left ventricle to act as a localiser. From this image an oblique section is prescribed through the long axis of the left ventricle. The caudal angle of the axis of the heart is measured from this oblique sagittal image and a horizontal long-axis view demonstrating the four chambers is prescribed. From this image, sections through the short-axis heart (at right angles to the long-axis) can be prescribed. In the short axis, the left ventricle appears like a doughnut with the right ventricle lying in front of it against the chest wall.

Each of these planes can be used as a pilot for multi-slice image acquisition and cine imaging in one plane.

*Multi-slice image acquisition*
As described, multi-slice images of the heart can be acquired which are either parallel to the horizontal long axis or short axis of the left ventricle. Using this approach, a series of 8 mm sections can be acquired through the left ventricle which will enable the physician to scroll through each individual image to assess morphology and combined with appropriate software to assess cardiac function. In these studies, cardiac gating and a gradient-echo sequence is required. This will make the blood pool appear white due to the high signal from flowing blood.

Coronary arteries can also be investigated using this method. After selection of the appropriate imaging plane, at least four 2 mm slices are acquired using a 14 s breath hold. Using this pulse sequence, combined with fat saturation and magnetisation transfer, background tissue is suppressed and the coronary arteries highlighted.

*Cine application*
Using a breath-hold technique a rapid sequence of images can be acquired of a particular slice to give a dynamic view of function throughout the cardiac cycle. Using this approach, images can be played back in a cine loop which will enable assessment of global and regional function. In these studies cardiac gating is essential. Up to two slices can usually be obtained simultaneously and the number of phases for each slice depends on the ECG R-to-R (RR) wave interval. The TR multiplied by the number of phases must fit into the ECG RR interval to ensure distinct phases throughout the whole cardiac cycle are obtained. A TR of 50 ms and a RR interval of 540 ms will facilitate a total of 16 phases. Slice thickness is variable, but around 8 mm is typical.

Using a flow-compensated gradient-echo type sequence to rephase only those protons moving with relatively uniform velocity, normal flow appears bright while turbulent or accelerated flow appear as signal voids. Application includes:

- In the case of the four-chamber view taken in the horizontal axis, flow disturbances associated with regurgitation can be seen such as those caused by mitral stenosis and atrial and ventricular septal defects.
- A coronal view of the thorax will show the aortic root and demonstrate any aortic stenosis and regurgitation.
- An oblique sagittal will show the aortic arch and is good for showing flow associated with coarctations.

*Echo planar imaging (EPI)*
This ultra-fast imaging protocol has potential for the future but requires extra gradient strength.

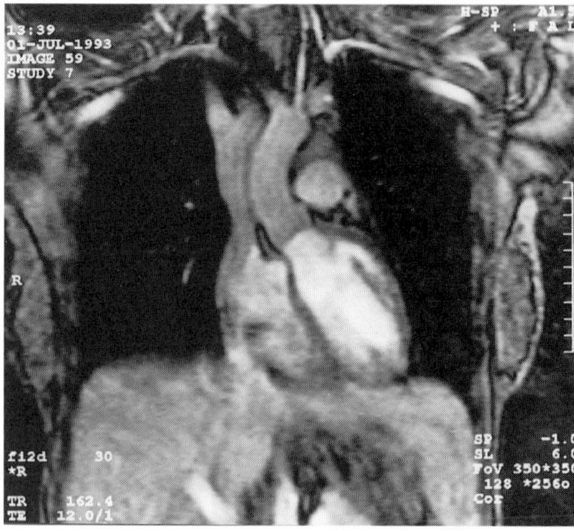


**Figure 8.23a** Gradient-echo coronal diastolic image through the left ventricle showing aortic route (high signal from flowing blood)

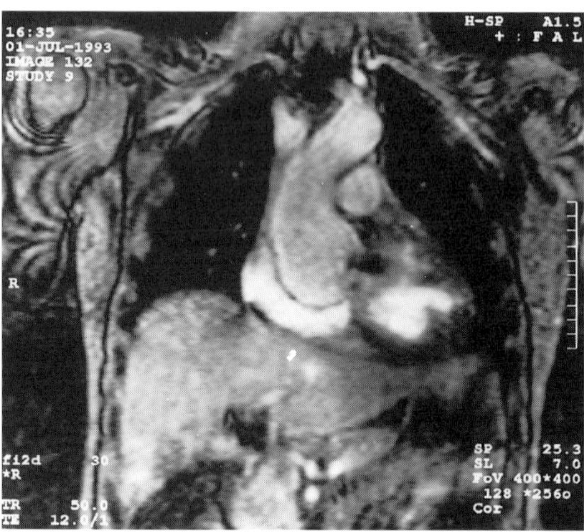


**Figure 8.23b** Gradient-echo coronal systolic image through the left ventricle showing aortic route (high signal from flowing blood)

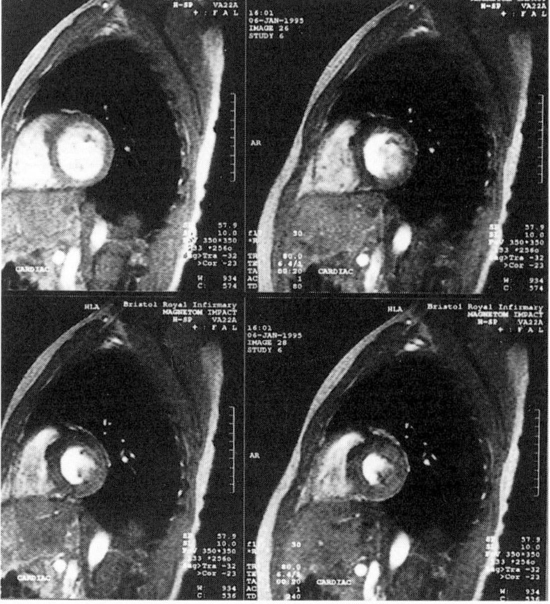

**Figure 8.23c** Gradient-echo cine images – short-axis view through the ventricles in different phases of the cardiac cycle

(a)

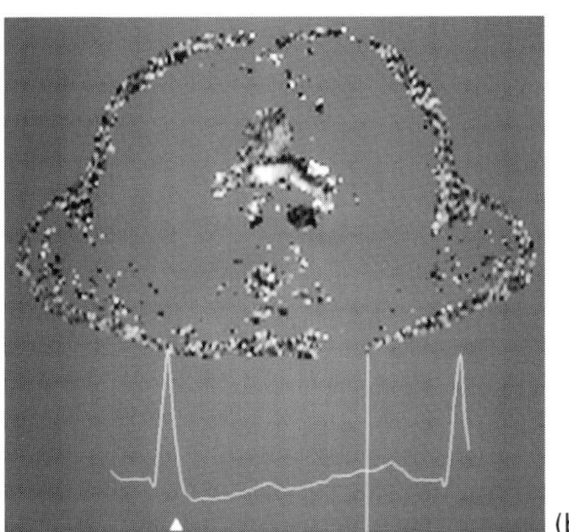

(b)

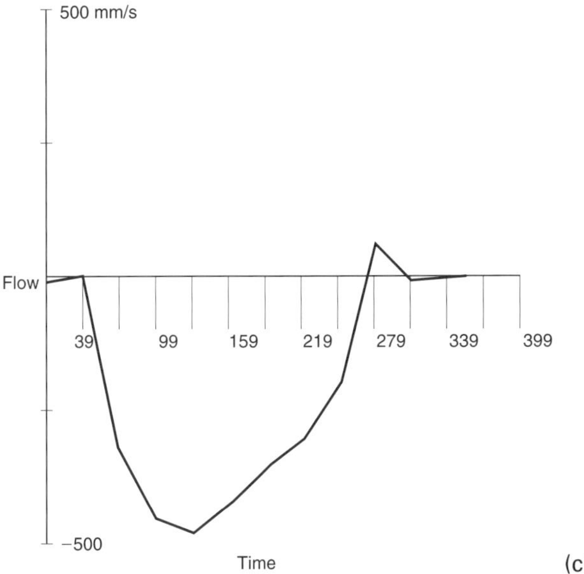


(c)

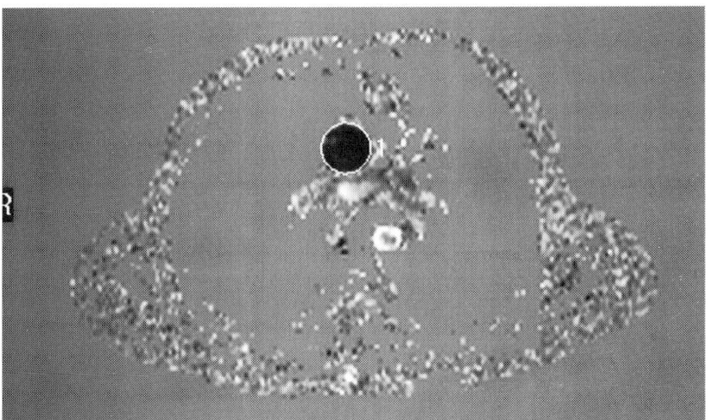

(d)

*Flow imaging and phase velocity*

Further developments using a spin-echo sequence enable blood flow and velocity through a vessel or heart chamber to be quantified.

One such method – phase velocity mapping – uses the phase component of the MR signal. This technique uses a spin-echo sequence which comprises a 90° and 180° pulse. The pulses, however, are applied in such a way that each pulse is applied to a different slice through the patient. As a result, only blood that has flowed between the two slices, and so experiences both pulses, will have signal. The time between the two pulses and the distance between the two slices dictate the particular velocity that is recorded.

This protocol delivers a 180° pulse to the imaging plane, causing saturation by reducing both longitudinal and transverse magnetisation within the plane. If a 90° pulse is applied to the saturated plane, no signal will be recorded as there is no residual magnetisation. If, however, blood with full magnetisation flows into the plane when a 90° pulse is delivered, it will give a strong signal and can be used to form an image. The intensity of the signal will be proportional to the velocity of flow as high velocities will lead to more magnetised blood within the slice.

This net magnetisation related to phase shift can be used to construct a phase shift image showing the direction and velocity of flow. This technique can be used to display the velocity of the flowing blood within the cardiac chambers and major vessels, the pixel intensity representing phase shift and therefore directly related to velocity of flow in the encoding direction. Stationary tissues with medium signal intensity are depicted grey, representing zero velocity, while high signal intensity, depicted white, represents caudal flow and low signal intensity, seen black, depicts cranial flow. This technique can be applied in the assessment of atrial septal defects, coarctation, bypass grafts and valve disease, etc.

With colour coding software this can be taken further to enable colour to be added based on the direction of flow, e.g. blue for veins and red for arteries.

The velocity data can also be integrated with lumen area to yield cross-sectional flow within a vessel and this can be displayed in the form of a graph with 'flow rate' plotted against 'time'. This facility can be used to determine velocity across the heart valves, to assess chamber pressures and in the ascending aorta to determine ventricular stroke volume. This technique has potential to be applied to coronary arteries, with increased velocity indicating stenosis.

**Figure 8.24** (a,b) Transaxial images at the same location showing pixel intensity as a function of velocity of protons (a) with the heart in systole (b) heart in distole; (c,d) blood flow study of the ascending aorta showing (c) blood flow in mm/s plotted against time and (d) an image derived approximately 30 ms after the start of the R wave

# 8 Heart

## Computed tomography

At the time of writing, CT systems which offer ultra-fast image acquisition times and the capability of performing ventricular functional assessment are not widely available. However, the majority of current CT scanners may be employed to assess the patency of coronary grafts using a dynamic scanning protocol. This procedure should be superseded eventually by MR angiography when MR becomes more readily available.

**Position of patient and imaging modality**

The patient lies supine, head first on the scanner table, with arms lifted above the head. The median sagittal plane is adjusted perpendicular to the centre of the table top, with the coronal plane parallel to the table top. The scan plane is perpendicular to the long axis of the body. The patient is then moved into the scanner and positioned so that the scan reference point is at the level of the sternal notch. The table height is adjusted so that the coronal alignment light is at the level of the mid-axillary line, to ensure the patient is in the centre of the scan field.

**Imaging procedure**

A postero-anterior scan projection radiograph is obtained, starting 5 cm above and ending, 28 cm below the sternal notch. From this scan image 10 mm contiguous sections are prescribed from the arch of the aorta to mid-ventricular level. These images are assessed to determine the location of each graft.

Further scanning following a bolus injection of a non-ionic contrast medium with normal saline chaser will demonstrate the patency of a graft. Dynamic scan mode is selected, with six sequential scans prescribed at each level, employing a 5 s preparation delay. Following deep inspiration, scanning takes place during suspended respiration which lasts 30 s.

*Contrast medium and injector data*

| *Volume* | *Concentration* | *Flow rate* |
|---|---|---|
| 25 ml* | 350 mgI/ml | 8 ml/s |

* Volume = 25 ml contrast + 35 ml normal saline. The contrast and saline mixture is layered in the syringe, with the contrast injected first, followed by the saline.

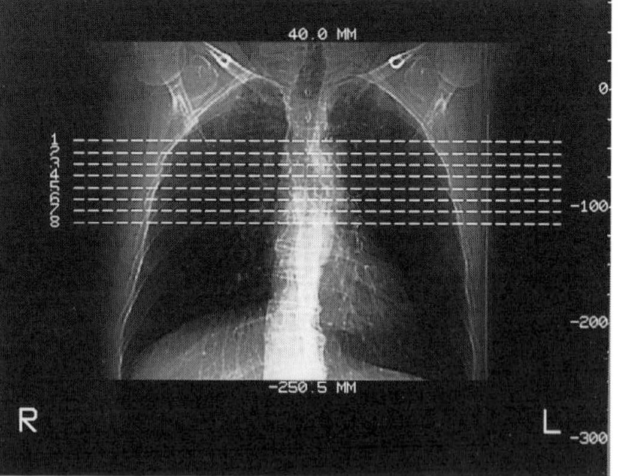


**Figure 8.25a** Scan projection radiograph showing prescribed transaxial levels

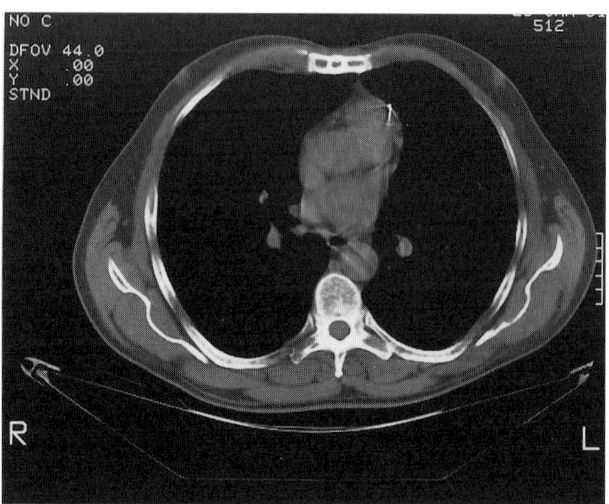


**Figure 8.25b** Pre-contrast transaxial image showing streak artefacts from surgical clip

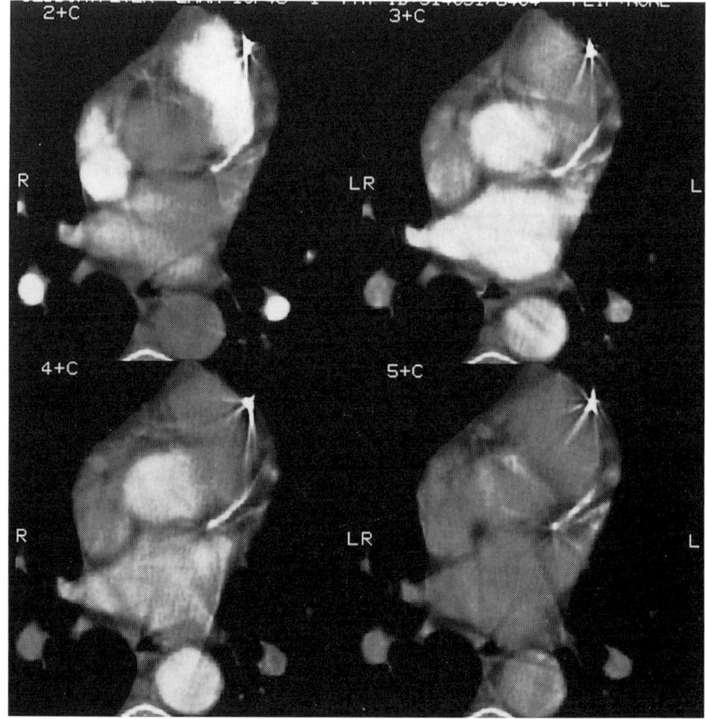


**Figure 8.25c** Series of images at one anatomical level showing different stages of contrast enhancement (note contrast enhancement in the bypass grafts)

# Aorta

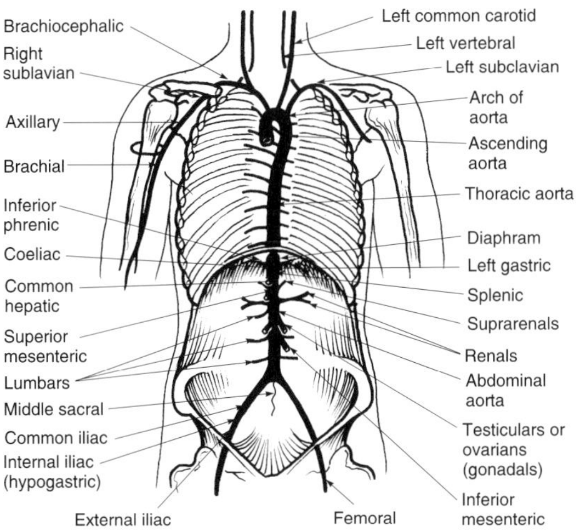

Figure 8.26a Principal branches of the aorta (anterior aspect)

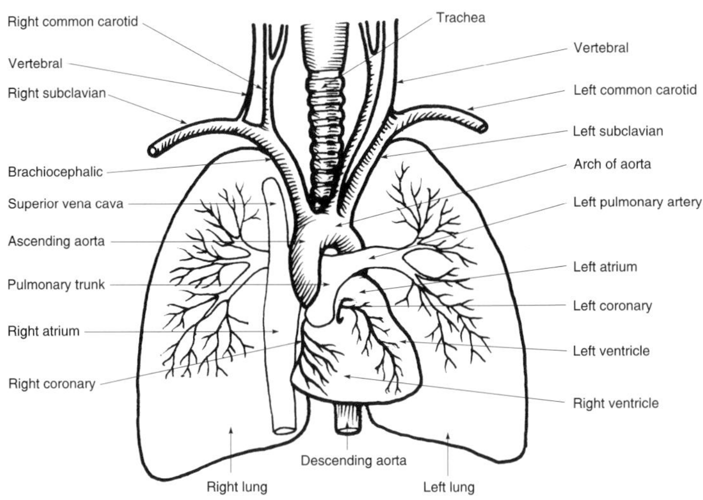


**Figure 8.26b** Aortic arch (anterior aspect)

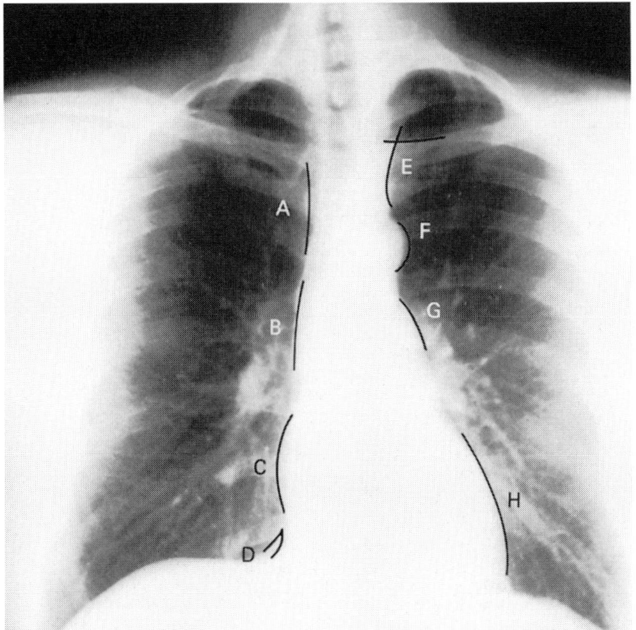


**Figure 8.26c** A, superior vena cava; B, ascending thoracic aorta; C, right atrium; D, inferior vena cava; E, left subclavian vein; F, aortic knuckle; G, main pulmonary artery; H, left ventricle

The aorta, which conveys oxygenated blood from the heart, is subdivided into four sections: ascending, arch, descending thoracic and abdominal aorta.

The descending thoracic aorta commences at the lower border of the fourth thoracic vertebra to the left of the midline and becomes the abdominal aorta as it passes below the crura of the diaphragm at the level of the 12th thoracic vertebra. There are many branches along its total length until it bifurcates into the common iliac arteries at the level of the fourth lumbar vertebrae to the left of the midline.

## Indications

Stenosis or occlusion of the vessel caused by atheromatous plaques, aneurysms/dissection, trauma effecting any level of the vessel. Location and extent of a dissecting aneurysm which will include an assessment of the renal arteries to exclude their involvement. Location of branches prior to selective arteriography. Coarctation of the thoracic aorta which is accompanied by severe hypertension in the upper limbs.

## Recommended imaging procedures

Postero-anterior and left lateral chest radiographs are useful in demonstrating the outline of the aortic arch and thoracic aorta, the presence of calcification of the vessel wall and any other major changes such as a widened mediastinum suggesting an aortic aneurysm.

Calcification in the abdominal aorta may be identified on anteroposterior and lateral abdominal radiographs.

Ultrasound is used routinely to demonstrate the abdominal aorta and may also be employed to visualise the thoracic aorta using a trans-oesophageal approach.

Computed tomography may be used to assess the aorta throughout its length, but is particularly useful in demonstrating the complications of aortic disease i.e. dissection, bleeding and retroperitoneal fibrosis.

Magnetic resonance imaging, when available, is used for the same indications as CT.

Angiography with or without digital imaging can be used at any level of the aorta.

# 8 Aorta

## Ultrasound

Ultrasound is a useful first-line imaging modality for examining the abdominal aorta – it is quick, cheap and non-invasive. Two-dimensional real-time scanning is employed using either a mechanical sector or a curved linear array probe. Colour flow Doppler is useful in identifying blood flow turbulence. Scans are normally performed after an 8 h fast to reduce bowel gas which, if present, reduces image quality.

**Indications**

Assessment of suspected abdominal aneurysms. Monitoring known aneurysms for changes in the diameter (surgical action is taken when the external diameter exceeds 5 cm).

**Position of patient and imaging modality**

The patient lies supine on the imaging couch and is examined normally with a 3.5 MHz transducer which is held against the anterior abdominal wall using a suitable coupling gel. A 5 MHz probe may be used if the patient is of slender build.

**Imaging procedure**

The full length of the abdominal aorta is scanned, from the diaphragm to the aortic bifurcation, both in longitudinal and transverse planes. Using the electronic calipers, measurements are taken of the maximum dimensions in all planes. When a saccular aneurysm is diagnosed, the diameter of the lumen is compared to the aorta's overall diameter and the total length of the lesion noted. Colour flow Doppler (see Plate 11) is useful in detecting blood flow turbulence associated with thrombosis at the site of the aneurysm. Both kidneys are also examined to assess renal blood flow and any change in renal size. Involvement of the renal arteries with associated chronic ischaemia causes a reduction in kidney size.

Hydronephrosis may be detected if a ureter is adherent to an inflammatory aneurysm.

Static images are best acquired on suspended respiration, choosing the most suitable phase of breathing to remove bowel from the region of interest.

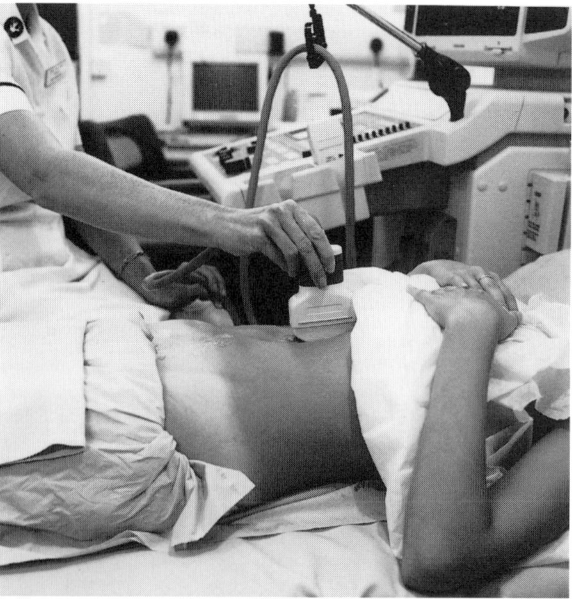

**Figure 8.27a** Patient and transducer

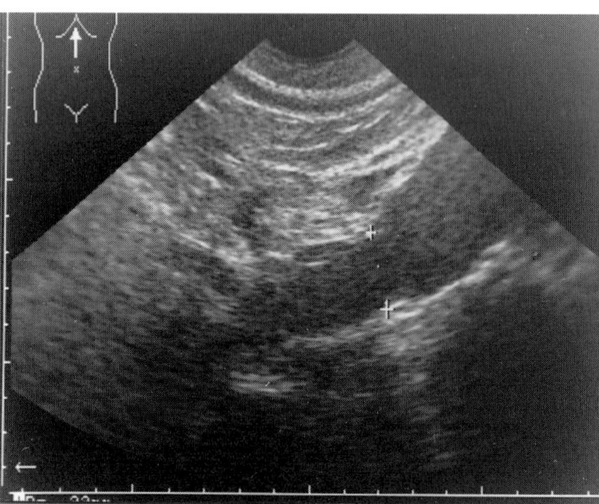

**Figure 8.27b** Longitudinal section in the midline demonstrating the origin of an aortic aneurysm. Calipers are shown across the lumen

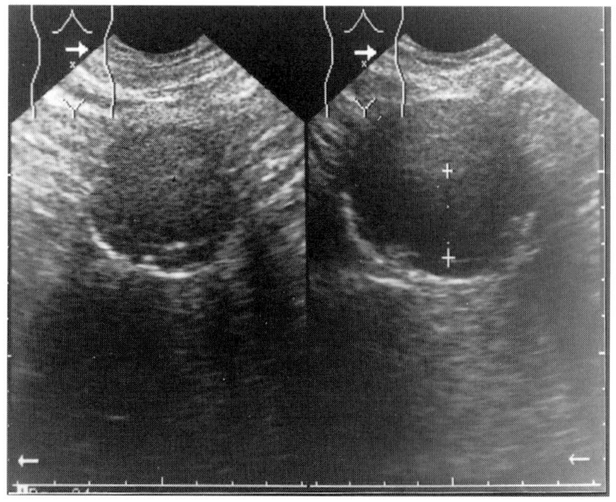

(i) (ii)

**Figure 8.27c** Transverse sections through an aorta with an aneurysm; (i) just below the renal arteries demonstrating dilatation and highly echogenic posterior aortic wall; (ii) mid-portion of the aneurysm showing echogenic thrombus and on-screen calipers measuring lumen size

## Computed tomography

Computed tomography may be used to locate the origin and extent of a dissecting aneurysm. It is also employed following trauma to identify the location of a tear. When an abdominal aneurysm is detected, it is necessary to visualise the renal arteries to exclude any involvement which could affect patient management. Routinely, only contrast-enhanced images are obtained during the infusion of a non-ionic contrast agent.

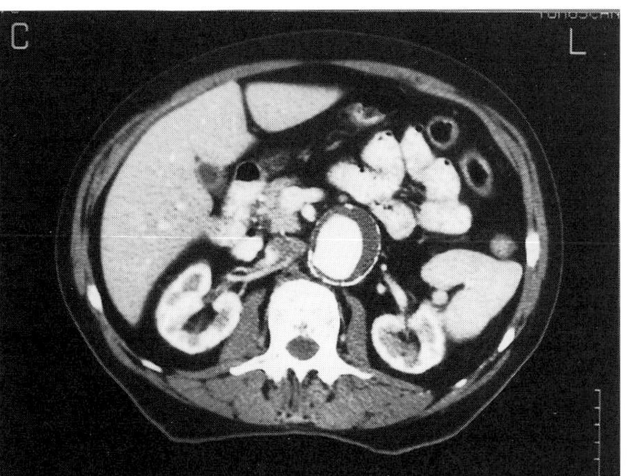

**Figure 8.28a** CT post-contrast image showing aortic aneurysm at the level of the renal vessels

### Indications

Aortic dissection and aneurysm.

### Position of patient and imaging modality

The patient lies supine, head first on the scanner table. Arms are raised and placed behind the head, out of the scan plane. The median sagittal plane is perpendicular and the coronal plane is parallel to the scanner table. The scanner table height is adjusted to ensure that the coronal plane alignment light is at the level of the mid-axillary line. The patient is then moved into the scanner so that the scan reference point is at the level of the sternal notch.

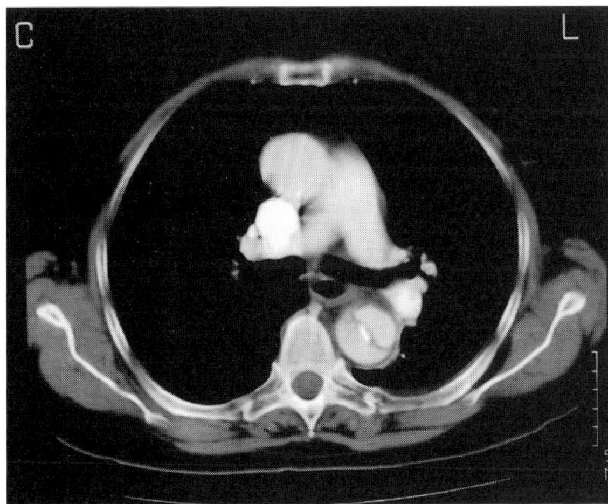

**Figure 8.28b** CT post-contrast image showing a dissecting aneurysm of the thoracic aorta with contrast in both the true and false lumen

### Imaging procedure

A postero-anterior scan projection radiograph is performed, starting at the sternal notch and terminating at a distance of 450 mm below this point to include the aortic arch, thoracic and abdominal aorta. From this scan image, 10 mm thick contrast enhanced scans of the aorta are prescribed at 15 mm table increments, commencing at the aortic arch and terminating at the level of the anterior iliac spines, to demonstrate the aortic bifurcation and femoral arteries. Images should be taken during gentle respiration using the shortest scan time. Image acquisition commences after a scan delay to ensure that the vessel is opacified; 30 s is normally adequate. In the acute situation, when spiral scanning is available, a volume acquisition technique is employed using a 10 mm slice thickness with a 20 mm table increment and a 10 mm reconstruction index. If further detail is required of a specific area of the aorta, e.g. renal arteries or postoperatively, volume scanning may be performed using a 5 mm slice thickness and a 5 mm table increment with a reconstruction index of 3 mm resulting in overlapping sections.

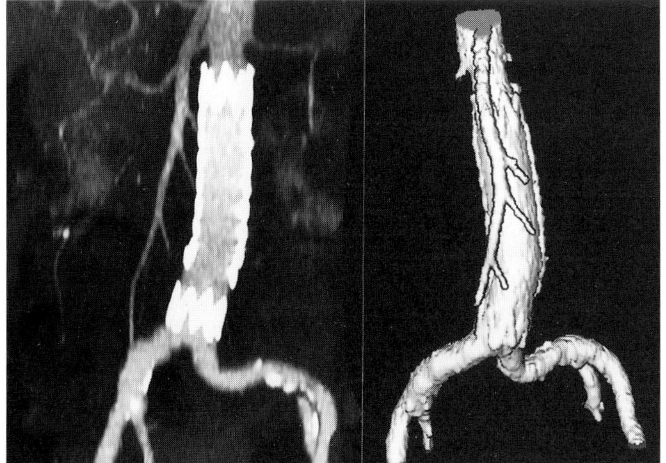

**Figure 8.28c** Three-dimensional reconstructed images of the aorta (postoperative) using (i) the MIP method, and (ii) the seed pixel method

### Image analysis

The typical CT finding for acute dissection of the aorta is the presence of two opacified channels with an intimal flap between them. The CT density within the false channel is less than the true channel because of the slower flow rate. The digital data can be reformatted in any anatomical plane or reconstructed in 3D by using a maximum intensity pixel (MIP) method or a surface rendering technique, e.g. seed pixel method.

*Contrast medium and injector data*

| *Volume* | *Concentration* | *Flow rate* |
|---|---|---|
| 100 ml | 140–300 mgI/ml | 3 ml/sec |

For the abdominal aorta, scanning commences after a scan delay of 30 s.

# 8 Aorta

## Angiography

Aortography is commonly performed by a Seldinger technique with retrograde catheterisation of a femoral artery, with the tip of the catheter positioned in the aorta under fluoroscopic control. The procedure is best performed using dedicated angiographic equipment with an image intensifier large enough (e.g. 40 cm) to accommodate the entire length of the abdominal or thoracic aorta. Alternatively, when digital imaging is unavailable, a 35 × 35 cm rapid film changer is selected. Cine radiography or rapid digital imaging acquisition is required to demonstrate the aortic arch. A non-ionic contrast agent is selected and administered using a contrast pressure injector and catheter with side holes near its tip.

Digital subtraction angiography (DSA) has the advantage that a smaller catheter can be selected for the procedure, thus enabling the after-care period following the procedure to be shortened. For optimal image subtraction, the use of a suitable drug to minimise bowel movement is essential. Intravenous DSA offers an alternative approach if the femoral arteries are occluded.

Translumbar aortography, when a catheter is inserted in the lumen of the aorta following direct needle puncture of the aorta, is only selected if the aorta is occluded and digital imaging is not available.

### Indications

Dissecting aneurysms of the thoracic aorta, abdominal saccular aneurysms and trauma when CT is not available or the results of CT are equivocal. Coarctation of the aortic arch and prior to selective angiography.

### Position of patient and imaging modality

The aortic arch is demonstrated in a similar way to the procedure described for left ventricular angiography on page 274. In this case a left anterior oblique 15° projection is selected to demonstrate the arch.

For the abdominal and thoracic aorta, postero-anterior projections are selected using dedicated angiographic equipment. Lateral or oblique projections may also be required for further detail as well as demonstrating the origin of any one of its branches.

The patient lies supine in the centre of the imaging couch, with the head raised on a shallow pillow. The image intensifier face is parallel to the imaging couch and positioned under fluoroscopic control at the level required. If a rapid film changer/image intensifier system is attached to the C-arm, the intensifier is rotated into position following fluoroscopy, immediately prior to permanent image acquisition.

### Direction and centring of the X-ray beam

For the postero-anterior projection the vertical ray is centred in the midline at the level required.

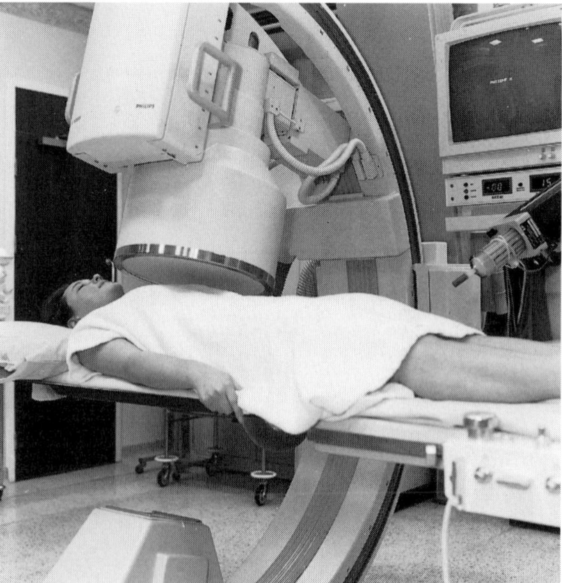

**Figure 8.29a** Image intensifier positioned for LAO 15° projection of aortic arch

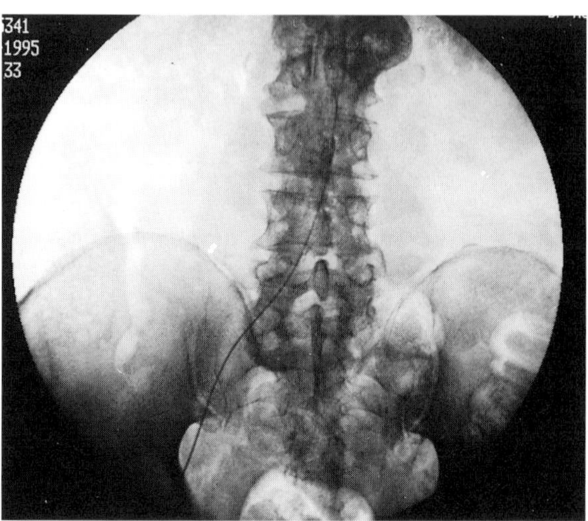


**Figure 8.29b** Pre-contrast image of abdomen showing guide wire positioned in aorta prior to bolus injection

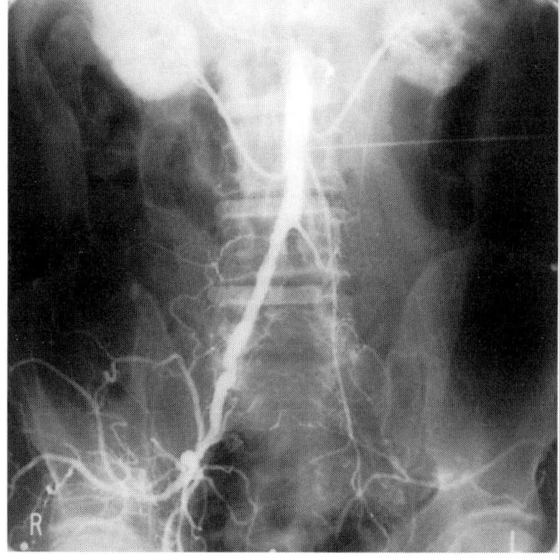


**Figure 8.29c** Translumbar aortography with direct needle puncture of the aorta showing occlusion of the left iliac system and the right common femoral which would preclude a Seldinger approach. NB. Aberrant renal arteries

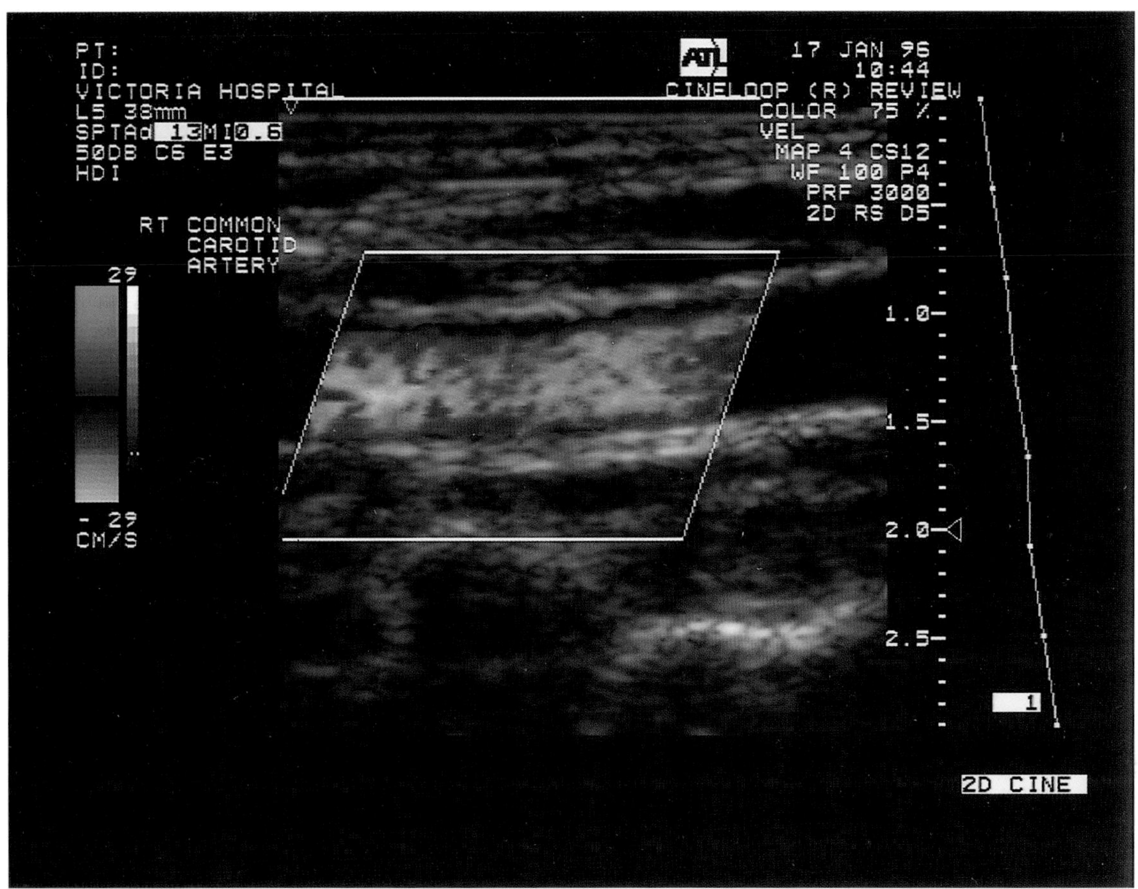


**Plate 4** Pulsed Doppler waveform from right common carotid artery (see text, page 271)

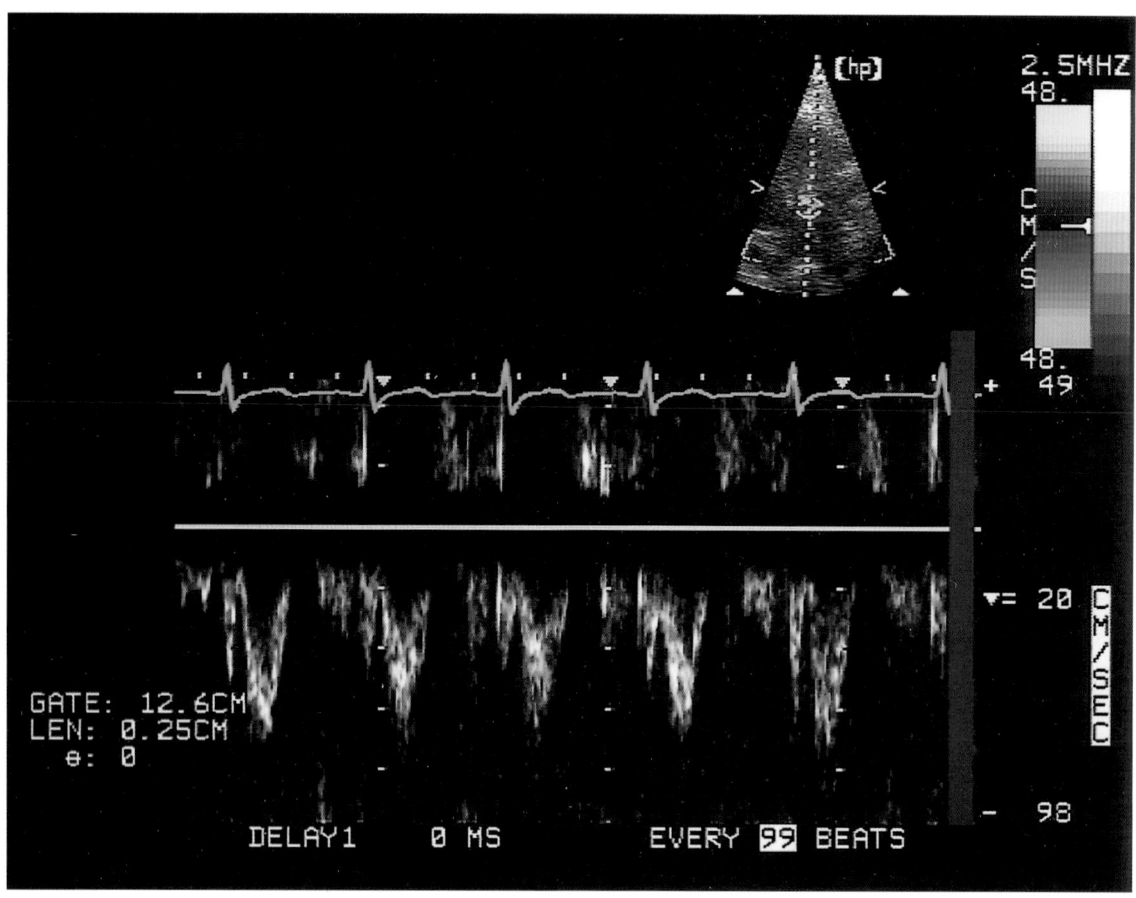


**Plate 5** Normal pulsed wave Doppler of left ventricular outflow tract (see text, page 281)

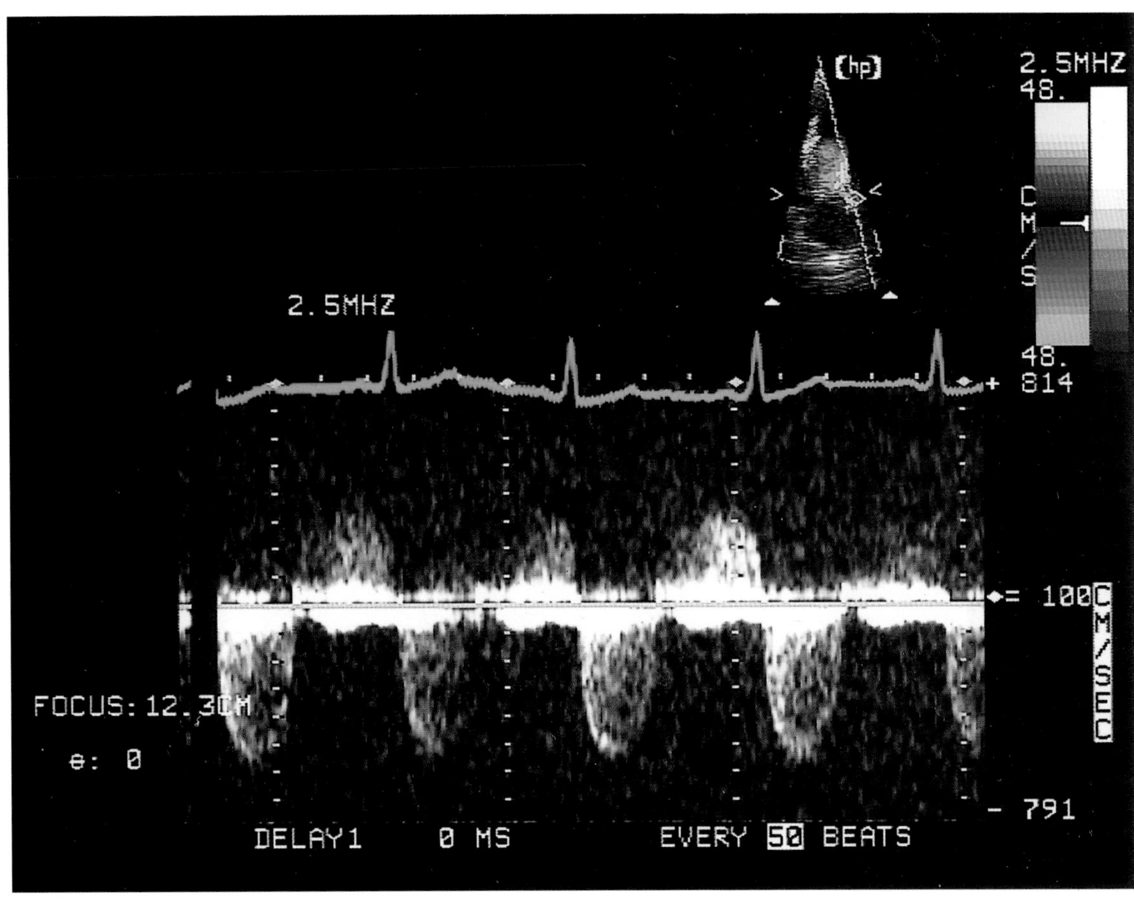


**Plate 6** Continuous wave Doppler demonstrating atrial stenosis and atrial regurgitation (see text, page 281)

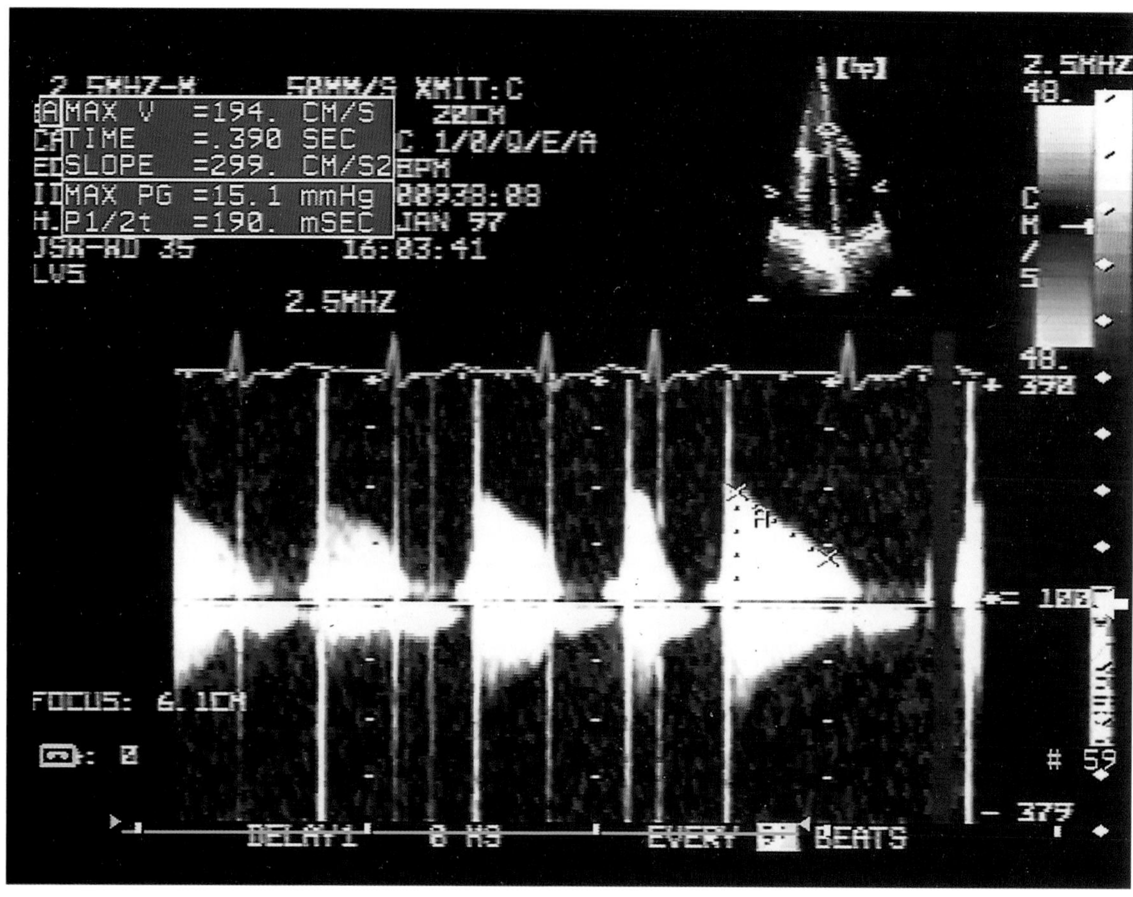


**Plate 7** CWD with calculation of 'pressure half-time' in a patient with mitral stenosis (see text, page 281)

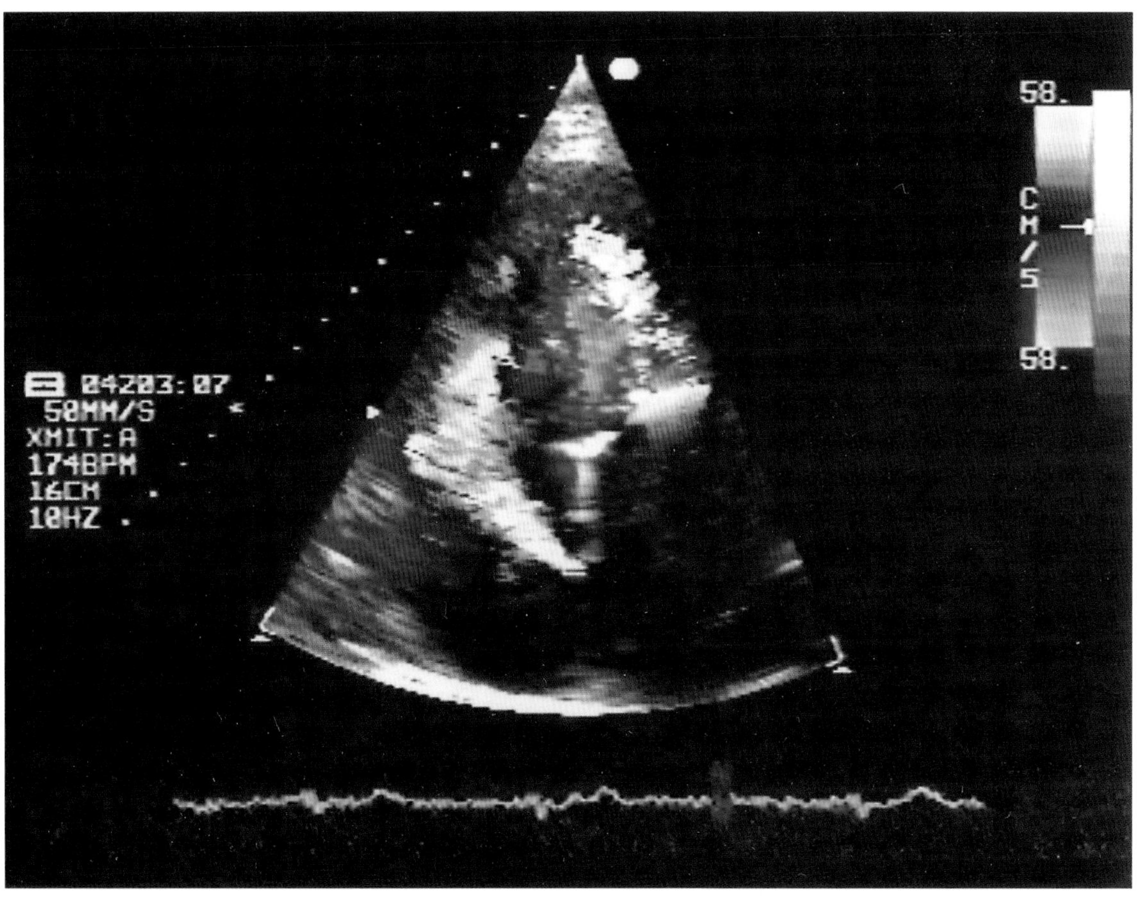


**Plate 8** Colour flow showing an atrial septal defect (see text, page 281)

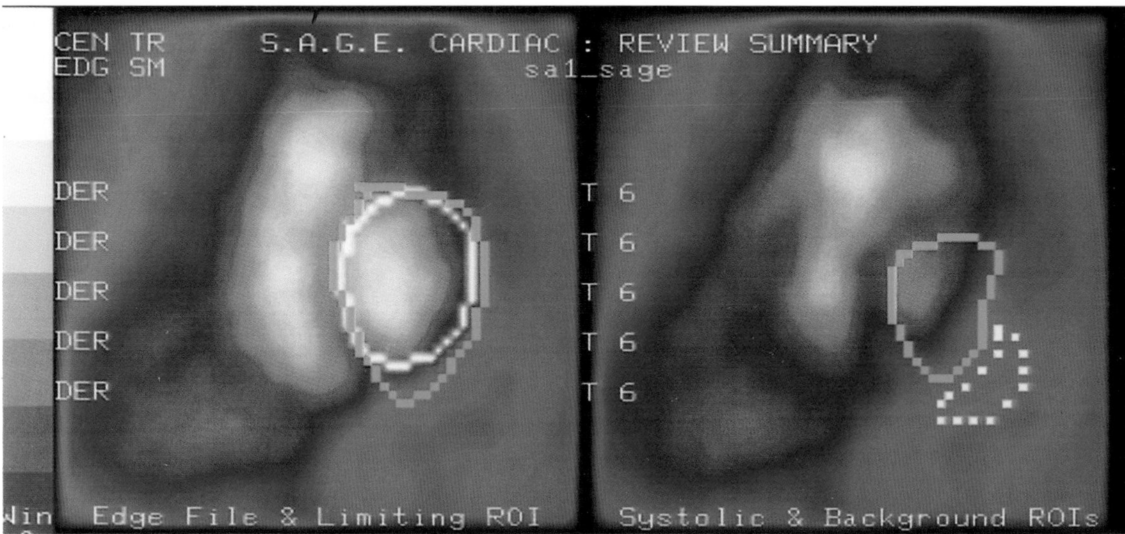


**Plate 9** MUGA cardiac review summary images; i) left ventricle in diastole, at its fullest, highlighted with the ROI shown in white; ii) left ventricle, in systole, at maximum contraction, with systolic (green) and background ROIs (see text, page 284)

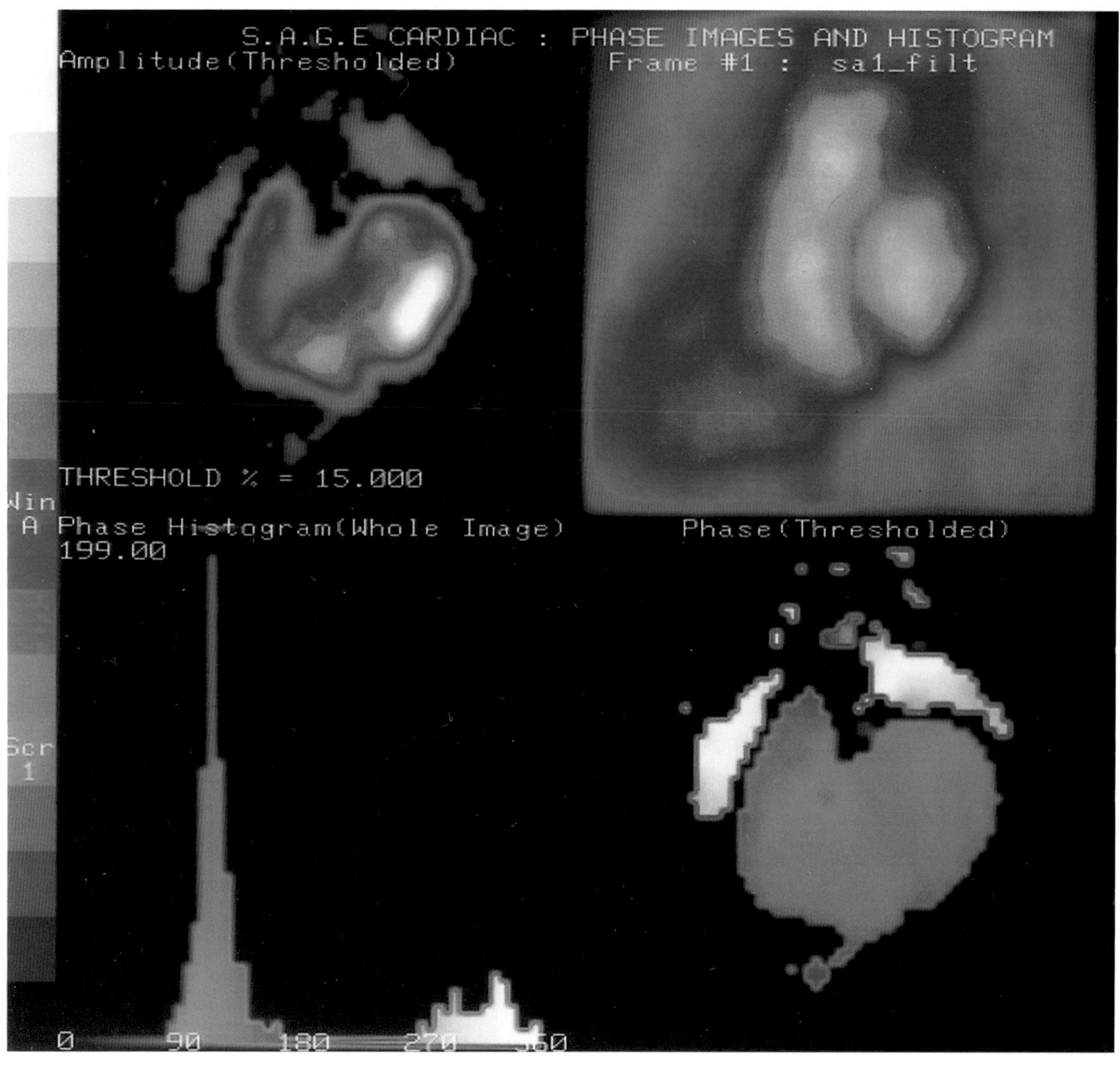


**Plate 10** Phase and amplitude images together with a phase histogram of a normal patient (see text, page 285)

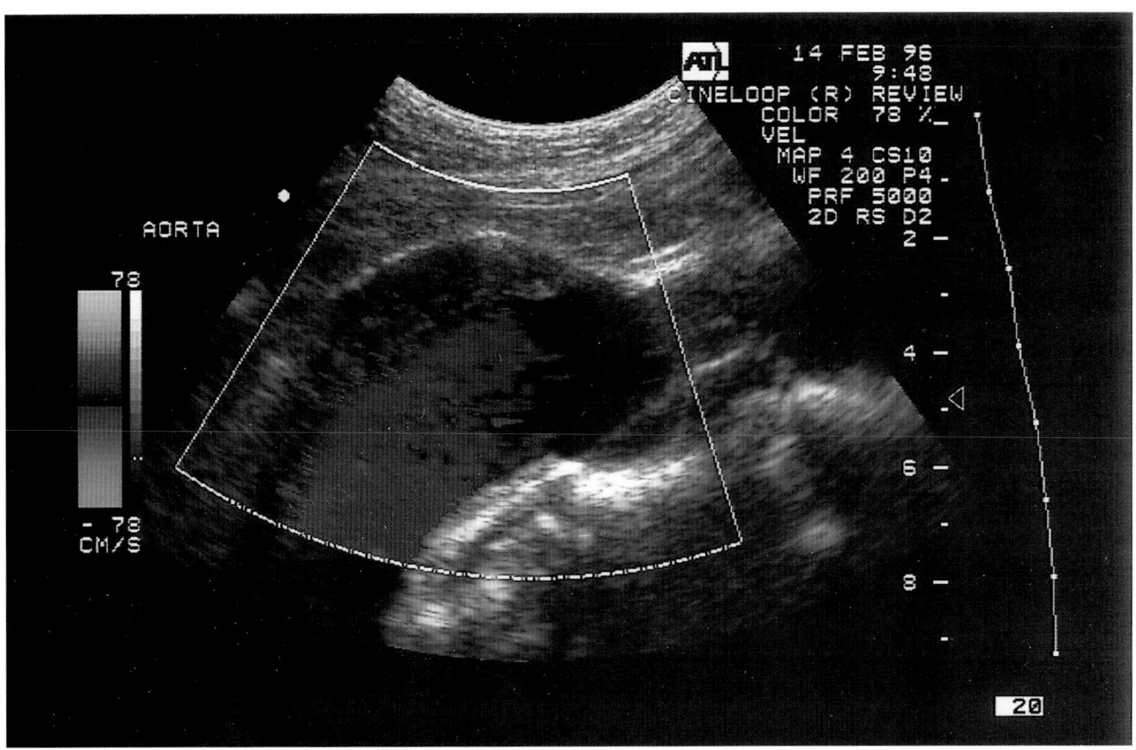


**Plate 11** Longitudinal colour flow image of aorta (see text, page 292)

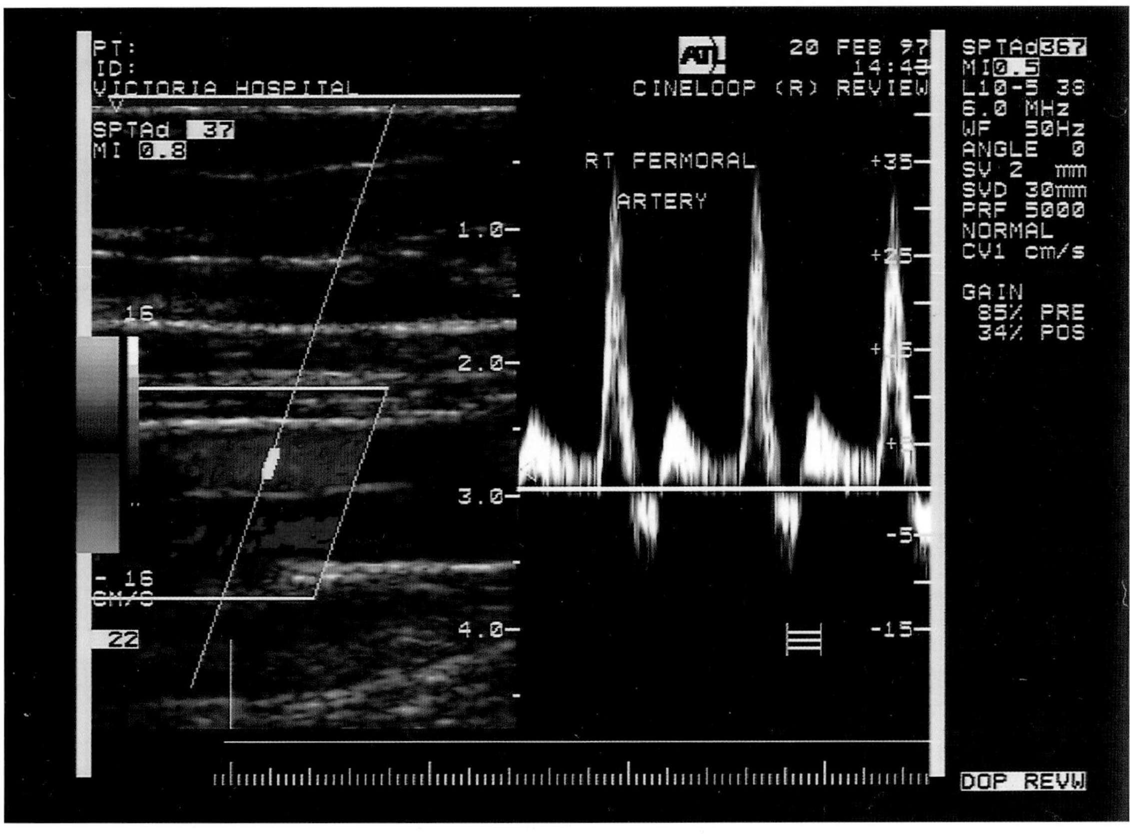


**Plate 12** Colour flow Doppler image of the femoral artery (seen in red) with typical blood flow waveform (see text, page 301)

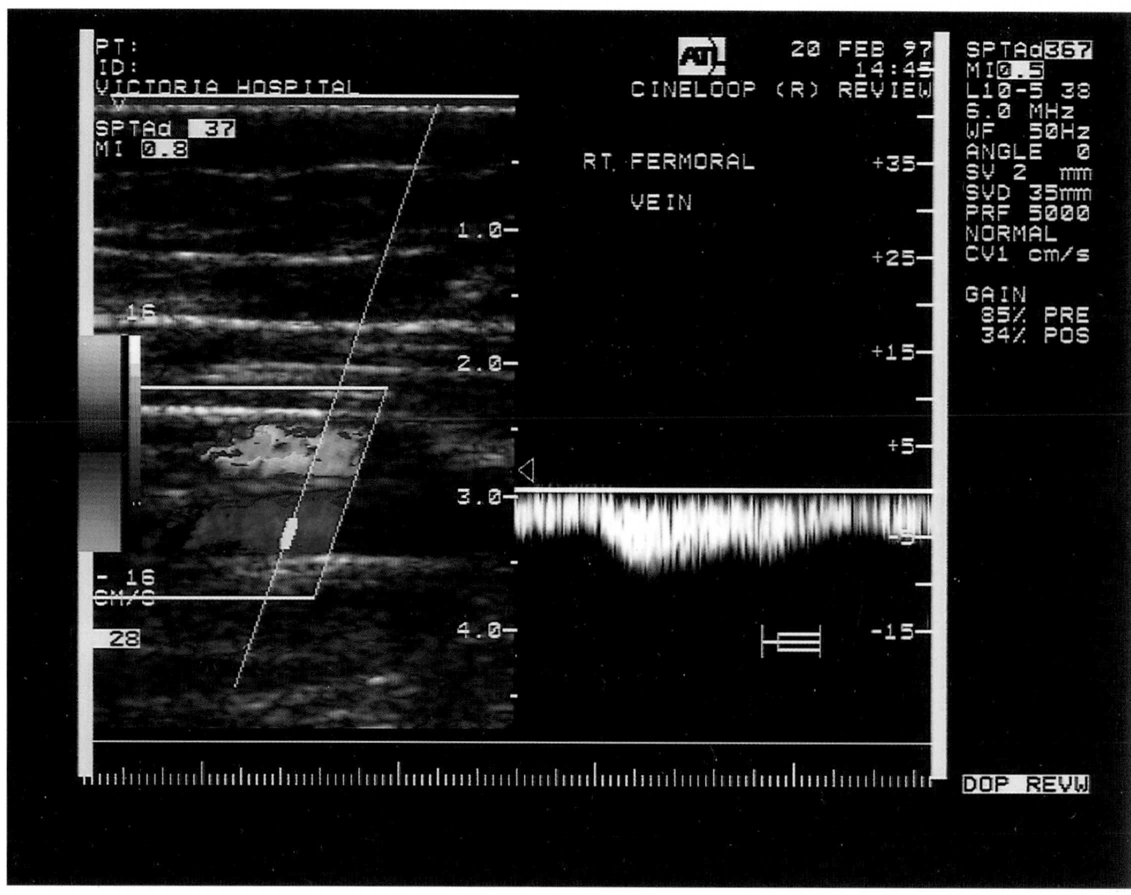


**Plate 13** Colour flow Doppler image of the right femoral vein (seen in blue) with typical blood flow waveform (see text, page 302)

## Angiography

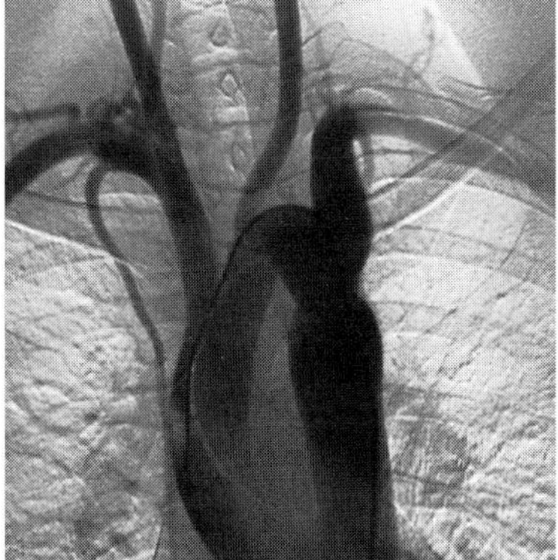

**Figure 8.30a** Aortic arch and descending aorta with coarctation of the aorta

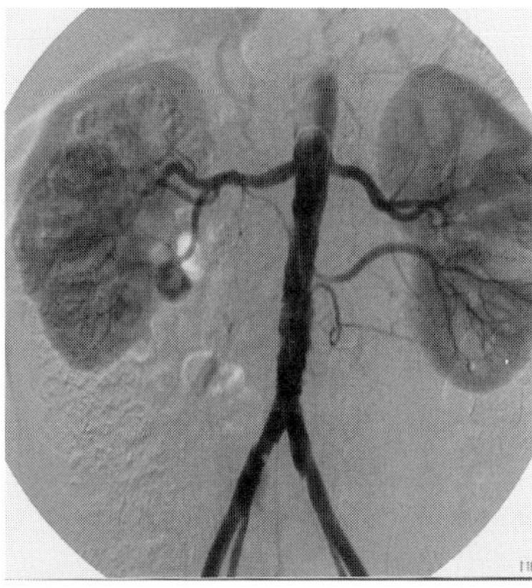

**Figure 8.30b** Abdominal aorta and renal arteries

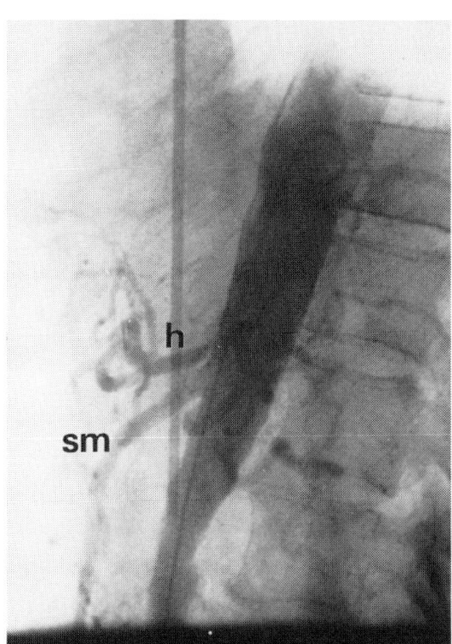


**Figure 8.30c** Lateral image of abdominal aorta at the level of the coeliac axis showing hepatic (h) and superior mesenteric (sm) arteries

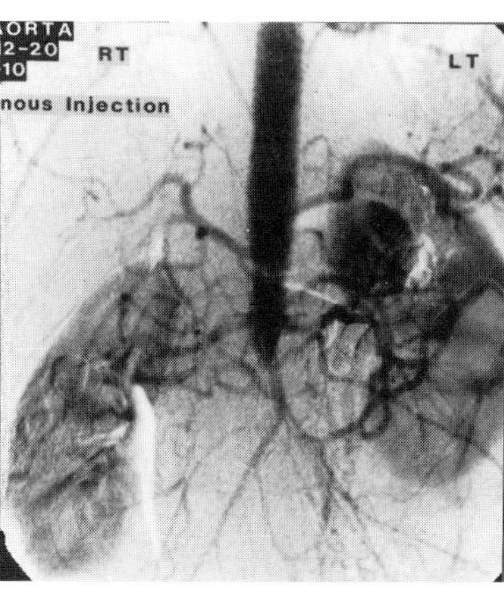


**Figure 8.30d** IVDSA image showing occlusion of the abdominal aorta immediately distal to the renal artery origins (Lericha syndrome)

### Imaging procedure

*Abdominal aorta*

A 6.5F polythene or 4 or 5F high-flow catheter is selected. The tip of the catheter is first manipulated under fluoroscopic control, so that it is above the level of the coeliac artery which is approximately at the level of the lower border of the 11th thoracic vertebrae. If a rapid film changer is used to acquire images, a single image may be made at this stage to check positioning for optimal field of view.

A bolus of contrast is then injected using a pressure injector and, following an exposure delay of 0.5 s, postero-anterior images are acquired at the level required, using a standard exposure sequence. If severe occlusive disease is found, the examination may be repeated using a modified exposure sequence.

Additional lateral or oblique projections may be required if stenosis of the coeliac or mesenteric arteries is suspected.

If required, the distal aorta and iliac vessels may be imaged by programmed movement of the couch top in conjunction with rapid serial radiography or manual movement with digital acquisition when the flow of contrast is observed on the image monitor.

The patient should be instructed to remain still during the whole procedure and images are acquired in suspended respiration.

*Thoracic aorta*

An 8F polythene catheter with five side holes near the tip or a pigtail catheter is selected. Alternatively, 5 or 6.5F high-flow catheters may be used.

The tip of the catheter is directed to the ascending aorta for demonstration of the arch, ascending and proximal descending aorta. Relocation of the catheter into the proximal descending aorta may be required.

Where coarctation is present, a brachial or right axillary approach may be required.

Following a bolus injection, LAO 15° images are acquired of the arch and proximal thoracic aorta. Further postero-anterior images of the distal thoracic aorta are acquired following another bolus injection. Additional lateral images may be acquired in cases of suspected aortic dissection.

*Imaging parameters*

| *Images/s* | *Run time* | *Total images* |
|---|---|---|
| 3 | 2 s | 6 |
| 2 | 3 s | 6 |

*Contrast medium and injection data*

| *Volume* | *Concentration* | *Flow rate* |
|---|---|---|
| 40 ml | 300 mgI/ml | 20 ml/s |

*Exposure delay* 0.5 s for abdominal aorta.
In DSA, the concentration may be reduced.

# 8 Aorta

## Magnetic resonance imaging

$T_1$ weighted spin-echo and gradient-echo sequences are used to demonstrate morphology and blood flow. Cardiac gating is necessary when imaging the thoracic region but is not necessary for assessing the abdominal aorta, although respiratory gating may be applied.

### Indications

Vessel patency, aneurysms, dissections and coarctation.

### Position of patient and imaging modality

The patient lies supine, head first on the scanner table, with the median sagittal plane perpendicular to the centre of the table, and if necessary with the cardiac gating applied. Using the transaxial alignment light, the external reference point is obtained either at the level of the manubrium for the aortic arch and the thoracic aorta or at the level of the xiphisternum for imaging the abdominal aorta. From this position the patient is moved the fixed distance into the isocentre of the magnet.

### Imaging procedure – thoracic aorta

Initially a transaxial spin-echo localiser scan is obtained to localise the ascending and descending aorta. From this image a series of compound oblique sagittal sections are selected to demonstrate the ascending aorta, aortic arch and descending aorta. A $T_1$ weighted spin-echo sequence is required to delineate morphology with a cine gradient-echo sequence, as described in MRI of the heart, necessary to demonstrate dynamic blood flow in cases of coarctation. A series of transaxial scans are also necessary to delineate the aorta in cross-section, to assess its diameter and to differentiate the true and false lumen of an aneurysm. A STIR sequence may be necessary to differentiate an infiltrating lesion from a static aneurysm.

### Imaging procedure – abdominal aorta

Initially a sagittal localiser scan is obtained to localise the abdominal aorta. From this image a series of coronal sections are prescribed through the aorta using either a $T_1$ weighted spin-echo or a flow-enhanced gradient-echo sequence. Sagittal and transaxial $T_1$ weighted images are also acquired. The diameter of the aorta is assessed from the transaxial images.

Contrast enhanced breath-hold $T_1$ weighted gradient-echo sequences may be used for delineating the renal arteries and the extent of any aneurysm or dissection. Phase contrast MRA may also be used for detailed study of the renal vessels.

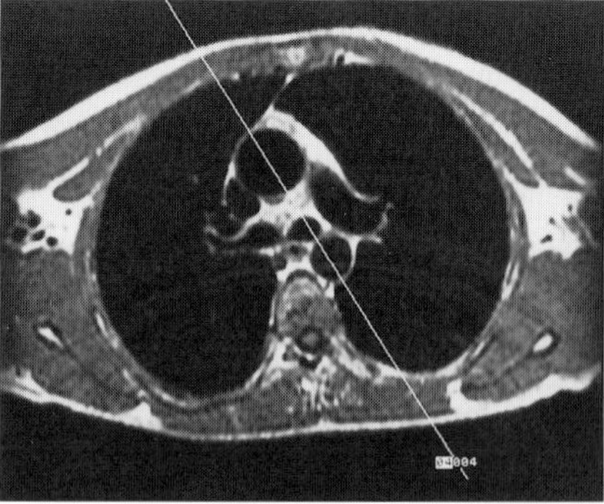

**Figure 8.31a** Transaxial spin-echo localiser scan showing the position of the sagittal oblique image through the ascending and descending aorta

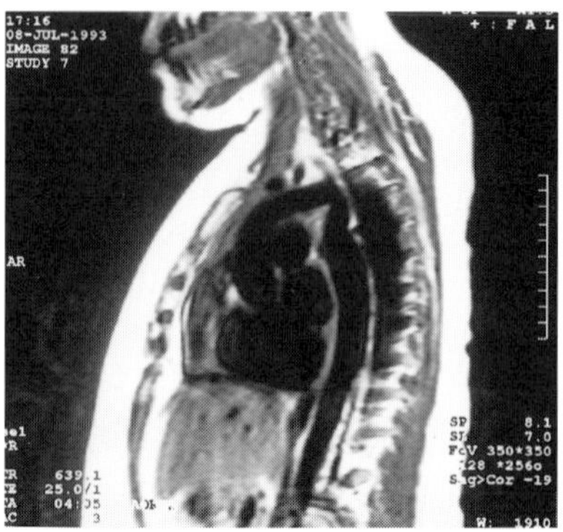

**Figure 8.31b** Sagittal oblique $T_1$ spin-echo scan showing coarctation of the thoracic aorta

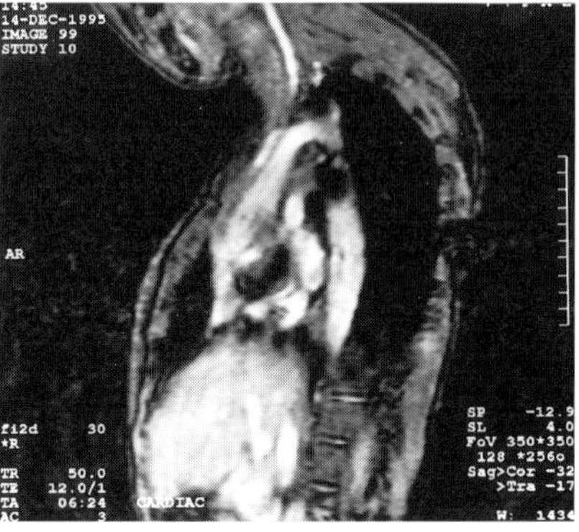

**Figure 8.31c** Sagittal oblique gradient-echo cine image showing severe coarctation of the aortic arch (NB. Jet of black blood indicating blood flow turbulence through the stenosis)

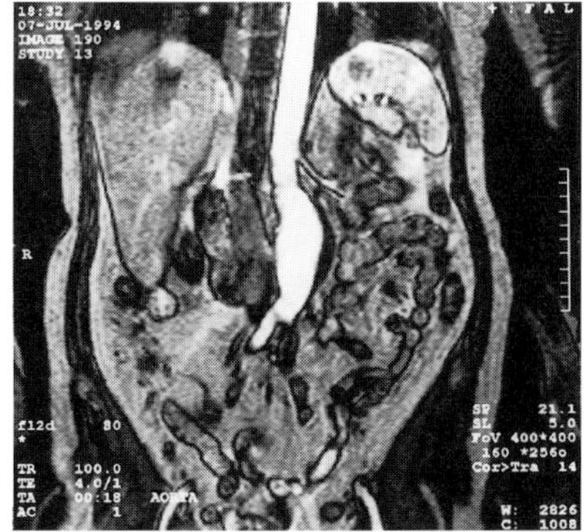

**Figure 8.31d** Coronal gradient-echo $T_1$ weighted post-contrast image using a breath-hold technique, showing an aneurysm of the abdominal aorta

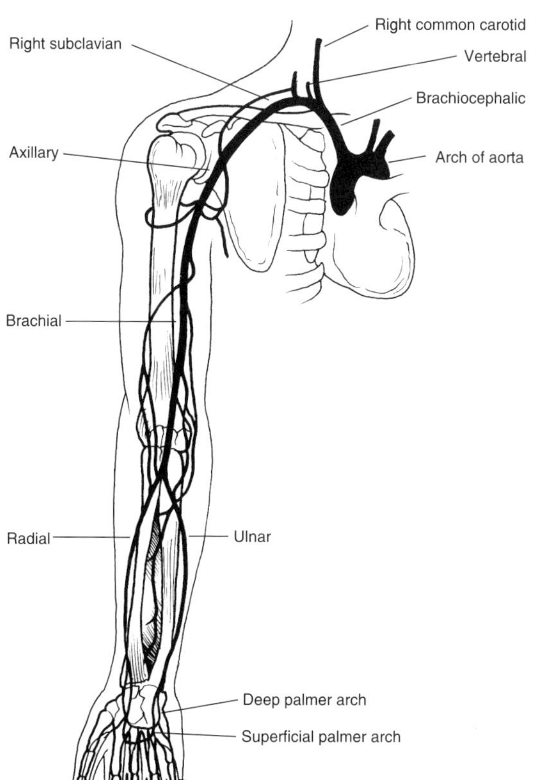


**Figure 8.32a** Arterial supply to upper limb (anterior aspect)

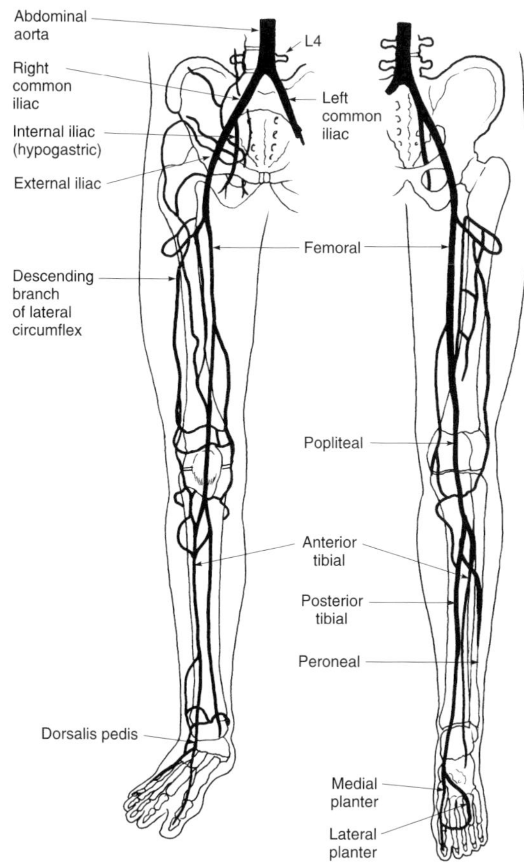


**Figure 8.32b** Arterial supply to lower limb (anterior and posterior aspects)



# Peripheral vessels, subclavian arteries and inferior vena cava

This section covers examination of the arterial and venous vessels of the upper and lower limbs including the subclavian arteries and inferior vena cava (IVC).

## Indications

*Arteries*
This will involve the detection of congenital abnormalities, investigation of narrowing and occlusion of vessels together with detailed blood flow analysis.

Such studies are undertaken prior to an following intervention.

*Veins*
Varicose veins, deep venous thrombosis and the location of arteriovenous malformations.

## Recommended imaging procedures

Soft tissue plain film radiography is limited to identification of calcification within a vessel wall.

Contrast angiography or venography using rapid serial radiography or digital imaging or digital substraction angiography (DSA) techniques will demonstrate both vessel anatomy and blood flow abnormalities. These procedures give excellent results but have the disadvantage of being invasive. The use of ionic contrast agents have been abandoned due to the high risk of inducing deep venous thrombus.

Continuous wave Doppler ultrasound, duplex ultrasound and colour flow imaging may all play a valuable non-invasive role in providing quantitative haemodynamic information and assessing vessels in the arms and legs. Overlying gas from abdominal structures, however, makes this an ineffective method for assessing the inferior vena cava below the liver and the iliac veins. Very low flow rates in the smaller calf veins make it difficult to visualise all the veins below the knee.

Magnetic resonance angiography and magnetic resonance venography make it possible to image vessels in the limbs and the abdomen. At the time of writing, the full diagnostic potential of these procedures has yet to be achieved.

# 8 Peripheral Vessels, Subclavian Arteries and Inferior Vena Cava

## Peripheral vessels

### Arteriography – lower limb

Bilateral lower limb arteriography is usually performed, except in trauma cases when the relevant leg is examined. It is most commonly performed by a Seldinger technique with retrograde catheterisation of a femoral artery, with the tip of the catheter positioned in the lower aorta. A non-ionic contrast agent is used.

The procedure is best performed using dedicated angiographic equipment with an image intensifier large enough (e.g. 40 cm) to accommodate both limbs and digital imaging facilities allowing image subtraction and blood flow analysis. Such equipment will provide motorised movement of the imaging couch or X-ray tube/image intensifier assembly to facilitate rapid digital image acquisition at predetermined positions along the length of the lower limbs. Images can also be acquired using a rapid serial film changer.

The examination, commencing at the pelvic region to demonstrate the lower aorta, is comprised of a series of images acquired at each of four or five staged positions along the length of the imaging couch terminating at the ankles. Alternatively, using a 'bolus chase' technique and digital fluoroscopy the injected contrast agent is observed using digital fluoroscopy as it flows along the arteries, with permanent images acquired as and when necessary. Intravenous DSA may be used as a procedure when arterial catheterisation is impossible.

*Indications*

Intermittent claudication due to atheromatous disease producing arterial narrowing or occlusion. Buerger's disease or other forms of arteritis. Trauma to a limb, with arterial involvement. Prior to and following interventional procedures or vascular surgery.

*Position of patient and imaging modality*

The patient lies supine in the centre of the imaging couch, with the head raised on a shallow pillow. Both knees are extended with the legs straightened and positioned together, with the feet pointing upwards and rotated slightly inwards to demonstrate the gap between the tibia and fibula. The feet are secured by a triangular wedge foam pad and restraining straps. The image intensifier is parallel to the imaging couch and positioned under fluoroscopic control over the pelvic area to ensure that the first image will include the distal aorta and proximal femoral arteries. For rapid serial radiography the film changer is rotated into position.

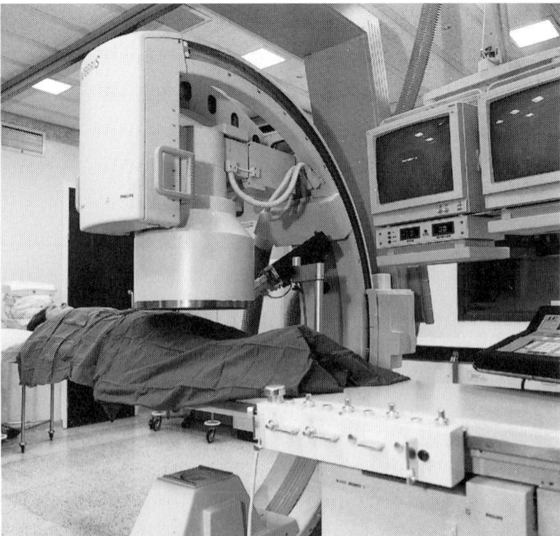

**Figure 8.33a** Patient and equipment

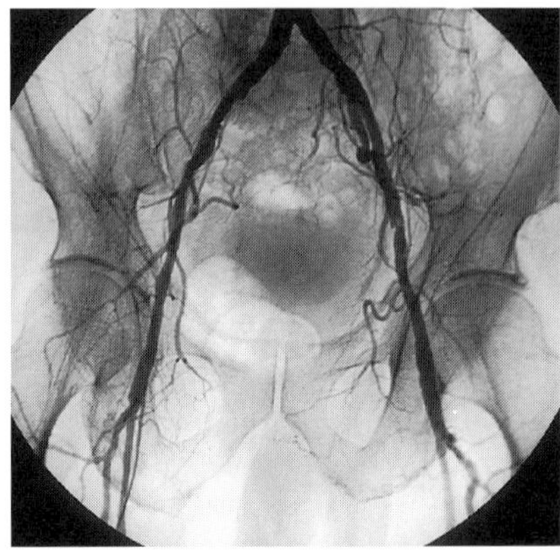

**Figure 8.33b** Image of the pelvic area showing the iliac and proximal femoral vessels

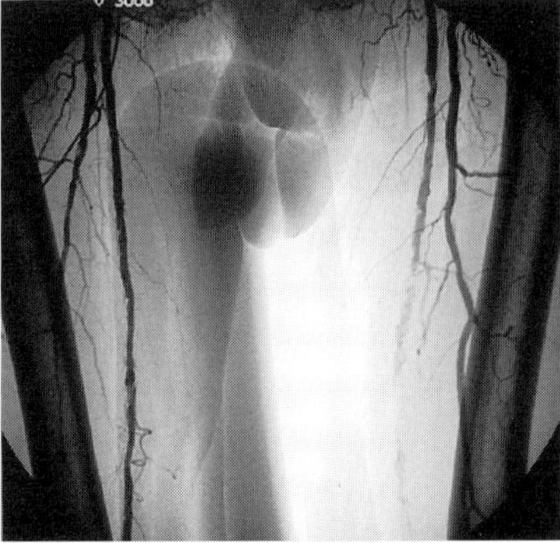

**Figure 8.33c** Image of superficial femoral and profunda femoris vessels with occlusive disease on the left

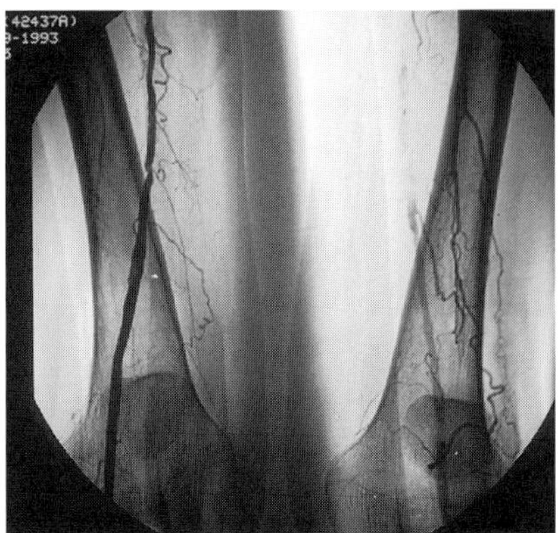

**Figure 8.33d** Image of the distal femoral and proximal popliteal vessels with occlusive disease, as shown in (c), and right-sided stenotic disease

## Peripheral vessels

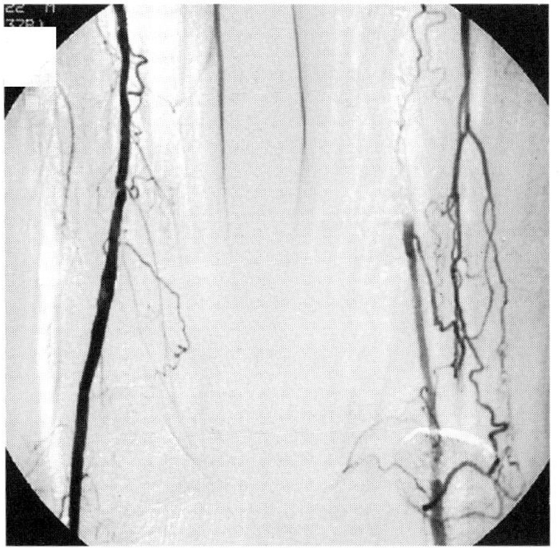

**Figure 8.34a** Subtracted image of (d) on preceding page showing collateral filling of distal left femoral beyond the occlusion

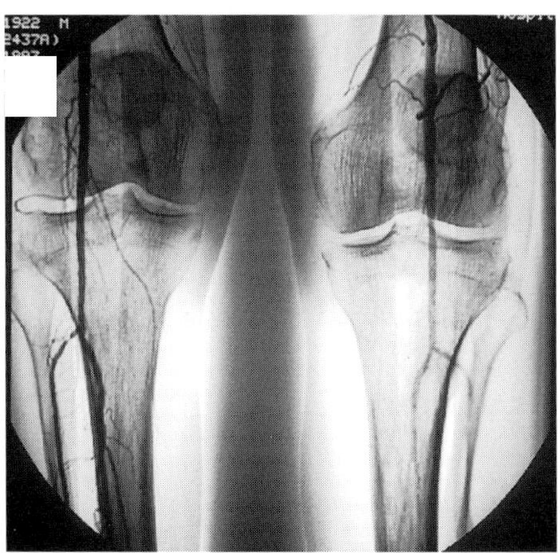

**Figure 8.34b** Image of knees showing popliteal and proximal tibial run-off

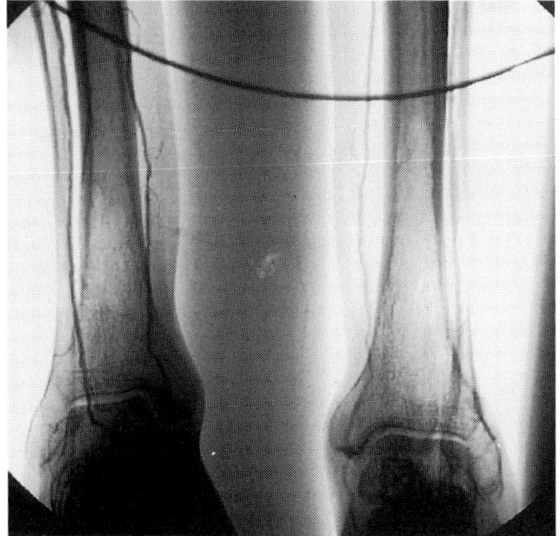

**Figure 8.34c** Image of both lower tibia and fibula showing distal anterior and posterior tibial and peroneal vessels

*Imaging procedure*

At this stage the couch top or image intensifier assembly is engaged at the start position. During the examination, postero-anterior projections of both thighs, knees and proximal lower legs, and distal lower legs and ankles, are taken. A bolus of contrast agent is delivered using a contrast pressure injector linked to the X-ray generator.

The tip of the catheter is positioned above the aortic bifurcation under fluoroscopic control. Prior to full examination of both limbs, a bolus of 10 ml of contrast agent is injected by hand into the aorta, and the flow of the contrast is observed and timed as it traverses the femoral arteries to the knees and lower down the limbs. An image acquisition protocol, incorporating an exposure delay following operation of the pressure injector, is prescribed to ensure complete visualisation of the arterial vessels for a single bolus injection of contrast, bearing in mind the timed arterial blood flow rate. The protocol, for each of the staged positions, will combine rapid serial image acquisition at a specific exposure rate for a predetermined run time, movement of the X-ray tube or imaging couch together with an appropriate reduction in kilovoltage for each position following the initial exposures of the pelvic area.

During digital image acquisition, image flare as a result of direct exposure of the image intensifier can be reduced by using either preshaped filters incorporated into the beam collimation device or a sword-shaped aluminium filter positioned between the legs.

When a 'bolus chase' technique is employed, movement of the image intensifier/X-ray tube assembly is under the direct control of the operator who is able to observe the filling of the vessels and control permanent image acquisition of these vessels using a predetermined and variable image acquisition rate.

For real-time DSA of a specific region, a bolus injection of contrast is given, with the image intensifier positioned over the affected vessels and an exposure sequence activated incorporating a mask image at the start of the sequence. Alternatively, some equipment is designed to enable a mask image to be taken at each position of a planned peripheral run prior to contrast medium being injected. The patient must not move until the complete exposure sequence is completed to avoid misregistration when the vessels are subtracted.

*Contrast medium and injector data*

| *Volume* | *Concentration* | *Flow rate* |
|---|---|---|
| 50 ml | 300 mgI/ml | 8 ml/s |

*Exposure delay* 2 s

In DSA, the concentration may be reduced

*Imaging parameters*

| *Position* | *Images/s* | *Run time* | *Total images* |
|---|---|---|---|
| 1 | 2 | 1 s | 2 |
| 2 | 2 | 1 s | 2 |
| 3 | 1 | 2 s | 2 |
| 4 | 1 | 2 s | 2 |
| 5 | 1 | 2 s | 2 |

# 8 Peripheral Vessels, Subclavian Arteries and Inferior Vena Cava

## Peripheral vessels

### Ultrasound – lower limb (arteries)

Doppler ultrasound is a quick, reproducible, painless and non-invasive technique, allowing assessment of the location and functional effect of vascular stenosis. Vessels are examined mainly using continuous wave Doppler (CWD) or alternatively using real-time B-mode imaging combined with pulsed wave Doppler (PWD) and colour flow Doppler.

*Indications*

Diagnosis and assessment of site and severity of occlusive arterial disease.

Before and after interventional procedures, e.g. angioplasty, to assess the effectiveness of the procedure and for monitoring the patency of a vascular graft.

**Continuous Wave Doppler**

Assessment of the lower limb arteries is made by sampling at specific palpable sites along both limbs to demonstrate the Doppler spectrum of the common femoral, popliteal, posterior tibial and dorsalis pedis arteries. The Doppler waveform produced from each location provides information on any blood flow impairment, the area of stenosis and the amount of disease that exists if the pulsatility index values are obtained and analysed. Normally both limbs are examined for comparison. Additionally, Doppler ultrasound is used to obtain 'segmental pressure measurements' at four different levels along both limbs to determine systolic pressure values and to determine the ankle systolic/brachial systolic pressure ratio index.

Further information may be obtained by repeating these measurements after exercising the patient.

*Recording procedure*

The arterial signals are bi-directional and are displayed as a waveform showing peak-to-peak frequencies over a period of time. Parameters should be set to calculate every 5 s, averaged over five cardiac cycles. A 4 MHz probe is used to evaluate the femoral and popliteal arteries and a 8 MHz probe for the tibial and dorsalis pedis arteries. The probe is assumed to be pointing towards the heart. The leg is examined by first locating the femoral pulse at the level of the inguinal ligament and applying warm coupling gel to the groin. The common femoral artery is then insonated, with the probe held at approximately 60° to the longitudinal axis of the artery. Both an audible Doppler signal and a Doppler waveform are obtained and the probe is adjusted to obtain the highest peak frequency possible. Using the freeze frame facility, a printout of the Doppler waveform and machine calculated results is obtained. The patient is turned prone and the probe is held at the level of the popliteal fossa to insonate the popliteal artery.

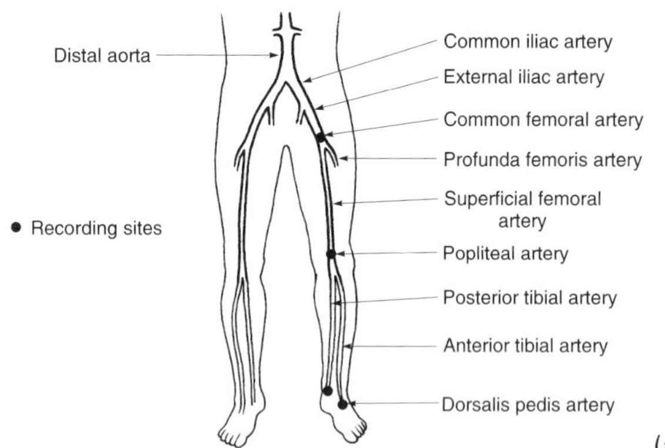


(a)

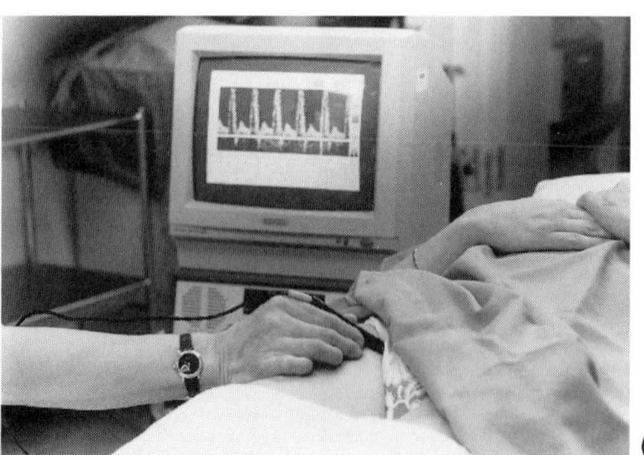

(b)

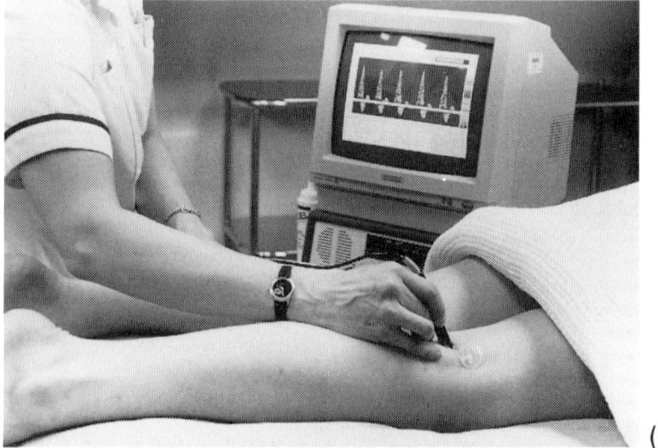

(c)

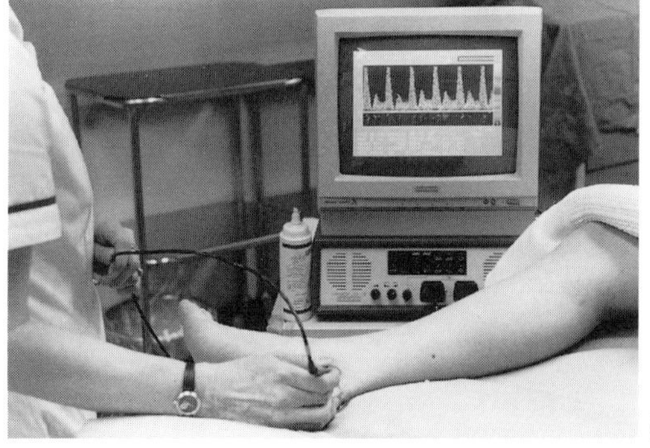

(d)

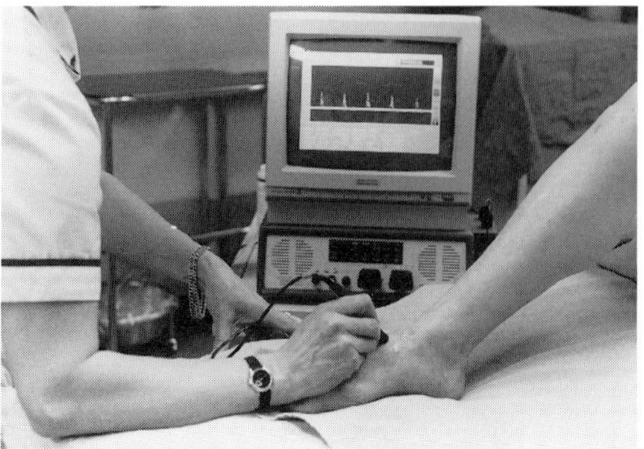

(e)

**Figure 8.35** (a) Lower limb recording sites; (b–e) Recording sites for (b) common femoral, (c) popliteal, (c) posterior tibial, and (e) dorsalis pedis arteries

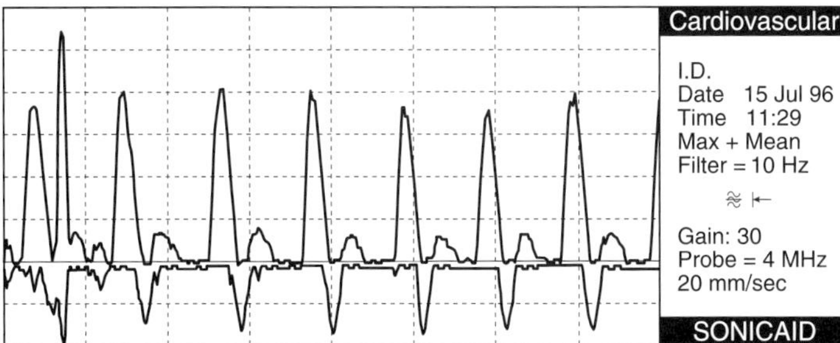


**Figure 8.36a** Common femoral Doppler waveform

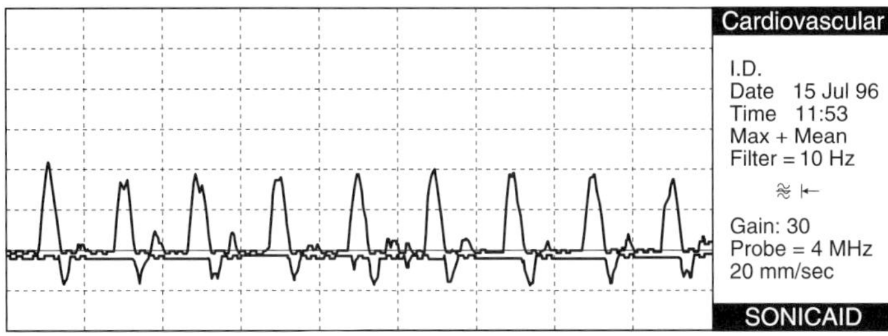


**Figure 8.36b** Popliteal Doppler waveform

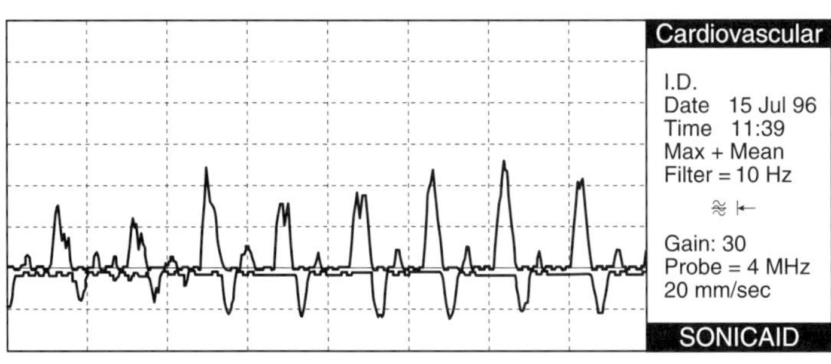


**Figure 8.36c** Posterior tibial waveform

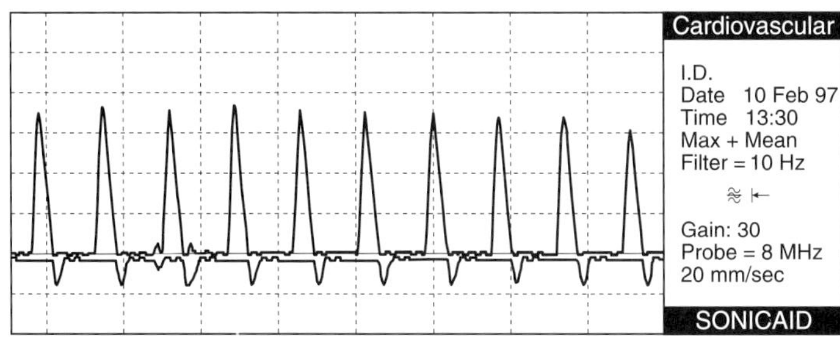


**Figure 8.36d** Dorsalis pedis Doppler waveform



## Peripheral vessels

The patient is turned supine, for examination of the posterior tibial artery, located just behind the medial malleolus, and dorsalis pedis artery located on the dorsum of the foot.

*Waveform parameters*

Doppler waveforms provide a means of analysing blood flow through the vessel immediately proximal to the site of insonation. The type of waveform pattern and parameters displayed are characteristic of where the vessel is monitored and will vary depending on the degree of arterial lumen constriction, peripheral dilatation or aneurysmal dilatation. A number of parameters can be used to quantify blood flow and the following are given as examples:

- *Pulsatility Index (PI)* is a measure of the amount of oscillatory energy contained within the pulse and provides quantitative information about disease proximal to the site of isonation, e.g. if the PI index is below the value of 4 for the femoral artery, this will indicate, with reasonable certainty, that the aorta or the iliac artery or both contain a stenosis with 75% diameter reduction.
- *Pulsatility index damping ratio* is used to quantify the degree of damping within an arterial segment. In healthy vessels, PI increases down the leg and is greatest at the ankle. In the presence of disease, the ratio decreases with increasing severity of disease.
- *Systolic velocity measurement* is used for determining the severity of arterial stenosis, with stenotic constriction causing localised increase in the peak systolic frequency.

Additionally, segmental pressure measurements along both limbs and measurement of the ankle systolic/brachial systolic pressure ratio index may be undertaken with CWD in order to diagnose occlusive disease. In the former, systolic pressures are obtained, using a sphygmomanometer cuff, at four locations on each leg: one at high thigh, one above the knee, one below the knee and one above the ankle. An 8 MHz probe is placed over the dorsalis pedis or the posterior tibial artery. A difference of 20–30 mmHg between each reading is borderline and greater than 30 mmHg difference indicates significant occlusive disease. In the latter a PI value of less than 1 indicates stenotic disease.

**Pulsed Wave Doppler/colour flow Doppler**

Using PWD a transverse scan is performed to locate the vessel which is then imaged in its longitudinal plane (see Plate 12). B-mode imaging is used to direct optimal placement of the pulsed wave Doppler sampling gate across the vessel. Colour flow Doppler will directly demonstrate stenosis and turbulence by nature of the colours displayed in the vessel and allow accurate placement of the Doppler sampling gate for analysis at the site of maximum stenosis.

# 8 Peripheral Vessels, Subclavian Arteries and Inferior Vena Cava

## Peripheral vessels

### Ultrasound – lower limb (veins)

Real-time B-mode imaging combined with colour flow is the preferred investigation for the diagnosis of deep venous thrombus in the common femoral and popliteal veins. It can also be used to diagnose the sites of incompetent perforating veins in varicose vein abnormalities.

*Imaging procedure*
With the patient supine, a 5–7 MHz linear transducer, covered with coupling gel, is positioned against the skin over the area of the affected vein and a transverse scan is performed to locate the vessel. Further imaging is performed in the longitudinal plane of the vessel, with the transducer moved both distally and proximally along the length of the vessel. As part of the imaging protocol, pressure is applied to the skin surface to observe if the section of vein is readily compressed or if it retains its dimensions which is indicative of the presence of a thrombus. Colour flow imaging is also employed, as it may demonstrate blood flow around a thrombus in the partly occluded vessel (see Plate 13).

When examining varicose veins the patient is asked to perform the Valsalva manoeuvre. The presence of any reflux is an indication of incompetent valves.

### Venography – lower limbs

Venography of the lower limb is normally confined to the demonstration of the deep leg veins by means of a suitably dilute non-ionic contrast agent (3 × 50 ml) which is injected by hand. This involves cannulation of a distal vein in the dorsum of the foot with a 19- or 21-gauge needle, if possible, directed distally. Contrast is prevented from entering the superficial veins of the leg being examined by the application of tourniquets around the leg – one above the ankle and the other above or below the knee.

The procedure is performed using fluoroscopic imaging equipment using either a conventional couch, with an overcouch image intensifier, or alternatively on a remote control system with an undercouch image intensifier. Permanent images are acquired using a serial cassette changer or with a digital imaging facility.

*Indications*
Deep venous thrombosis. Patency of deep veins prior to varicose vein surgery. Varicose veins for the detection of incompetent perforating veins and incompetent venous valves. Congenital vascular malformations involving the venous system.

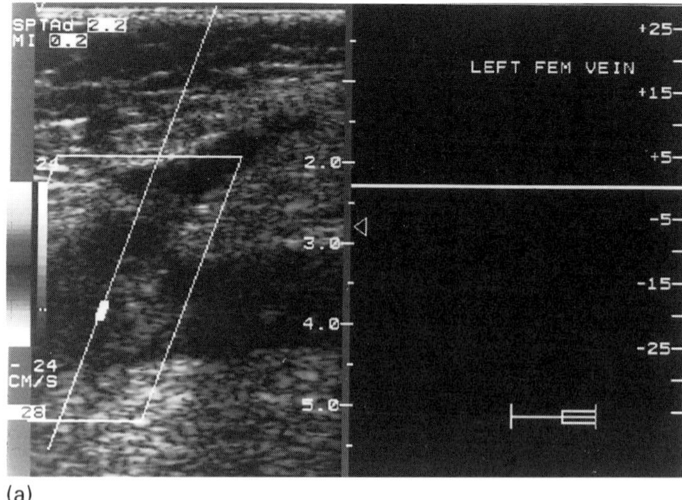


(a)

(b)

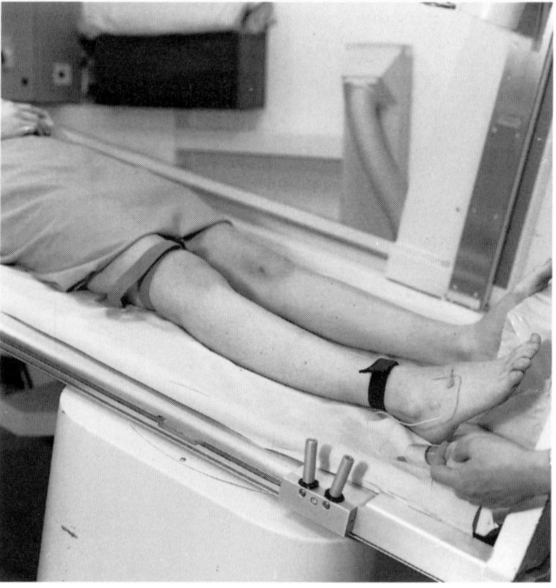

(c)

**Figure 8.37** (a,b) Duplex study showing (a) left femoral vein with thrombus and no blood flow demonstrated, and (b) left femoral vein with compression with the vein retaining its dimensions confirming thrombus. (c) Patient positioned for venography of lower limbs

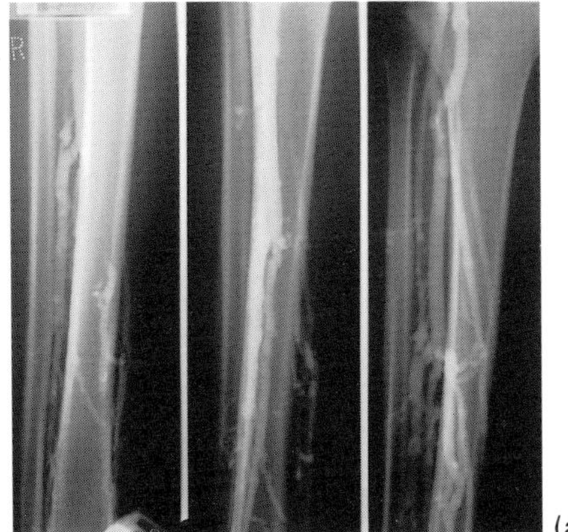
(a)

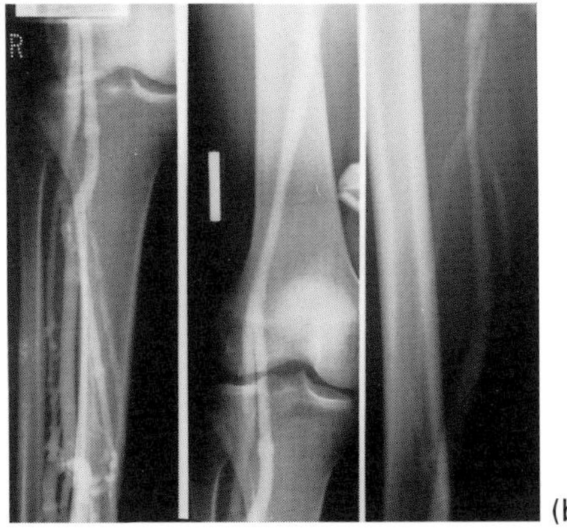
(b)

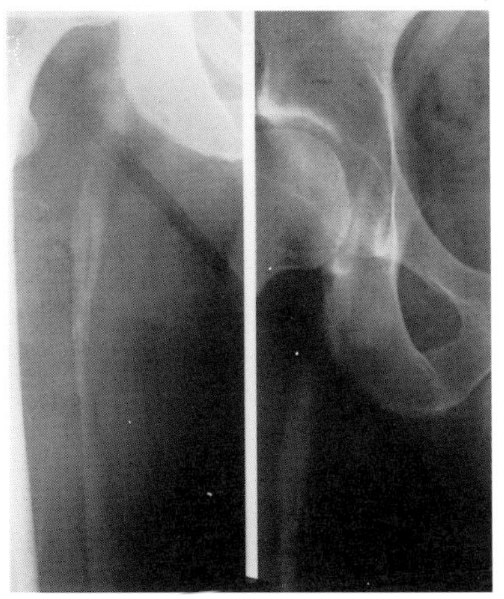
(c)

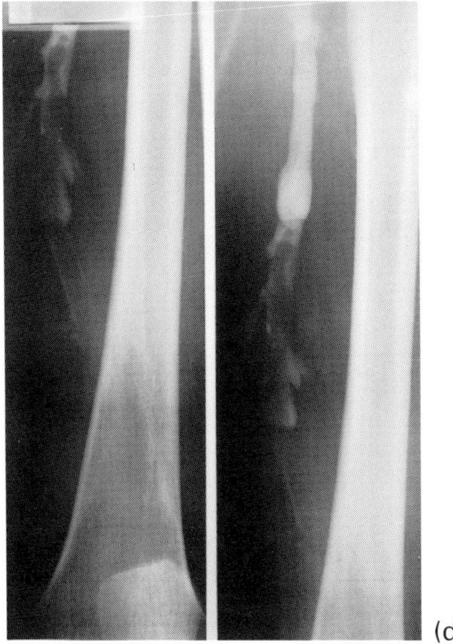
(d)

Figure 8.38 (a–c) Series of images from a right lower limb venogram; (d) example of left femoral vein thrombus

# Peripheral Vessels, Subclavian Arteries and Inferior Vena Cava 8

## Peripheral vessels

### Venography – lower limbs

*Position of patient and imaging modality*

The technique described assumes the use of a conventional imaging couch, with the patient supine and head raised on a shallow pillow. A series of images are taken of the affected limb, with the lower leg positioned for postero-anterior, oblique and lateral projections in order to demonstrate the deep calf veins. The upper leg is positioned for a series of postero-anterior projections to demonstrate the popliteal, femoral and iliac veins. As contrast is observed to flow through the veins, optimal positioning of the limb is aided by fluoroscopy to avoid overlapping of the vessels.

For the lower leg, postero-anterior projections are acquired, with the limb under examination extended and the ankle dorsiflexed and the limb rotated medially until the medial and lateral malleoli are equidistant from the table top. For oblique projections, the limb is rotated laterally approximately 45°. Lateral projections are acquired with the patient turned completely onto the affected side so that the medial and lateral malleoli are superimposed and the tibia parallel to the image receptor.

Postero-anterior projections of the upper leg and pelvic area are acquired with the leg extended and rotated slightly inwards.

For all projections the image intensifier is positioned above the relevant section of limb, parallel to the imaging table.

*Imaging procedure*

Contrast is injected into a vein in the dorsum of the foot. To make a vein prominent for cannulation, the lower tourniquet is tightened and with the couch tilted erect the patient is supported on the unaffected leg. The application of local heat to the dorsum of the foot, using a hot water bottle or water bath, may also be required. The tourniquet above the knee is also tightened prior to cannulation. After venous cannulation, with the table semi-erect, contrast medium is injected under fluoroscopic control, during which postero-anterior, oblique and lateral images are acquired of the calf veins filled with contrast. As the injection continues, the contrast medium is observed as it flows proximally through the popliteal and femoral veins. Permanent postero-anterior images are acquired at different levels of the upper leg with the table horizontal. The tourniquet above the knee is then released and to aid filling of the iliac veins, which may be assisted by gentle calf pressure. Permanent images of the iliac vein usually completes the investigation.

Incompetent valves are demonstrated by retrograde flow of contrast medium which may be accentuated by using the Valsalva manoeuvre which slows the flow of contrast and accentuates the demonstration of the venous valves.

*Contrast medium and injection data*

| *Volume* | *Concentration* | *Flow rate* |
|---|---|---|
| 50–150 ml | 150 mgI/ml | Hand injection |

# 8 Peripheral Vessels, Subclavian Arteries and Inferior Vena Cava

## Upper limbs and subclavian arteries

### Arteriography

Imaging is performed using dedicated angiographic equipment combined with digital imaging, thus enabling digital subtraction angiography, or alternatively with a rapid serial film changer.

The procedure is most commonly performed by a Seldinger technique, with retrograde catheterisation of a femoral artery. A non-ionic contrast agent and pressure injector are selected for the procedure.

*Indications*

There are a number of indications, which include: trauma with associated arterial involvement, investigation of tumours, aneurysms and arteriovenous malformations. The procedure is also used in the investigation of Raynaud's disease affecting the arteries of the hand and fingers, suspected occlusive disease and congenital anomalies of the subclavian artery (causing varied symptoms), before, during and following interventional procedures such as dilatation of occluded arteries and the embolisation of the blood supply to arteriovenous malformations.

*Position of patient and imaging modality*

Postero-anterior images are acquired of the upper thorax and neck region and limb under investigation. The patient is supine with the arms normally positioned alongside the trunk, with the palms of the hand facing upwards. In some cases an arm may be raised above the head to investigate the effects on arterial circulation, e.g. cervical ribs. The image intensifier/film changer is positioned parallel to the imaging couch and above the region under investigation.

*Imaging procedure*

An arch aortogram is performed initially, using a 5F pigtail catheter, to outline the vascular anatomy. Selective catheterisation of the right or left subclavian artery, using a Headhunter catheter, is then performed prior to separate examination of different regions of the arm. A small amount of contrast may be injected and observed as it traverses the limb, to determine the location of any abnormality prior to an imaging sequence. Following a bolus injection of contrast medium, images are then acquired, in rapid succession, at the predetermined region.

*Imaging parameters*

| *Images/s* | *Run time* | *Total images* |
|---|---|---|
| 1 | 8–10 s | 8–10 |

*Contrast medium and injector data*

| *Volume* | *Concentration* | *Flow rate* |
|---|---|---|
| 20 ml | 300 mgI/ml | 8–10 ml/s |

In DSA, the concentration may be reduced



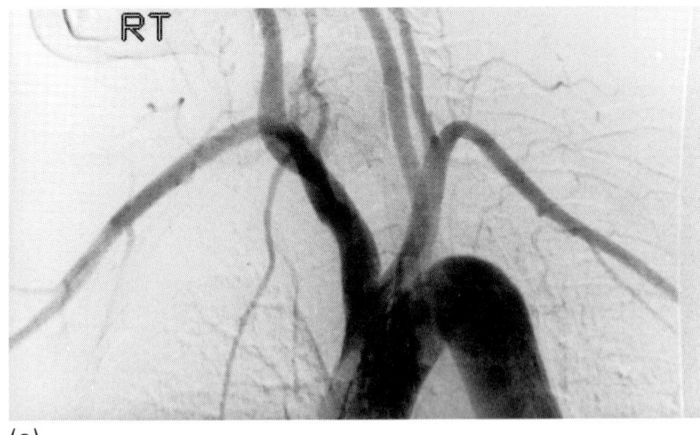


(a)

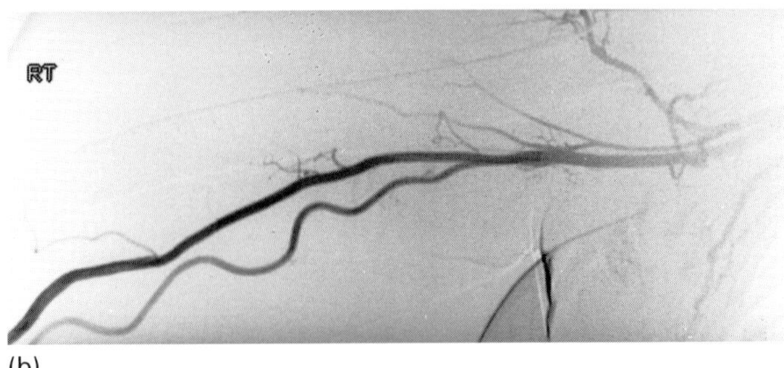


(b)

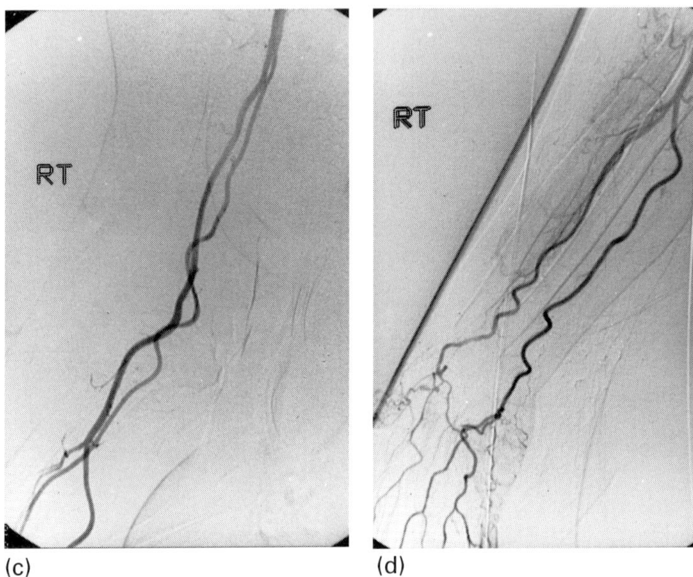


(c) (d)

**Figure 8.39a** Arch aortogram demonstrating neck vessels and both subclavian arteries; (b) right subclavian artery and axillary artery; (c) brachial artery; (d) radial, ulnar and digital arteries

## Upper limbs and subclavian arteries

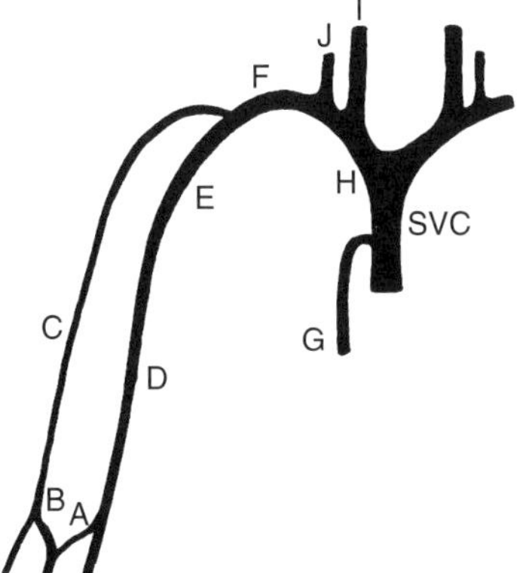


**Figure 8.40a** Schematic diagram of upper limb and SVC venous system (A, median basilic vein; B, median cephalic vein; C, cephalic vein; D, basilic vein; E, axillary vein; F, subclavian vein; G, azygos vein; H, innominate vein; I, interior jugular vein; J, exterior jugular vein; SVC, superior vena cava)

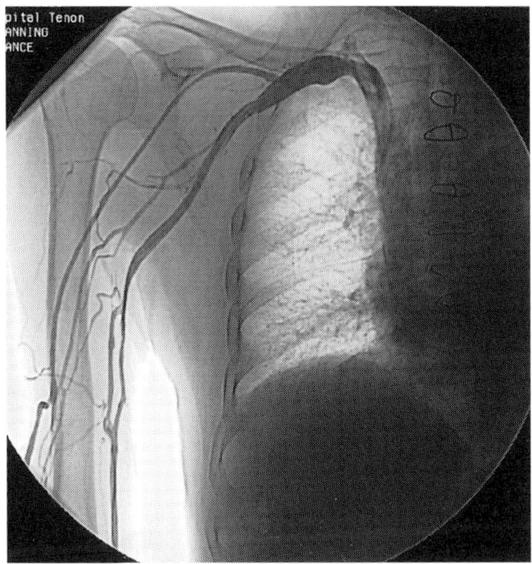

**Figure 8.40b** Image of upper limb and SVC venous system

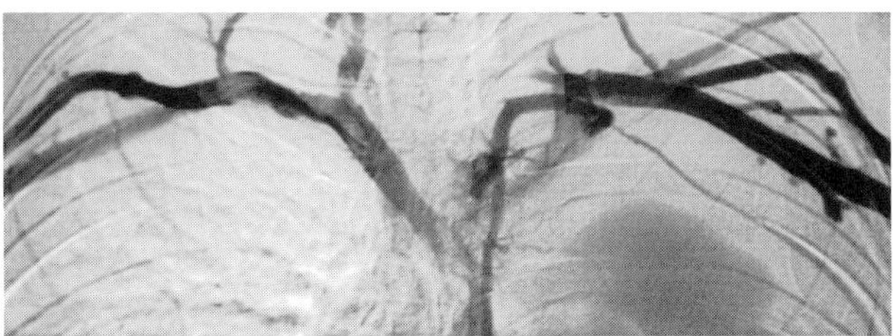

**Figure 8.40c** Venogram demonstrating poor contrast media filling both brachiocephalic veins with drainage via azygos and hemiazygos vein systems

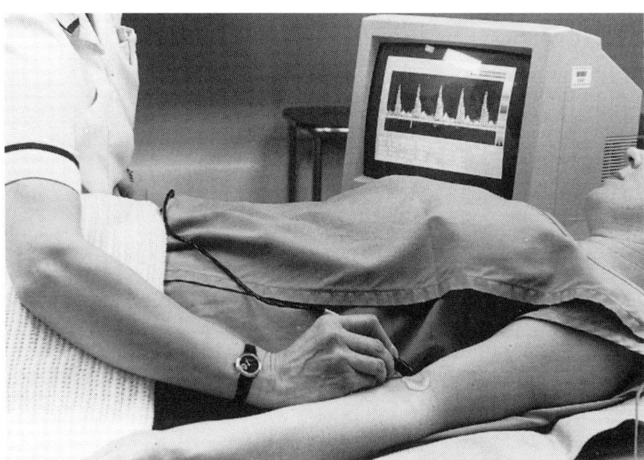

**Figure 8.40d** Recording site for brachial artery with typical continuous wave Doppler waveform

### Venography

Venography is performed using fluoroscopic imaging equipment or alternatively with dedicated angiographic equipment. The examination is usually confined to the shoulder region to determine the site of an obstruction.

Permanent images are acquired using either a serial cassette/film changer or with a digital imaging facility. The procedure involves cannulation of a distal vein, e.g. an antecubital vein, and a non-ionic contrast medium injected slowly under fluoroscopic control.

*Indications*
This includes investigation of upper limb oedema and suspected venous thrombosis of the upper limb.

*Position of patient and imaging modality*
The patient lies supine with head raised on a shallow pillow. The affected arm is extended, slightly abducted and externally rotated. The image intensifier is positioned parallel to the imaging couch over the shoulder region.

*Imaging procedure*
After venous cannulation, contrast medium is injected under fluoroscopic control and observed as it flows proximally through axillary and subclavian veins. Permanent images are acquired as and when necessary to demonstrate the vessels and the site of any pathology. The Valsalva manoeuvre may be performed to slow the flow of contrast and accentuate demonstration of the veins and the superior vena cava. Additional images may be taken, with the patient's arm abducted to 90° to determine if blood flow is affected by arm position.

*Contrast medium and injector data*

| *Volume* | *Concentration* | *Flow rate* |
|---|---|---|
| 20–50 ml | 150 mgI/ml | Hand injection |

### Ultrasound

Ultrasound examination of upper limb arteries and veins is rarely undertaken. However continuous wave Doppler examination of the arterial supply may be undertaken to investigate arterial disease in a similar way to that described on page 300. With the patient supine, sampling is undertaken of the subclavian, brachial, radial, ulnar and digital arteries. For thoracic outlet syndrome, spot measurements are taken over the brachial artery, first with the patient standing or sitting with arms by the side of the thorax. Additional readings are then taken, with shoulders held back and down, with head turned towards the affected side and then with the arm hyperabducted at 90° and 180°, to determine loss of signal as the result of compression of the subclavian artery.

# 8 Peripheral Vessels, Subclavian Arteries and Inferior Vena Cava

## Inferior vena cava

### Venography

Vena cavography (or venography) is commonly performed by a Seldinger technique with retrograde catheterisation of both femoral veins. A non-ionic contrast agent is selected and administered using a contrast pressure injector. Before contrast is administered, a test injection is given to see if contrast flows readily into the IVC, excluding the presence of a large loose thrombus and ensuring that the catheter tip is not wedged in a lumbar vein.

The procedure is best performed using dedicated angiographic equipment with a large image intensifier (e.g. 40 cm) combined with digital imaging facilities or alternatively with rapid serial radiography using an automatic film changer.

*Indications*
Occlusion of the vessel by thrombus, infiltration or narrowing by carcinoma such as a hypernephroma. It is also performed prior to and following the insertion of an umbrella-type filter in the vessel which is designed to trap emboli originating from pelvic or leg veins.

*Position of patient and imaging modality*
Postero-anterior images are acquired of the abdomen and lower thorax.

The patient is supine on the imaging couch, with head raised on a shallow pillow. The image intensifier or film changer is positioned parallel to the couch top and positioned under fluoroscopic control over the abdominal or thoracic area. Lateral images with the image intensifier parallel to the sagittal plane may also be taken to show the relationship of the vessel to the azygos venous system which may fill with contrast if the cava is occluded.

*Imaging procedure*
Two 6.5F catheters, one for each leg, with side holes near their tip, are selected for catheterisation. The tip of each catheter is manipulated, in turn, under fluoroscopic control to the junction of the common iliac veins. The procedure commences with a test injection to establish free flow of blood within the IVC. Once this is established a bolus of contrast is injected, using a pressure injector, following a short exposure delay. Prior to the injection the patient may be asked to perform the Valsalva manoeuvre, which has the effect of holding back the flow of contrast to allow filling of the vessel and opacification of the renal veins. Postero-anterior images are acquired at the level required, using a standard exposure sequence.

In cases when the femoral and iliac veins are obstructed, adequate images can be obtained using a digital subtraction technique following simultaneous injections into a distal vein in both feet associated with the application of a tourniquet above each knee to fill the deep veins.

The IVC may also be imaged by MRI, using a two-dimensional time of flight (TOF) protocol.

*Imaging parameters*

| *Images/s* | *Run time* | *Total images* |
|---|---|---|
| 1 | 10 | 10 |

*Contrast medium and injector data*

| *Volume* | *Concentration* | *Flow rate* |
|---|---|---|
| 40 ml | 300 mgI/ml | 15 ml/s |

*Exposure delay* 1 s

In DSA, the concentration may be reduced

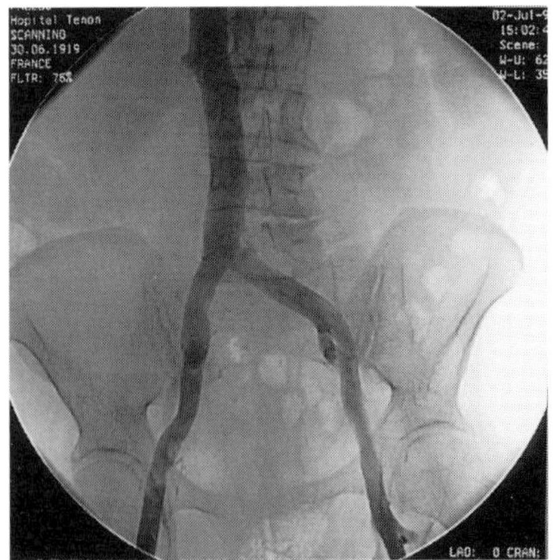

**Figure 8.41a** Iliac veins and distal IVC following injection into distal veins in both feet

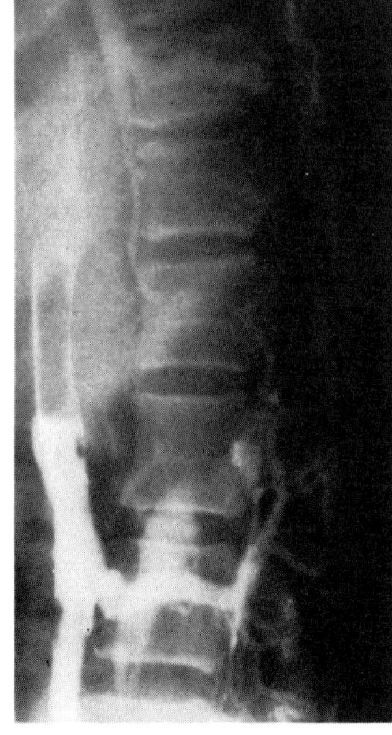

**Figure 8.41b** Thrombus in the IVC with contrast entering the azygos vein

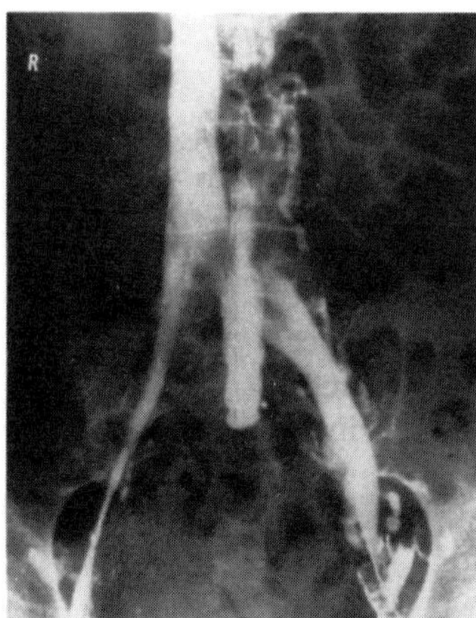

**Figure 8.41c** IVC with bilateral catheters in the iliac veins. Note contrast medium in the lymph nodes from previous lymphogram and contrast in the spinal theca from a previous myelogram

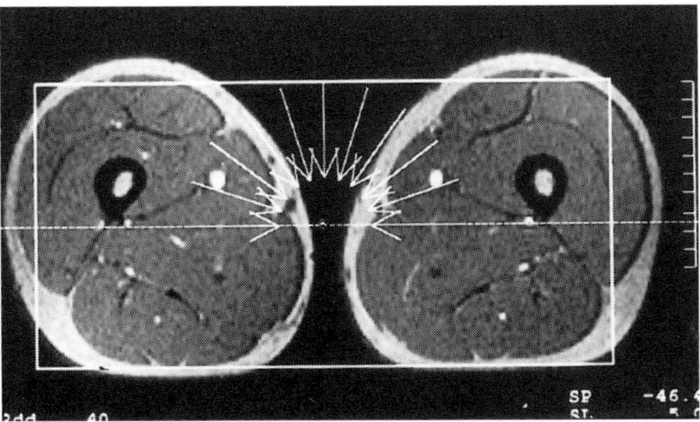

**Figure 8.42a** Transaxial image showing location of targeted MIP and angles of reconstruction

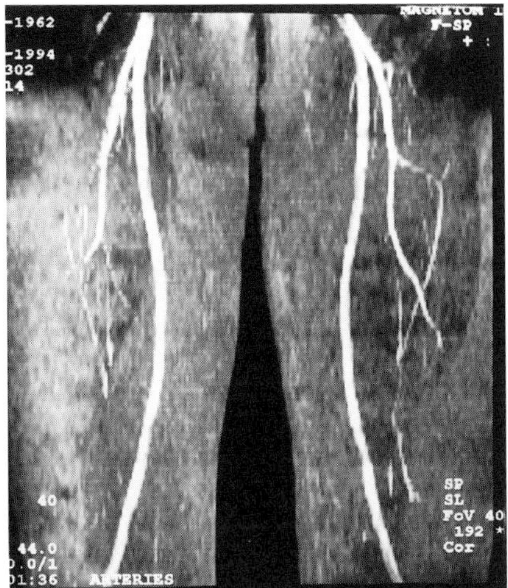

**Figure 8.42b** Coronal reconstructed MIP image of superficial femoral and profunda arteries

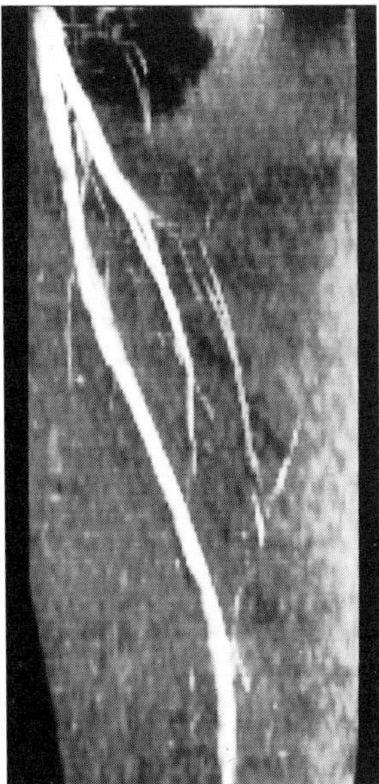

**Figure 8.42c** Lateral reconstructed MIP image of superficial femoral and profunda arteries

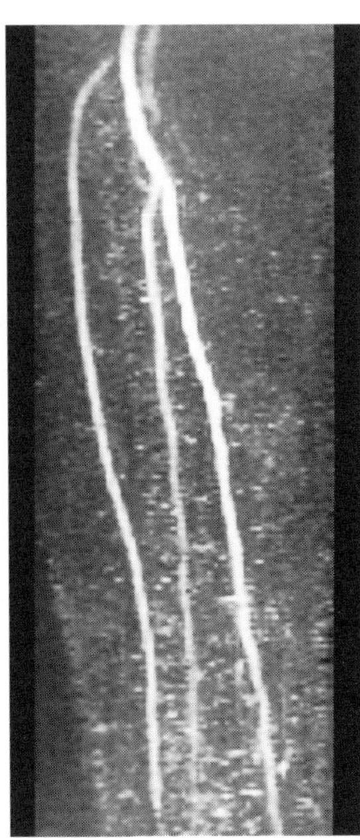

**Figure 8.42d** Reconstructed MIP image of calf arteries with leg in a surface coil

At the time of writing, magnetic resonance angiography (MRA) is used mainly to examine lower limb vessels. This is performed using a two-dimensional TOF imaging protocol and may be followed by phased velocity mapping of a diseased vessel, as described on page 289. Two- and three-dimensional phase contrast imaging, as described in Chapter 1, may also usefully be employed.

**Indications**
Arterial or venous abnormalities.

**Position of patient and imaging modality**
The patient lies supine, feet first, on the imaging couch. The body transmit/receive coil is used to image the pelvic vessels and longer anatomical areas. This permits coverage up to 50 cm in length and allows the comparison of the vessels of the other limb. Detailed examination of a single area may be achieved using a surface coil wrapped around the limb. If the body coil is used the table is adjusted to bring the external reference point to the centre of the affected anatomical area, if a surface coil is used the table is moved until the external reference point is at the centre of the coil.

From the selected external reference point the patient is driven to the isocentre of the magnet.

**Imaging procedure**
A coronal localiser scan, giving bilateral reference, is performed to obtain reference points for image acquisition in the transaxial plane. A TOF pulse sequence is selected, combined with a presaturation band either superior or inferior to the slice, to suppress arterial or venous flow selectively. An inferior saturation band will yield arterial flow and a superior saturation band venous flow. The use of an inversion pulse or fat saturation before slice selection can also help suppress the signal intensity of stationary tissue. Contiguous axial slices as thin as 1.5–3 mm, using flow compensation, are acquired to cover the desired region. The number prescribed will affect the total scan time and this must be kept within reason.

A phase velocity mapping protocol is prescribed in the transaxial plane of the site of any stenosis. This is performed using ECG gating to obtain 16 frames per cardiac cycle. The phase of proton spins is modulated using a bipolar gradient pulse for velocity encoding in the slice select direction. Regions of interest are drawn within the vessel in each of the phase images to determine the mean pixel value and thus the mean velocity. A velocity waveform for the vessel is generated, plotting the mean velocity against each image in the cardiac cycle.

When three-dimensional phase contrast imaging is used, velocity encoding is employed in all three directions. Care has to be taken, however, to select the velocity encoding carefully to avoid aliasing.

Maximum intensity pixel analysis is selected to demonstrate the vessels within the selected volume and to identify any lesions.

# 8 Cardiovascular System

## Interventional Procedures

The ability to gain access to organs and the vascular system has led to the rapid development of interventional techniques. This, in conjunction with improved imaging, has enlarged the role of radiology from a purely diagnostic service to encompass therapeutic management of the patient in specific cases. The principal areas of vascular intervention associated with arteries may be considered as percutaneous transluminal angioplasty, artherectomy, thrombolysis and stenting. Additionally, embolisation of the arterial supply to organs, arteriovenous malformations and bleeding vessels and the placement of special filters in the IVC are some of the interventional procedures commonly employed in a vascular laboratory.

### Percutaneous transluminal angioplasty

Percutaneous transluminal angioplasty (PTA) is undertaken following a diagnostic angiogram which demonstrates a stenotic lesion. It is a well-recognised procedure in peripheral vessels but, as improvements are made in balloon catheters and guide wires, it can now be applied to high-risk areas such as mesenteric, renal and carotid arteries.

The balloon is inflated to crack and break the diseased artherosclerotic intima of the vessel wall and to dilate the medial and adventitial layers, allowing expansion of the lumen. The balloon should not be over-inflated, to avoid distending the vessel and separating plaque from the vessel wall and risking either a distal embolus or a tear of the outer layer, causing bleeding or a pseudoaneurysm.

To reduce the risk of acute thrombus, platelet inhibitors, anticoagulants and vasodilators are administered prior to, during and after angioplasty.

#### Imaging procedure

A catheter is introduced into the vessel under treatment and advanced to the level of the stenosis. The length and location of the lesion are marked with either radio-opaque markers or a 'road-mapping' device. A suitable guide wire is advanced through the catheter and across the stenosis. The catheter is now advanced over the guide wire which is now withdrawn. A heavy duty guide wire is then introduced through the catheter and positioned to enable it to be visible on fluoroscopy. The conventional catheter is removed and replaced with the balloon catheter, of which the balloon matches the diameter of the vessel and length of the diseased segment. The balloon is positioned at the centre of the lesion and slowly inflated using a 10 ml syringe or inflation device. The balloon is inflated the minimum number of times necessary to dilate the full length of the stenosis. After the final inflation, a repeat angiogram is performed in the same projection as that which optimally demonstrated the lesion.

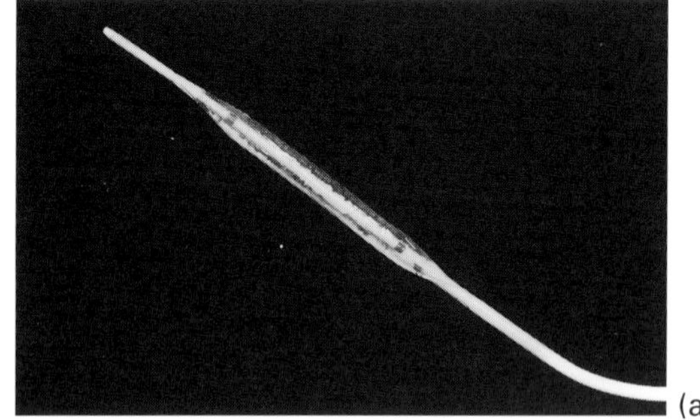
(a)

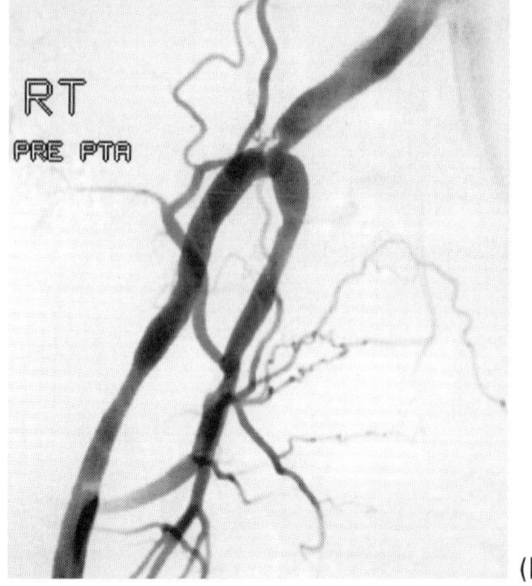

(b)

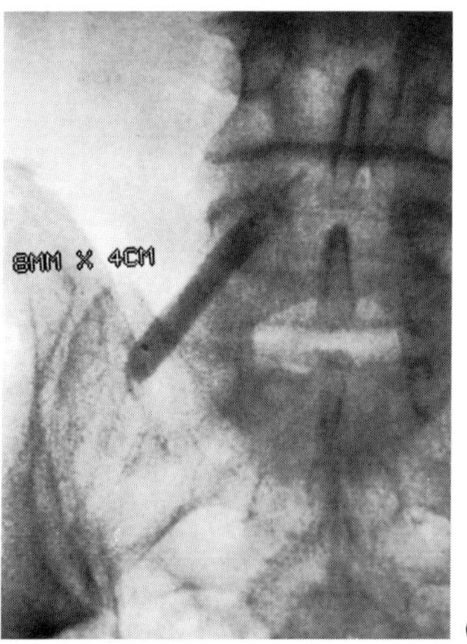

(c)

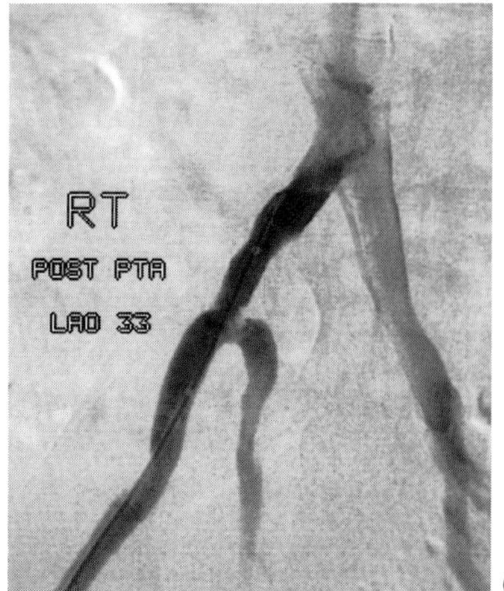

(d)

**Figure 8.43** (a) Typical balloon catheter; (b–d) selected images from a PTA procedure of the common iliac artery at the level of its bifurcation

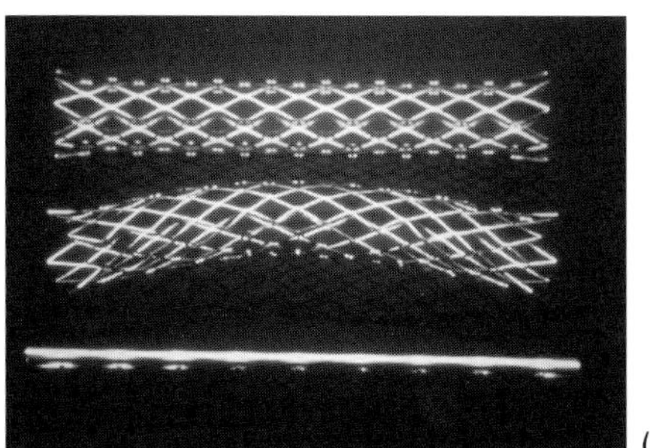
(a)

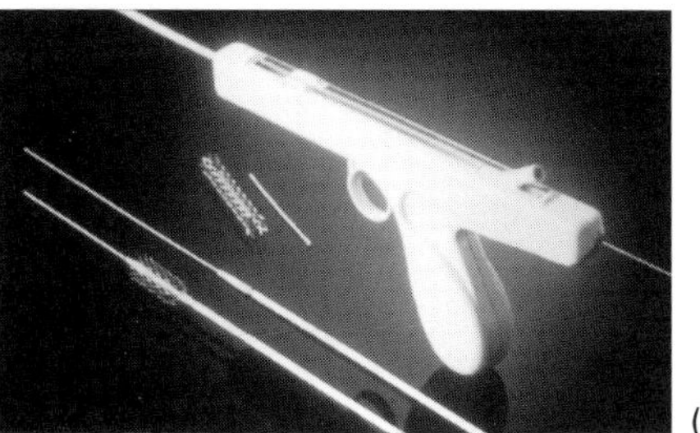
(b)

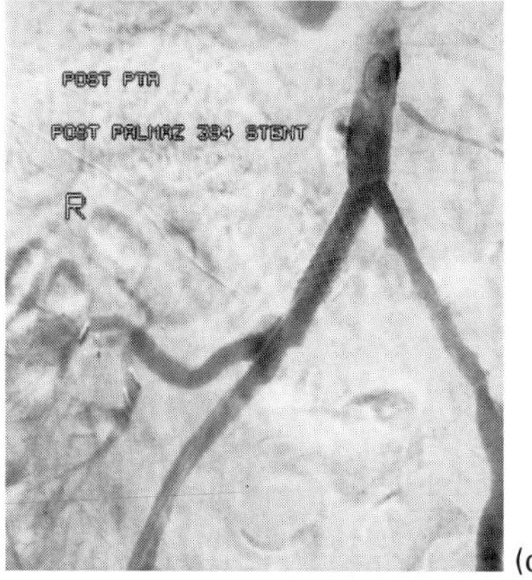

(c)

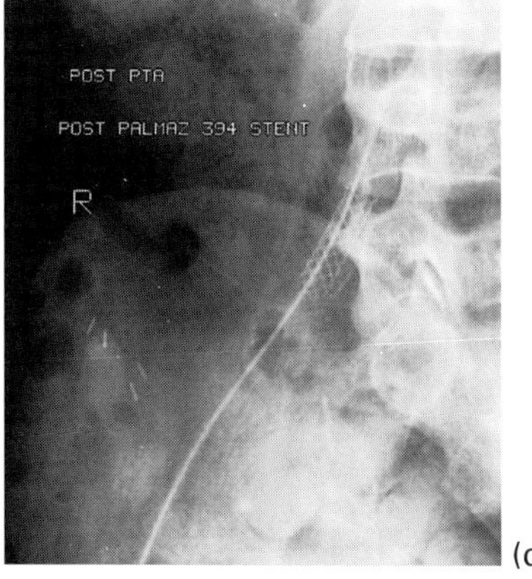

(d)

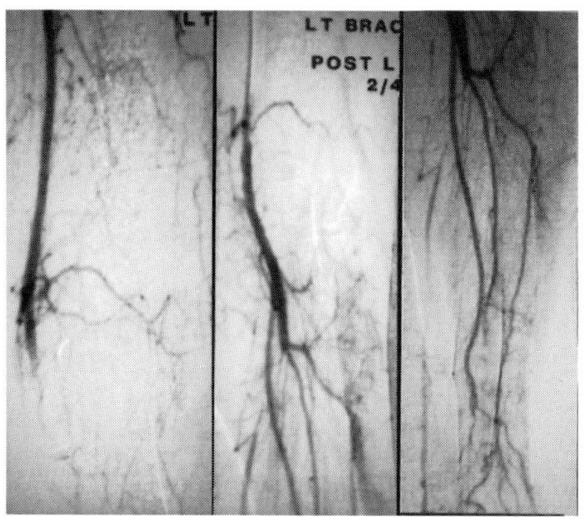

(e)

## Vascular stents

Stents are used as a follow-up procedure if percutaneous angioplasty has not fully dilated a vessel or re-stenosis has occurred. These metallic devices, e.g. tantalum and nitinol, are constructed in the form of a cylindrical wire net. They are flexible and expandable and are made in an assortment of lengths and diameters to cater for the requirements of different lesions and vessels, e.g. leg and iliac arteries and aorta. Two types of stents are available: (a) self-expanding stents loaded in the end of a special introducer catheter, and (b) balloon expandable stents consisting of continuous tubular mesh fitted around a deflated angioplasty balloon. Both devices have radio-opaque markers to identify the distal and proximal ends of the stent. The stent with its delivery catheter is introduced into a femoral artery, following puncture of the vessel using the Seldinger technique. The catheter is advanced under fluoroscopic control to the site of the dilated stenosis and upon ejection from the catheter the stent expands to the internal diameter of the vessel and straddles the stenotic region.

## Thrombolysis

Thrombolysis involves the introduction of a pharmaceutical substance which dissolves a thrombus. The procedure is usually performed in patients who present with acute ischaemic limbs and when emergency embolectomy is not considered suitable.

A diagnostic angiogram is performed initially to outline the arterial distribution in the limb and to determine the location of any blockage and the nature of any flow distal to a blockage. If there is a defined blockage with normal vessels distally, i.e. three-vessel run-off in the leg, then embolectomy is the treatment of choice. If no run-off is identified, it is unlikely that embolectomy will prove curative and thrombolysis is therefore the method of choice. A catheter with an end hole and side holes is advanced under fluoroscopic control to the site of blockage. Lysis is best achieved by impaction of the catheter within the thrombus. Passage of a slide wire through the block, if achievable, will increase the surface area and therefore improves the efficiency of the lysis. Once positioned, the catheter is connected to an infusion pump containing the lysis agent. When Actilyse (rt-PA) is selected, the typical dose prescribed is 20 mg dissolved in 50 ml of heparin saline which is infused at the rate of 1 mg/h which equates to 2.5 ml/h. This volume generally allows overnight lysis. A repeat angiogram may be performed to assess the effect of treatment. Depending on the degree of resolution obtained, an angioplasty procedure may also be performed to ensure that the vessel is left with a viable channel if an underlying stenosis is shown following lysis.

**Figure 8.44** (a,b) Typical metallic stents with applicator for deployment from the catheter sheath; (c) stent in common iliac artery; (d) stent in right common iliac artery (NB. Renal transplant kidney); (e) thrombus in brachial artery relieved by thrombolysis

## Embolisation

The use of embolisation techniques may be applied to blood vessels that are either supplying tumours or arteriovenous (AV) malformations.

Embolisation of tumour vessels may be temporary or permanent. Where the tumour is to be surgically resected, the purpose of embolisation is to minimise the blood loss at surgery and reduce tumour mass. If surgery is to be performed within 48–56 h, the embolisation may adequately be achieved using the patient's own blood in the form of an autologeous blood clot. If the tumour is not to be resected, permanent embolisation will be required. Among the materials for permanent embolisation are metal coils, polystyrene balls/polystyrene sheet (to be cut) and chemical agents.

Metai coils are supplied in a cartridge which allows the coil, secured in the compressed position, to be fed into the catheter and advanced by use of a guide wire, into position in the vessel of interest. The coil is released from the end of the catheter and expands within the lumen of the vessel. The coil of wire has fibres attached which act as a thrombus focus. Clot is thus formed, which leads to the effective embolisation of the vessel. It may be necessary, in the case of a large vessel, that a number of coils are required before complete occlusion is achieved.

The efficacy of the coils is monitored by the use of contrast media injections in conjunction with fluoroscopy.

Polystyrene balls or the particles are utilised by first suspending the material in contrast media in order to render them visible under fluoroscopy and then the suspension is drawn into a syringe and then injected via the catheter into the target vessel. There is a tendency for the particles to flocculate in the syringe, making them difficult to expel.

The problem presented by AV malformations is that there are usually multiple feeding vessels of varying diameters which require embolising and therefore a mixture of the available materials may have to be utilised.

The use of chemical agents such as cyanoacrylate glue (superglue) may be of value in vessels of very small diameter. However, extreme care has to be exercised in the use of these agents as there is the possibility of the catheter adhering to the vessel wall.

Considerable interest has been shown in the application of interventional techniques to the treatment of cerebral vascular anomalies such as AV malformations and aneurysms (see page 355). The most important criteria for the success of these techniques, as indeed for all interventional procedures, are in the accurate positioning of the catheter, and to ensure that there is no risk of the catheter moving from the region of interest.

## Atherectomy devices

Atherectomy devices are used to debulk and remove as much atherosclerotic material from the lumen of a diseased vessel. The artherectomy catheter, e.g. Simpson's, has a cylindrical stainless steel housing with a longitudinal side window at its distal tip. A rotary cup-shaped cutter, activated through a cable by battery power, slides back and forward within the metal cylinder to scrape away the atheromatous plaque and increase the luminal calibre of the vessel.

This material is then removed either by the spiral action of the device or, in some cases, by suction that is applied to the lumen of the catheter. It is also the case that in some systems the fragmentation of the material is such that the particles are so small as to be allowed to circulate freely without risk of vascular occlusion.

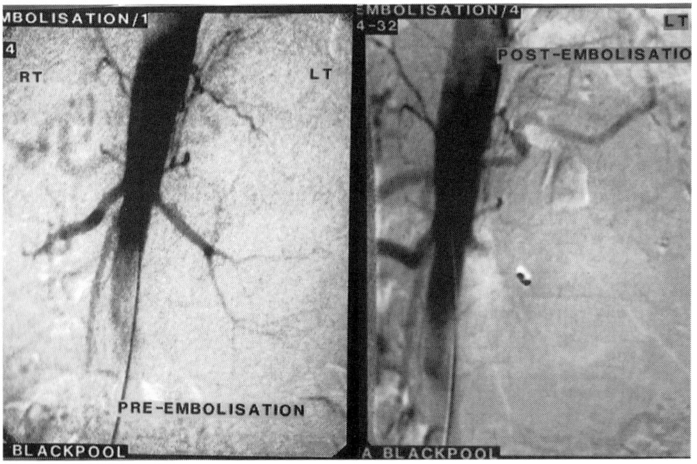


**Figure 8.45a** Pre- and post-coil embolisation images of a renal artery

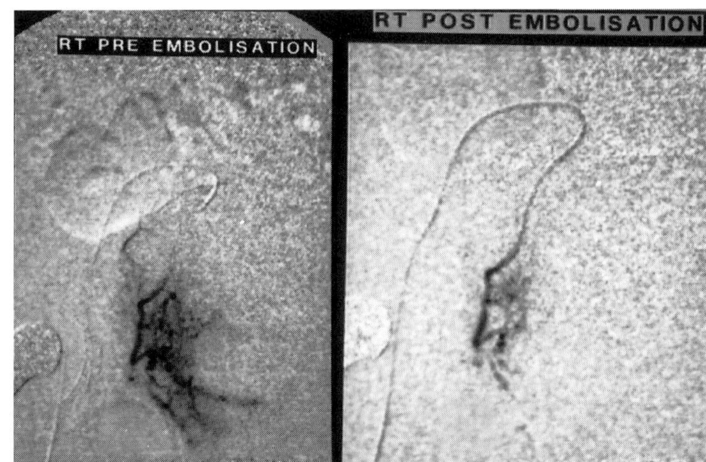


**Figure 8.45b** Pre- and post-embolisation images of an adenocarcinoma of the prostate, using plastic spheres, following selective angiography of the right internal iliac artery

## Vena cava filters

Vena cava filters are used extensively to reduce the risk of pulmonary embolism. There are basically two types of implants: (a) temporary otherwise known as removable filters, and (b) permanent filters.

Such devices are made from titanium or an alloy of nickel and titanium and come in a variety of designs and sizes. Their purpose is to fit exactly in the lumen of the IVC, below the level of the lower renal veins, and to capture thrombi for natural and gradual lysis.

The introduction of permanent filters is by means of a special catheter delivery system which is unique to the design of filter selected. Access to the IVC is via the right or left femoral vein or alternatively the left subclavian vein or the right or left jugular veins. Temporary filters are introduced via the right jugular vein and are attached to a tethering catheter which is used to extract the filter. During the period of implantation, the proximal end of the catheter is located in a subcutaneous pocket of skin.

### Indications

*Temporary filter*

This type of filter is implanted for a period of no more that 6 weeks and may be used in patients with contraindications to anticoagulant therapy who are to undergo major surgery, or during pregnancy where there is a major risk of pulmonary embolism.

Before removal of temporary filters, serial vena cavograms are performed and lysis undertaken if thrombi are present in the filter.

*Permanent filter*

These filters may be employed in patients who have a recurrent risk of pulmonary embolism and when anticoagulant therapy is contraindicated. They are also employed when adequate anticoagulation has failed to prevent recurrent embolism and following an episode of massive pulmonary embolism.

### Imaging procedure

For the right femoral route, which is the most popular, the femoral vein is punctured using a modified Seldinger technique, following which a J-tipped guide wire is advanced into the distal vena cava or iliac vein. Following removal of the needle, an introducer catheter, usually with a radiographic marker at its tip, and dilator are advanced under fluoroscopic control into the iliac vein or distal vena cava, at which point the guide wire and dilator are removed. A vena cavogram is performed (see page 306) to assess patency and vessel anatomy and to locate the level of the renal veins, in order that they can be identified by a radio-opaque marker or graded ruler. At this stage the diameter of the cava is assessed to select the correct size of filter. The guide wire and dilator are reintroduced to advance the introducer catheter so that the tip is 1 cm below the level of the lower renal veins. Following removal of the guide wire and dilator, the filter in its delivery set is introduced into the catheter and advanced under fluoroscopic control until it reaches the tip of the catheter. At this point the filter is delivered into the vessel by following the filter manufacturer's instructions, which vary depending on the type of delivery mechanism supplied. As soon as the filter is in the vessel it will expand to take up its designed shape.

The introducer catheter is removed into the iliac vein and the vena cavogram is repeated to confirm the position of the filter.

During the procedure the introducer catheter must be flushed through frequently with heparinised saline to prevent thrombus formation.

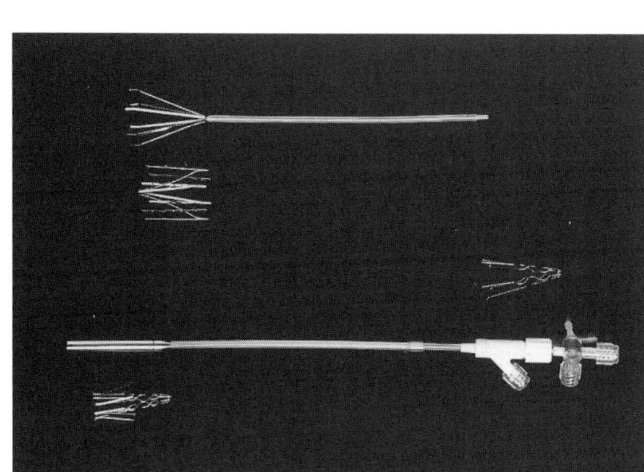

**Figure 8.46a** Sample of filters available

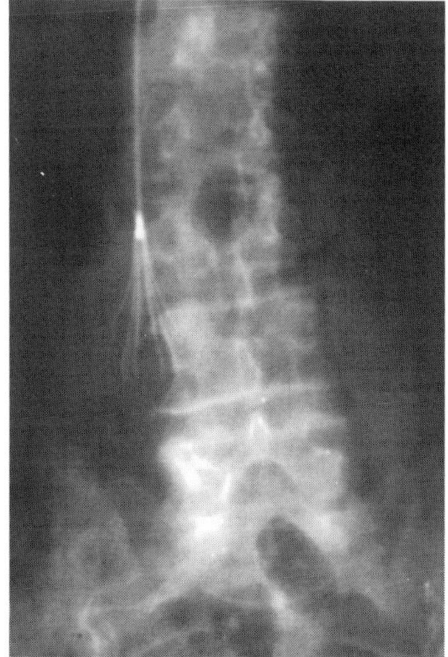

**Figure 8.46b** Image of temporary filter in position

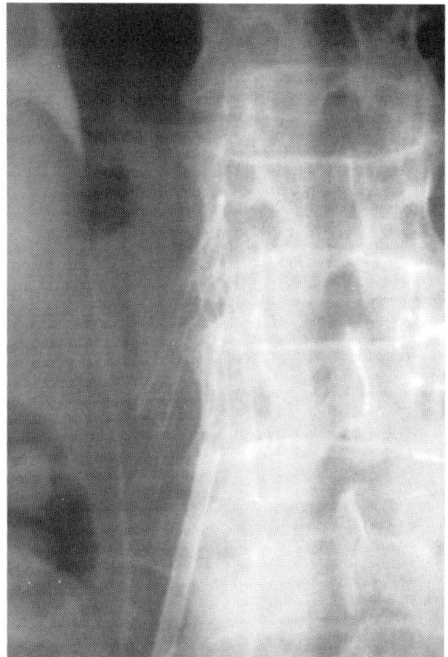

**Figure 8.46c** Image of permanent filter in position following cavogram (note kidney function)

# 9

# ENDOCRINE SYSTEM

## CONTENTS

# 9 Endocrine System

## Introduction

The endocrine system consists of several ductless glands, many of which are anatomically sited remotely from one another. For the purpose of this chapter the specialised imaging procedures for the following glands are described:

- pituitary gland
- parathyroid glands
- thymus
- thyroid gland
- adrenal (suprarenal) glands.

Imaging of the pancreas, ovaries and testes and the pineal gland are described elsewhere in this book.

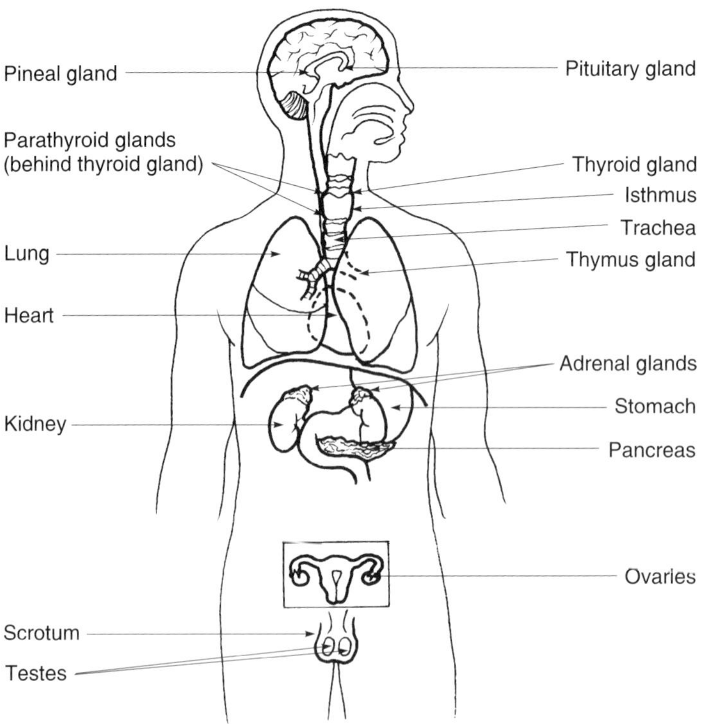


**Figure 9.1** Location of endocrine gland

### Indications

Hormonal imbalance resulting from either an overactive or an underactive gland can affect the activity of target organs situated remotely from the gland. The most common reason for radiological investigation is to assess the size and shape of the gland and to detect the presence of any tumour within the gland.

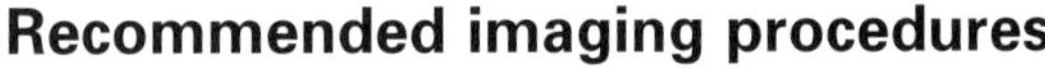

### Recommended imaging procedures

The imaging methods selected depend upon the gland being investigated; in certain situations, several complementary techniques may be required to provide maximum diagnostic information (Table 9.1).

**Table 9.1 Imaging modalities for glands to be investigated**

| *Endocrine gland imaging modality* | *Pituitary* | *Parathyroid* | *Thyroid* | *Adrenal* | *Thymus* |
|---|---|---|---|---|---|
| Computed tomography | ✓ | ✓ | | ✓ | ✓ |
| Ultrasound | | ✓ | ✓ | ✓ | |
| Radionuclide imaging | | ✓ | ✓ | ✓ | |
| Magnetic resonance imaging | ✓ | | | | |
| Radiography/fluorography | ✓ | | ✓ | | |

## Pituitary Gland

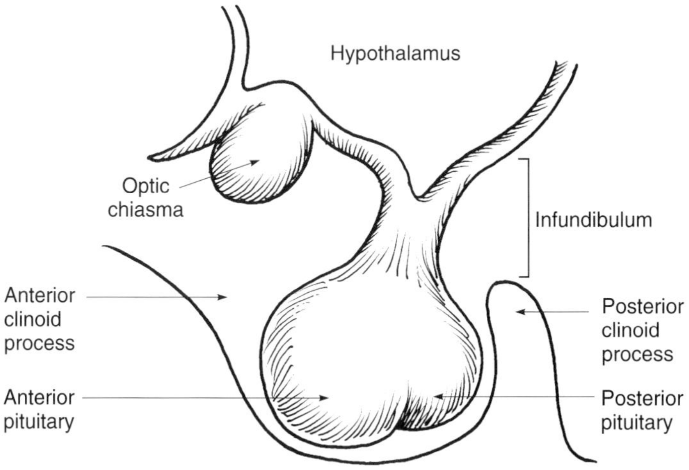

Figure 9.2a Pituitary gland (diagrammatic)

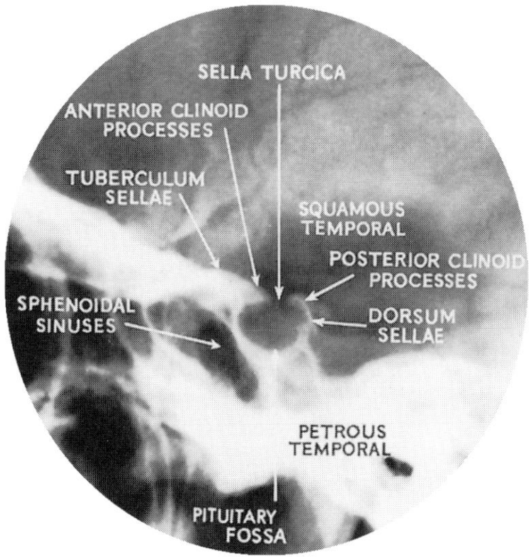

Figure 9.2b Collimated lateral projection radiograph – sella turcica

The pituitary gland lies in the sella turcica of the sphenoid bone. The infundibulum (pituitary stalk) connects the gland to the hypothalamus of the brain. The gland is divided both functionally and anatomically into anterior and posterior lobes.

The hormones contained in the anterior lobe are released into the blood stream after stimulation by the hormone-releasing factors of the hypothalamus, while those stored in the posterior lobe are released after direct stimulation by the hypothalamus (Table 9.2).

### Recommended imaging procedures

A lateral radiograph of the skull may be performed. This projection will demonstrate gross changes through bone erosion in the size and shape of the sella turcica. The sella is generally enlarged in conditions such as acromegaly and chromophobe adenoma; it is usually normal in size in Cushing's disease.

Further detailed investigation of the gland will be undertaken by either CT (coronal and transaxial scanning) or MRI.

### Indications

Imaging is undertaken to detect the presence of a tumour within the gland and its relationship to the surrounding anatomical structures.

**Table 9.2 Hormones in the pituitary gland and their function**

| *Pituitary gland* | *Hormone* | *Function* |
|---|---|---|
| Anterior lobe | Human growth hormone | Increase growth rate of body tissue |
| | Thyroid-stimulating hormone | Stimulate synthesis and secretion of thyroxine |
| | Adrenocorticotrophic hormone | Control production and secretion of (a) glucocorticoids, (b) mineralocorticoids, (c) sex hormones |
| | Follicle-stimulating hormones | Stimulate oestrogen<br>Initiate sperm production |
| | Luteinising hormone | Stimulate (a) release of developed ovum, (b) uterus to accept fertilised ovum |
| | Prolactin | Initiate and maintain milk secretion |
| | Melanocyte-stimulating hormone | Increase pigmentation of skin |
| Posterior lobe | Oxytocin | Stimulate the muscle cells of pregnant uterus to contract |
| | Antidiuretic hormone | Stimulate kidneys to reabsorb water |

# 9 Pituitary Gland

## Computed tomography – coronal plane

Coronal plane imaging reduces the radiation dose to the lens of the eye and avoids the cross-hatch artefact from the petrous ridges associated with scans obtained in the transaxial plane.

Images are obtained immediately following the intravenous injection of an iodine-based contrast medium. A non-ionic contrast medium is preferred, to reduce the incidence of allergic reaction and movement artefact.

**Position of patient and imaging modality**

*Method 1*

The patient lies prone on the scanner table. The neck is extended and the chin rests on the head support. Ideally, the coronal plane is positioned parallel to the scan plane, with the median sagittal plane and the transaxial plane perpendicular to the scan plane. The patient is then moved into the scanner and positioned so that the scan reference point is at the level of the external auditory meatus. This position may be uncomfortable for some patients and it may be impossible to extend the neck adequately to obtain the optimum coronal plane. This can be compensated for by angulation of the gantry. This position may be associated with respiratory movement artefact.

*Method 2*

The patient lies supine on the scanner table. The neck is extended and the vertex of the skull supported on a coronal head rest. The coronal plane is positioned parallel to the scan plane and the scanner gantry angled to compensate for any positioning difficulties. Although still uncomfortable for the patient, this position is tolerated better than method 1 and results in less movement artefact.

**Imaging procedure**

A lateral scan projection radiograph is obtained, starting 10 cm posterior to the scan reference point and ending 10 cm anterior to the reference point. From this scan projection radiograph, 1.5 mm contiguous sections are prescribed, starting immediately behind the posterior clinoid process and ending just in front of the anterior margin of the sella, with the scanner gantry angled to obtain sections perpendicular to the floor of the pituitary sella turcica.

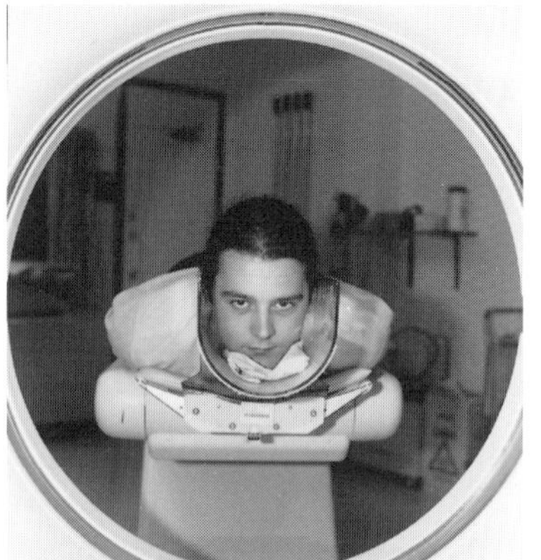

**Figure 9.3a** Method 1 – patient prone

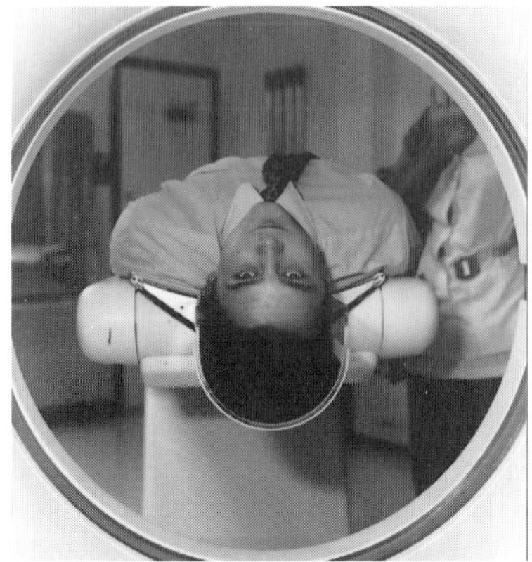

**Figure 9.3b** Method 2 – patient supine

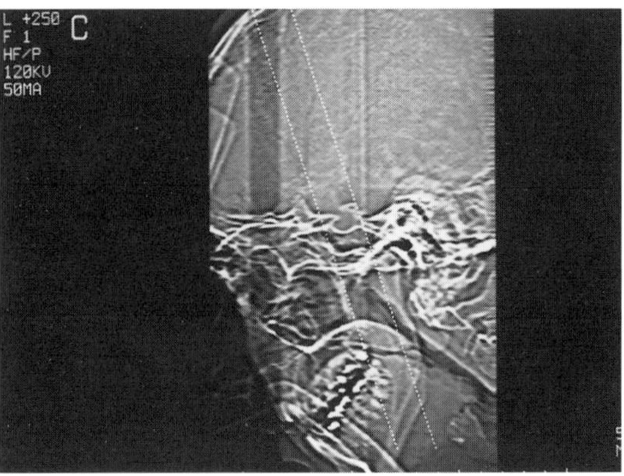


**Figure 9.3c** Scan projection radiograph showing start and end locations

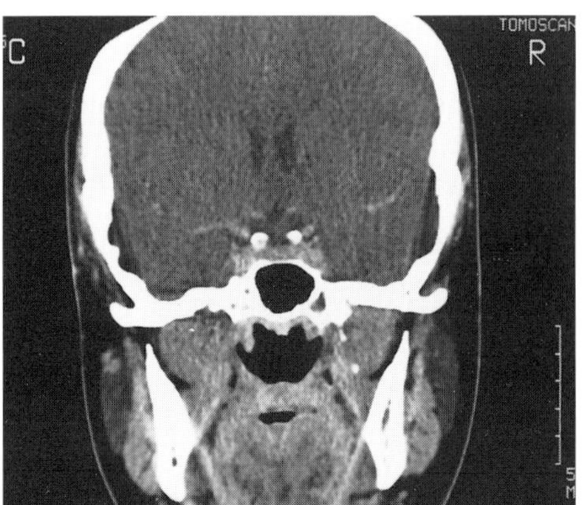


**Figure 9.3d** Coronal image through the pituitary gland

# Pituitary Gland 9

## Computed tomography – transaxial plane

Figure 9.4a Patient and equipment

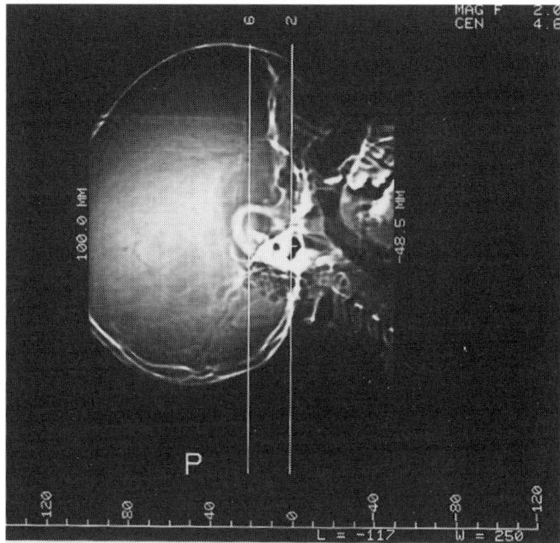


**Figure 9.4b** Lateral scan projection radiograph showing start and end locations

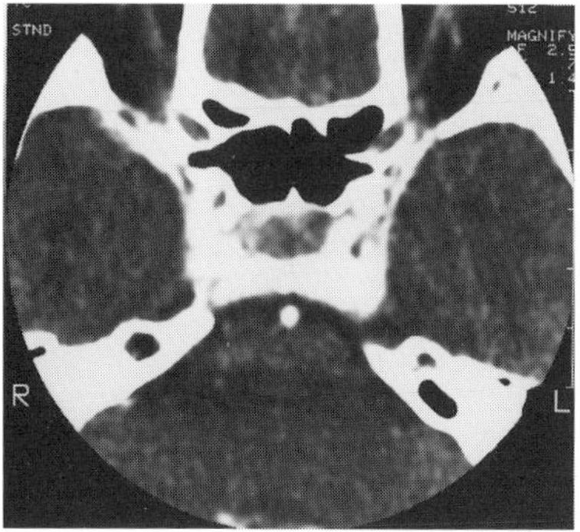


**Figure 9.4c** Magnified transaxial image at the level of the pituitary gland

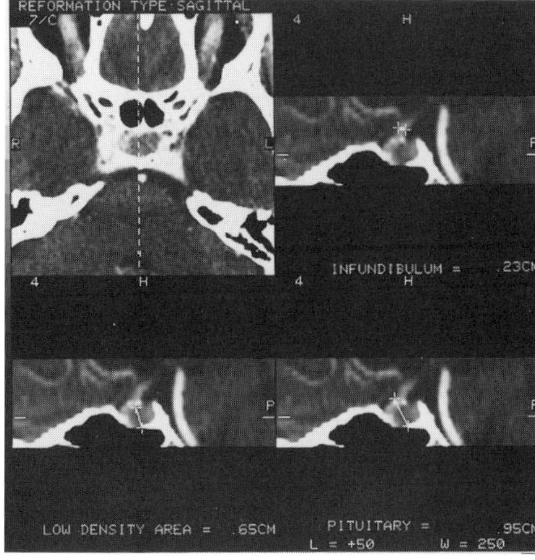


**Figure 9.4d** Sagittal re-formations with measurements

Transaxial plane imaging may be necessary when the patient's physical condition makes it impossible to obtain or maintain the coronal position. Again, images are acquired after the intravenous administration of a suitable iodinated contrast agent.

### Position of patient and imaging modality

The patient lies supine on the scanning table, with head resting in the transaxial head support. Positioning is aided by external alignment lights. The radiographic baseline is positioned parallel to the transverse alignment light. The median sagittal plane is perpendicular to the table and coincident with the sagittal alignment light. To ensure that the skull is symmetrically positioned, the external auditory meatuses must be equidistant from the head support and the interorbital (interpupillary) line parallel to the scan plane. The patient is moved into the scanner so that the scan reference point is at the level of the external auditory meatus.

### Imaging procedure

A lateral scan projection radiograph is performed, starting 4 cm below the radiographic baseline and ending 10 cm above the baseline. From the scan projection radiograph, 1.5 mm contiguous sections are prescribed from immediately below the floor of the sella turcica to approximately 10 mm above the anterior clinoid process of the sphenoid bone. The scanner gantry is angled to obtain sections parallel to the floor of the pituitary fossa (+10° above the orbitomeatal line), to reduce radiation dose to the lens of the eye.

### Image analysis

The digital data derived from either scanning method can be reformatted to produce images in the sagittal plane. From the transaxial images reformations can also be obtained in the coronal plane.

Measurements can be made of:

- vertical height of the pituitary gland
- anteroposterior diameter of the infundibulum
- size/dimensions of any adenoma.

*Contrast medium and injector data*

| *Volume* | *Concentration* | *Flow rate* |
|---|---|---|
| 100 ml | 340–370 mgI/ml | Hand injection |

# 9 Pituitary Gland

## Magnetic resonance imaging

A combination of high-resolution and 3D imaging has enabled MRI to be used in the assessment of both pituitary and parasellar abnormalities.

$T_1$ weighted sequences give excellent anatomical definition of this region, showing the optic chiasm and infundibulum within the low signal intensity of the cerebrospinal fluid.

$T_2$ weighted sequences and contrast enhanced $T_1$ weighted scans may be used to give further information on the size and extent of any tumour which may be present.

Because of the lack of signal from cortical bone on MRI, CT may better demonstrate erosion of the sellar floor.

**Contraindications**

These centre on the presence of metallic objects. Patients with surgical aneurysmal clips must not be scanned.

Torque forces on the clips from the magnetic field can result in movement of the clips and rupture of the vessel walls. Foreign bodies in the eye, due to occupational injury, other trauma or surgery, are also a contraindication as are patients with cardiac pacemakers.

**Position of patient and imaging modality**

The patient lies supine on the scanner table, head resting in the head support of the head coil. Positioning is aided by external alignment lights. The medial sagittal plane is parallel to the sagittal alignment light and the transaxial alignment light parallel to the anthropological baseline.

The table is now adjusted until the external reference point is at the centre of the head coil. From this position the patient and head assembly are driven the fixed distance to the isocentre of the magnet.

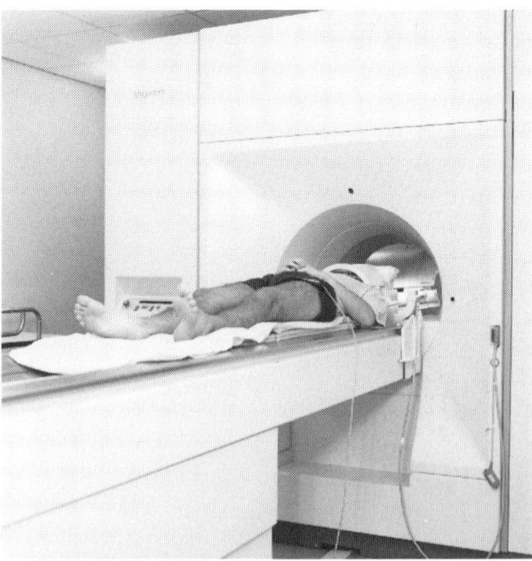

**Figure 9.5a** Patient in the head rest

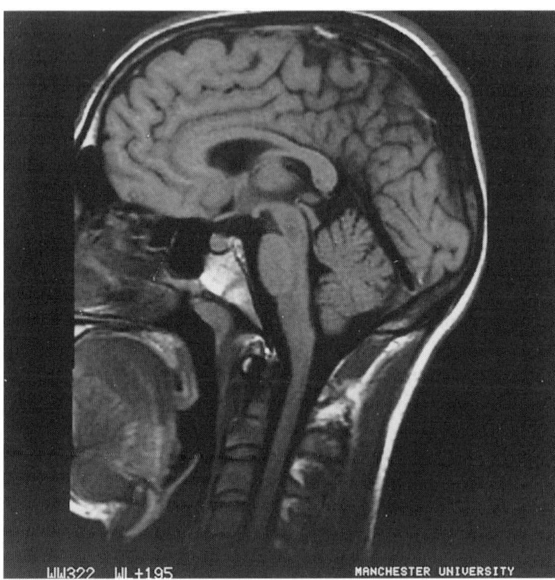


**Figure 9.5b** Midline sagittal $T_1$ weighted image showing pituitary gland

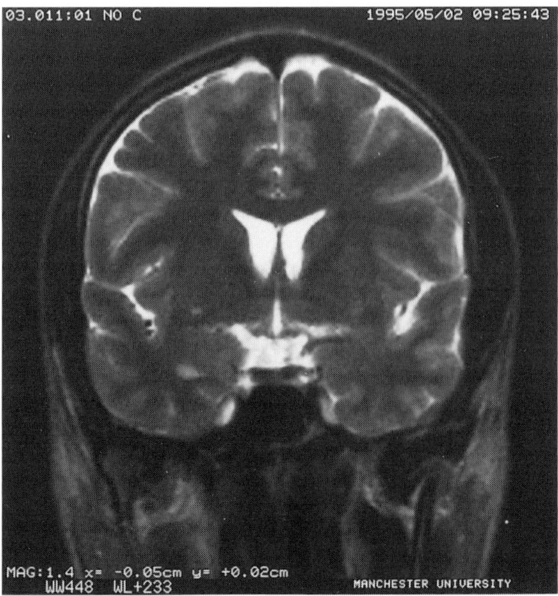


**Figure 9.5c** Coronal $T_2$ weighted image showing pituitary gland

## Magnetic resonance imaging

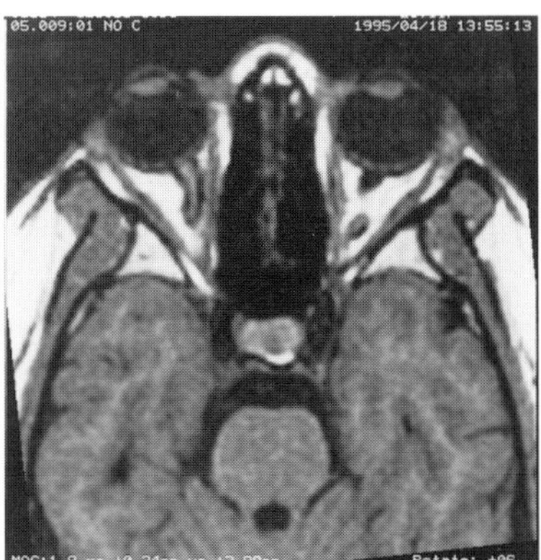

**Figure 9.6a** Pre-contrast transaxial $T_1$ weighted image

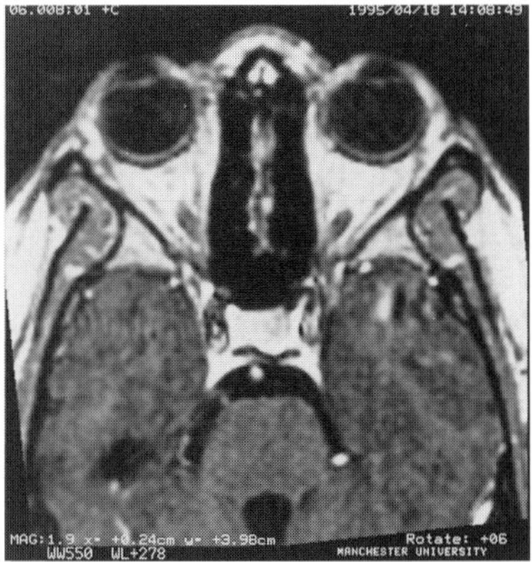

**Figure 9.6b** Post-contrast transaxial $T_1$ weighted image

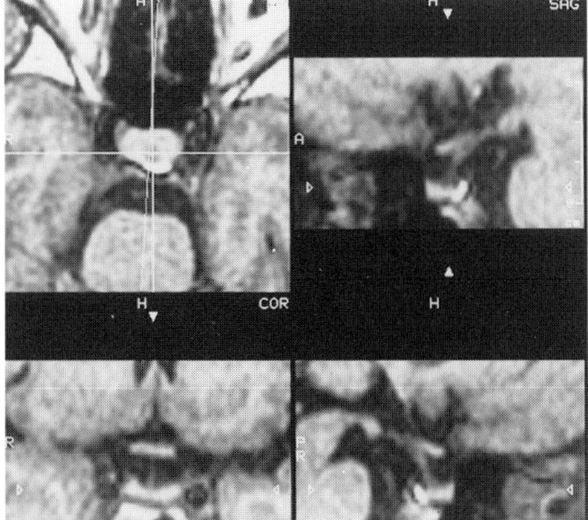

**Figure 9.6c** Three-dimensional image set

**Imaging procedure**

A midline localiser scan in the sagittal plane is initially obtained. From this image, $T_1$ and $T_2$ weighted sequences in the coronal plane are prescribed, perpendicular to the floor of the sella turcica, commencing immediately behind the posterior clinoid process and ending immediately in front of the anterior clinoid process. For large tumours extending beyond the sella, sagittal or transaxial $T_1$ weighted images may be necessary.

After review, it may be necessary to repeat the $T_1$ weighted sequences following the intravenous administration of gadolinium DTPA. For the repeat scans it is essential that the decibel level is identical to that set for the pre-contrast scans. This ensures that any enhancement is real and not merely machine related.

Further advances have enabled high-resolution 3D images to be produced. This technique allows information to be obtained from a volume of tissue. The number of sections required to obtain the volume depends on the size of the region to be sampled. Contiguous 1.25 mm sections are obtained in the transaxial plane using a gradient-echo sequence and the digital data reconstructed retrospectively to give high-resolution images in any anatomical plane.

This sequence may be repeated during the infusion of gadolinium DTPA. However, as the normal pituitary enhances more rapidly than micro-adenomas, the scan sequence and the injection should start simultaneously and the scan time should not exceed 4 min. If scanning is delayed, it may be impossible to visualise separately the tumour from the remainder of the gland.

*Contrast and injection data*

| *Volume* | *Pharmaceutical* | *Flow rate* |
|---|---|---|
| 0.2 ml/kg body weight | Gadolinium DTPA | Hand injection |

**Table 9.3 Imaging parameters**

| *Imaging plane* | *Imaging sequence* | *TR* | *TE* | *Field of view* (cm) | *No. of NEX* | *Slice width/ gap* (mm) | *Matrix (horizontal–vertical)* |
|---|---|---|---|---|---|---|---|
| Coronal | Fast spin-echo $T_2$ weighted (echo train length – 12) | 6000 | 102 | 25 | 3 | 3/1 | 192 × 256 |
| Coronal, sagittal and transaxial | Spin-echo $T_1$ weighted | 500 | 25 | 25 | 2 | 3/1 | 192 × 256 |
| 3D volume with flip angle 45° (pre- and post-contrast) | SPGR | 50 | 12 | 25 | 1 | 1.25 (35 slices) | 192 × 256 |

# 9 Endocrine System

## Parathyroid Glands

There are four parathyroid glands, normally in close proximity to the posterior aspect of the thyroid gland. Generally there are two in a superior position and two in an inferior position. They produce the parathyroid hormone which regulates the plasma calcium level. Occasionally (5%), glands are ectopic in site, usually in the mediastinum.

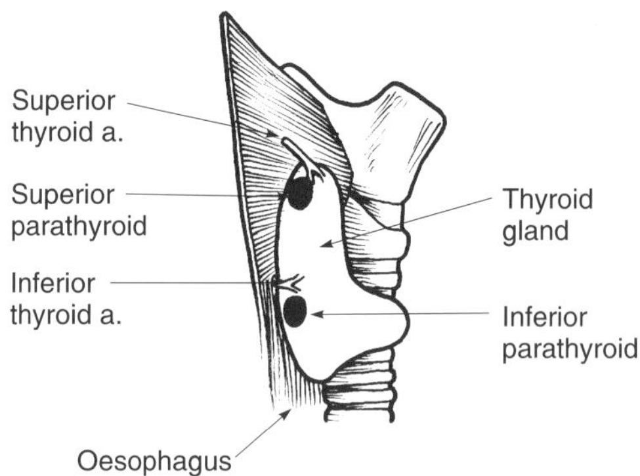


**Figure 9.7a** Location of parathyroid glands

### Recommended imaging procedures

Detailed investigation of the parathyroid glands is principally undertaken by CT and RNI.

Ultrasound is not generally used as a routine investigation and if attempted must be performed by an experienced sonographer. When performed, it is carried out in a similar way to that described for the thyroid gland on page 324.

Normal glands, because of their size and position, are not visualised by any imaging technique. The role of imaging is a preoperative procedure to locate an adenoma.

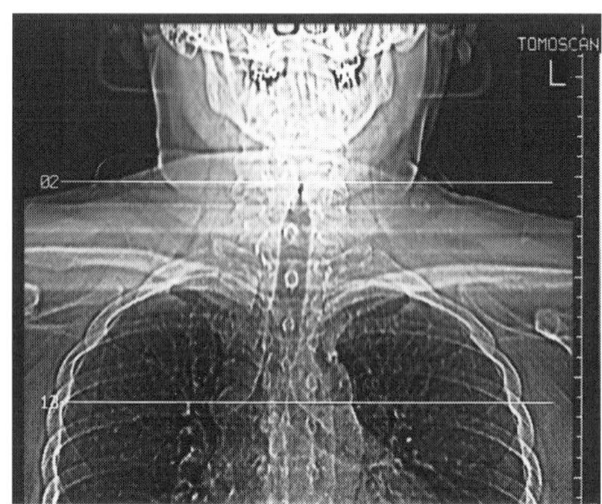


**Figure 9.7b** AP scan projection radiograph showing start and end locations

### Indications

Raised plasma calcium level with detectable parathyroid hormone indicating the presence of tumour within one or more glands (adenoma 83%, hyperplasia 12%, carcinoma 5%).

### Computed tomography

Transaxial images are obtained before and during the infusion of a non-ionic contrast medium. A non-ionic contrast medium is preferred to reduce patient movement (and swallowing) during scanning and incidence of adverse reactions. All scans are taken on suspended inspiration.

#### Position of patient and imaging modality

The patient lies supine, head first on the scanner table, with neck extended and supported on a positioning pad. Positioning is aided by external alignment lights. The median sagittal plane is perpendicular and the coronal plane is parallel to the scanner table. The scan plane is perpendicular to the long axis of the body to enable transaxial cross-sectional imaging to be performed. The scanner table height is adjusted to ensure that the coronal plane alignment light is approximately 5 cm posterior to the angle of the mandible. The patient is moved into the scanner until the scan reference point is at the level of the sternal notch.

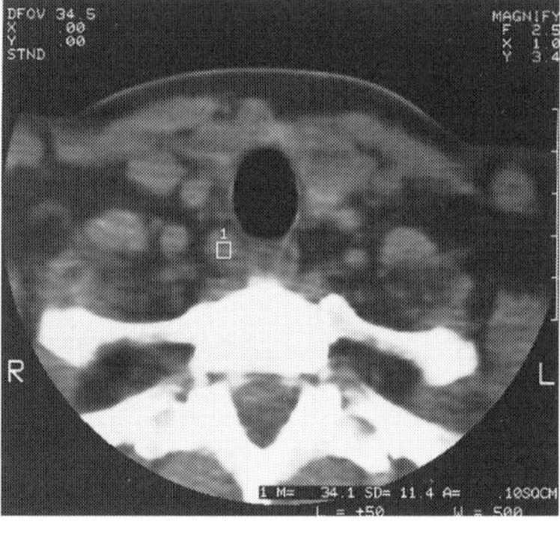


**Figure 9.7c** Pre-contrast section showing a parathyroid mass (note ROI with a CT number of 34.1 HU)

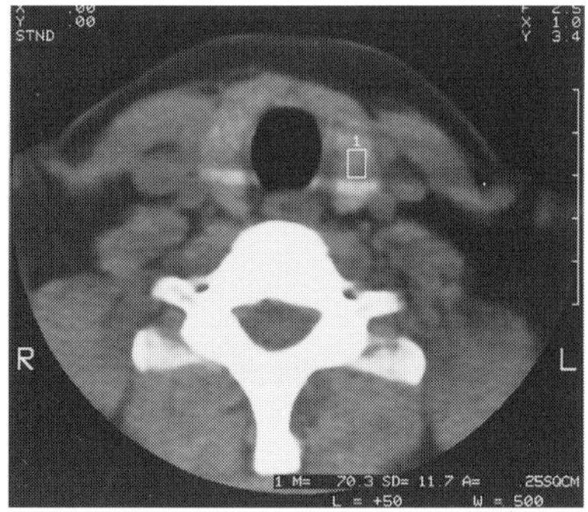


**Figure 9.7d** Further pre-contrast image at a different level with a ROI over the thyroid gland (note CT number is higher for thyroid tissue – 70.3 HU compared with 34.1 HU)

## Computed tomography

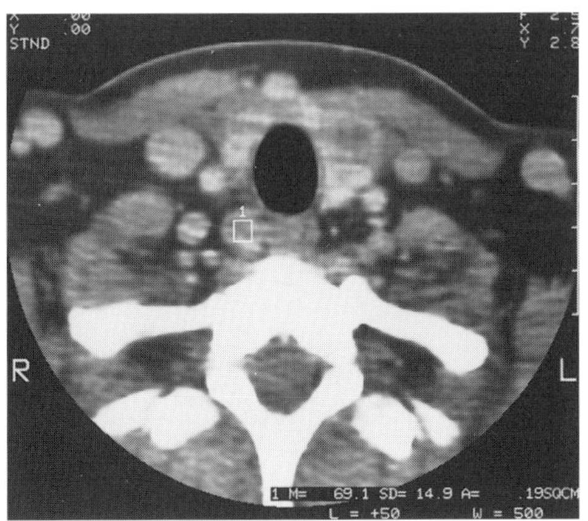

**Figure 9.8a** Post-contrast image with ROI over parathyroid tissue (CT number = 69.1)

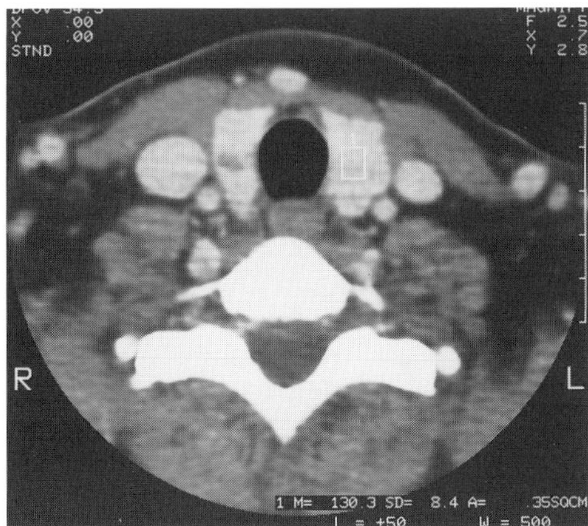

**Figure 9.8b** Post-contrast image with ROI over thyroid tissue demonstrating greater enhancement in the thyroid gland compared to the parathyroid (CT number = 130.3)

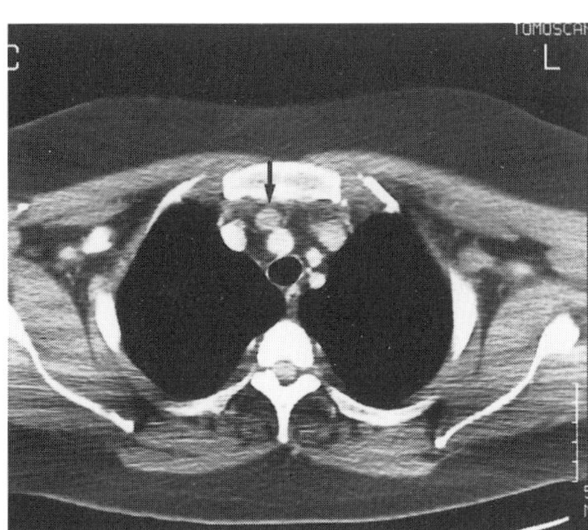

**Figure 9.8c** Post-contrast section showing retrosternal parathyroid tissue

### Imaging procedure

An anteroposterior scan projection radiograph is performed, starting 12 cm above and ending 12 cm below the reference point. From this image, 10 mm contiguous sections are prescribed from the hyoid bone to the bifurcation of the trachea, with all images acquired on suspended respiration. These pre-contrast images are reviewed and the relevant anatomical area to be rescanned during the injection of the contrast medium is determined. Narrower 5 mm contiguous sections are prescribed and performed during contrast infusion, increasing the spatial resolution and decreasing the scan time. Approximately 18 contiguous sections are necessary to cover the relevant area. Contrast enhanced scans should begin at the hyoid and progress inferiorly, to avoid streak artefacts from undiluted contrast medium passing through the subclavian vein during scanning and degrading image quality.

If spiral scanning options are available these images may be acquired with a volume acquisition, using a 5 mm slice thickness and 5 mm table increments, but with a 3 mm reconstruction index to give overlapping sections.

*Contrast medium and injector data*

| *Volume* | *Concentration* | *Flow rate* |
|---|---|---|
| 100 ml | 240 mgI/ml | 2 ml/s |

A 25 s pre-scan delay is chosen, allowing 50 ml of contrast to be injected before the start of scanning.

### Image analysis

Images are interrogated using the region-of-interest (ROI) facility to aid interpretation. The CT number of thyroid is higher pre-contrast than parathyroid tissue because of the iodine content of the gland. By comparing the attenuation values, both pre-contrast and post-contrast, it is possible to establish whether a lesion is thyroid or parathyroid in origin.

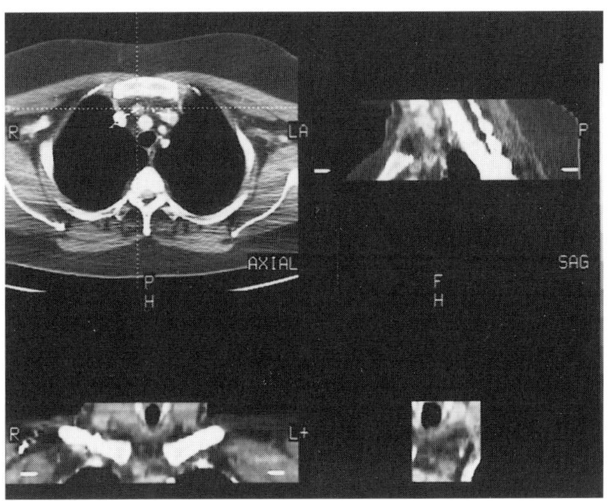

**Figure 9.8d** Set of reformatted images through the abnormality demonstrated in (c) showing its relationship to normal vascular structures

# 9 Parathyroid Glands

## Radionuclide imaging

Due to the close anatomical relationship of the parathyroid glands and the thyroid gland, and because both take up the tracer substances, a static image subtraction technique involving two radiopharmaceuticals is necessary to obtain images of the parathyroid glands.

Technetium-99m pertechnetate ($^{99m}$Tc) is taken up by the thyroid gland. Thallium chloride ($^{201}$Tl) is taken up by both the thyroid gland and the parathyroid glands. Computer processing enables the $^{99m}$Tc images to be subtracted from the $^{201}$Tl images to produce residual $^{201}$Tl images of a parathyroid tumour. Tumours have increased uptake of the radiopharmaceutical and are identified as localised 'hotspots'.

If CT is contemplated, radionuclide imaging must be done first, as iodinated contrast agents will block the $^{99m}$Tc uptake for 6–8 weeks, preventing the study from working.

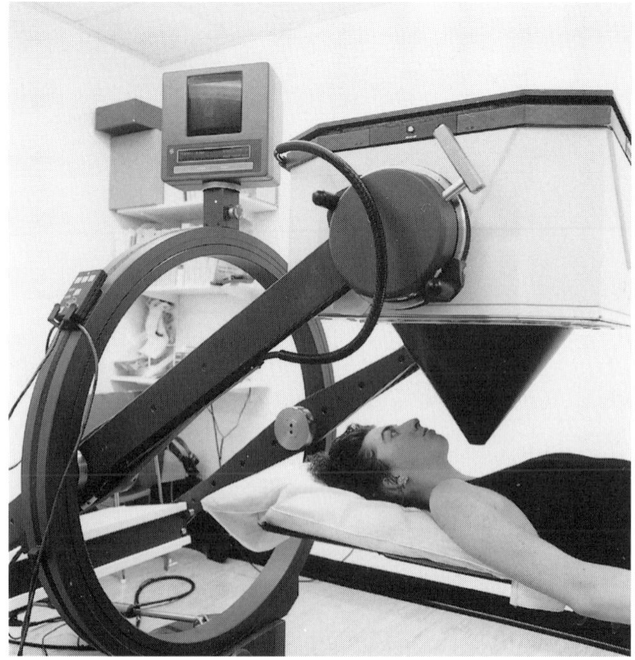

**Figure 9.9a** Patient in position

### Position of patient and imaging modality

The patient lies supine on the scanning table, neck extended and head supported by pads and a head band to restrict movement. The gamma camera is positioned over the neck region, parallel to the table, ensuring that the thyroid gland is in the centre of the imaging field. The camera is lowered as close as possible to the patient before image acquisition.

### Imaging procedure

A pinhole camera for magnification is preferred and a dual acquisition technique employed.

At the operator's console, energy windows corresponding to the energy levels for $^{99m}$Tc and $^{201}$Tl are selected.

Initially $^{99m}$Tc is injected intravenously. A delay of 12 min then allows maximum uptake of the radiopharmaceutical within the thyroid gland. After this period, $^{201}$Tl is injected and with a delay of 1–2 min, to allow clearance from the subclavian vein and carotid arteries, image acquisition commences. The total image acquisition time is 18 min. Subsequent computer processing enables the $^{99m}$Tc image to be gradually subtracted from the $^{201}$Tl image, thus producing images of the parathyroid tumour. The subtraction is correct when the thyroid activity equals the background activity in the neck.

To complete the study, a parallel hole collimator is used to image the lower neck and upper mediastinum to check for ectopic glands.

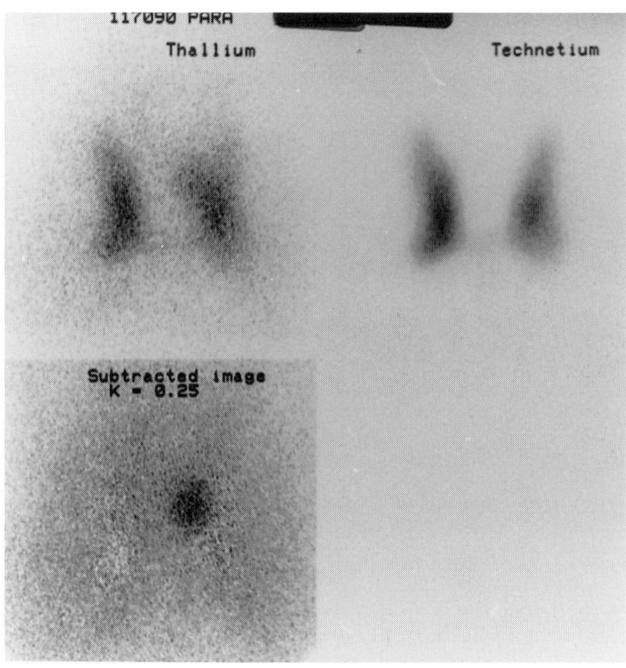


**Figure 9.9b** Series showing thallium and technetium images together with a subtracted image. The subtracted image shows a localised area of increased activity (hot spot) consistent with the presence of a tumour

*Imaging and radiopharmaceuticals parameters*

| *Type* | *Administered activity* | *Principal energy* |
|---|---|---|
| $^{99m}$Tc pertechnetate | 40 MBq | 140 keV |
| $^{201}$Tl thallium chloride | 80 MBq | 72 keV |

| *Window width* | *Acquisition time/counts* |
|---|---|
| 20% | 18 min |

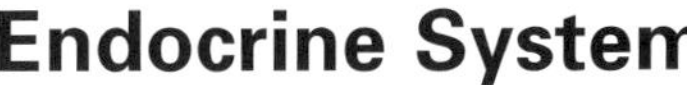



## Thymus Gland

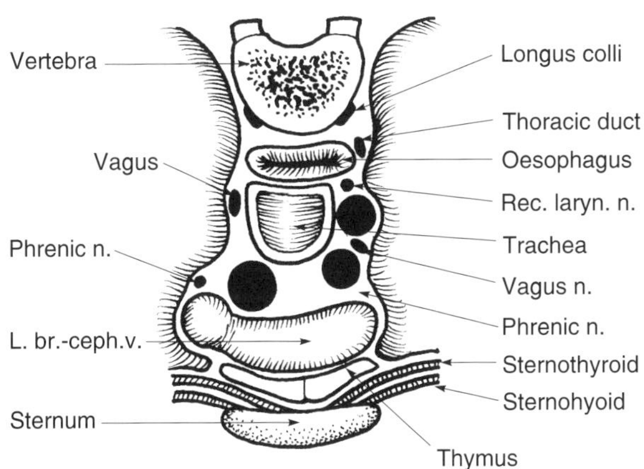


**Figure 9.10a** Transverse section through the mediastinum

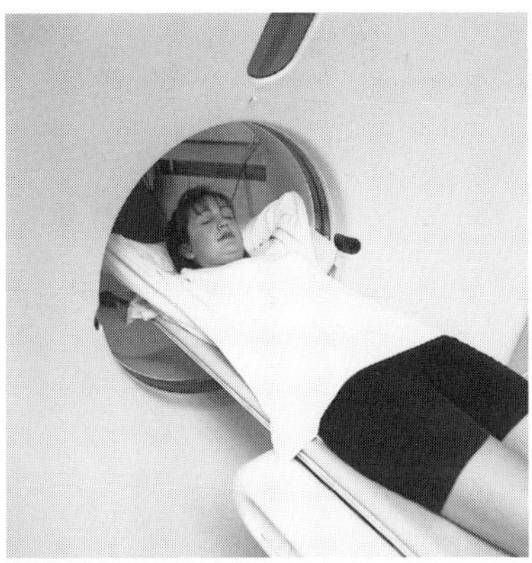

**Figure 9.10b** Patient in position

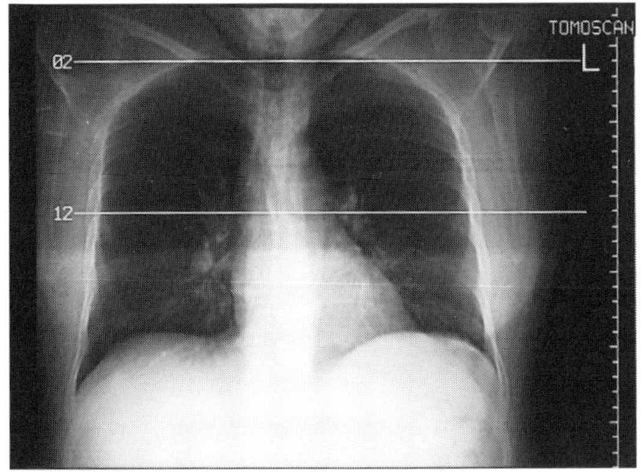


**Figure 9.10c** Scan projection radiograph showing start and end locations

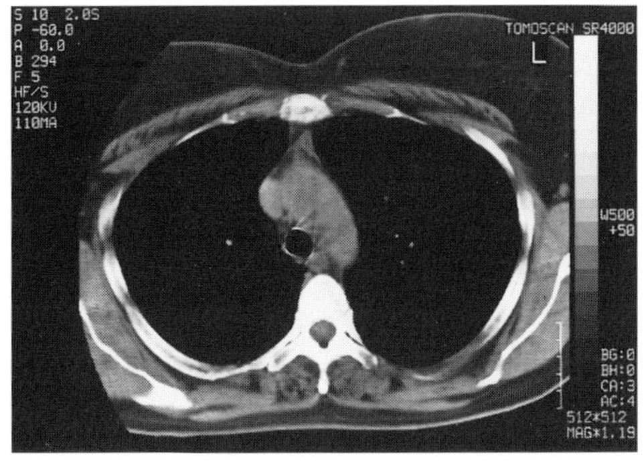


**Figure 9.10d** Transaxial image showing the anterior mediastinum

The thymus gland is situated in the anterior mediastinum and is more prominent in children than in adults. By producing T-cell lymphocytes, the gland plays an important role in immunological mechanisms.

### Recommended imaging procedures

Computed tomography is the method of choice.

### Indications

To determine the presence, nature and extent of any anterior mediastinal mass evident on chest radiographs.

Thymic tumours (thymoma) must be excluded in patients presenting with autoimmune or neurological conditions.

Patients with myasthenia gravis have a high incidence of thymic abnormality.

### Computed tomography

Transaxial images are performed through the mediastinum. A thymoma is usually well defined and surrounded by mediastinal fat, so that post-contrast scans are seldom required. All scans are performed on suspended respiration.

#### Position of patient and imaging modality

The patient lies supine, head first on the scanner table, with neck extended and supported on a positioning pad. Arms are raised and placed behind the patient's head, out of the scan plane. Positioning is aided by transaxial, coronal and sagittal alignment lights. The median sagittal plane is perpendicular and the coronal plane is parallel to the table. The scan plane is now perpendicular to the long axis of the body to enable transaxial cross-sectional imaging to be undertaken.

The scanner table height is adjusted to ensure that the coronal plane alignment light is at the level of the mid-axillary line. The patient is then moved into the scanner so that the scan reference point is at the level of the sternal notch.

#### Imaging procedure

An anteroposterior scan projection radiograph is performed, starting 6 cm above and ending 12 cm below the reference point. From this scan image, 10 mm contiguous sections are prescribed, from 3 cm above the sternal notch to the bifurcation of the trachea.

# 9 Endocrine System

## Thyroid Gland

The thyroid gland lies in the neck, anterior to the third to sixth cervical vertebrae. Ectopic tissue may be found in the mediastinum and the lingual region. Two hormones are produced: thyroxin and calcitonin.

### Recommended imaging procedures

Investigation of the thyroid gland is usually undertaken by RNI and ultrasound. Computed tomography and MRI have a limited role in the detection of thyroid disease and at present are not the imaging methods of choice.

Ultrasound is important in differentiating solid from cystic disease.

### Indications

To assess the site of origin and characteristics of a mass in the neck or mediastinum.

### Ultrasound

Two-dimensional real-time ultrasound is routinely performed. This is used to differentiate solid from cystic lesions, both of which can be 'cold spots' on the radionuclide scan image and to assess the size of each lobe and isthmus.

**Position of patient and imaging modality**

The patient lies supine on the scanning table, neck slightly extended, all clothing and jewellery removed from the neck. Because of the superficial anatomical position of the gland a 7.5–10 MHz linear array probe is selected.

**Imaging procedure**

Images are obtained initially in the transaxial and longitudinal planes. Visual comparison of the texture and dimensions of each lobe is made. From these images it is determined whether further images in the oblique plane are required. In suspected cases of hypoglossal cysts, ultrasound should be repeated with the tongue extended to assess movement of the cyst.

Colour flow Doppler may be useful in assessing blood flow to masses demonstrated within the thyroid gland.

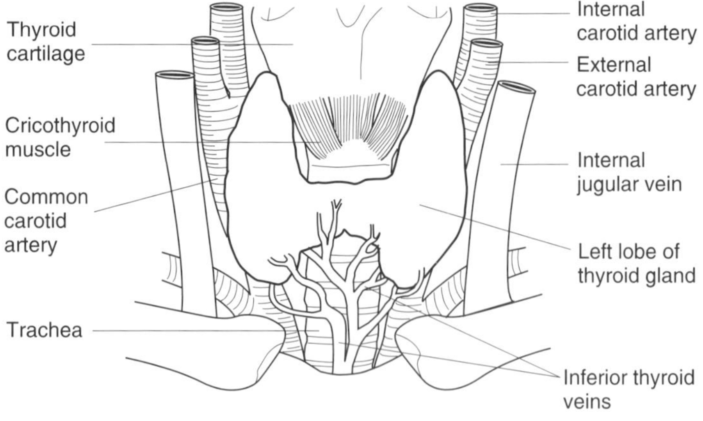


**Figure 9.11a** Thyroid gland (anterior aspect)

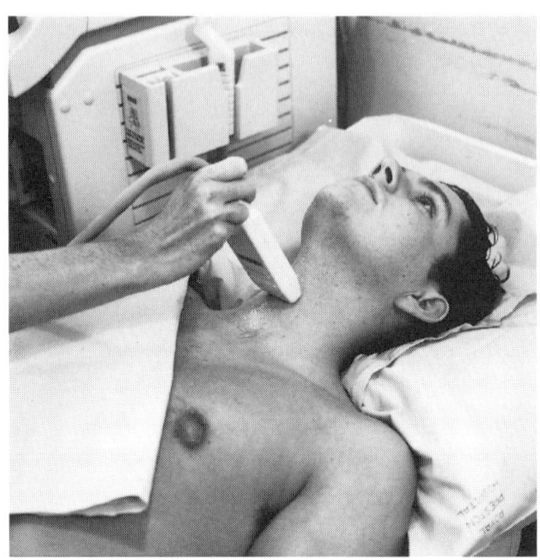

**Figure 9.11b** Patient and transducer

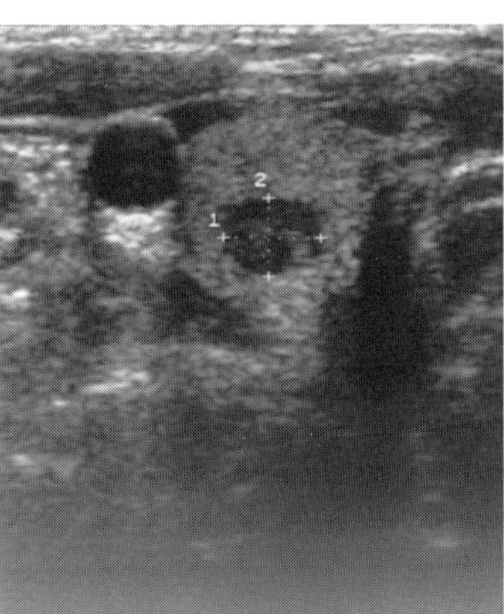

**Figure 9.11c** Transverse image demonstrating the upper pole of the right lobe of the thyroid containing a mass indicated by calipers

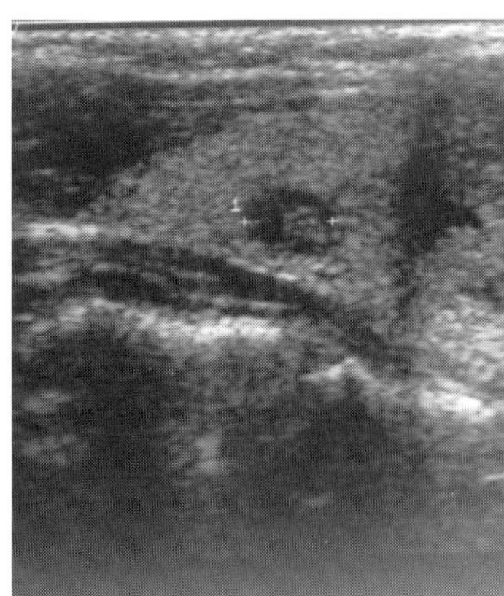

**Figure 9.11d** Longitudinal image showing the same mass as demonstrated in (c)

## Radionuclide imaging

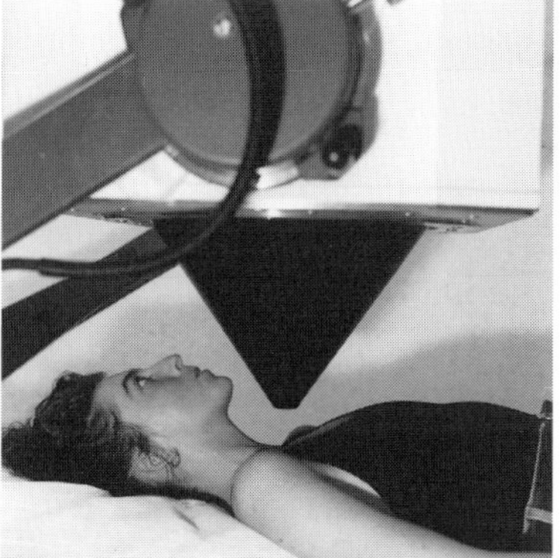

**Figure 9.12a** The pinhole camera

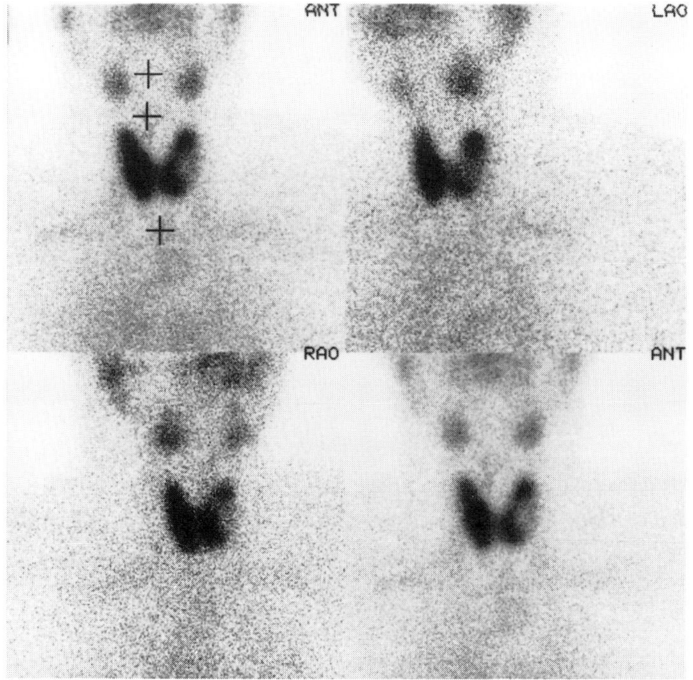


**Figure 9.12b** Series of different views. Note in the anterior view (top left) the symphysis menti of the mandible, cricoid cartilage and top of the sternum are identified in descending order

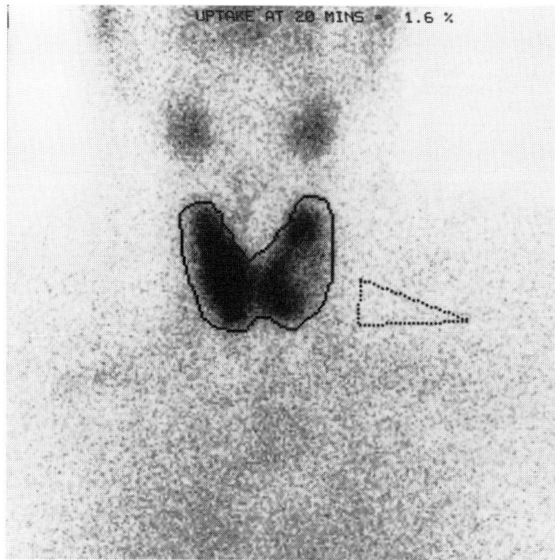


**Figure 9.12c** Anterior image at 20 min post-injection. A ROI is shown drawn around the thyroid gland and a triangular ROI identified to measure background and calculate percentage uptake in the thyroid gland, calculated here at 1.6%

Because the thyroid is capable of taking up iodine and iodine analogues, several radiopharmaceuticals may be used for imaging, the most common of which is $^{99m}$Tc pertechnetate, and this technique is described below. Radionuclide ($^{123}$I) taken orally 2 h prior to scanning can also be used. A functional nodule which may be benign or malignant will appear as a 'hot spot' compared with the normal gland, owing to increased uptake of the radiopharmaceutical. Nodules which show low inactivity are described as 'cold spots' and will require ultrasound examination to establish the diagnosis and differentiate between solid and cystic lesions. Before the start of the examination it is necessary to confirm that the patient is not taking any thyroid blocking agents such as potassium or thyroxin, or that no recent X-ray examination involving iodinated contrast agents has been performed. It is also worth noting the patient's diet, as certain health foods have a high iodine content. All these have an adverse effect on the uptake of the tracer substance within the gland.

### Position of patient and imaging modality

After the radiopharmaceutical is injected intravenously, the patient lies supine on the scanning couch, neck extended and head may be supported by pads and a head band to limit movement. Radioactive spot markers are placed on the sternal notch, thyroid cartilage and either the left or right side of the neck to aid image interpretation. The gamma camera is positioned over the neck region, parallel to the scanning couch, ensuring that the thyroid gland is at the centre of the imaging field. The camera is lowered as close as possible to the patient immediately before imaging.

### Imaging procedure

Image acquisition begins after a delay of 15–20 min to allow uptake of the radiopharmaceutical within the gland. A static acquisition technique is used throughout the examination. Initially, a single anterior view is taken with a parallel hole collimator to give a general view of the neck and to identify any ectopic or retrosternal thyroid tissue. Following this image, a pinhole collimator for magnification is selected and the anterior view repeated. Several additional views may be required to visualise the abnormality suspected clinically. To visualise solitary nodules, supplementary right and left anterior oblique views are taken with the camera rotated to each side in turn, while maintaining position of the gland in the middle of the imaging field. If functional thyroid tissue is suspected in the lingual region, an additional lateral view may be necessary with the camera rotated through 90° and repositioned so that the thyroid is again central in the field.

Analysis of thyroid uptake is performed using data collected at a set time. Normal uptake is in the region of 1–2%.

*Imaging and radiopharmaceutical parameters*

| *Type* | *Administered activity* | *Principal energy* |
|---|---|---|
| $^{99m}$Tc pertechnetate | 75 MBq | 140 keV |
| *Window width* | *Acquisition counts/time* | |
| 20% | 150 000 | |

# 9 Endocrine System

## Adrenal Glands

These are paired glands situated anteromedially to the upper pole of the kidneys. Each gland consists of a cortex and a medulla. The adrenal cortex secretes aldosterone, cortisol and various sex hormones. The chromaffin cells of the medulla contain adrenaline and noradrenaline. Such tissue can also be found in ectopic sites, the most common being near the aortic bifurcation or in relation to the bladder.

### Recommended imaging procedures

Computed tomography and ultrasound have replaced the more invasive techniques of angiography and venography with venous hormone sampling. Although small (5 g), the glands are well demonstrated on CT because of surrounding fat in Gerota's fascia. Radionuclide imaging has been used to locate tumours.

### Indications

To identify the cause of biochemically proven adrenal dysfunction. Cortical disorders can result in Cushing's syndrome (hypercortisolism) and Conn's syndrome (aldosteronism). Phaeochromocytomas are tumours arising from chromaffin cells and can be found either within the medulla of the glands or in any ectopic chromaffin tissue.

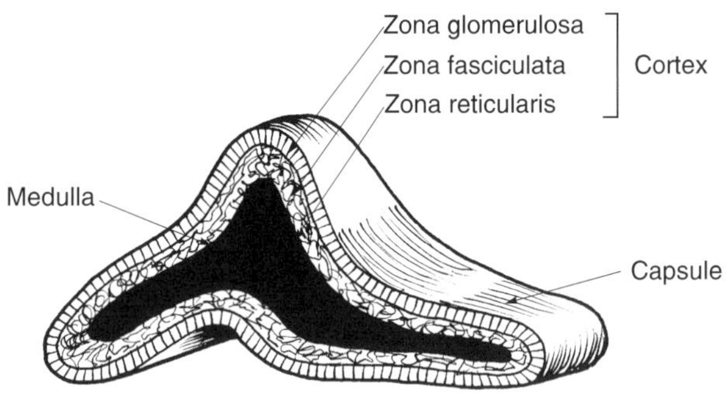

Zona glomerulosa
Zona fasciculata
Zona reticularis
Cortex
Medulla
Capsule

**Figure 9.13a** Section through adrenal gland (diagrammatic)

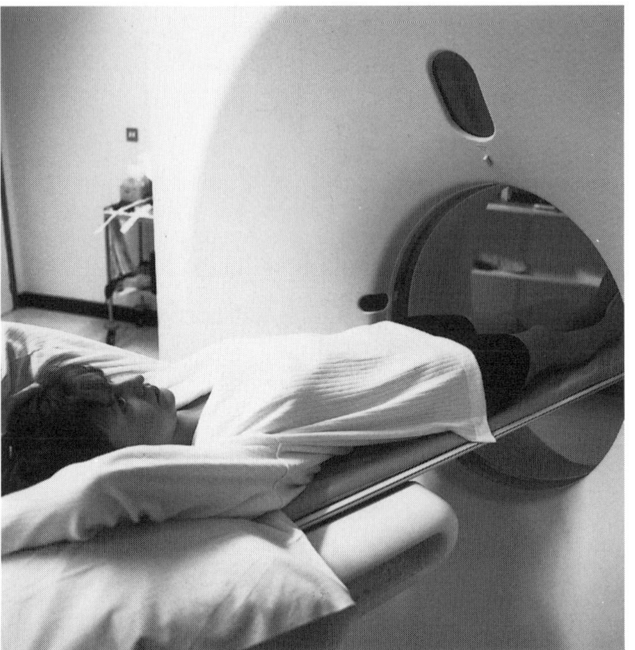

**Figure 9.13b** Patient in scanner

59.7 MM
32.0
-48.0
80
40
0
-40
-80
-120
R
L
154.4 MM

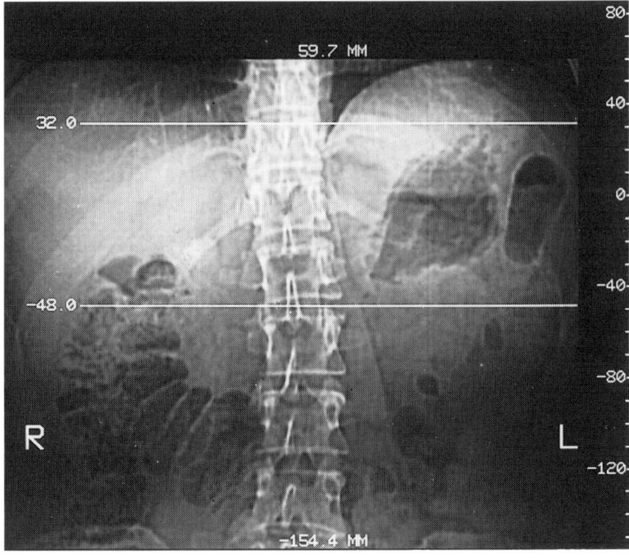

**Figure 9.13c** AP scan projection radiograph showing start and end locations

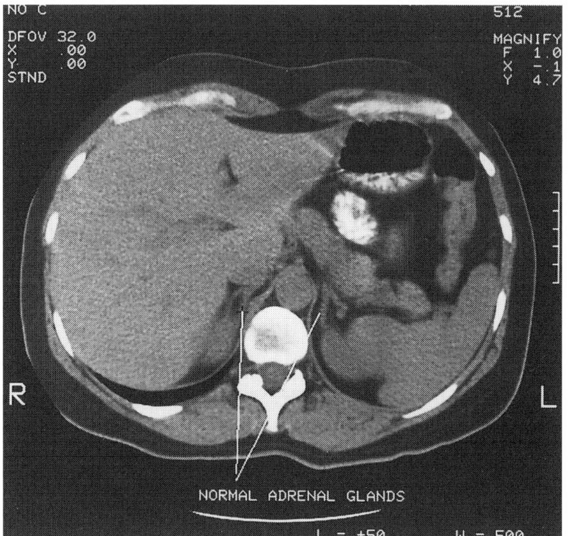


**Figure 9.14a** Pre-contrast image showing normal adrenal gland

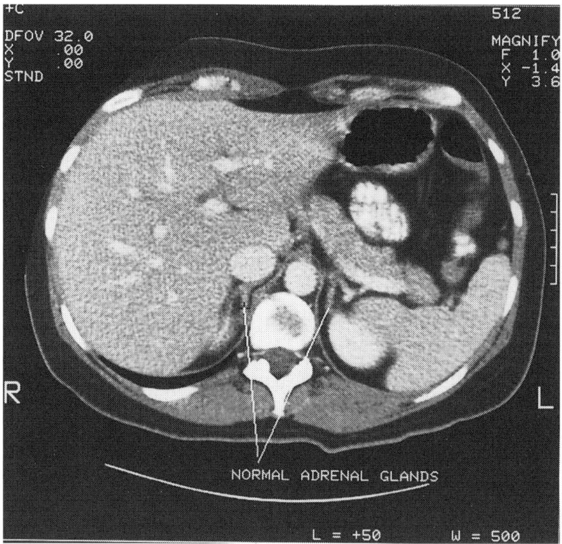


**Figure 9.14b** Post-contrast image showing normal adrenal gland

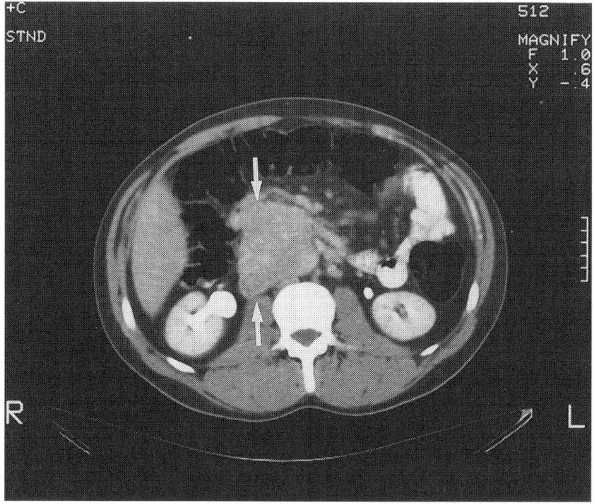


**Figure 9.14c** Post-contrast image showing a large ectopic phaeochromocytoma

# Adrenal Glands



## Computed tomography

Transaxial images are obtained before and during infusion of a non-ionic contrast agent to determine the site, size, vascularity and anatomical relationship of a tumour. Oral contrast medium in the form of dilute Gastrografin or barium is required to identify the small bowel. This is particularly important when a phaeochromocytoma is clinically suspected, as it may be necessary to continue scanning into the pelvis to detect an ectopic tumour.

### Position of patient and imaging modality

The patient lies supine, feet first on the scanner table. Arms are raised and placed behind the patient's head, out of the scan plane. Positioning is aided by external alignment lights. The median sagittal plane is perpendicular and the coronal plane is parallel to the scanner table. The scan plane is now perpendicular to the long axis of the body to enable transaxial cross-sectional imaging to be undertaken. The scanner table height is adjusted to ensure that the coronal plane alignment light is at the level of the mid-axillary line. The patient is then moved into the scanner so that the scan reference point is at the level of the xiphisternum.

### Imaging procedure

An anteroposterior scan projection radiograph is performed, starting approximately 6 cm above and ending 15 cm below the reference point. From this image, 10 mm contiguous sections are prescribed through the adrenal area from the 11th thoracic vertebra to the third lumbar vertebra, with all images taken on suspended respiration. If the adrenal glands are clearly identified and normal, no further scanning is necessary. If this is not the case, or an adrenal tumour is present, narrower 5 mm contiguous sections are prescribed and performed during contrast infusion, increasing spatial resolution and decreasing scan time. Approximately 15 contiguous sections are necessary to cover the relevant area.

If spiral scanning options are available, both pre- and post-contrast enhancement images may be acquired with a volume acquisition, using a 5 mm slice thickness and 5 mm table increments, but with a 3 mm reconstruction index to give overlapping sections. Image acquisition for both sets of images is performed using a single breath hold to ensure that the full extent of the glands are demonstrated.

### Ectopic tumours

If the suspected clinical diagnosis is phaeochromocytoma and the adrenals are well seen and normal, post-contrast scans are continued through the abdomen and pelvis to identify a tumour in an ectoptic site. The prescribed technique is 10 mm sections at 20 mm table increments.

*Contrast and injector data*

| *Volume* | *Concentration* | *Flow rate* |
|---|---|---|
| 100 ml | 300 mgI/ml | 2 ml/s |

A 30 s pre-scan delay is chosen, allowing 60 ml of contrast to be injected before the start of scanning.

# 9 Adrenal Glands

## Ultrasound

Ultrasound can be used to detect abnormalities of the adrenal glands only if the examination is undertaken by an experienced ultrasonographer using high-quality equipment. As the glands are situated high in the abdomen adjacent to the spine, they can easily be obscured by the ribs, bowel gas, the transverse processes of the vertebrae and perinephric fat.

The sensitivity and specificity of ultrasound in the detection of adrenal lesions is much less than CT, which is the preferred imaging technique.

**Position of patient and imaging modality**

The right adrenal gland is examined with the patient either supine or turned 45° onto the left side with the right side uppermost. The left adrenal gland can also be examined with the patient supine or more usually in the lateral position with the patient turned onto the right side.

**Imaging procedure**

Ultrasound gel is applied to the upper abdomen. To image the right adrenal gland, the liver is used as an acoustic window. The transducer is positioned at the ninth and 10th intercostal space in the mid-axillary line. By rotating the transducer, a series of transverse images are produced from the renal hilum, below, to a level several centimetres above the kidney to completely cover the adrenal gland. Further longitudinal images are produced by rotating the transducer through 90°.

To image the left adrenal gland, the spleen is used as the acoustic window. The transducer is placed at the eighth and ninth intercostal space in the posterior axillary line and a coronal image is obtained showing the left kidney. From this position the transducer is angled slightly to identify the left adrenal gland in the perirenal space between the kidney, spleen and the left crus of the diaphragm. Further images in the right decubitus position may also be necessary to identify the gland.

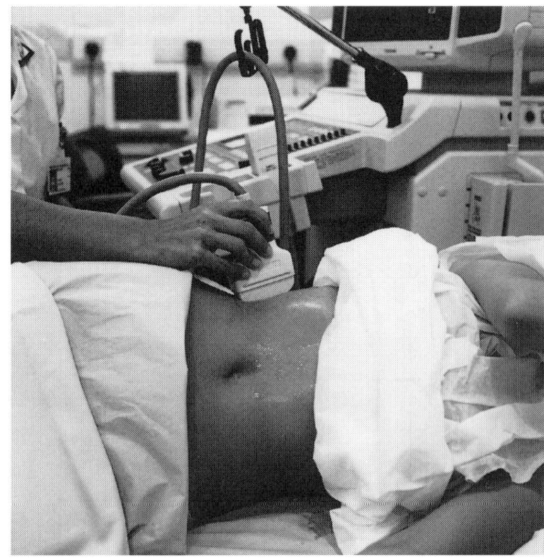

**Figure 9.15b** Patient positioned for examination of right adrenal

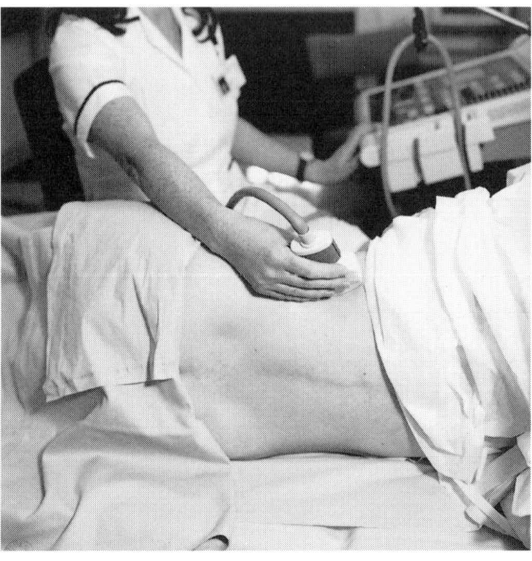

**Figure 9.15c** Patient positioned for examination of left adrenal

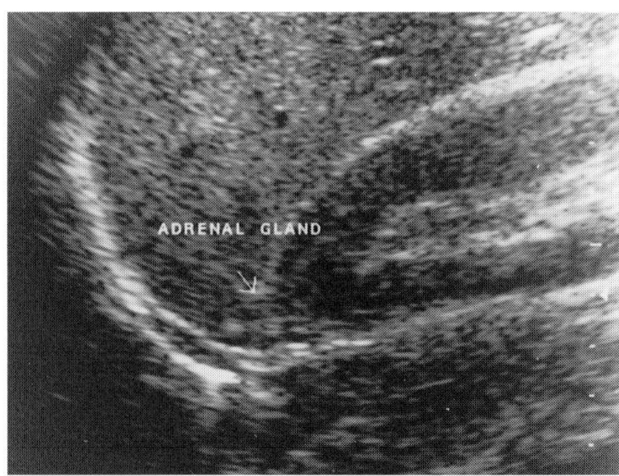


**Figure 9.15a** Longitudinal section of right kidney showing adrenal gland

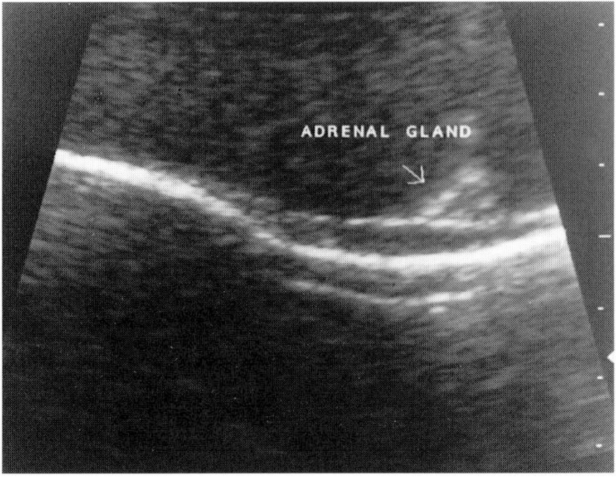


**Figure 9.15d** Oblique abdominal scan showing right adrenal gland

## Radionuclide imaging

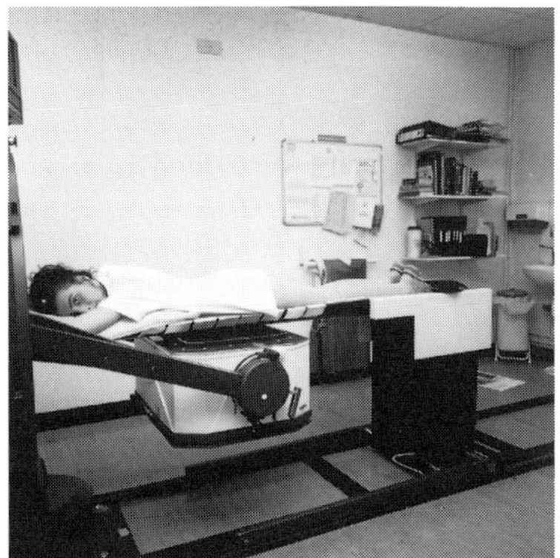

**Figure 9.16a** Patient prone for anterior view of abdomen and pelvis

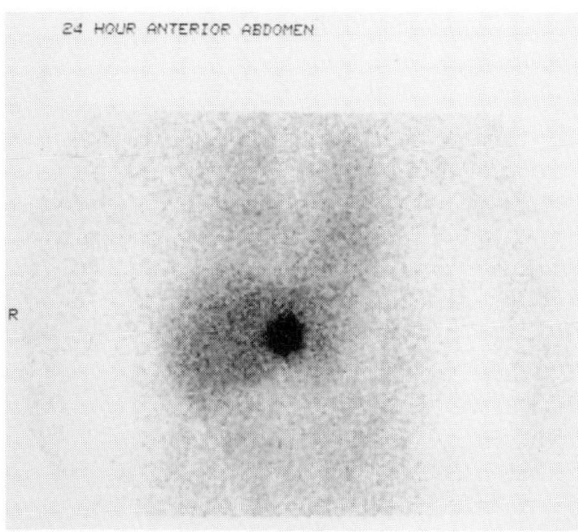


**Figure 9.16b** Twenty-four-hour posterior whole-body scan showing intense area of uptake consistent with a phaeochromocytoma

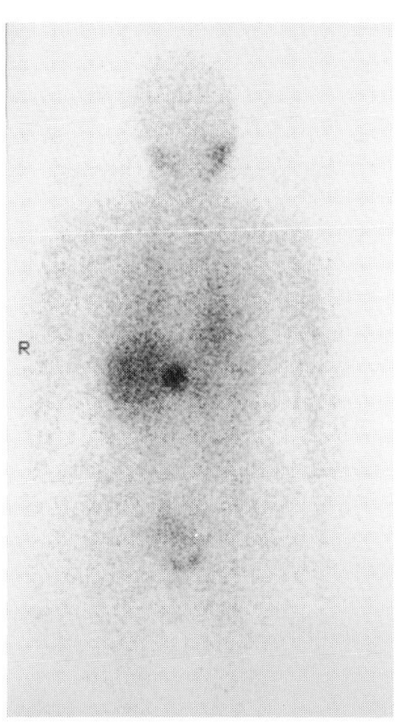


**Figure 9.16c** Twenty-four-hour anterior abdomen scan of patient shown in (b)

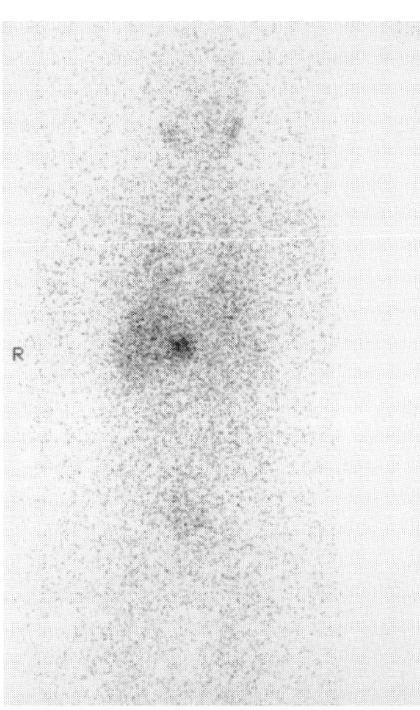


**Figure 9.16d** Forty-eight-hour posterior whole-body scan showing same area of intense uptake

Radionuclide imaging is used mainly to identify tumours of the adrenal medulla. Imaging of the cortex has been performed using labelled cholesterol ($^{79}$SE cholesterol) and images acquired daily for up to 5 days after injection. This technique is seldom used and is not described here.

Tumours of the medulla are imaged using radioiodine, either $^{131}$I or $^{123}$I labelled to MIBG (metaiodobenzylguanidine). The former is more widely available and less expensive than the latter, but has the disadvantage of a longer half-life – 8.1 days compared with 13 h. Scanning continues up to 72 h post-injection $^{131}$I MIBG, but ends after 48 h if using $^{123}$I MIBG. The technique described uses $^{123}$I MIBG. Either whole body scanning or additional images of the head/neck, thorax, abdomen and pelvis must be obtained if either an ectopic tumour or metastases from malignant phaeochromocytoma are suspected.

### Preparation of the patient

Potassium iodide tablets (120 mg/day) are given orally, starting 1 day before and ending 3 days after the examination to block uptake of free iodine in the thyroid gland. Also some antidepressant and antihypertensive drugs must be discontinued as they interfere with norepinephrine uptake and therefore hamper MIBG uptake. Immediately prior to the injection the patient must micturate to aid identification of areas of increased uptake around the bladder. As there is a risk of an increase in blood pressure, monitoring should be done during the i.v. injection of the radiopharmaceutical and appropriate emergency drugs available.

### Position of patient and imaging modality

Anterior and posterior views are acquired routinely and can be performed in either the erect, prone or supine position. The imaging field of the gamma camera is positioned as close to the patient as possible, parallel to the scanning table and centred over the adrenal areas.

### Imaging procedure

A high-energy general-purpose parallel-hole collimator is selected and a static acquisition technique used. The radiopharmaceutical is injected intravenously and image acquisition commenced for the anterior and the posterior views. In addition to the routine images, lateral and oblique views of the adrenal area may be necessary. Further images of ectopic sites should then be acquired. Image acquisition time is 10 min per image on day 1 of the examination. These images are repeated daily for up to 48 h, with an increased acquisition time of 20 min.

*Imaging and radiopharmaceutical parameters*

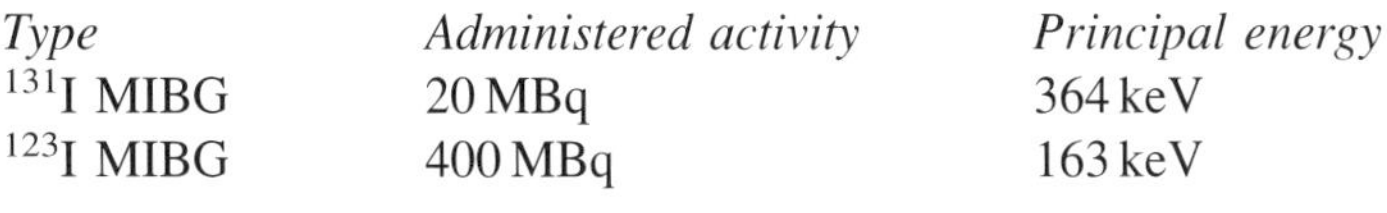

| *Type* | *Administered activity* | *Principal energy* |
|---|---|---|
| $^{131}$I MIBG | 20 MBq | 364 keV |
| $^{123}$I MIBG | 400 MBq | 163 keV |

| *Window width* | *Acquisition counts/time* |
|---|---|
| 20% | 20 min |

# 10

## CENTRAL NERVOUS SYSTEM

### CONTENTS

# 10 Central Nervous System

## Brain

### Introduction

The central nervous system comprises the brain and the spinal cord.

The brain develops from a simple tube along which three swellings grow. These develop into the forebrain, comprising the cerebrum, thalamus and hypothalamus, the midbrain, comprising the cerebral peduncles, and the hindbrain, comprising the cerebellum, pons and medulla oblongata.

The cerebrum is the largest part and occupies the anterior and middle cranial fossae. It is divided into the right and left cerebral hemispheres by the longitudinal fissure which contains the falx cerebri. The two hemispheres are joined below the falx by the corpus callosum.

Each hemisphere is divided into four lobes – frontal, parietal, temporal and occipital – which correspond to the overlying bony structure.

The surface layer or cortex is composed of nerve cells (grey matter). In order to accommodate as large an area as possible, it is folded and has a wrinkled appearance, with gyri and sulci. The most important of these are the central sulcus (fissure of Rolando) which separates the frontal and parietal lobes, the lateral sulcus (fissure of Sylvius) which separates the temporal lobe from the frontal and parietal lobes, and the pre- and post-central gyri which lie in front of and behind the central sulcus, respectively.

Certain areas are identified with specific brain functions. The pre-central gyrus is known as the motor cortex and is the origin of all voluntary movements. The post-central gyrus is known as the sensory cortex and receives and appreciates all general sensations.

Other important areas include the auditory area which receives impulses from the auditory nerve and is situated in the cortex of the temporal lobe immediately below the lateral sulcus; the visual area, situated in the cortex of the occipital lobe and receives impulses via the optic chiasm; and the motor speech area (Broca's area) which initiates tongue movements and is situated in the cortex of the frontal lobe just above the anterior end of the lateral sulcus. The sensory speech area which interprets the written and spoken word is situated in the lower part of the parietal cortex.

Each hemisphere is responsible for movement and sensations from the opposite side of the body. For example, in right-handed people highly developed skills such as writing are a function of the left cerebral hemisphere.

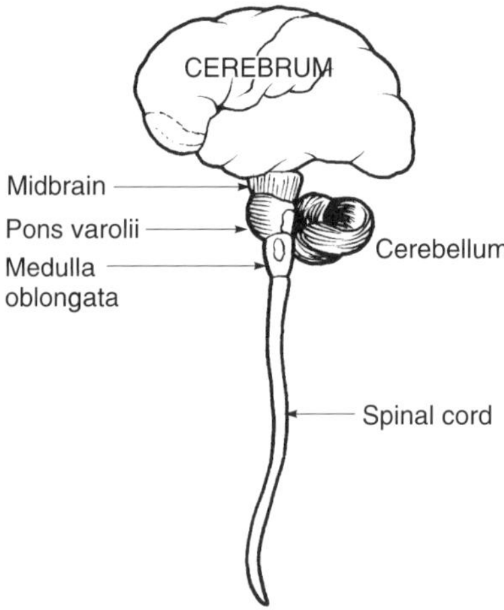


**Figure 10.1a** Schematic representation of central nervous system

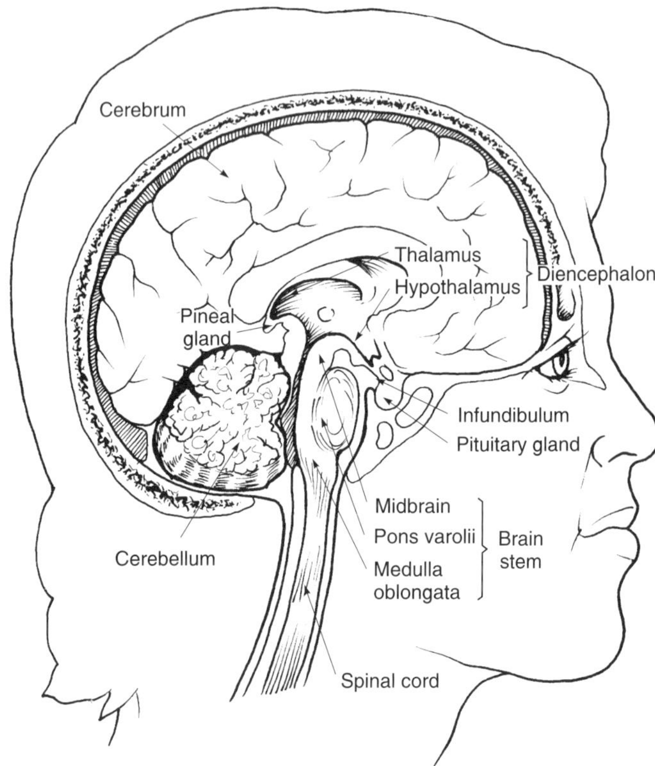


**Figure 10.1b** Midline sagittal section through brain

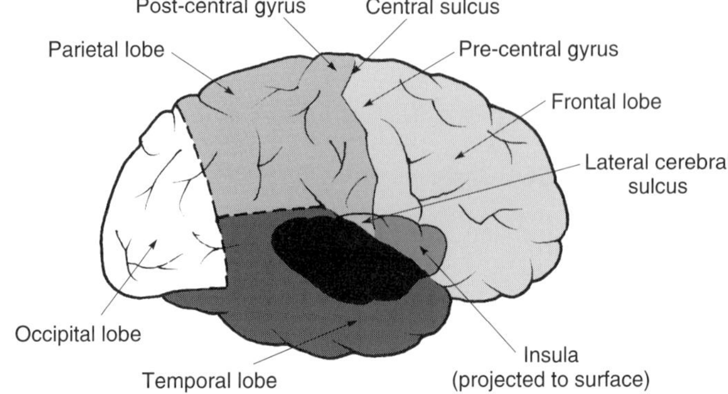


**Figure 10.1c** Lateral aspect of cerebrum showing various lobes and sulci

## Brain

Corpus callosum
Cerebrum
Lateral ventricle
Thalamus
Caudate nucleus
Corpus striatum
Putamen
Globus pallidus
Lentiform nucleus
Insula
Third ventricle
Claustrum
Hypothalamus
Optic tract
Infundibulum
Internal capsule
Pituitary gland

**Figure 10.2a** Coronal section through the brain

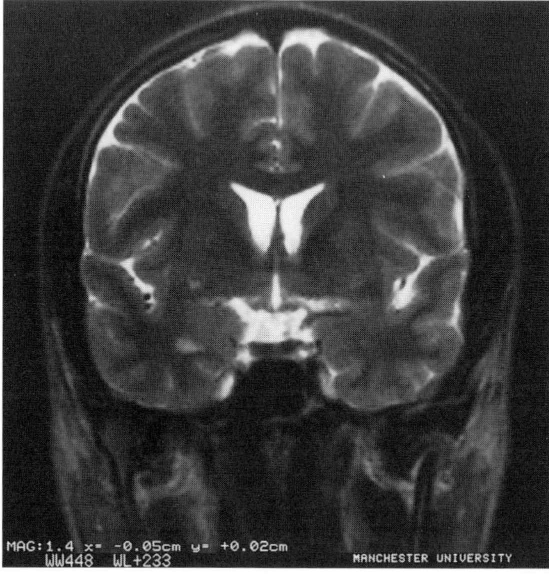


**Figure 10.2b** Coronal $T_2$ weighted MR image of the brain

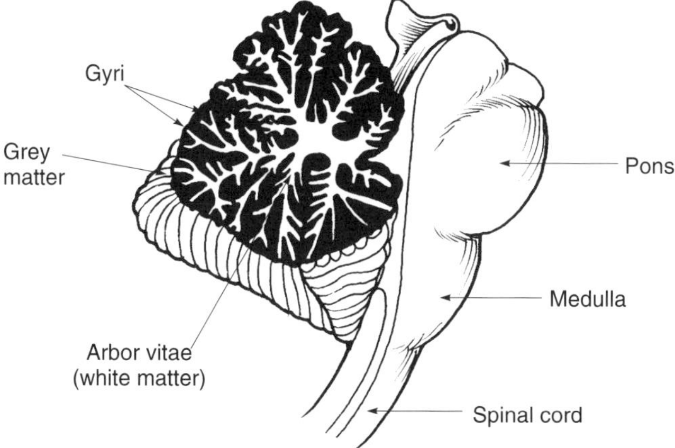


**Figure 10.2c** Sagittal section through the cerebellum

The interior of the cerebral hemispheres is composed mainly of nerve fibres (white matter) and contains two cavities, the lateral ventricles which are filled with cerebrospinal fluid. There are, however, three important areas of grey matter in the interior of the cerebral hemispheres. The basal ganglia lie on the anterior and central parts of the lateral walls of the lateral ventricles, and influence skeletal muscle tone. The thalamus, which is situated below the corpus callosum, forms the lateral wall of the third ventricle and acts as a relay station for peripheral nerve impulses passing from the spinal cord to the sensory cortex. The hypothalamus which lies below the thalamus forms the floor of the third ventricle. It is attached to the post-pituitary gland and acts as a control centre for bodily functions such as the regulation of body temperature, sleep and metabolism of fats and carbohydrates.

The midbrain is situated between the cerebrum and the pons. The ventral portion contains two cerebral peduncles which are composed mainly of fibres passing between the forebrain and the hindbrain. The dorsal portion contains four groups of cells, the corpora quadrigemina which serve as reflex centres for movements of the eye, head and trunk, in response to visual and auditory stimuli. There is a narrow canal within the midbrain, termed the aqueduct of Sylvius, which communicates with the third ventricle above and the fourth ventricle below.

The hindbrain consists of the pons, medulla oblongata and the cerebellum. The pons is situated in front of the cerebellum and above the medulla oblongata. It is composed mainly of nerve fibres passing from the cerebral hemispheres to the spinal cord and between the cerebral hemispheres themselves. The anatomical structure of the pons is the reverse of the fore- and midbrain in that the nerve cells lie deep and the nerve fibres are superficial.

The medulla oblongata is 2.5 cm long and is triangular in shape (▽). It is situated in the posterior cranial fossa above the foramen magnum and extends from the pons above and is continuous with the spinal cord inferiorly. The anterior and posterior surfaces are marked by a central fissure.

The anatomical structure is similar to that of the pons and the deep nerve cells provide the origin for some of the cranial nerves; others are vital centres for cardiac, respiratory, vasomotor and reflex functions.

The cerebellum is situated in the posterior cranial fossa behind the pons and the medulla. It consists of two hemispheres joined by a narrow median strip, termed the vermis. The grey matter lies on the surface and its internal structure forms a branch-like pattern known as the arbor vitae. Cerebellar functions are below the level of consciousness and include the maintenance of balance and posture and co-ordination of voluntary muscle movement.

# 10 Central Nervous System

## Brain

### Spinal cord

The spinal cord is an elongated section of the central nervous system. It is approximately 45 cm long and cylindrical in cross-section. It is continuous with the medulla oblongata superiorly extending from the upper border of the atlas to the lower border of the first lumbar vertebra. It presents swellings in the cervical and lumbar regions which correspond to the brachial and lumbar sacral plexus.

It is surrounded by dura, arachnoid and pia mater. Cerebrospinal fluid (CSF) is present in the central canal and in the subarachnoid space.

### Spinal nerves

Thirty-one pairs of spinal nerves arise from the spinal cord and derive their name from the area from which they originate. The lumbar, sacral and coccygeal nerves leave the cord before its termination and extend inferiorly through the subarachnoid space to form the cauda equina.

The spinal cord is incompletely divided by the anterior median fissure and the posterior median septum. The grey matter lies deep in an 'H' pattern and the white matter lies superficially. The central canal contains CSF and is continuous with the fourth ventricle.

The posterior horns are stimulated by sensory impulses and the anterior horns originate motor impulses. The white matter comprises three tracts, one ascending carrying sensory information, one descending carrying motor information and one intersegmental carrying information from one level to another.

### Cranial nerves

There are twelve pairs of cranial nerves attached to the brain. They are numbered i–xii, from anterior to posterior. Some contain motor fibres, some sensory fibres and some are mixed. Motor fibres originate as nuclei in the brain stem, whereas sensory fibres originate externally, e.g. in special sense organs such as the eye, ear or nose.

Nerve fibres enter and leave the brain through foramina in the floor of the anterior, middle and posterior cranial fossae. Table 10.1, detailing the cranial nerves by number, name, function and passage through base of skull, appears on the facing page.

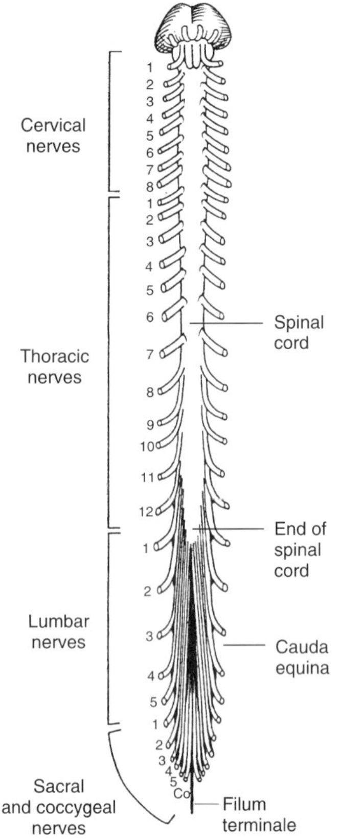


**Figure 10.3a** Spinal cord and nerves

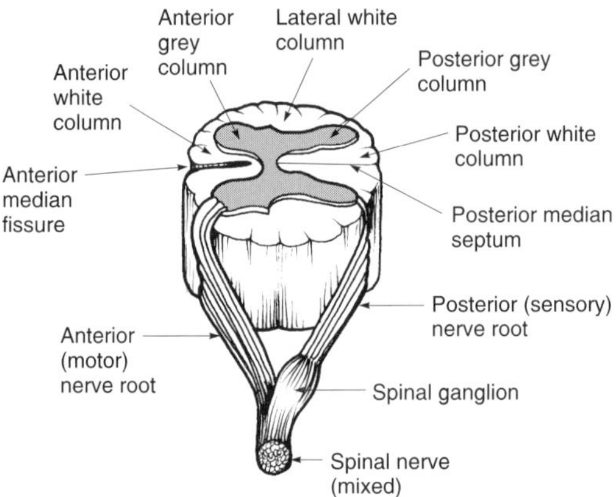


**Figure 10.3b** Section through spinal cord showing nerve roots

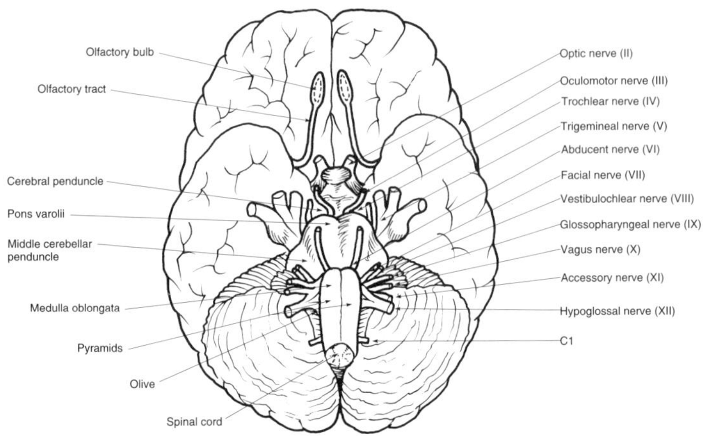


**Figure 10.3c** Inferior aspect of brain

# Central Nervous System 10

## Brain

**Table 10.1 Summary of the cranial nerves**

| *No.* | *Name/type* | *Route through base of skull* | *Function* |
|---|---|---|---|
| i | Olfactory (sensory) | Cribriform plate of ethmoid | Sense of smell |
| ii | Optic (sensory) | Optic foramen | Sense of sight<br>Balance |
| iii | Oculomotor (motor) | Superior orbital fissure | Movements of the eyeball and pupil |
| iv | Trochlear (motor) | Superior orbital fissure | Movements of the eyeball |
| v | Trigeminal (mixed): | | |
| | (i) ophthalmic | (a) Superior orbital fissure (s) | Cornea, nasal mucosa, skin |
| | (ii) maxillary | (b) Foramen rotundum (s) | Skin, mouth, teeth, tongue |
| | (iii) mandibular | (c) Foramen ovale (m) | Mastication |
| vi | Abducens (motor) | Superior orbital fissure | Movements of the eyeball |
| vii | Facial (mixed) | Internal auditory meatus/ styloid foramen | Facial movements, taste |
| viii | Auditory/vestibulocochlear (sensory) | Internal auditory meatus | Balance, hearing |
| ix | Glossopharyngeal (mixed) | Jugular foramen | Taste, saliva secretion, pharangeal movements |
| x | Vagus (mixed) | Jugular foramen | Larynx, pharynx, oesophagus, heart, lungs, stomach, small intestine, large intestine (part) |
| xi | Accessory (motor) | Jugular foramen | Movements of head, neck, larynx, pharynx |
| xii | Hypoglossal (motor) | Hypoglossal canal | Tongue movements |

# 10 Central Nervous System

## Brain

The ventricular system comprises a fluid-filled system within the brain containing CSF which is normally a clear colourless alkaline fluid. There are four cavities, known as the right and left lateral ventricles, the third ventricle and the fourth ventricle, which communicate with each other and are continuous with the central canal of the spinal cord.

The lateral ventricles are roughly 6 cm long and lie in the cerebral hemispheres either side of the midline below the corpus callosum. Each comprises an anterior horn, posterior horn and temporal horn situated in the frontal lobe, occipital lobe and temporal lobes of the brain, respectively. In the posterior part of the anterior horn is the interventricular foramen which joins the two ventricles and communicates inferiorly to open into the third ventricle through the foramen of Monro. The single third ventricle is a narrow midline structure situated between the two thalami. The floor is formed by the hypothalamus and an anterior projection forms the infundibular recess of the pituitary gland. It communicates posteriorly and inferiorly through the aqueduct of Sylvius to the fourth ventricle.

The fourth ventricle is a midline structure situated behind the pons and in front of the cerebellum. It is diamond shaped from above and presents two lateral recesses on either side which pass inferiorly and anteriorly. It is continuous inferiorly with the central canal of the spinal cord.

The fourth ventricle communicates with the subarachnoid space via three foramen, one central, one in the roof which is known as foramen of Magendie and one in the roof of each of the lateral recesses, known as foramen of Luschka.

The ventricular system is lined with ciliated epithelium, termed ependyma.

### Circulation of cerebrospinal fluid

The walls of the lateral ventricles and the roof of the third and fourth ventricles are lined with a highly vascular membrane, termed the choroid plexus. This produces CSF from the blood and secretes it into the ventricular system.

It passes from the lateral ventricles through foramen of Monro into the third ventricle and through the aqueduct of Sylvius into the fourth ventricle. From the fourth ventricle it passes down the central canal and through the foramen of Magendie and Luschka into the subarachnoid space.

It passes forwards and laterally over the cerebral hemispheres and is reabsorbed back into the blood stream through arachnoid granulations in the superior sagittal sinus and lateral sinus.

The absence of granules or obstruction of the aqueduct (aqueduct stenosis) can result in hydrocephalus.

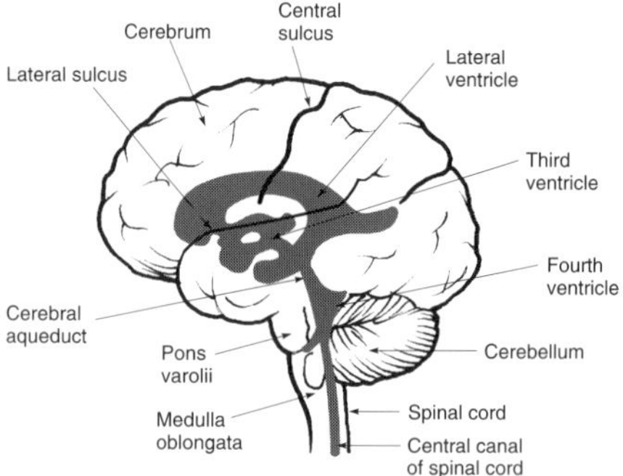


**Figure 10.4a** Lateral aspect of brain showing position of ventricles

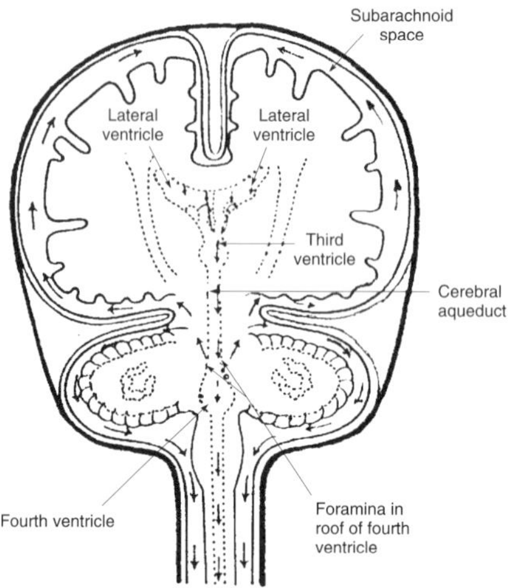


**Figure 10.4b** Circulation of cerebrospinal fluid

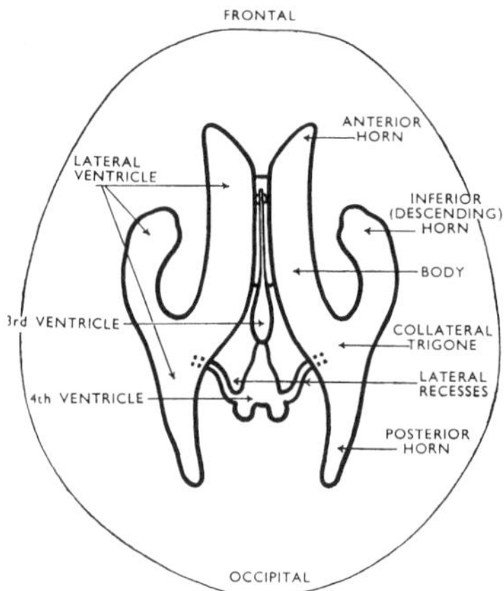


**Figure 10.4c** Ventricular system (supero-inferior aspect)

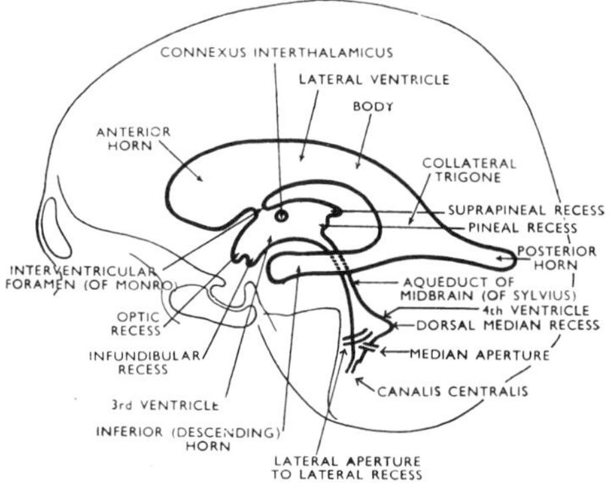


**Figure 10.4d** Ventricular system (lateral aspect)

## Recommended imaging procedures

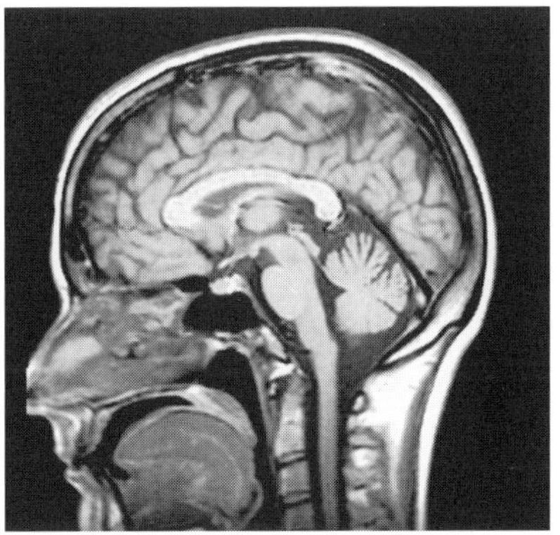
Figure 10.5a Midline sagittal $T_1$ weighted MR image

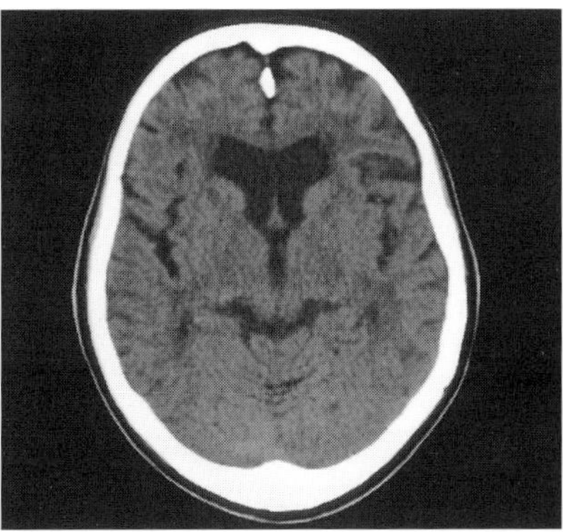
Figure 10.5b Transaxial CT image

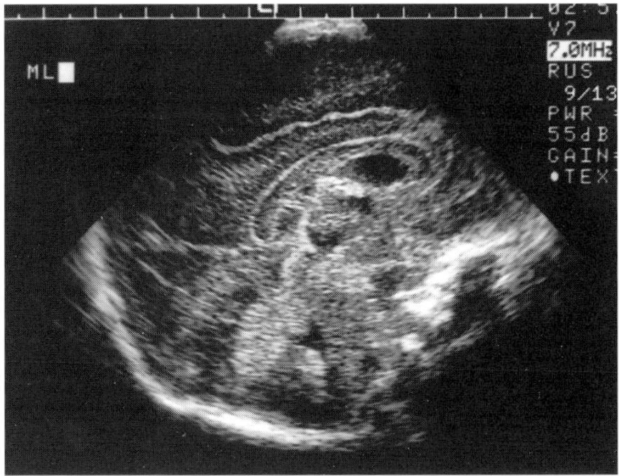

Figure 10.5c Midline sagittal ultrasound image

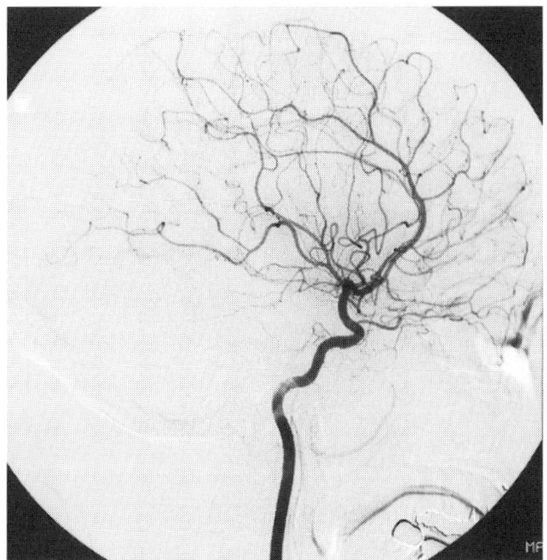
Figure 10.5d Cerebral angiogram (carotid vessels)

The multiplanar, non-invasive, non-ionising properties and the high inherent contrast of MRI have made this technique, where available, the examination of choice for disorders of the central nervous system. Because there is no MR signal from bone, it has a further advantage over CT scanning in producing high-definition images of the posterior cranial fossa without the streak artefacts arising from the mastoid air cells and surrounding dense bone (present in CT scans of the posterior cranial fossa). Computed tomography is the preferred technique in cases of acute haemorrhage and trauma, but MRI may be extremely useful after the acute phase.

However, CT does have the advantage over MRI in the assessment of bony abnormalities, e.g. trauma, bone destruction due to tumour and congenital abnormalities. Also, MRI may be contraindicated in certain cases, e.g. claustrophobia, the presence of pacemakers, aneurysmal and surgical clips.

Because of the radiosensitivity of the lens of the eye, it is important in CT head scanning to minimise radiation dose to the patient. This may be achieved by limiting the number of sections required to achieve diagnosis, avoiding overlapping sections, adjusting the patient position or angling the scanner gantry to avoid directly irradiating the lens, and lastly reducing radiographic technique parameters.

Direct coronal CT sections are useful in imaging the pituitary gland (see Chapter 9) and the orbital cavity, although artefacts from dental fillings may degrade the image quality. To overcome this, it may be necessary to acquire transaxial images and reformat the digital data into the desired anatomical plane. Spatial resolution is less in reformations than directly acquired images.

Image enhancement agents play a significant role in both MRI and CT, helping to assess abnormalities and their relationship to surrounding structures.

Non-tomographic RNI has a limited role and has now been superseded by CT and MRI; however, SPECT scanning has an important role in assessing function.

Ultrasound examinations are limited because of the surrounding bony structures, but it is the imaging modality of choice in young children with patent fontanelles.

Cerebral angiography using either a venous or arterial approach is undertaken using specialised digital angiographic equipment and may lead to interventional procedures such as embolisation.

# 10 Brain

## Magnetic Resonance Imaging

### Standard brain protocol

Magnetic resonance imaging offers many imaging options, e.g. type of sequence and anatomical plane, but the examination time is always a limiting factor and not all options can be undertaken. A combination of $T_1$ and $T_2$ weighted sequences in selective planes is necessary. A $T_2$ weighted sequence allows most intracranial lesions to be identified against normal isointense brain tissue and is usually obtained in the first instance. $T_1$ weighted images in the appropriate anatomical plane are acquired next and repeated using contrast enhancement if necessary. By scanning in this order, the same imaging parameters can be used without further machine 'set-up', thus ensuring that the decibel level is the same as that used for non-enhanced scan. The following imaging procedure offers a guideline; sequences will vary between machines and the best anatomical plane can only be decided after the initial images have been viewed. Contrast enhancement is used to further delineate suspected abnormalities.

**Indications**

Intracranial haemorrhage (non-acute), tumour, aneurysm, trauma, metastases, multiple sclerosis.

**Contraindications**

These centre on the presence of metallic objects. Patients with surgical aneurysmal clips should not be scanned, as torque forces on the clips from the magnetic field can result in movement of the clips and rupture of the vessel walls. However, new non-ferromagnetic clips are now available, but it is imperative that the operator ascertains which type of clip has been used before scanning a postoperative patient. Foreign bodies in the eye due to occupational injury, other trauma or surgery are also contra-indicated, as are patients with cardiac pacemakers and cochlear implants.

**Position of patient and imaging modality**

The patient lies supine on the scanner table, head resting in the head support of the head coil. Position is aided by external halogen alignment lights. The median sagittal plane is parallel to the sagittal alignment light and the transaxial alignment light parallel to the anthropological baseline. The table is now adjusted until the external reference point is at the centre of the head coil. From this position the patient and the head coil assembly are driven the fixed distance to the isocentre of the magnet.

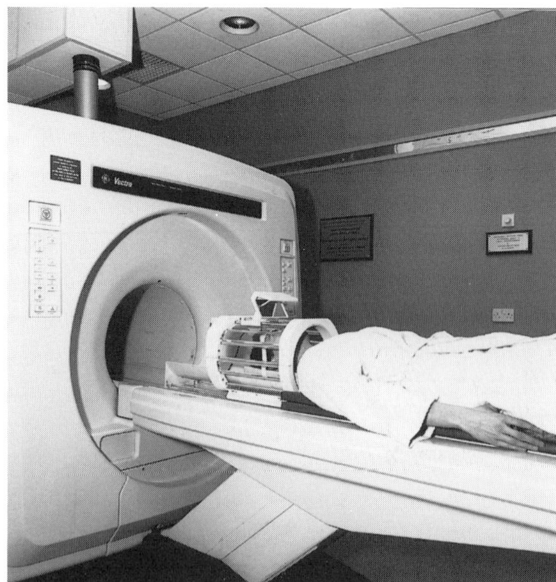

**Figure 10.6a** Patient supine in head coil

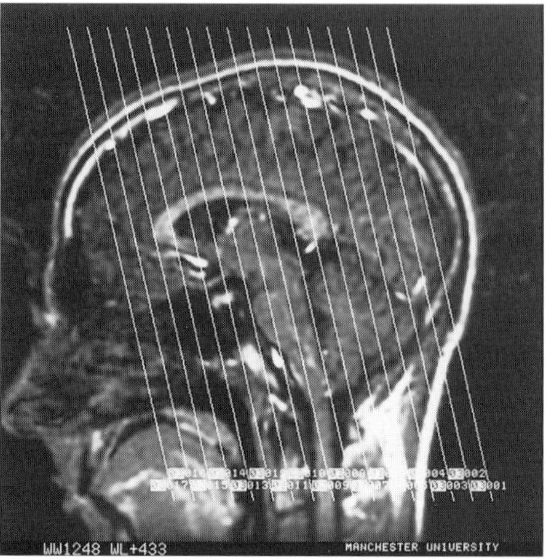


**Figure 10.6b** Midline sagittal localiser image showing prescribed coronal sections

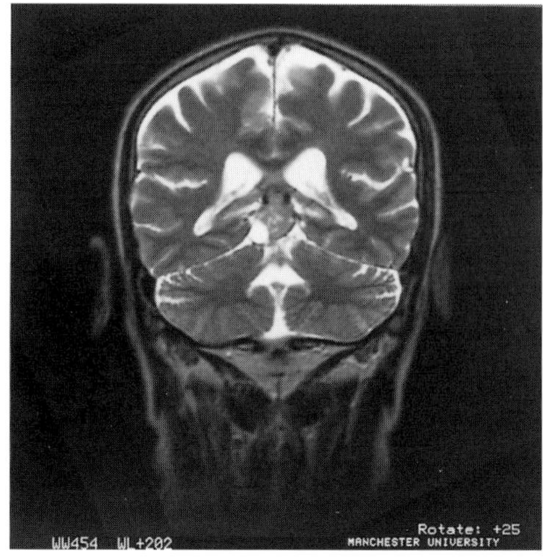


**Figure 10.6c** Coronal $T_2$ weighted image

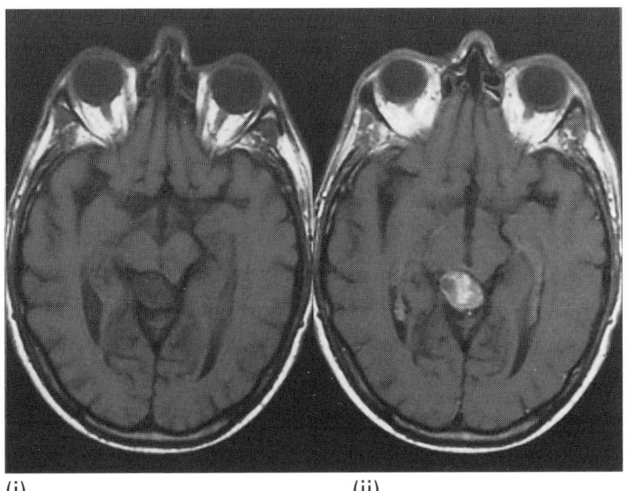

(i) (ii)

**Figure 10.7a** Transaxial $T_1$ weighted pre-contrast (i) and post-contrast (ii) enhancement images showing high signal lesion in the post-contrast image

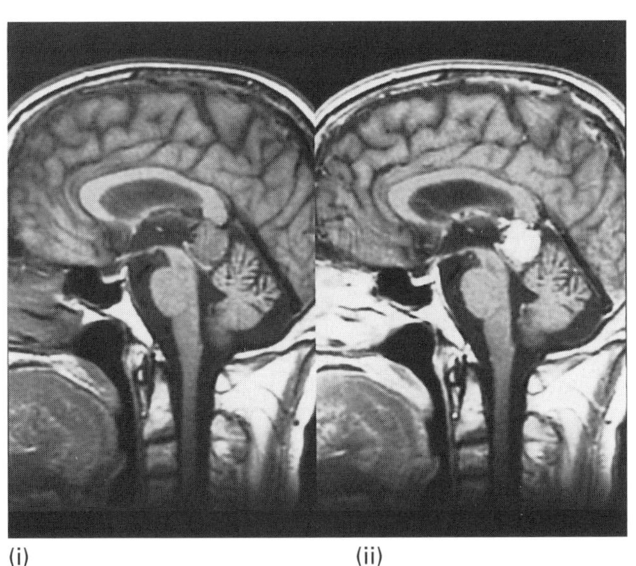

(i) (ii)

**Figure 10.7b** Sagittal $T_1$ weighted pre-contrast (i) and post-contrast (ii) enhancement images showing high signal lesion in the post-contrast image

## Magnetic Resonance Imaging

### Imaging procedure

Initial midline sagittal and transaxial localiser scans are obtained. From the sagittal image, $T_2$ weighted sections in either the coronal plane or transaxial plane are acquired using a 7 mm slice, with a 2 mm gap between each image. The transaxial images are aligned parallel to the hard palate. The coronal images are then aligned at 90° to the transaxial imaging plane.

Further $T_1$ weighted scans are prescribed in either the sagittal or transaxial plane to cover any area of suspected abnormality. The section width and gap may be reduced, depending on the area to be scanned. After review, $T_1$ weighted scans may be repeated following the injection of a suitable image enhancement agent (gadolinium DTPA). For the repeat scans it is important that the decibel level is identical to that of the pre-contrast scans to ensure that any enhancement is real.

*Contrast medium and injection data*

| *Volume* | *Pharmaceutical* | *Flow rate* |
|---|---|---|
| 0.2 ml/kg body weight | Gadolinium DTPA | Hand injection |

**Table 10.2 Imaging parameters**

| *Imaging plane* | *Imaging sequence* | *TR* | *TE* | *Field of view* (cm) | *No. of NEX* | *Slice width/ gap* (mm) | *Matrix (horizontal – vertical)* |
|---|---|---|---|---|---|---|---|
| Coronal or sagittal | Fast spin-echo $T_2$ weighted (echo train length –12) | 6000 | 102 | 25 | 2 | 5–7/1–2 | 192 × 256 |
| Transaxial | Spin-echo $T_1$ weighted | 500 | 25 | 25 | 2 | 5/2 | 192 × 256 |
| Sagittal | Spin-echo $T_1$ weighted | 500 | 25 | 25 | 2 | 5/2 | 192 × 224 |
| Transaxial Post-contrast | Spin-echo $T_1$ weighted | 500 | 25 | 25 | 2 | 5/2 | 192 × 256 |

# 10 Brain

## Posterior cranial fossa

Magnetic resonance is the preferred imaging modality for lesions of the posterior cranial fossa, brain stem and internal auditory meatuses.

In the clinical diagnosis of acoustic neuroma, contrast enhancement $T_1$ weighted scans may suffice. For other lesions, initial $T_1$ and $T_2$ scans are required and may be followed by contrast enhanced $T_1$ weighted images.

### Indications

Tumours of the seventh and eighth cranial nerves, posterior fossa and brain stem, bony destruction, trauma and congenital anomalies.

### Position of patient and imaging modality

The patient position is that described for routine MRI brain scanning.

### Imaging procedure

Initial coronal, sagittal and transaxial localiser scans are performed. From the sagittal image, $T_2$ weighted scans are prescribed in either the coronal or transaxial plane to cover the entire posterior cranial fossa. Section width equals 5 mm and there is a 1 mm gap between each scan. Further high-resolution images in the appropriate anatomical plane may be required through any area of abnormality. These may be either $T_2$ weighted fast spin-echo images or a $T_1$ weighted 3D volume acquisition prior to and repeated after the intravenous injection of a paramagnetic enhancement agent.

*Contrast medium and injector data*

| *Volume* | *Concentration* | *Flow rate* |
|---|---|---|
| 0.2 ml/kg body weight | Gadolinium DTPA | Hand injection |

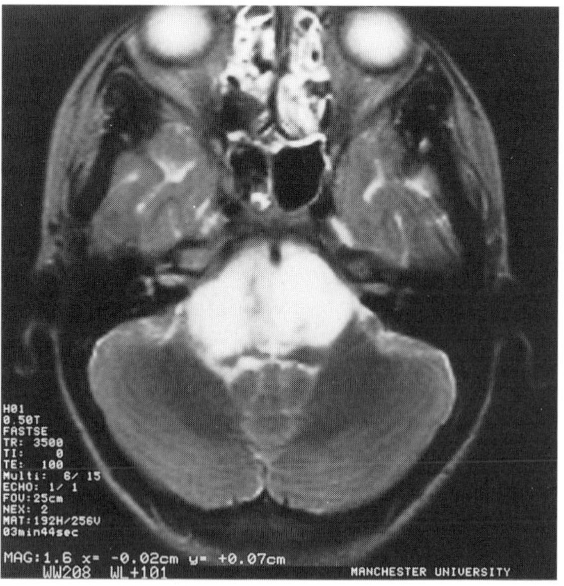


**Figure 10.8a** Transaxial $T_2$ weighted image showing high signal from a low-grade glioma (tumour)

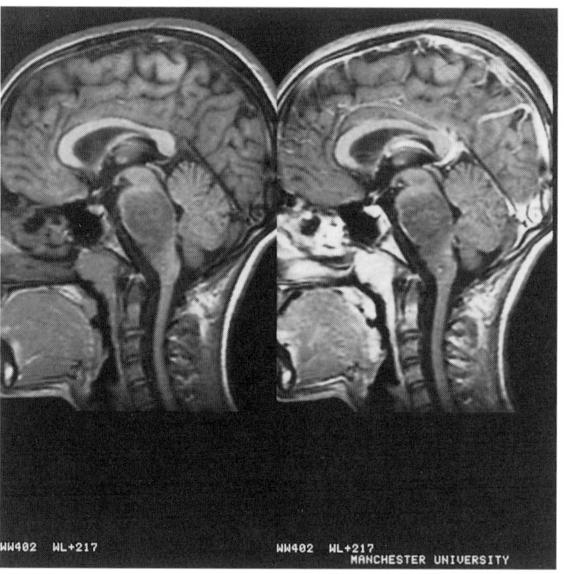


**Figure 10.8b** Pre- and post-contrast $T_1$ weighted images in the same patient as above – note lack of contrast enhancement in the tumour typical of low-grade gliomas

**Table 10.3 Imaging parameters**

| *Imaging plane* | *Imaging sequence* | *TR* | *TE* | *Field of view* (cm) | *No. of NEX* | *Slice width/ gap* (mm) | *Matrix (horizontal – vertical)* |
|---|---|---|---|---|---|---|---|
| Coronal or transaxial | Fast spin-echo $T_2$ weighted (echo train length –12) | 6000 | 102 | 25 | 2 | 5/1 | 192 × 256 |
| Transaxial or sagittal (pre- and post-contrast if needed) | Spin-echo $T_1$ weighted | 500 | 25 | 25 | 2 | 5/1 | 192 × 256/224 |
| 3D volume with flip angle 45° (pre- and post-contrast if needed) | SPGR | 50 | 12 | 25 | 1 | 1.25 (no gap) 35 slices | 192 × 256 |

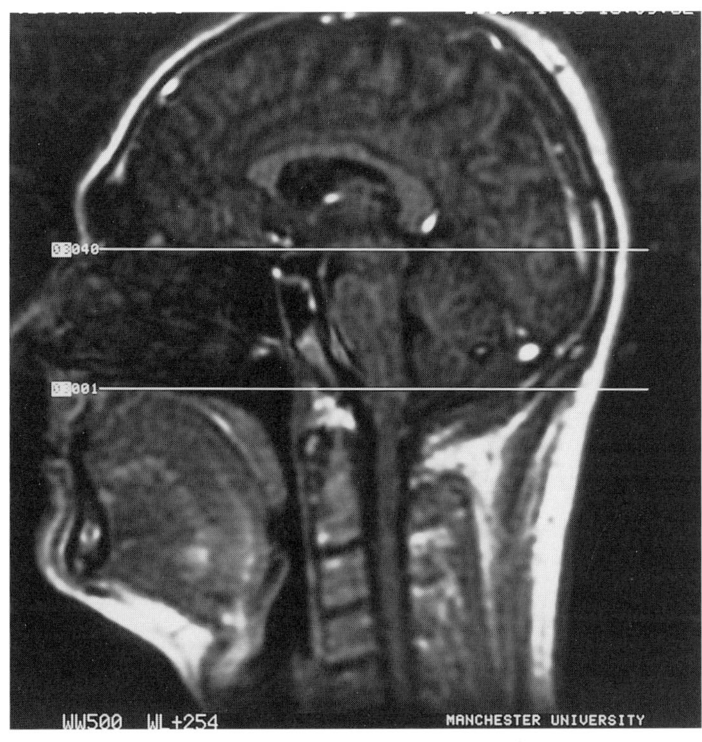


**Figure 10.9a** Sagittal localiser scan showing the position of a 3D data set

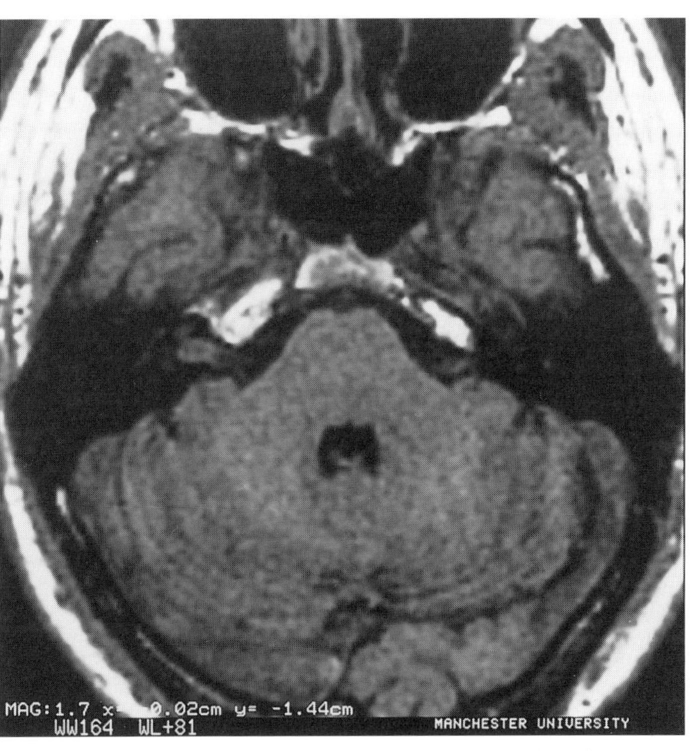


**Figure 10.9b** Transaxial $T_2$ weighted image showing the seventh and eighth cranial nerves

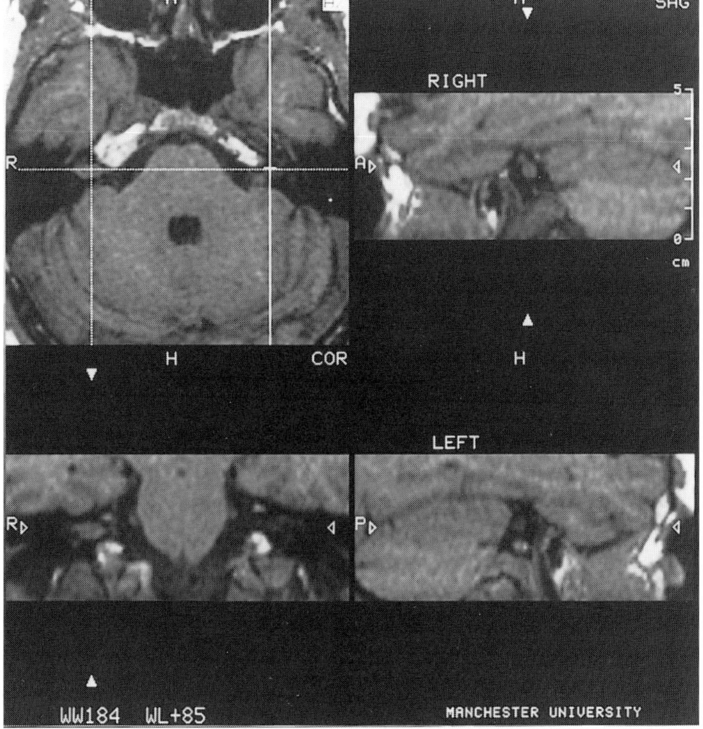


**Figure 10.9c** 3D image set showing the seventh and eighth cranial nerves in the various orthogonal planes

# 10 Brain

## Computed Tomography

### Standard brain protocol

In routine CT brain scanning, various transaxial scan planes are acceptable. The baseline from the external auditory meatus (EAM) to the superior orbital margin is often used to avoid unnecessary irradiation of the lens of the eye. The anthropological baseline can be chosen to produce sections in a similar anatomical plane to that used during stereotaxic surgery. This also demonstrates the posterior and middle cranial fossae.

General guidelines for the use of contrast enhancement in CT are widely accepted. In cases of atrophia, trauma, intracranial haemorrhage, stroke, hydrocephalus and some congenital abnormalities, contrast enhancement is not usually required to make a diagnosis. In lesions which either obstruct the blood–brain barrier (e.g. infective diseases and tumours) or are vascular in nature (e.g. aneurysm, arteriovenous malformations), pre- and post-contrast scans are desirable to increase diagnostic accuracy. Ideally, all initial scans should be clinically assessed before administrating a contrast medium.

#### Indications

The indications are similar to those listed for MRI scanning and include trauma, cerebrovascular accident and infection.

#### Position of patient and imaging modality

The patient lies supine on the scanner table, head resting in the head support and positioning is aided by alignment lights. The orbitomeatal baseline is positioned parallel to the transverse alignment and the median sagittal plane is perpendicular to the table and coincident with the sagittal alignment light. To ensure that the skull is symmetrically positioned, the external auditory meatuses must be equidistant from the skull support and the interorbital (interpupillary) line is parallel to the scan plane. The head is secured in position with the aid of Velcro straps. The patient is moved into the scanner and the table is raised to bring the scan reference point to the level of the EAM.

#### Imaging procedure

A lateral scan projection radiograph is obtained, starting 5 cm below and ending 12 cm above the baseline. From this image, 5 mm contiguous sections are prescribed from the foramen magnum, the superior border of the petrous bone, parallel to the orbitomeatal baseline. Further 10 mm contiguous sections are prescribed from the superior border of the petrous bone to the vertex. After review, sections may be repeated immediately after intravenous injection of a non-ionic contrast medium.

*Contrast medium and injection data*

| *Volume* | *Concentration* | *Flow rate* |
|---|---|---|
| 50–100 ml | 300–370 mgI/ml | Hand injection |

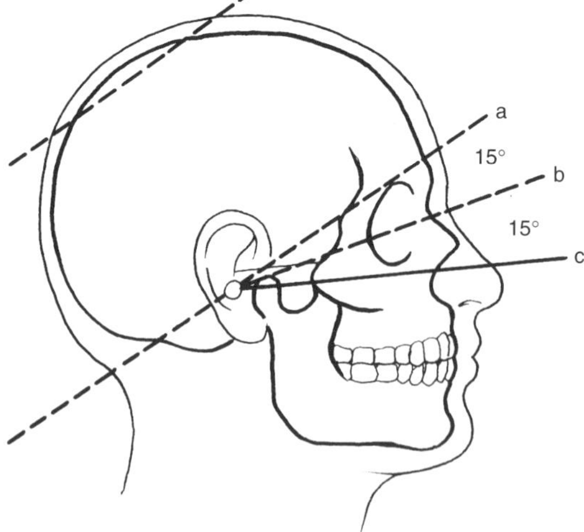


**Figure 10.10a** Lateral skull diagram showing different baselines: (a) EAM to superior orbital margin; (b) orbitomeatal (radiographic) baseline; (c) anthropological baseline

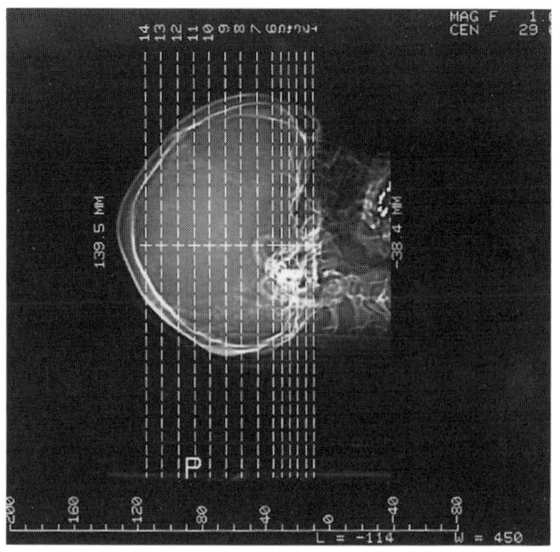

**Figure 10.10b** Lateral scan projection radiograph showing prescribed sections parallel to baseline (EAM to superior orbital margin)

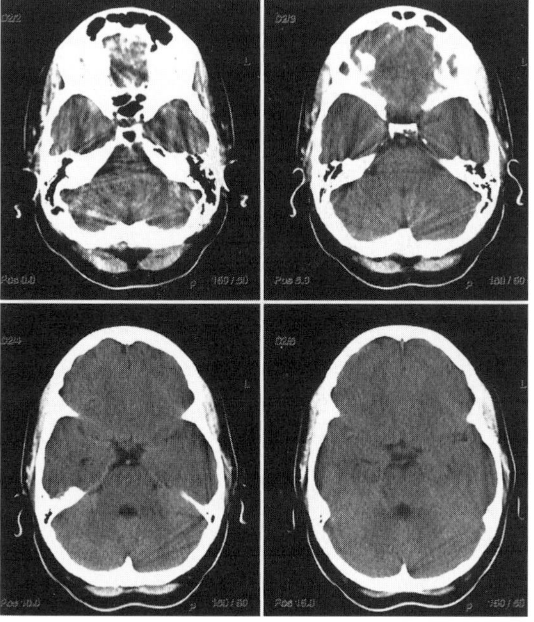

**Figure 10.10c** Initial images from a standard brain protocol

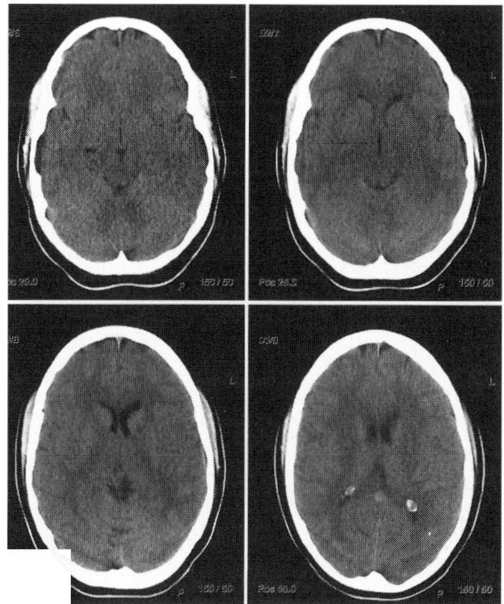

**Figure 10.11a** Further images from a standard brain protocol

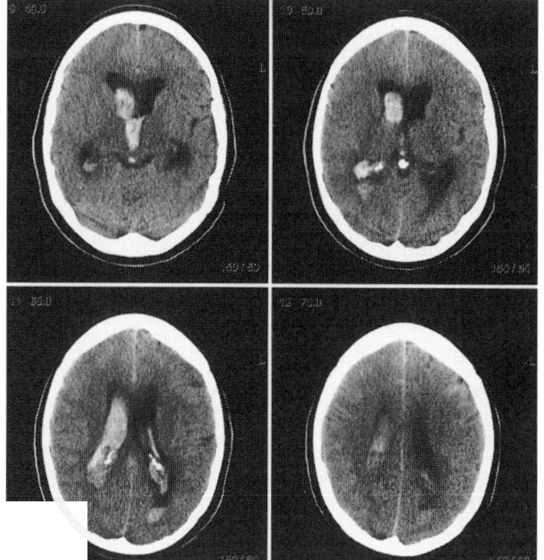

**Figure 10.11b** Example of subarachnoid haematoma

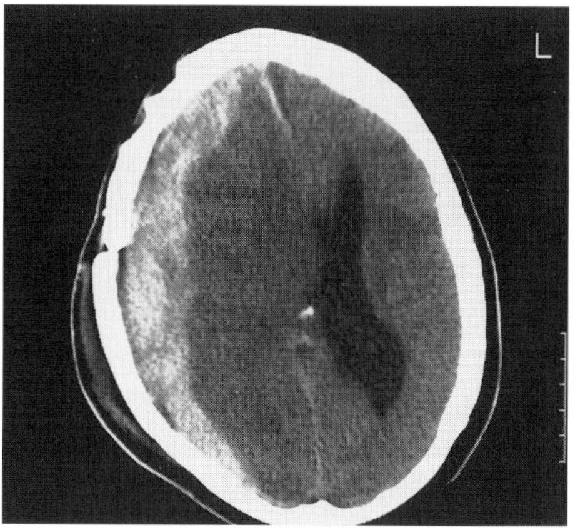


**Figure 10.11c** Example of subdural haematoma

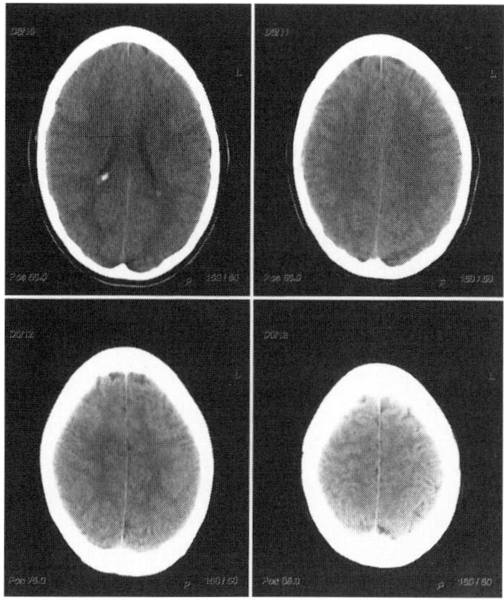

**Figure 10.11d** Final images from a standard brain protocol

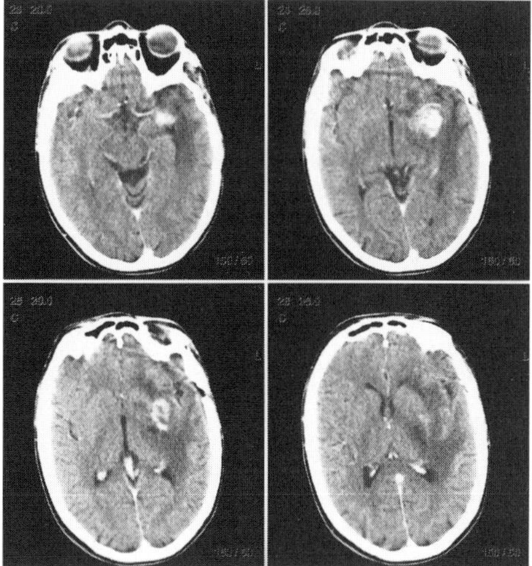

**Figure 10.11e** Selected sections demonstrating a contrast enhancing lesion and surrounding oedema in the left hemisphere

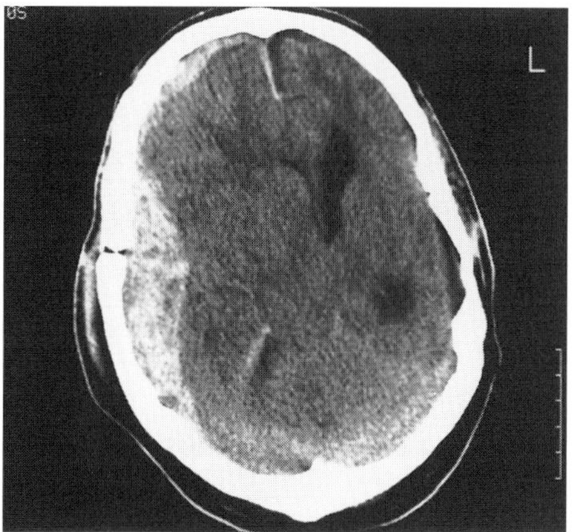


**Figure 10.11f** Example of extradural haematoma

## Posterior cranial fossa

In general CT images of this region are degraded by streak artefacts from surrounding air-filled bony structures. This can be reduced by decreasing the section width and increasing the number of sections acquired. CT is, however, the preferred modality for imaging bony abnormalities. The sections can be obtained in either the transaxial or coronal planes.

Transaxial imaging is more comfortable for the patient, with less risk of artefacts from movement or dental fillings.

Coronal imaging may be helpful in assessing abnormalities of the petrous bone. However, with the growth in MRI, this procedure is not routinely performed. The procedure, if required, is performed in a similar way to that described for the pituitary gland in Chapter 9.

A narrow section width (1.5–3 mm) is necessary, combined with a 'bone edge' algorithm. Images may be targeted either prospectively or retrospectively to produce large images of the affected area without a decrease in spatial resolution.

The digital data may be reformatted to produce images in different anatomical planes.

**Position of patient and imaging modality**

The position of the patient and imaging modality is the same as that described for the standard brain CT protocol.

**Imaging procedure**

A lateral scan projection radiograph is taken, starting 5 cm below and ending 10 cm above the scan reference point. If a soft tissue abnormality is suspected, 5 mm contiguous scans are prescribed, starting at the foramen magnum and ending just superior to the petrous bone, using a standard algorithm. After review, contrast enhanced scans are obtained for the area of the suspected abnormality.

Section width and table increment are reduced to 3 mm and again a standard algorithm is used.

If a bony abnormality is clinically suspected, 1.5 mm contiguous sections are prescribed through the petrous bone using a high resolution algorithm.

*Contrast medium and injection data*

| *Volume* | *Concentration* | *Flow rate* |
|---|---|---|
| 50–100 ml | 340–370 mgI/ml | Hand injection |

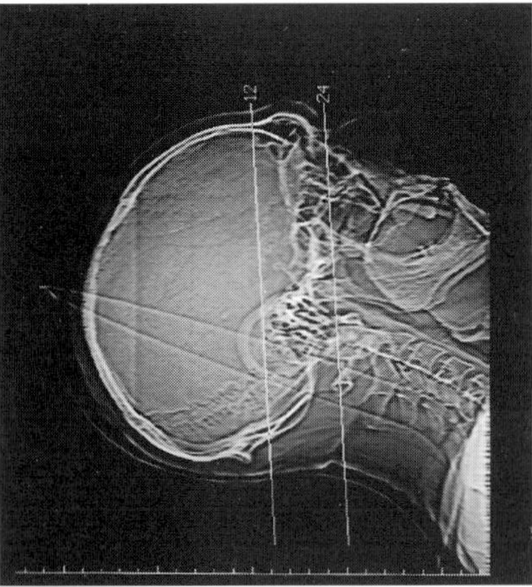


**Figure 10.12a** Scan projection radiograph showing start and end locations

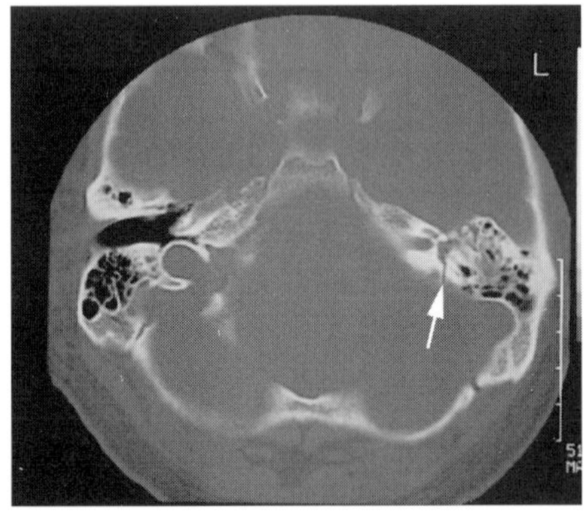


**Figure 10.12b** High-resolution reconstructed image using a bone algorithm, showing a fracture through the left petrous bone

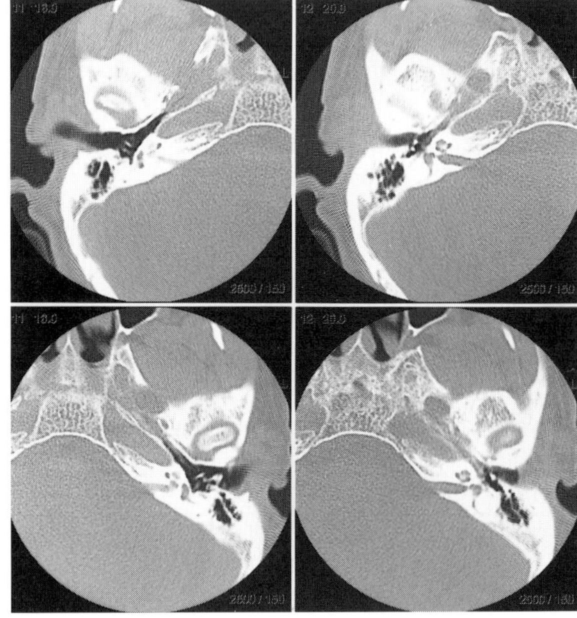

**Figure 10.12c** High-resolution transaxial sections through the right and left internal auditory meatuses showing the ear ossicles

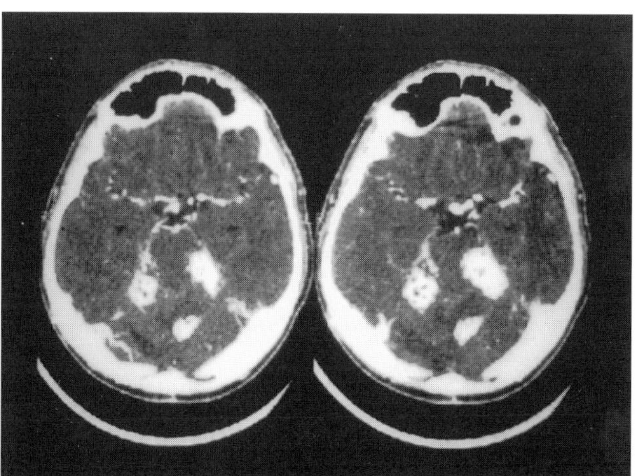

**Figure 10.13a** Post-contrast enhancement images showing bilateral acoustic neuromas

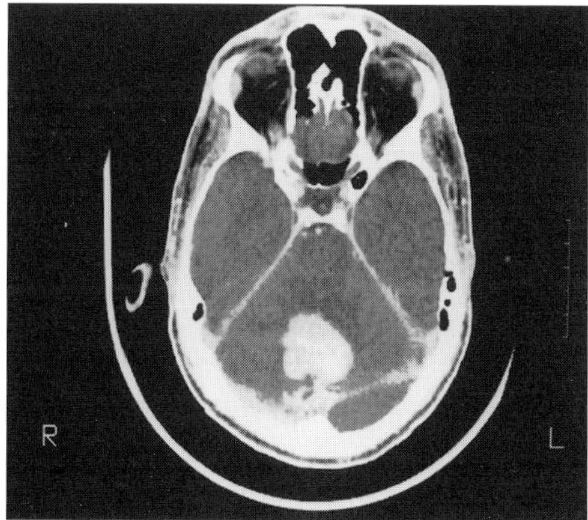


**Figure 10.13b** Post-contrast enhancement image showing a large tumour mass in the posterior fossa compressing the fourth ventricle

## Air meatography

This is undertaken if conventional CT is equivocal in clinically suspected tumours of the eighth cranial nerve and MR is unavailable or contra-indicated.

*Position of patient and imaging modality*

The patient lies in the lateral decubitus position with the affected side uppermost, head supported in the head rest or on support pads. The head is adjusted into the true lateral position, with the medial sagittal plane parallel to the table top. The table is adjusted until the coronal alignment light is in the midline of the patient and the scan reference point is at the level of the external auditory meatus.

*Imaging procedure*

In this position 2–3 ml of air is injected via lumbar puncture into the subarachnoid space. A lateral scan projection radiograph is taken from 5 cm below to 10 cm above the scan reference point. From this image, 1.5 mm contiguous sections, using a standard algorithm, are prescribed to the internal auditory meatus and cerebellopontine angle. If a tumour is present, air will be unable to pass into the meatus.

*Contrast medium and injection data*

| *Volume* | *Concentration* | *Flow rate* |
|---|---|---|
| 2–3 ml | Air | Lumbar puncture |

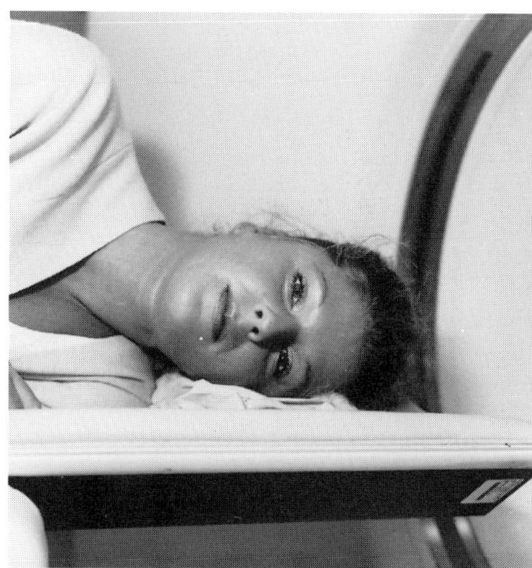

**Figure 10.13c** Patient in position for air meatography

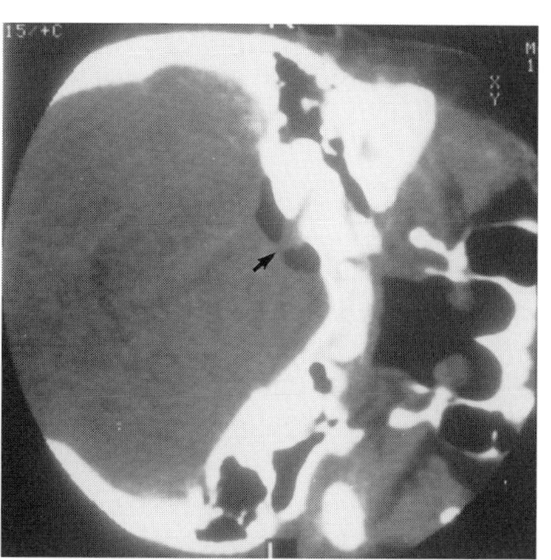

**Figure 10.13d** Transaxial CT image showing air surrounding small acoustic lesion

# 10 Brain

## Radionuclide Imaging

### Conventional procedure

Radionuclide imaging is performed either by utilising the breakdown of the blood–brain barrier or an intact blood–brain barrier.

The assessment of intracerebral disease, using a standard brain protocol, is based on the fact that any breakdown in the blood–brain barrier will allow the passage of a radiopharmaceutical previously injected into the blood stream to cross into the affected brain. This procedure, however, has been superseded by MRI and CT which are now used primarily to investigate intracerebral disease. When employed it also facilitates assessment of carotid and cerebral blood flow. To assess the vascular supply, a dynamic series of images are acquired immediately following a bolus intravenous injection of the radiopharmaceutical, followed by a further series of static images acquired 1–2 h post-injection, to image abnormalities associated with the breakdown of the blood–brain barrier. Diethylene triamine penta-acetic acid (DTPA) labelled with $^{99m}$Tc is selected.

### Corebral blood flow

Radionuclide imaging is used in the assessment of regional cerebral blood flow by employing a radiopharmaceutical which is capable of crossing the intact blood–brain barrier. The pattern of the isotope distribution associated with this mechanism in both normal and abnormal brain tissue is therefore assessed.

An amine compound such as hexamethylproplene-amine-oxime (HM-PAO) labelled with $^{99m}$Tc is selected. These lipophilic compounds cross the blood–brain barrier and are extracted into the grey and white matter in proportion to the blood flow, and are almost all extracted on the first pass through the cerebral circulation following injection. Image acquisition is normally planned 15–30 min after intravenous injection employing SPECT. If required, dynamic images can be acquired showing blood flowing in the two carotid arteries in a similar way to the standard brain protocol. However, because the uptake of the radiopharmaceutical in the brain, the superior sagittal sinus and jugular veins are not visualised.

#### Indications

Dementia and Alzheimer's disease. Chronic cerebrovascular disease, epilepsy and Huntingdon's disease.

#### Position of patient and imaging modality

The patient lies supine on the imaging couch, using a radiolucent head support extension which is clipped onto the table end. The patient's head is adjusted so that the sagittal plane is perpendicular to the imaging couch and the head centralised relative to the isocentre of the circular movement. The gamma camera is initially positioned parallel to the imaging couch, and above the patient's head.

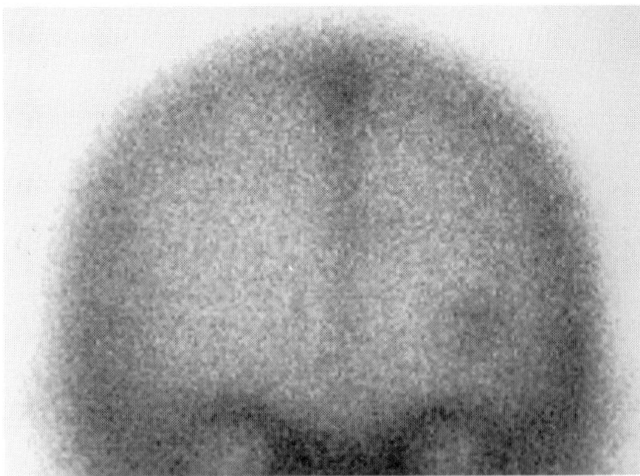

**Figure 10.14a** Standard AP brain protocol image showing abnormal uptake consistent with a lesion affecting the blood–brain barrier

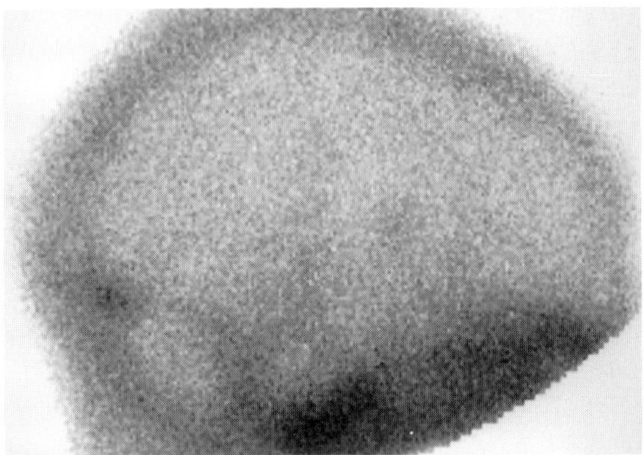

**Figure 10.14b** Standard lateral brain protocol image again showing abnormal uptake

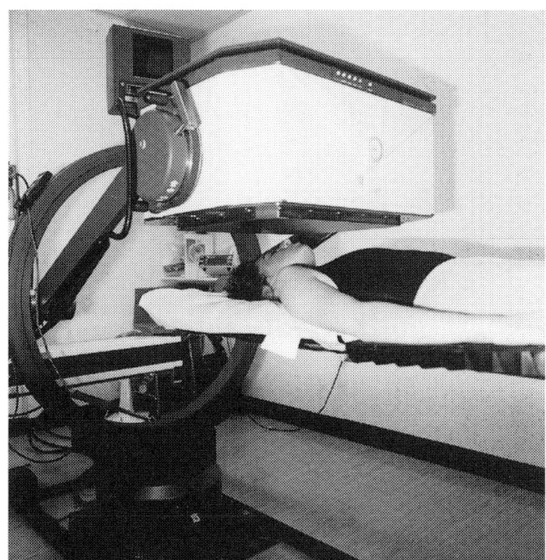

**Figure 10.15a** SPECT imaging using a single gamma camera

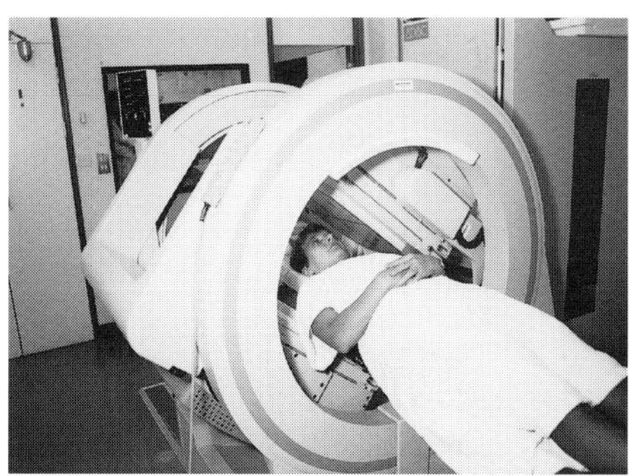

**Figure 10.15b** SPECT imaging using a twin-headed gamma camera

### Imaging procedure

A high-resolution collimator is preferred, but this will increase imaging time, and if the patient's condition is such that they cannot remain still for the procedure, a general-purpose collimator is selected. Using a single gamma camera, a 360° circular tomogram is selected. From the anterior start position an image acquisition protocol is selected which rotates the camera for a total of 64 individually staged view positions. Image acquisition time is set at 30 s per view, with the total procedure lasting 32 min.

For some patients this period is too extensive to maintain a fixed and motion-free position. To overcome this difficulty a dedicated brain SPECT imaging system incorporating three camera units is available in some centres which reduces acquisition time to a third, making this system more suitable for sick and confused patients. Alternatively, a twin camera unit may be employed to reduce acquisition time.

### Image analysis

Following data acquisition, a series of reconstructed images of the brain using filtered back-projection techniques are employed for subjective assessment on the colour monitor.

Depending on the computer software, simultaneous display of transaxial, sagittal and coronal sections are available on the monitor for a preselected area of the brain (see Plates 14–16). Abnormal differences in uptake of the radiopharmaceutical can be assessed in terms of lower or higher uptake than normal. Ischaemic cortex is characterised by under-perfusion, while certain tumours and cerebral haemorrhage show no uptake. In cases of epilepsy, during the ictal phase epileptogenic centres can be demonstrated as areas of increased uptake.

*Imaging and radiopharmaceutical parameters*

| *Type* | *Administered activity* | *Principal energy* |
|---|---|---|
| $^{99m}$Tc HM-PAO | 500 MBq | 140 keV |
| *Window width* | *Acquisition counts/time* | |
| 20% | 64 views at 30 s per view | |

# 10 Brain

## Ultrasound

Ultrasound examination of the brain is only possible in infants prior to closure of the anterior fontanelle. It is non-invasive, causes minimal disturbance to the baby, and is cheap and portable compared with other means of brain imaging. It is usually performed on neonates who are at high risk, e.g. under 32 weeks' gestation, low birth weight, problems at delivery or with respiratory distress.

As these babies are most likely to be nursed on a neonatal unit, a strict protocol should be set, limiting the scan time to ensure the baby is not unnecessarily stressed and to minimise the risk of cross-infection. If feasible, a dedicated ultrasound unit should be housed in the ward. This should be cleansed and tested frequently as part of a quality assurance programme. Care must be taken to use the correct electrical sockets. Other apparatus must never be switched off without the permission of the nursing/medical staff. If the baby is on a life support system, again medical advice must be sought before moving the equipment/monitors. The operator must wash his/her hands thoroughly before and after contact with the infant and the transducer cleansed with an alcohol swab immediately before and after use.

Images are routinely obtained in the coronal and sagittal planes using a two-dimensional real-time sector scanner with a 5–7.5 MHz transducer. The anterior fontanelle is used as an acoustic window for the coronal and sagittal scans. Additionally, transaxial scans are useful for evaluating and measuring enlarged ventricles in cases of gross hydrocephalus. Transaxial images are obtained through the temporoparietal bone.

### Indications

Congenital abnormalities, hydrocephalus, intracranial haemorrhage, periventricular haemorrhage, ischaemic cerebral lesions and intracranial cysts.

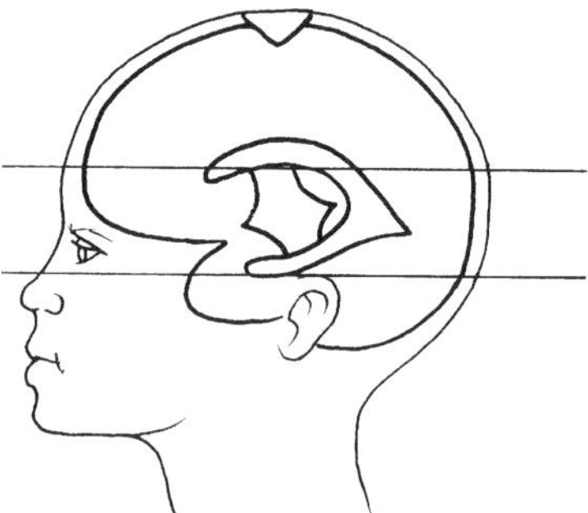

**Figure 10.16a** Schematic diagram of lateral skull showing defined area for transaxial scanning

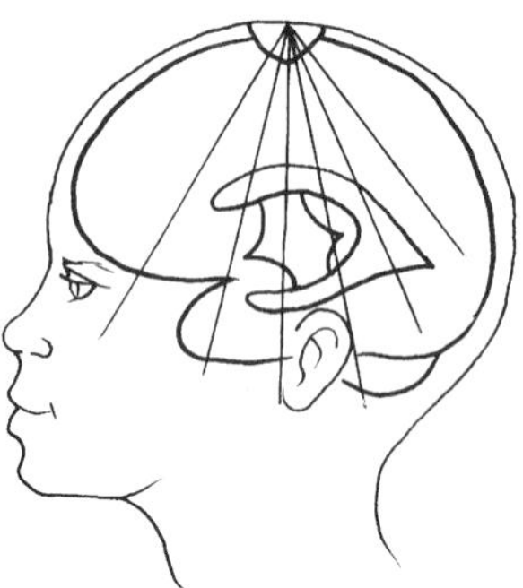

**Figure 10.16b** Schematic diagram of lateral skull showing range of transducer angulations for coronal plane imaging

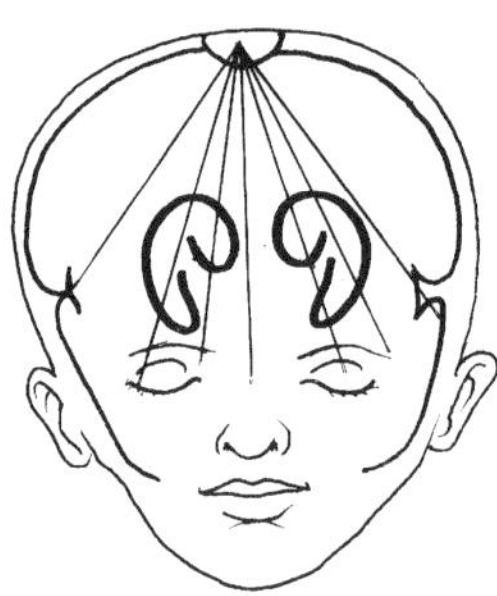

**Figure 10.16c** Schematic diagram of AP skull showing range of transducer angulations for sagittal and parasagittal plane imaging

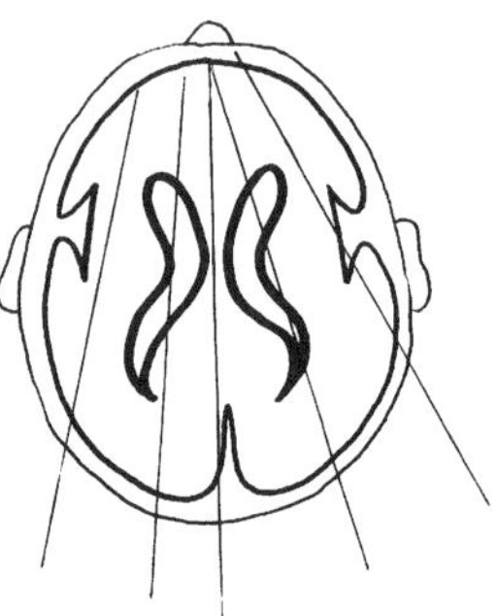

**Figure 10.16d** Schematic diagram of axial skull showing range of transducer angulations for sagittal and parasagittal plane imaging

## Imaging procedure

After applying an ultrasound coupling gel, the transducer is placed gently on the anterior fontanelle along the coronal axis and angled sequentially anteriorly and posteriorly to obtain a series of coronal images of the brain. The series must contain images of the frontal lobes, frontal horns, the foramen of Monro and the third ventricle, the bodies of the lateral ventricle, trigone of the third ventricles and the occipital lobes.

The transducer is now rotated 90° into the sagittal plane. The midline sagittal section is acquired, showing the corpus callosum, third and fourth ventricles and the cerebellar vermis. Parasagittal images of each hemisphere are obtained by angling the transducer to the left and right towards the Sylvian fissures. These images demonstrate the lateral ventricles and brain parenchyma.

For transaxial imaging, the transducer is placed against the temporoparietal bone to acquire two sections in the transaxial plane, one at the level of the cerebral peduncles, the second showing the lateral ventricles.

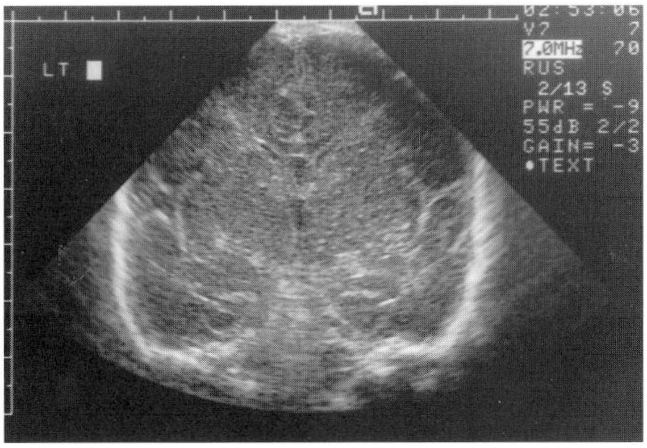

**Figure 10.17a** Mid-coronal image showing the third ventricle

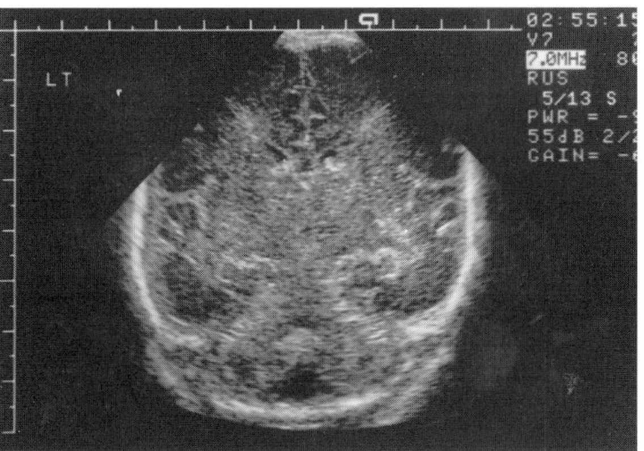

**Figure 10.17b** Coronal image through the posterior fossa showing the fourth ventricle

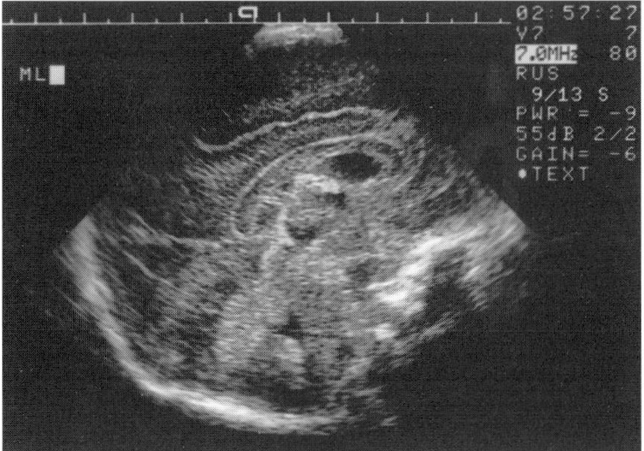

**Figure 10.17c** Midline sagittal image showing the corpus callosum and the fourth ventricle

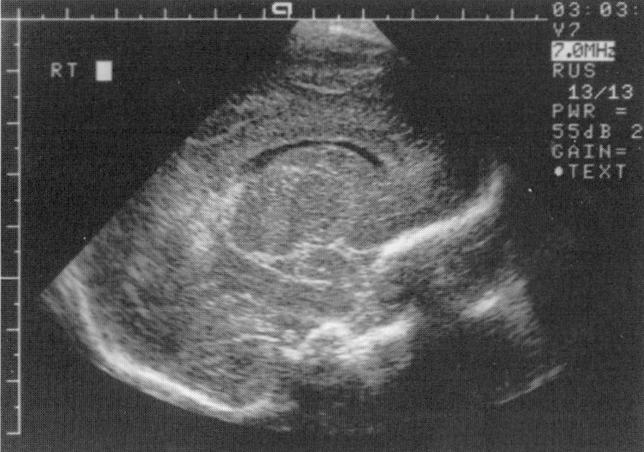

**Figure 10.17d** Right parasagittal image showing lateral ventricle and choroid plexus

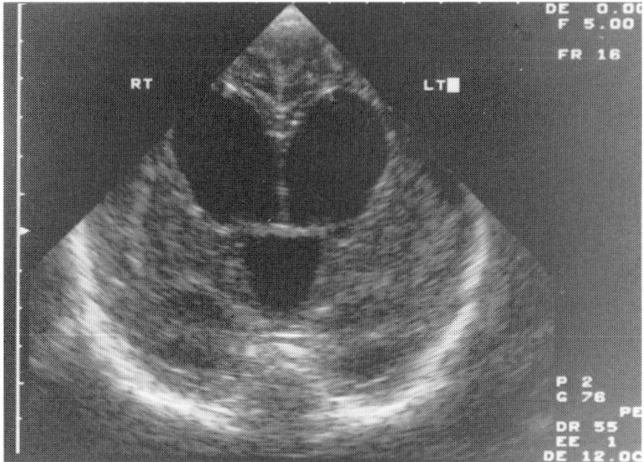

**Figure 10.17e** Coronal image showing hydrocephalus

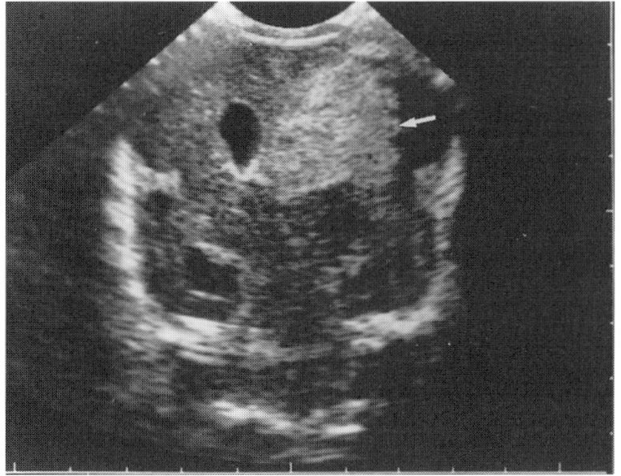

**Figure 10.17f** Coronal image showing intraventricular haemorrhage

## Angiography

Angiography may be performed using either intravascular contrast media or by employing MRI.

Cerebral angiography demonstrates the cerebral blood vessels by opacifying them with a suitable contrast agent. Intra-arterial angiography is normally carried out following selective placement of an angiographic catheter in either a carotid or vertebral artery, following catheterisation of a femoral artery using the Seldinger method.

A contrast injector may be employed which enables a bolus of contrast to be injected in a controlled and repeatable fashion. Hand injection is also acceptable, as sufficient pressure can be applied to overcome the patient's blood supply. However, close co-operation with the radiologist is necessary to obtain optimal timing between injection and the first exposure.

Direct percutaneous puncture of the carotid arteries, below the bifurcation of external and internal carotid artery in the neck, may be used when catheterisation of the arteries is unsuccessful. The vertebral arteries are difficult to puncture directly and such a procedure is normally only carried out using a general anaesthetic due to the discomfort to the patient.

The advent of digital image subtraction facilities has allowed intravenous angiography (IVDSA) to be undertaken using a peripheral vein site. However, the spatial resolution of IVDSA has proved to be inadequate for most conditions and this technique is now used mainly as a screening tool for cerebral vascular arteriosclerosis and to assess aneurysmal clips.

A variety of interventional procedures may be carried out in specialist centres. These include: embolisation of tumours, dilatation of arteries and administration of cytotoxic drugs used in the treatment of tumours and the occlusion of anteriovenous malformations by liquid polymerising agents.

Specialised isocentric equipment, with image intensification and the facility to record images either digitally or by automatic film changer, is necessary. Digital image subtraction is used to aid visualisation of small vessels free from overlying bony structures.

Conventional radiographic subtraction is employed when DSA is unavailable.

Careful use of immobilisation bands together with beam collimation will aid in the production of high-quality images. Magnification techniques may also be employed to demonstrate small details. A small legend should be included on all imaging projections to identify which side of the head is being examined.

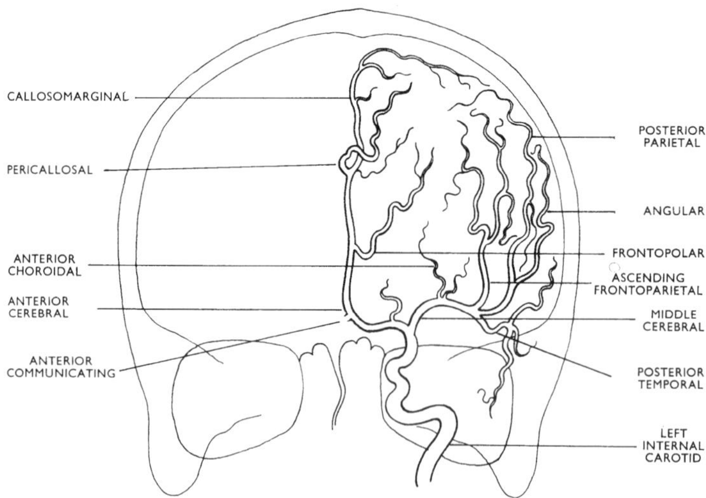


**Figure 10.18a** Internal carotid artery circulation – anterior aspect

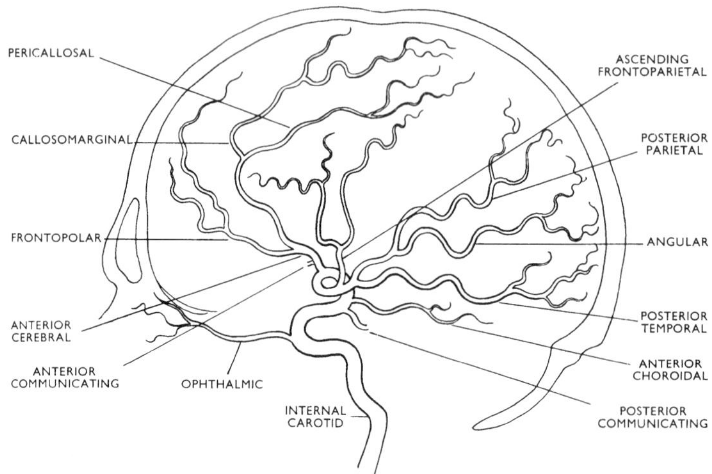


**Figure 10.18b** Internal carotid artery circulation – lateral aspect

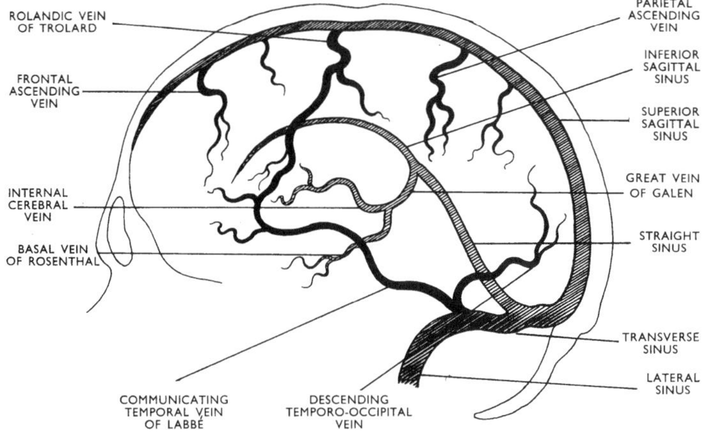


**Figure 10.19a** Venous drainage of brain – lateral aspect

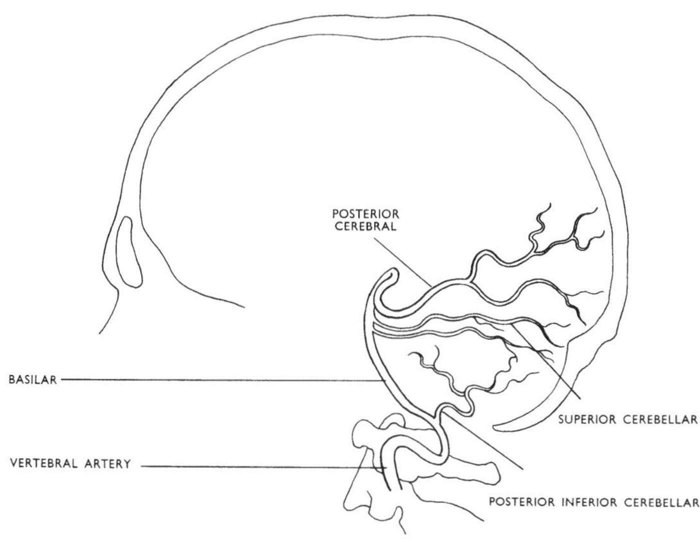


**Figure 10.19b** Vertebral artery circulation – lateral aspect

## Indications

This examination is undertaken to demonstrate the blood supply to a tumour and its relationship to surrounding tissues, to confirm the presence of an aneurysm, showing its position and size, to diagnose arteriosclerosis and to confirm the location of an angioma or arteriovenous malformation with subsequent treatment which may include embolisation.

## Contraindications

The onset of weakness in the arm or leg of one side of the body, suggesting that the arteries may have gone into spasm and blood pressure has dropped.

## Recommended projections

The projections and procedures for cerebral angiography will vary from department to department, depending on the radiologist's preference and the clinical condition of the patient.

Projections will normally include a standard routine which will be supplemented by additional projections as and when necessary to demonstrate the full extent of any disease process. It must be emphasised that patients are not stereotyped; therefore, projection angulation, suggested contrast data and exposure sequences given can vary from patient to patient and are meant as a general guide.

- **Carotid angiography**
  *Standard projections*
  Occipitofrontal 15° cephalad lateral.

  *Supplementary projections*
  Anterior oblique (cephalad angulation)
  Occipitofrontal 20° caudad
  Anterior oblique (caudad angulation)
  Submentovertical (basal)
  Occipitofrontal (per orbital)
  Anterior oblique (per orbital oblique)

- **Vertebral angiography**
  *Standard projections*
  Occipitofrontal 30° cephalad
  Lateral (collimated)

  *Supplementary projections*
  Anterior oblique (cephalad angulation)
  Submentovertical (basal)

# 10 Carotid vessels

## Angiography

### Occipitofrontal 15° cephalad

This projection demonstrates the anterior and middle cerebral arteries and the deep cerebral veins. Angulation of the beam is necessary to ensure that the orbits and petrous ridges are superimposed, leaving the cranial vessels clear of overlying structures.

*Position of patient and imaging modality*

The patient is supine, with the head raised on a non-opaque pad. The head is positioned to bring both the median sagittal and anthropological planes at right angles to the imaging couch, with the external auditory meatuses equidistant from the couch top. The head is immobilised with a head binder. The automatic film changer or image intensifier is initially positioned above the patient's head and parallel to the imaging couch. The head is also centred in respect to the image receptor selected.

*Direction and centring of the X-ray beam*

The central ray is angled cranially so that it makes an angle of 15° to the anthropological plane, with the middle of the image receptor positioned approximately 4 cm above the glabella. The image receptor is adjusted into its final position after reference to the fluoroscopic image.

*Imaging procedure*

An image acquisition protocol is selected to ensure that the arterial, capillary and venous circulation is demonstrated. A 0.5 s inject delay allows a mask film to be taken.

*Imaging parameters*

| *Image/s* | *Run time* | *Total images* |
|---|---|---|
| 2 | 2 s | 4 |
| 1 | 6 s | 6 |

*Contrast medium and injector data*

**Common carotid**

| *Volume* | *Concentration* | *Flow rate* |
|---|---|---|
| 8 ml | 300 mgI/ml | Hand injection |

**Selective carotid**

| *Volume* | *Concentration* | *Flow rate* |
|---|---|---|
| 6 ml | 300 mgI/ml | Hand injection |

In DSA, the concentration may be reduced

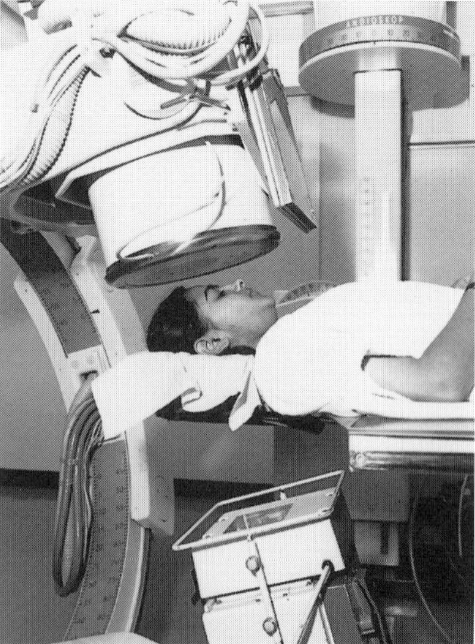

**Figure 10.20a** Patient and equipment

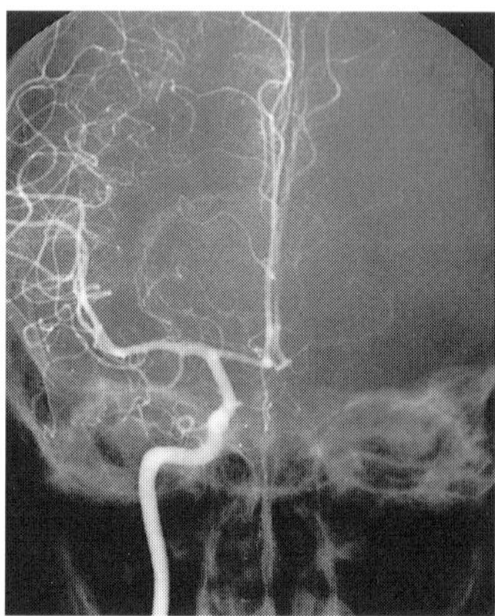

**Figure 10.20b** Unsubtracted image showing filling of arteries and bony landmarks

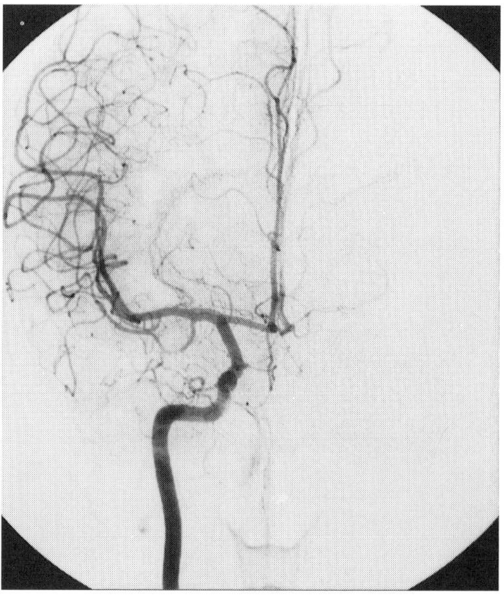

**Figure 10.20c** Subtracted image of vessels shown in (b)

Figure 10.21a Patient and equipment

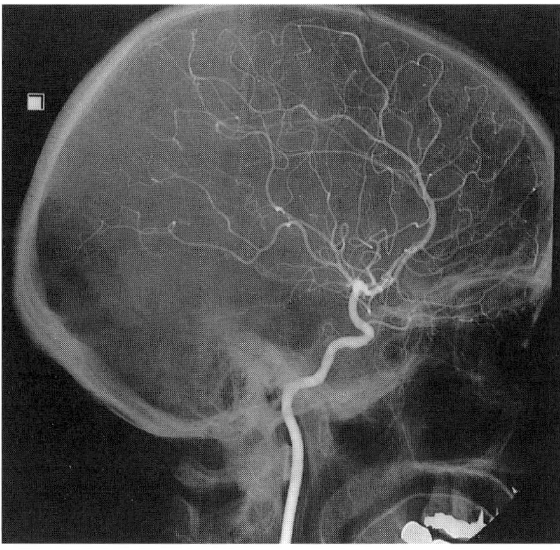

Figure 10.21b Unsubtracted image showing filling of arteries and bony landmarks

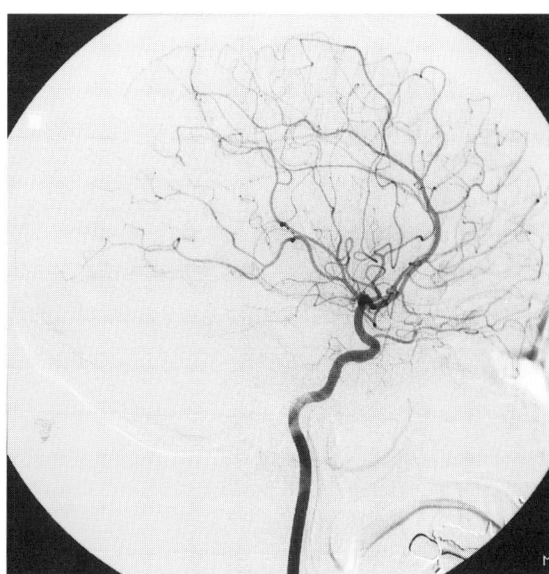

Figure 10.21c Subtracted image of vessels shown in (b)

## Lateral

This projection demonstrates the entire intracranial vascular network supplied by the carotid artery.

*Position of patient and imaging modality*
The position is supine, with the head raised to rest on a non-opaque pad. The head is positioned to bring both the median sagittal and anthropological planes at right angles to the imaging couch, ensuring that the external auditory meatuses are equidistant from the couch top. The head is immobilised in this position. The automatic film changer or image intensifier is then positioned against the lateral side of the head under investigation so that it is parallel to the median sagittal plane and at right angles to the interpupillary line.

*Direction and centring of the X-ray beam*
The horizontal central ray is directed parallel to the interorbital line so that it is at right angles to the median sagittal plane and the image receptor and centred to a point 2 cm anterior and superior to the external auditory meatus.

*Imaging procedure*
An image acquisition protocol is selected to ensure that the arterial, capillary and venous circulation is demonstrated. A 0.5 s inject delay allows a mask film to be taken.

*Imaging parameters*

| *Image/s* | *Run time* | *Total images* |
|---|---|---|
| 2 | 2 s | 4 |
| 1 | 6 s | 6 |

*Contrast medium and injector data*

**Common carotid**

| *Volume* | *Concentration* | *Flow rate* |
|---|---|---|
| 8 ml | 300 mgI/ml | Hand injection |

**Selective carotid**

| *Volume* | *Concentration* | *Flow rate* |
|---|---|---|
| 6 ml | 300 mgI/ml | Hand injection |

In DSA, the concentration may be reduced

# 10 Carotid vessels

## Angiography

### Anterior oblique (cephalad angulation)

This projection is employed to demonstrate the anterior and middle cerebral arteries as well as showing small aneurysms on the anterior and posterior communicating arteries.

*Position of patient and imaging modality*

The patient is supine, with the head raised on a non-opaque pad. The head is positioned to bring both the median sagittal and anthropological planes at right angles to the imaging couch ensuring that the external auditory meatuses are equidistant from the couch top. The head is immobilised in this position. The central ray is first angled cranially 25° and then 15–20° away from the side being injected with contrast. The face of the image receptor is then brought close to the orbit of the side being examined so that its centre is positioned approximately 3 cm above the middle of the supraorbital margin. The image receptor may be adjusted into its final position after reference to the fluoroscopic image.

*Imaging procedure*

An image acquisition protocol is selected to ensure that the arterial, capillary and venous circulation is demonstrated. A 0.5 s inject delay allows a mask film to be taken.

*Imaging parameters*

| *Image/s* | *Run time* | *Flow rate* |
|---|---|---|
| 2 | 2 s | 4 |
| 1 | 6 s | 6 |

*Contrast medium and injector data*

| *Volume* | *Concentration* | *Flow rate* |
|---|---|---|
| 8 ml | 300 mgI/ml | Hand injection |

In DSA, the concentration may be reduced

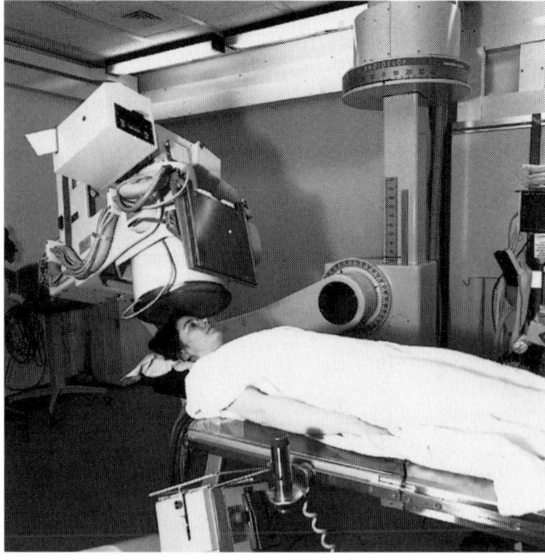

**Figure 10.22a** Patient and equipment

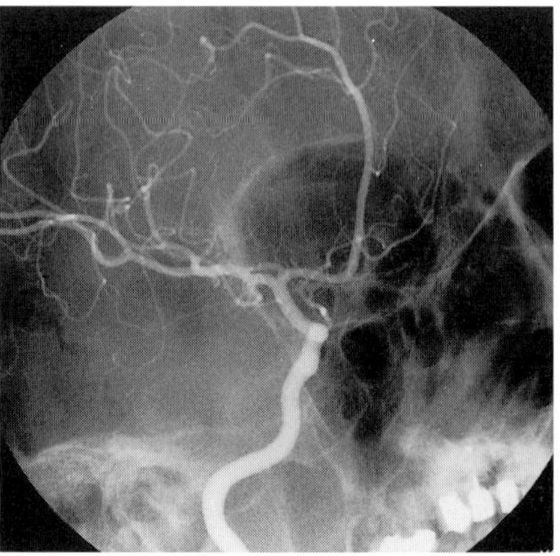

**Figure 10.22b** Unsubtracted image showing filling of arteries and bony landmarks

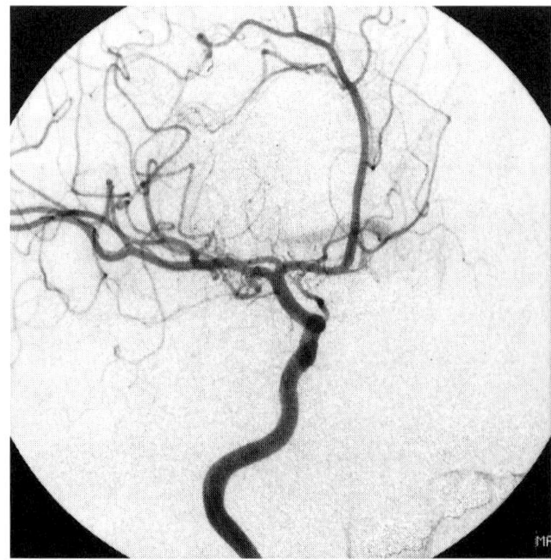

**Figure 10.22c** Subtracted image of vessels shown in (b)

## Supplementary projections and embolisation procedures

Additional supplementary projections may be employed in order to locate the precise position on an aneurysm or to reveal the neck of an aneurysm which will be clipped off during surgery or obliterated using an embolisation technique.

Additional projections include:

- occipitofrontal 20° caudad
- anterior oblique (caudad angulation).

The exact degree of rotation of the X-ray tube will be determined by fluoroscopy.

For embolisation of a cerebral artery, using special coils to occlude the blood supply to a cerebral aneurysm, routine angiography projections are performed initially and then at various stages throughout the procedure to monitor vessel occlusion (see page 310 for further information).

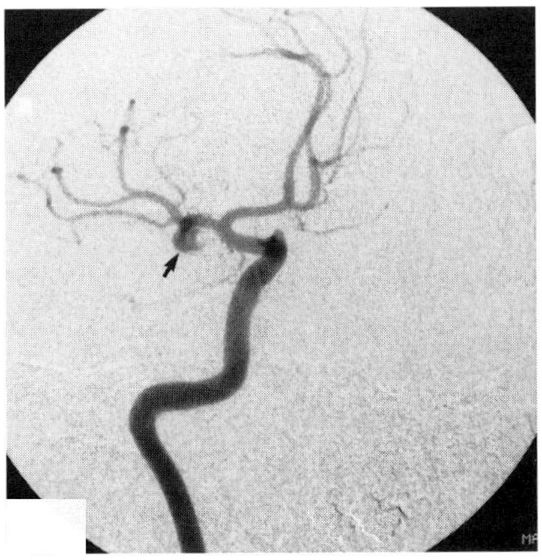

(a)

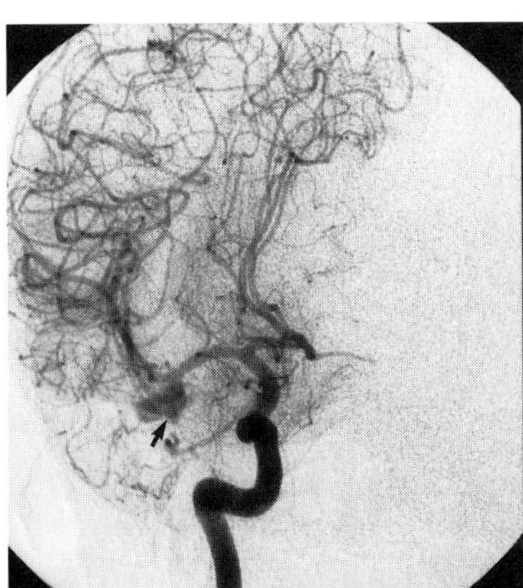

(b)

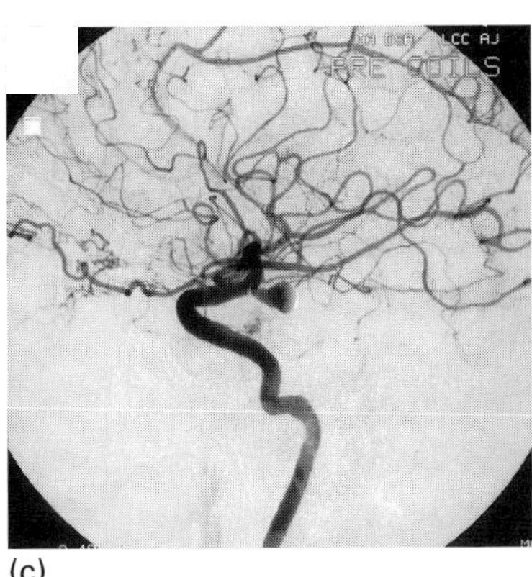

(c)

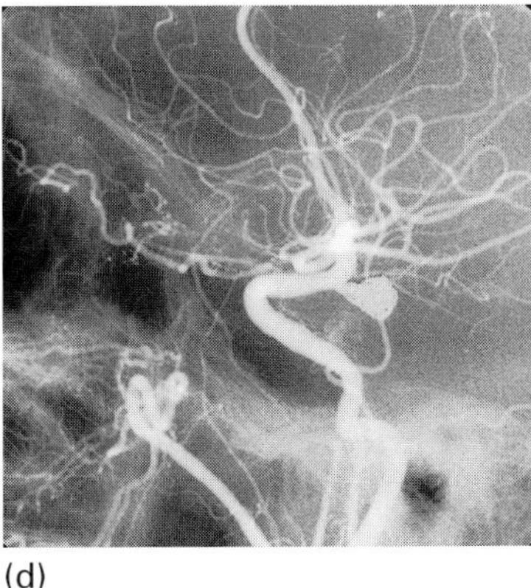

(d)

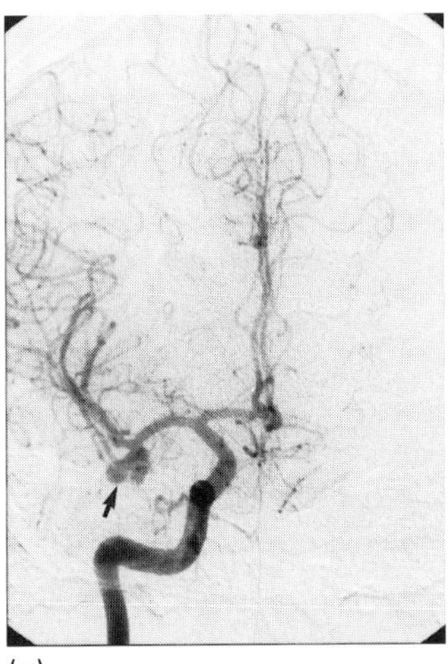

(e)

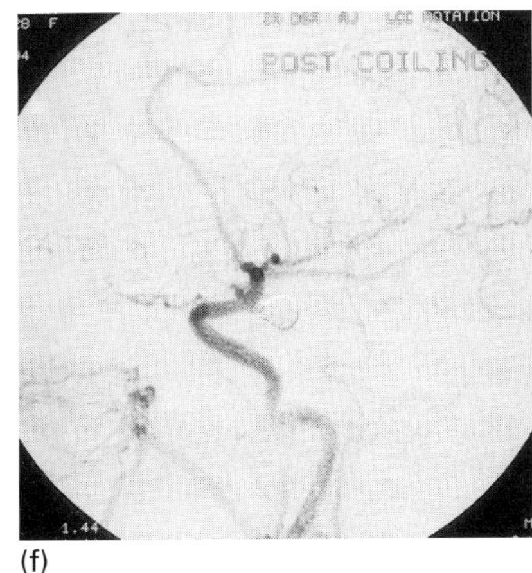


(f)

**Figure 10.23** (a) Standard anterior oblique showing middle cerebral aneurysm; (b) modified anterior oblique (20° × 20°) subtracted image showing neck of an aneurysm; (c,d,f) embolisation procedure showing (c) aneurysm pre-embolisation, (d) image during the procedure, and (f) post-coil embolisation showing occlusion of the aneurysm; (e) occipitofrontal 20° caudad subtracted image showing aneurysm seen in (b)

# 10 Vertebral vessels

## Angiography

### Occipitofrontal 30° cephalad

This projection demonstrates the vertebral arteries and the basilar artery, together with the posterior cerebral arteries and the corresponding branches of the basilar artery. The procedure normally involves catheterisation of one vertebral artery only to visualise arteries on both sides of the head. Occasionally, catheterisation of the opposite vertebral artery is required when the posterior inferior cerebellar artery of that side is not demonstrated on the first injection.

*Position of patient and imaging modality*

The patient is supine, with the head raised on a non-opaque pad so that the median sagittal and anthropological planes are at right angles to the imaging couch. The external auditory meatuses should be equidistant from the couch top. The head is immobilised. Initially, the automatic film changer or image intensifier is positioned above the patient's head and parallel to the imaging couch, with the head centred in respect to the image receptor selected.

*Direction and centring of the X-ray beam*

The central ray is angled cranially so that it makes an angle of 30° to the anthropological plane and positioned so that the centre of the image receptor is opposite a point 6 cm above the glabella in the midline.

*Imaging procedure*

An image acquisition protocol is selected to ensure that the arterial, capillary and venous circulation is demonstrated. A 0.5 s inject delay allows a mask film to be taken.

*Imaging parameters*

| *Image/s* | *Run time* | *Total images* |
|---|---|---|
| 2 | 2 s | 4 |
| 1 | 6 s | 6 |

*Contrast medium and injector data*

| *Volume* | *Concentration* | *Flow rate* |
|---|---|---|
| 4–5 ml | 300 mgI/ml | Hand injection |

In DSA, the concentration may be reduced

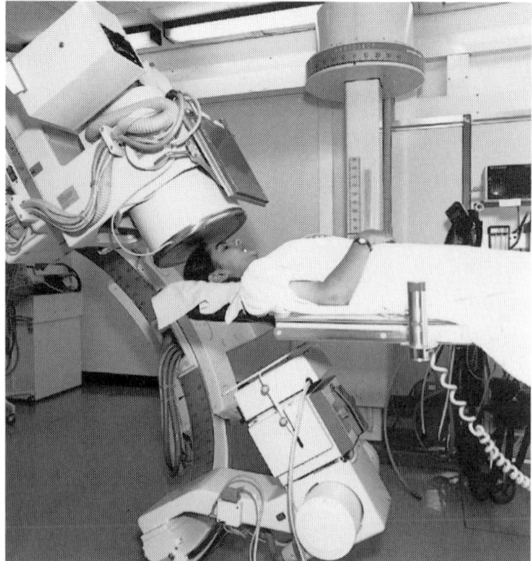

**Figure 10.24a** Patient and equipment

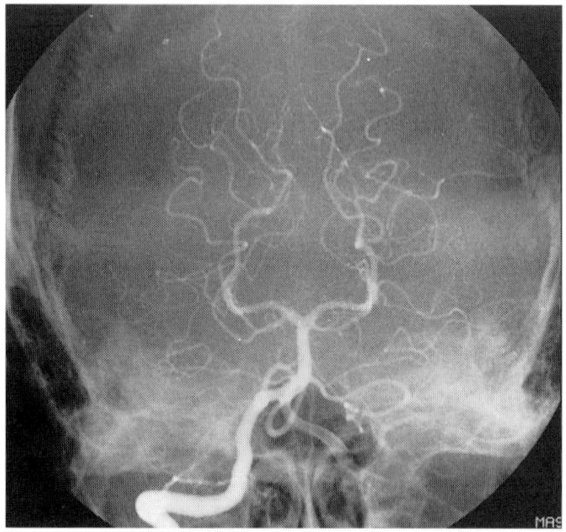

**Figure 10.24b** Unsubtracted image showing filling of arteries and bony landmarks

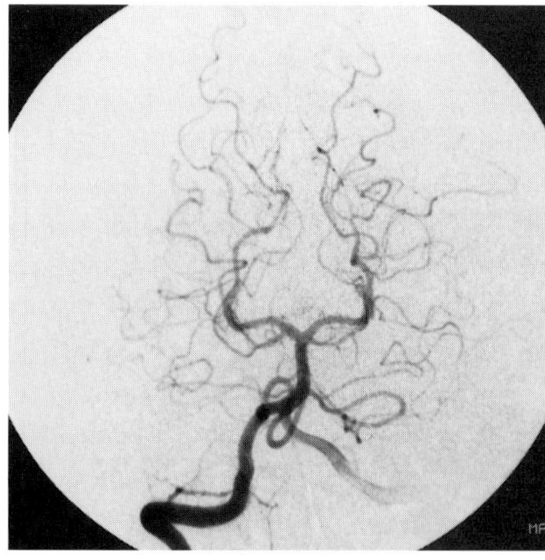

**Figure 10.24c** Subtracted image of vessels shown in (b)

Figure 10.25a Patient and equipment

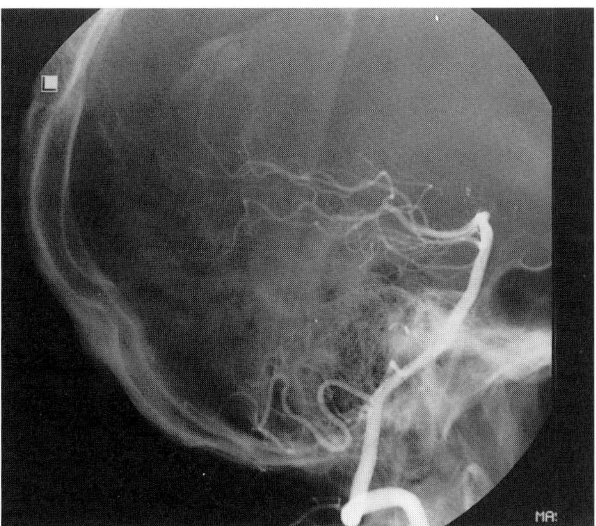

Figure 10.25b Unsubtracted image showing filling of arteries and bony landmarks

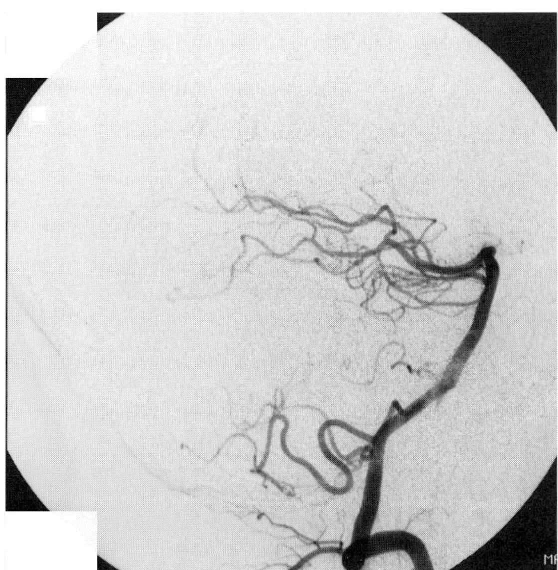

Figure 10.25c Subtracted image of vessels shown in (b)

## Lateral (collimated)

This projection complements that of the occipitofrontal 30° cephalad.

*Position of patient and imaging modality*
The patient is supine, with the head raised on a non-opaque pad and positioned to bring both the median sagittal and anthropological planes at right angles to the imaging couch.

The external auditory meatuses should be equidistant from the couch top, with the head immobilised in this position. The automatic film changer or image intensifier is then positioned against the side of the head under investigation so that it is parallel to the median sagittal plane and at right angles to the interpupillary line.

*Direction and centring of the X-ray beam*
The horizontal central ray is directed parallel to the interorbital line so that it is at right angles to the median sagittal plane and the image receptor and centred 2 cm above the external auditory meatus in the auricular line. The radiation field is collimated to the region of the vertebral blood supply.

*Imaging procedure*
An image acquisition protocol is selected to ensure that the arterial, capillary and venous circulation is demonstrated. A 0.5 s inject delay allows a mask film to be taken.

*Imaging parameters*

| *Image/s* | *Run time* | *Total images* |
|---|---|---|
| 2 | 2 s | 4 |
| 1 | 6 s | 6 |

*Contrast medium and injector data*

| *Volume* | *Concentration* | *Flow rate* |
|---|---|---|
| 4–5 ml | 300 mgI/ml | Hand injection |

In DSA, the concentration may be reduced

## Submentovertical (basal)

This supplementary projection may be used to visualise the precise location of an aneurysm and to reveal the neck of an aneurysm prior to surgery. Imaging parameters together with contrast medium and injector data are similar to the standard projections already described.

## Magnetic resonance angiography

Magnetic resonance angiography enables non-invasive investigation of the cerebral blood vessels by means of either two- or three-dïmensional time of flight (TOF) and two- or three-dimensional phase contrast (PC) imaging protocols. Such procedures may be carried out at the same time as the standard brain protocol when the brain parenchyma is being assessed for the effects of vascular disease or trauma.

The preferred protocol will depend on many factors such as the size, nature and location abnormality being investigated, the direction, velocity and flow pattern of blood, and whether or not intra- or extracranial vessels are being investigated.

Protocols may also include flow compensation parameters to take account of the fact that blood in a vessel will be moving at different velocities.

Flow imaging is discussed in more detail in Chapter 1. For the purpose of this section, 3D TOF and 3D PC protocols are briefly described.

MR contrast agents that shorten the relaxation time of blood can be used to improve signal when the velocity of blood is slow.

### Indications

Intracranial aneurysms, e.g. circle of Willis, cerebral ischaemia or infarction and follow-up of arteriovenous malformations.

### Contraindications

See Chapter 1 for general details. Patients with surgical aneurismal metallic clips must not be scanned, as torque forces on the clips from the magnetic field can result in movement of the clips and rupture of the vessel walls. New non-ferromagnetic clips are now available, but it is imperative to ascertain which type of clip has been used before scanning a postoperative patient.

*Position of patient and imaging modality*

The patient lies supine on the scanner table, head resting in the head support of the head coil. Position is aided by halogen alignment lights. The median sagittal plane is positioned parallel to the sagittal alignment light and the anthropological baseline parallel to the transaxial alignment light. The table is now adjusted until the external reference point is at the centre of the head coil. From this position the patient and head coil assembly are driven the fixed distance to the isocentre of the magnet.

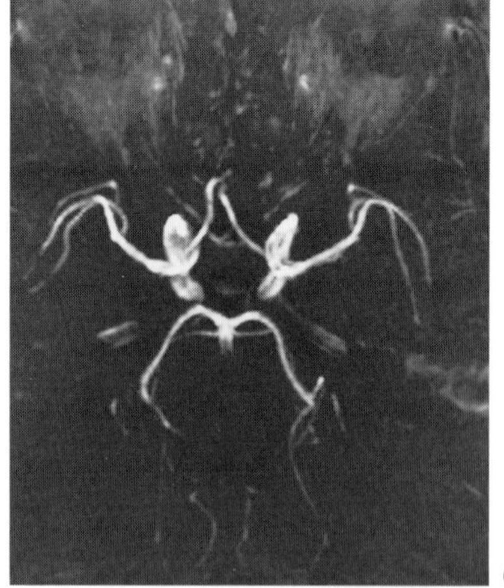
(a)

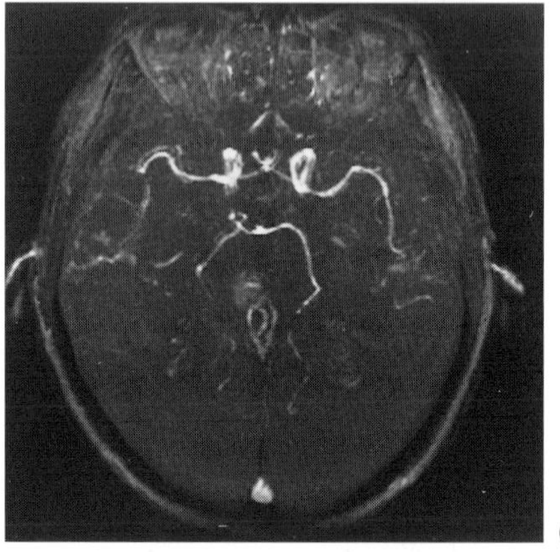
(b)

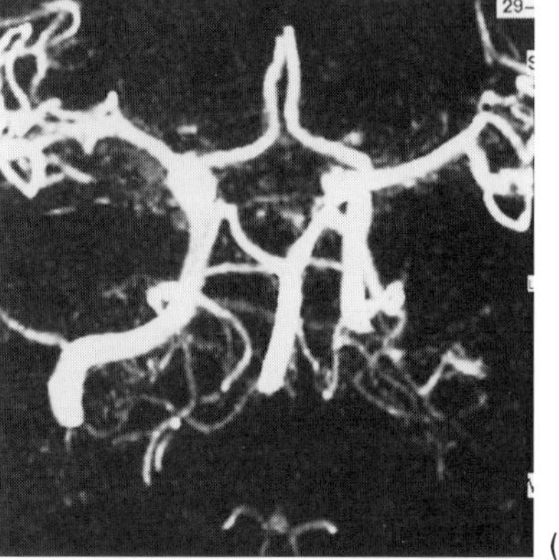
(c)

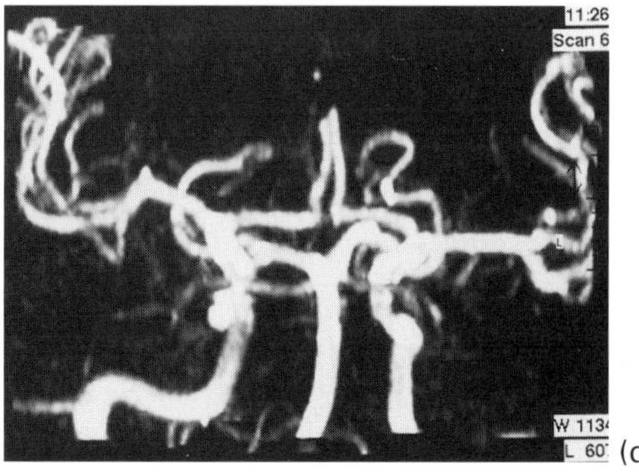

(d)

**Figure 10.26** (a) Magnified time of flight MIP image of the circle of Willis; (b) standard time of flight MIP image of the circle of Willis showing a small vertebral aneurysm; (c,d) further magnified time of flight image of the circle of Willis in different degrees of rotation around the *x*-axis

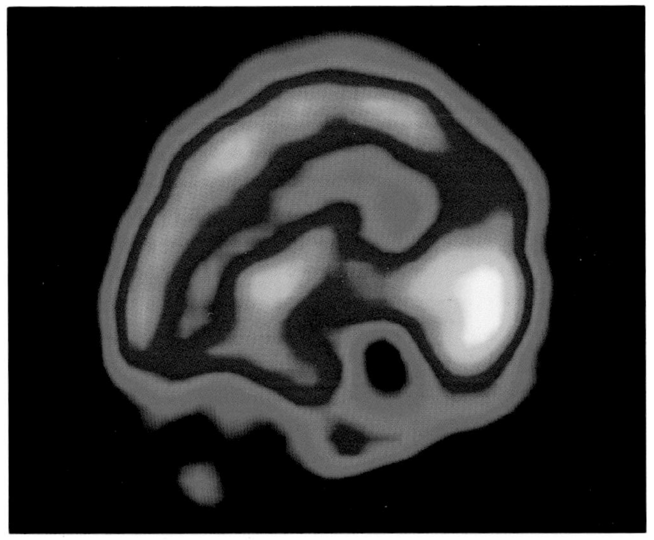

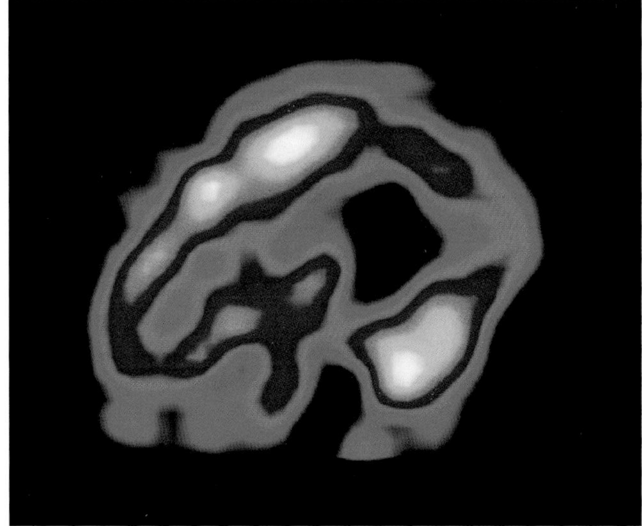

**Plate 14** Sagittal images showing (i) normal and (ii) abnormal HM-PAO brain scan (see text, page 347)

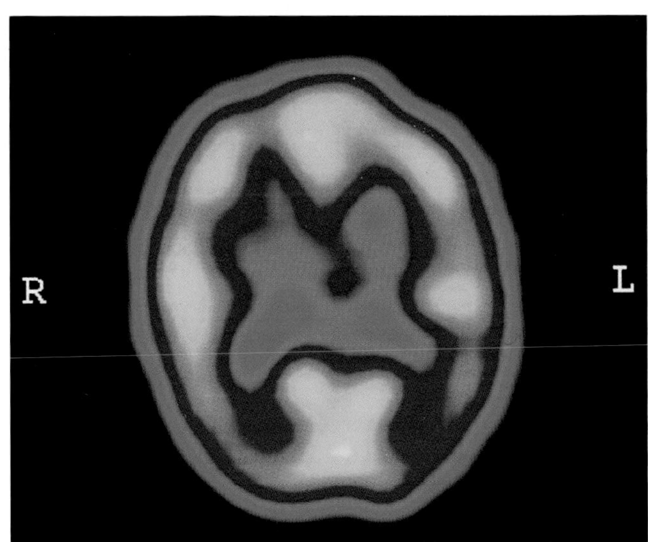


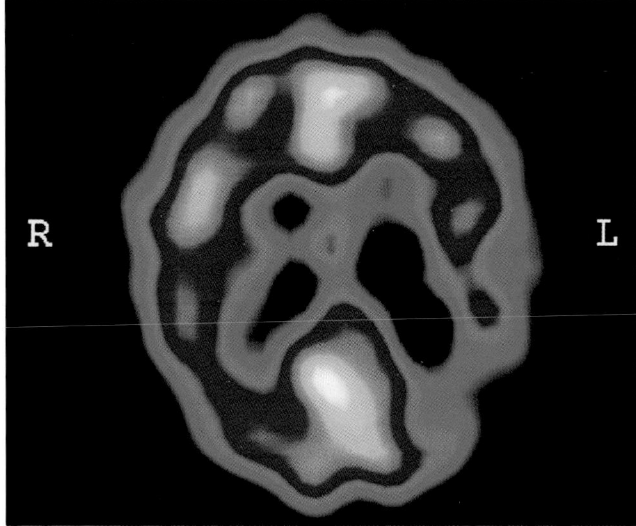


**Plate 15** Transaxial images showing (i) normal and (ii) abnormal HM-PAO brain scan (see text, page 347)

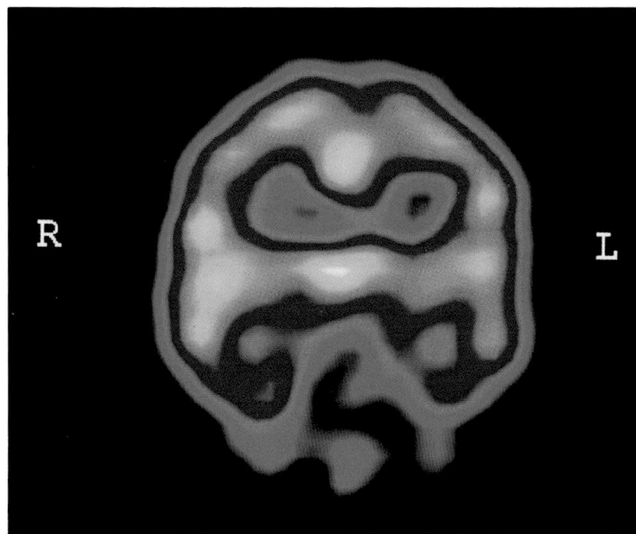


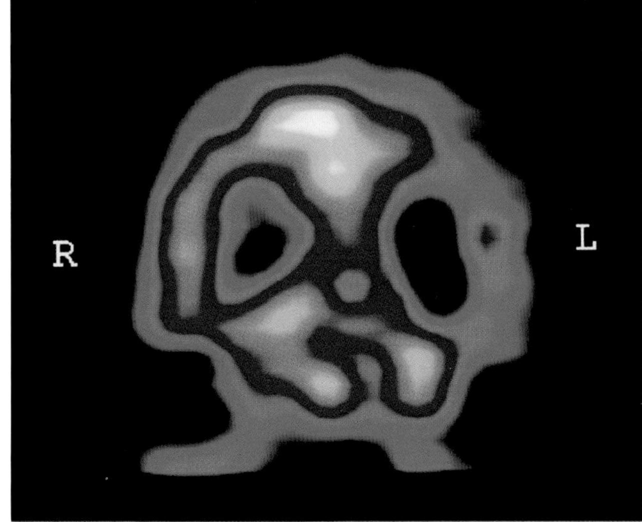


**Plate 16** Coronal images showing (i) normal and (ii) abnormal HM-PAO brain scan (see text, page 347)

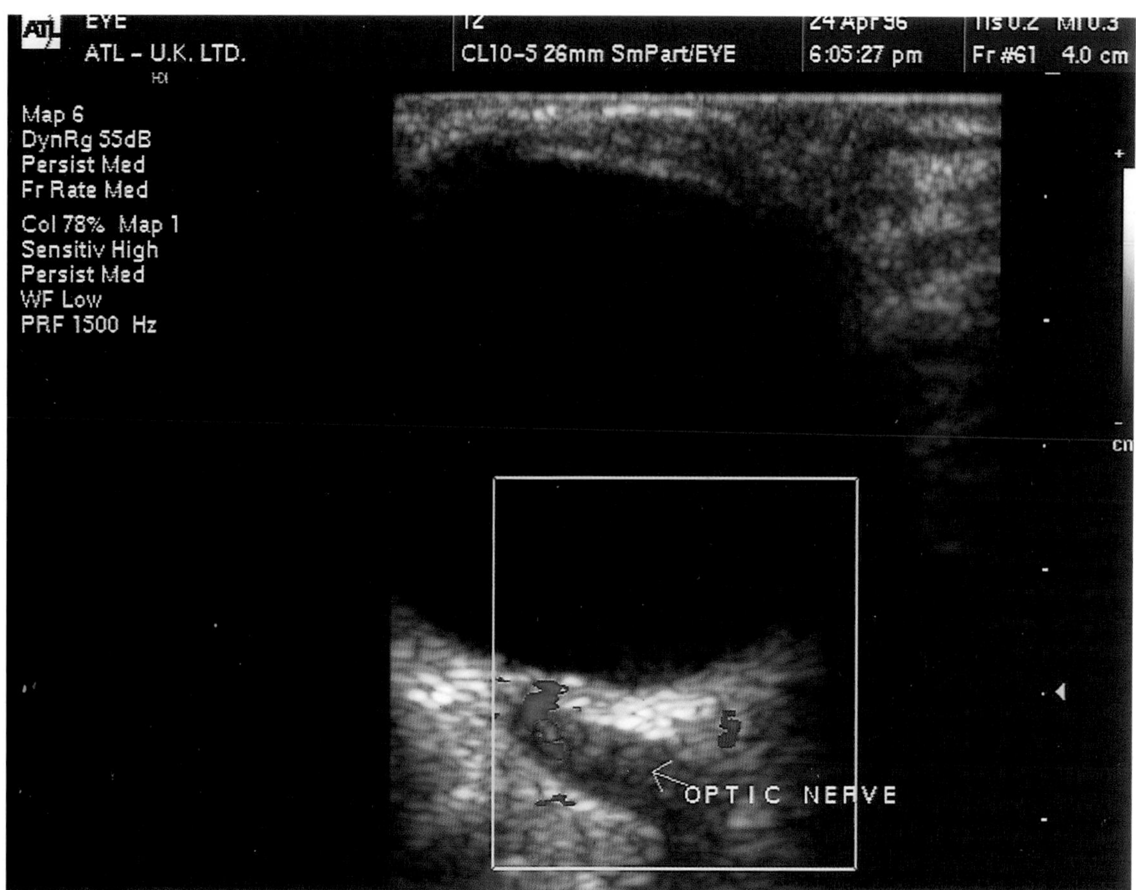


**Plate 17** Normal transverse section with colour Doppler showing optic nerve and blood vessels (see text, page 378)

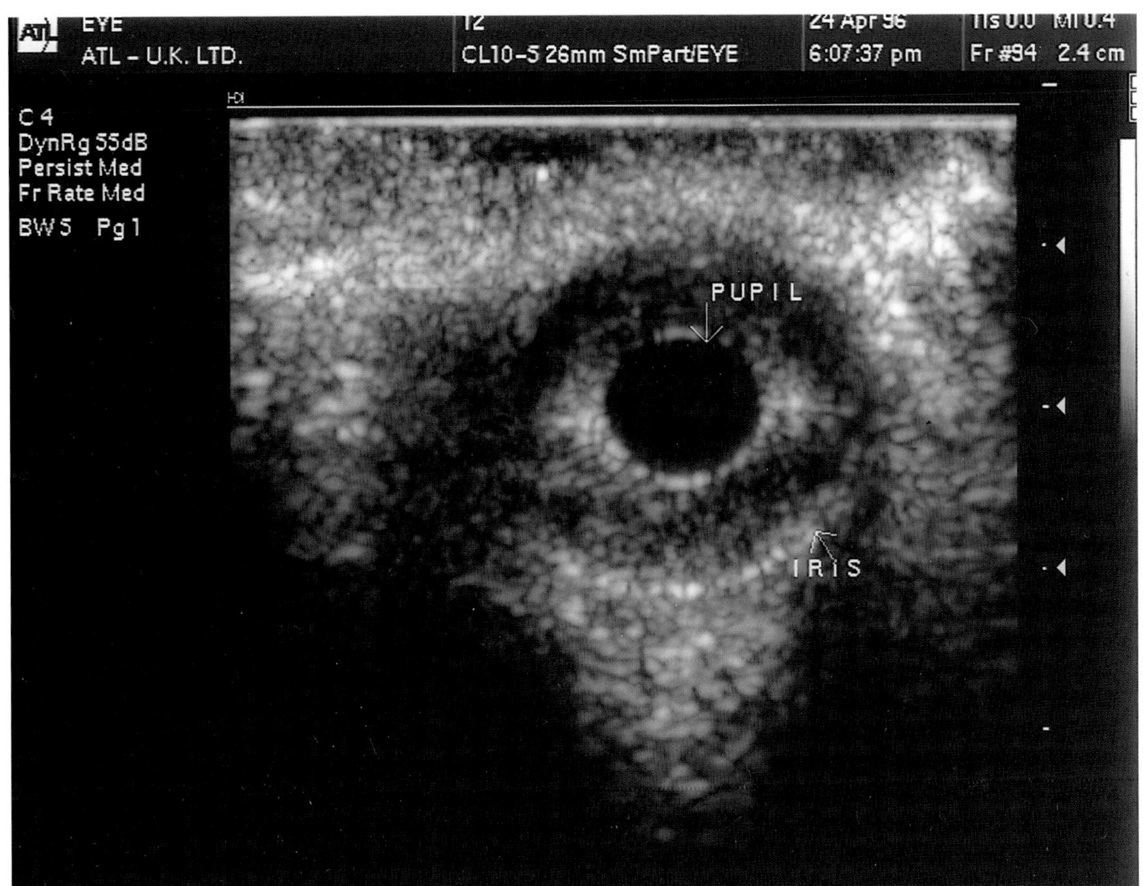


**Plate 18** Anterior coronal view showing pupil and iris (see text, page 378)

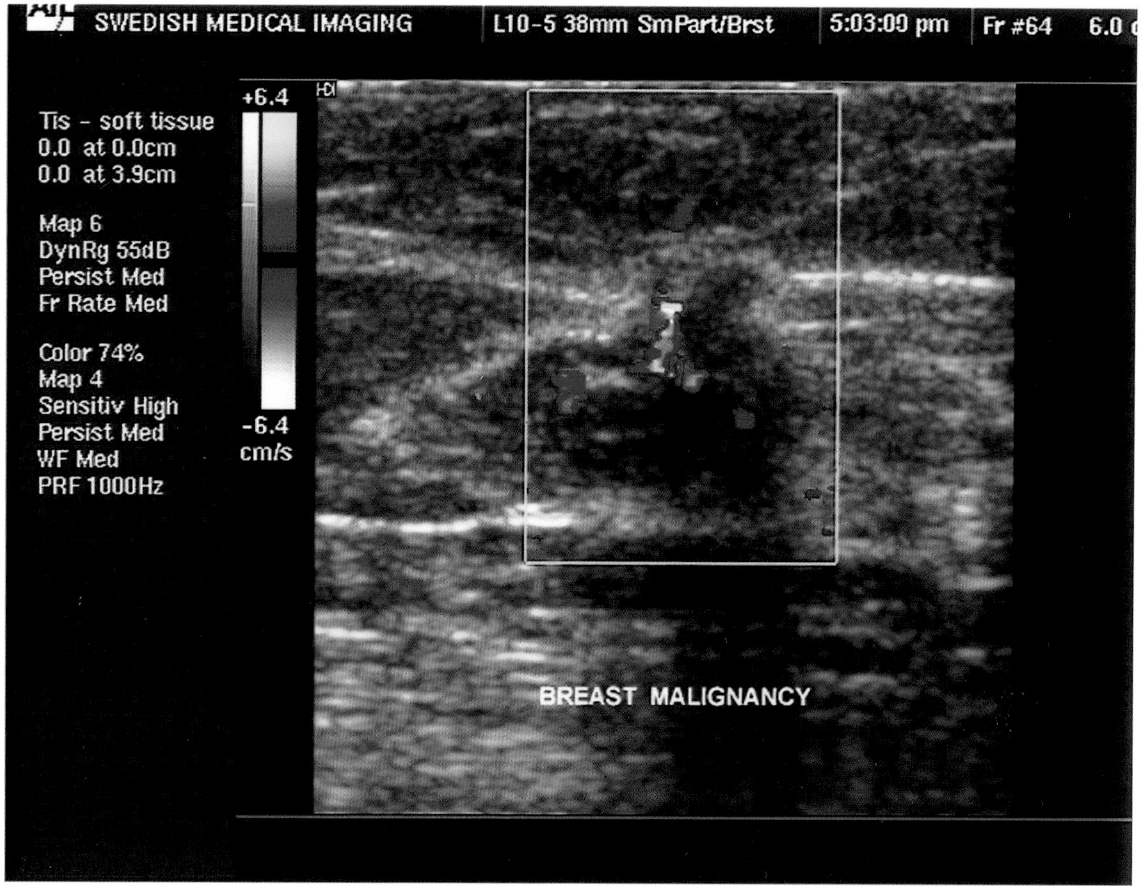


**Plate 19** Example of a malignant tumour which presents with an irregular and ill-defined margin, acoustic shadowing and an abnormal blood flow (see text, page 385)

## Magnetic resonance angiography

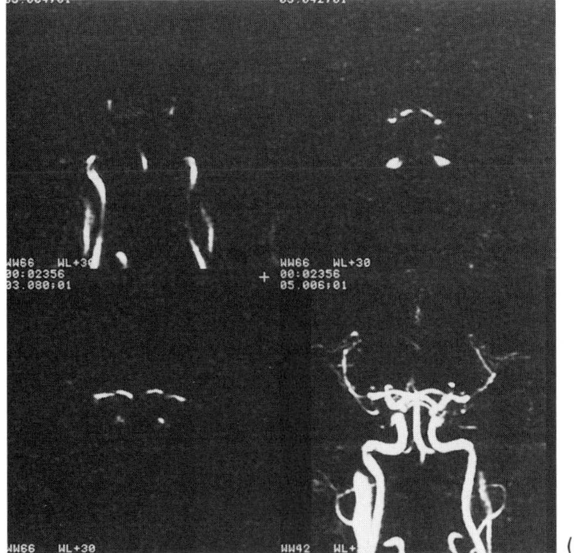
(a)

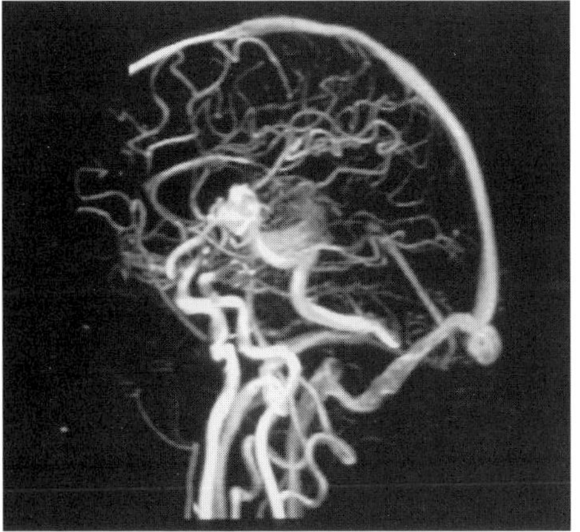
(b)

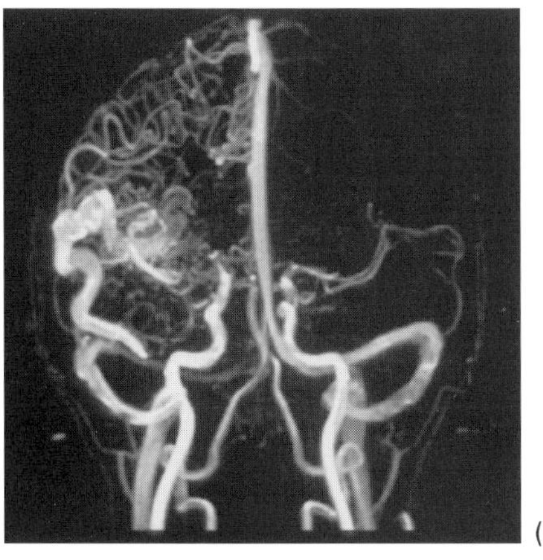
(c)

**Figure 10.27** (a) Phased contrast study showing three phase directions: top left – head to feet; top right – anteroposterior; bottom left – left to right; bottom right – a final MIP image displayed in the coronal plane. (b,c) Sagittal and phase contrast images demonstrating a large arteriovenous malformation in the right hemisphere associated with the right middle cerebral artery

### 3D time of flight

This protocol is ideal for imaging aneurysms of the circle of Willis and intracranial vascular occlusive disease.

A 28–60 slice 3D volume is obtained of the region of interest. A 60 slice, 5–7 cm slab, is generally used for imaging arterial structures without severe loss of vascular signal due to saturation effects. Slice thickness is typically 0.7–1.0 mm, with a FOV of 16–20 cm, depending on patient size and region of interest. A repetition time (TR) of 40–55 ms and a flip angle of 15–20° are usually sufficient to suppress stationary spins. Echo time (TE) as short as 5 ms can be achieved with flow compensation.

Depending on the desired resolution and acquisition time, the acquisition matrix and number of excitations may be varied, e.g. from $128^2$ to $512^2$ with 1 NEX.

### 3D phase contrast imaging

This protocol is useful for large-volume image acquisitions such as the whole head, assessing intracranial aneurysms, demonstrating venous occlusions and malformations, examining vascular components of congenital malformations and evaluating traumatic intracranial vascular injuries. Phase contrast imaging, however, has the disadvantage of longer scan times and therefore may be susceptible to movement artefacts.

Using 15–20° flip angles, large volumes can be imaged without serious loss of signal intensity due to saturation effects. As a result of the reduced saturation dependency, short TRs may be used, e.g. 25–28 ms, with minimal saturation of moving spins.

Further reductions in saturation may be achieved by using intravenous contrast agents which shorten the $T_1$ of blood.

A 28–60 slice 3D volume is obtained using a 18–20 cm FOV and 0.7–1.5 mm slice thickness at minimal TEs which are system dependent. Acquisition time and resolution is based on a 128 × 256 matrix and 1 NEX.

### Image viewing

Once the 3D data set has been acquired it is initially displayed as a series of slices, usually in the axial plane. The 3D volume is then subjected to a maximum intensity pixel (MIP) ray projection to create a series of projections to rotate the vascular structures around the *x*, *y* or *z* axis. A cine loop display can provide the perception of depth.

# 10 Central Nervous System

## Vertebral Column

### Introduction

The vertebral column consists of 33 irregular ring-shaped bones (vertebrae) which articulate with each other. Their function is to provide support for the head and trunk and to permit a degree of movement. They transmit the weight of the upper torso to the pelvis, provide articulation for the ribs and attachment for muscles. They also transmit and protect the spinal cord and its coverings. The column comprises 7 cervical, 12 thoracic, 5 lumbar, sacrum and coccyx. The vertebrae are separated by discs of fibrocartilage. The vertebrae increase in size downwards. Although the vertebrae in each region are characteristic, most share common or typical features.

The body is roughly cylindrical and forms the anterior part of the bone. The superior and inferior surfaces are flat and covered by hyaline cartilage. The anterior posterior and lateral surfaces are slightly concave.

The vertebral arch forms the posterior part of the bone and is formed by the pedicles and the laminae. The pedicles are short and thick, projecting backwards from the junction of the lateral and posterior surfaces of the body. On the superior and inferior surfaces of the pedicles are the intervertebral notches which in the articulated column form the intervertebral foramen for transmission of nerves entering and leaving the neural canal. The laminae are flattened plates of bone which project backwards and medially from the posterior end of the pedicles. They unite to form the vertebral arch.

The vertebral foramen is bounded by the posterior aspect of the body, the pedicles, and the laminae and transmits the spinal cord and coverings. In the articulated skeleton the intervertebral discs and ligaments form the neural canal. The spinous processes project backwards in the midline from the junction of the laminae. They are frequently palpable and visible.

The transverse processes project laterally from the junction of the pedicles and laminae. The superior articular process projects upwards from the junction of the pedicle and lamina and presents an articular facet which faces posterolaterally. The inferior articular process projects downwards and presents an articular facet which faces antero-medially. Typical vertebrae from each of the regions of the vertebral column are illustrated opposite.

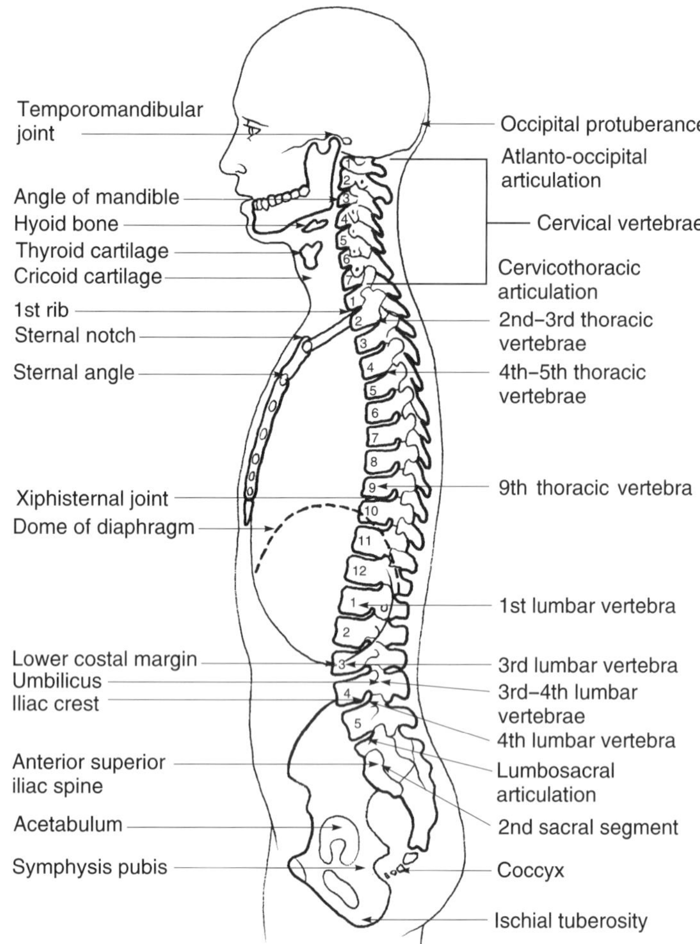


**Figure 10.28** Vertebral levels

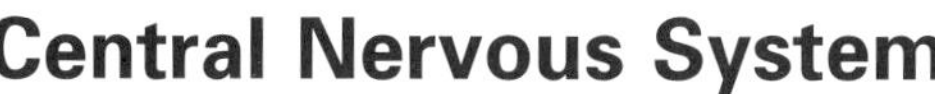



## Vertebral Column

Body
Anterior tubercle
Posterior tubercle
Foramen transversarium
Superior articular facet
Vertebral foramen
Bifid spinous process

**Figure 10.29a** Cervical vertebra

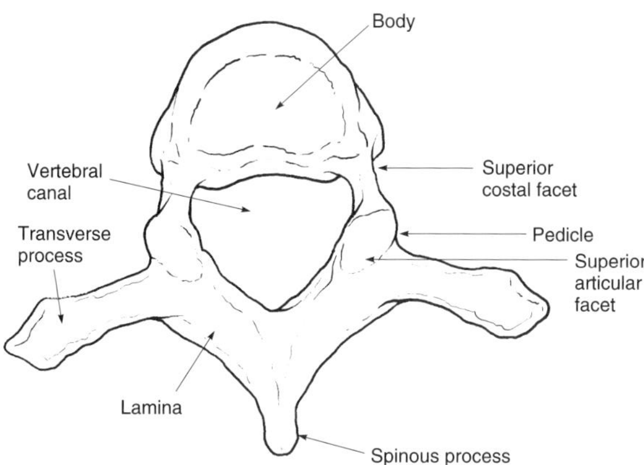


**Figure 10.29b** Thoracic vertebra

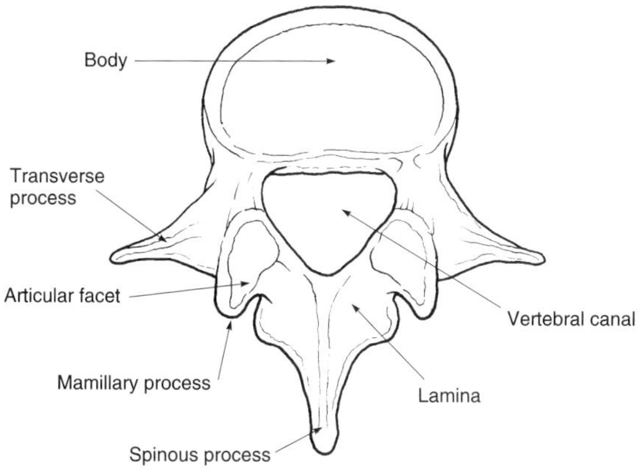


**Figure 10.29c** Lumber vertebra

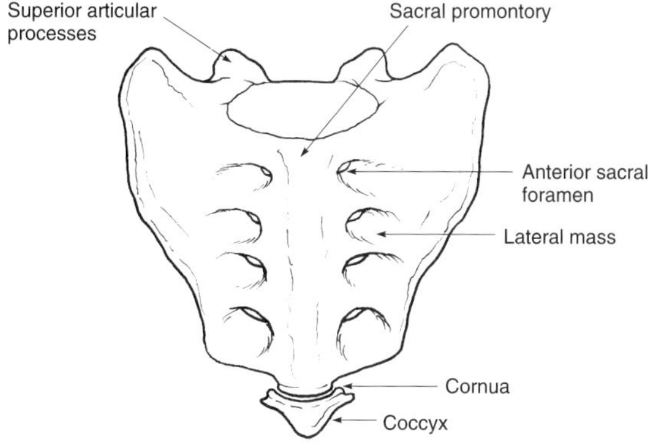


**Figure 10.29d** Anterior aspect of the sacrum and coccyx

Individual vertebrae articulate with each other posteriorly between the vertebral arches and anteriorly between the vertebral bodies. Although the degree of movement between adjacent vertebrae is small, the cumulative effect permits a considerable range of movement of the vertebral column as a whole.

The joints between the vertebral arches are synovial plane joints. They are supported by ligaments running the length of the vertebral column and others which attach to adjacent vertebral arches.

The joints between the vertebral bodies are cartilaginous. Adjacent bodies articulate with each other through intervertebral discs and are supported by anterior and posterior longitudinal ligaments which run along the anterior and posterior aspects of the vertebral bodies, respectively.

The intervertebral discs constitute approximately 20% of the length of the vertebral column and increase in thickness from upper thoracic to the lower lumbar region. In the cervical and lumbar regions the discs are wedge shaped (thickest anteriorly) and hence contribute to the anterior convexity of the column.

The discs themselves comprise a tough outer laminated portion known as the annulus fibrosus and an inner gelatinous core, the nucleus pulposus.

Initially, the nucleus pulposus has a high water content which progressively reduces, being replaced by fibrous tissue. This reduces the elasticity of the disc and diminishes the overall length of the vertebral column.

Degenerative changes or trauma to the vertebral column may result in the prolapse of the nucleus pulposus, usually postero-laterally, into the vertebral canal. This occurs most commonly at the level of L4/5 or L5/S1. It can also occur in the lower cervical area at C5/6 or C6/7 or less frequently in other areas.

### Recommended imaging procedures

Both MRI and CT have drastically altered the approach to spinal imaging, superseding more invasive techniques. MRI should now be the first method of choice, but machine access is still a limiting factor. Computed tomography is now widely available and is routinely used either with or without intrathecal or intravenous contrast media.

Myelography and air meatography, although described in this chapter, are now performed less frequently and usually in conjunction with CT and only if MRI is unavailable.

Intravenous contrast agents are used in MRI and CT to further delineate tumours and to differentiate between fibrosis and disc tissue in postoperative recurrent disc disease.

# Magnet Resonance Imaging

Magnetic resonance imaging, using surface coils, produces high-quality images of the entire spine, spinal canal and spinal cord in any anatomical plane. Surface coil designs do vary from manufacturer to manufacturer. Two techniques are described. The first technique to be described uses a phased array spinal coil. This assembly consists of six coils arranged in a row. Any four adjacent coils can be selected at any one time, giving a maximum field of view of 48 cm. This method allows the entire spinal cord to be imaged without repositioning either the patient or the surface coil. The second technique uses a dedicated cervical spine surface coil and a Bucky design quadrature coil for thoracic and lumbar spinal imaging. In the Bucky design, the coil moves a limited distance within a frame, allowing different areas to be imaged without repositioning the patient. When using this method, it is imperative that there is a degree of overlap to ensure that the vertebrae are correctly identified.

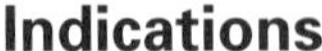

## Indications

Tumours of the spine and spinal cord plaques associated with multiple sclerosis. Complex spinal anomalies, prolapsed intervertebral discs and syringomyelia, trauma with cord compression, acute cord compression.

## Position of patient and imaging modality

**Method 1 – cervical/thoracic/lumbar spines**

The patient lies supine, head first, with the median sagittal plane perpendicular to the scanner table and the spine positioned centrally over the phased array surface coil. A band is placed over the forehead to minimise patient movement and the knees are flexed to reduce lumbar curvature.

Usually the upper, middle or lower four coils are selected to scan, respectively, from the mid-posterior fossa of the brain to T12, C4–L3, T3 to mid-sacrum. The appropriate scan reference point is obtained using the external alignment lights. The sternal notch is used for cervical and thoracic imaging and the xiphisternum for thoracolumbar imaging. From the reference point, the patient and the surface coil are advanced the fixed distance to the isocentre of the magnet.

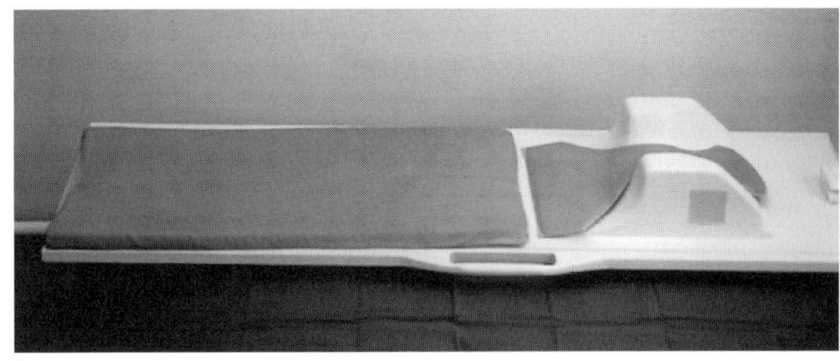

(a)

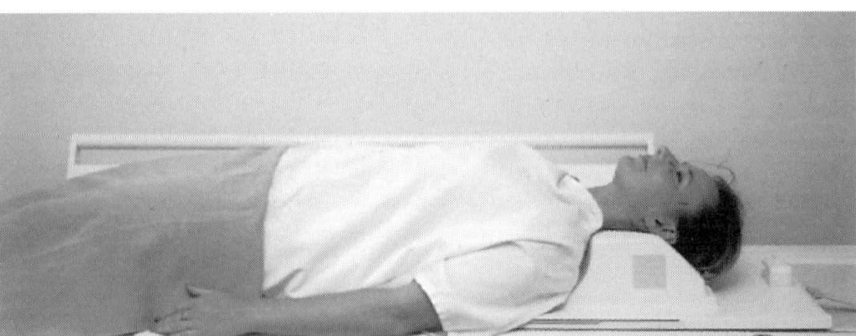

(b)

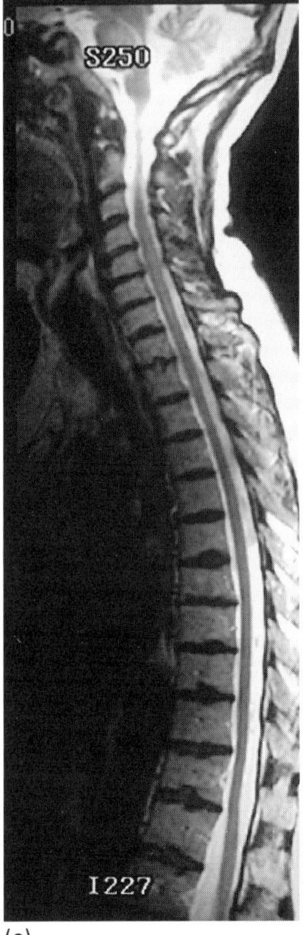



(c)

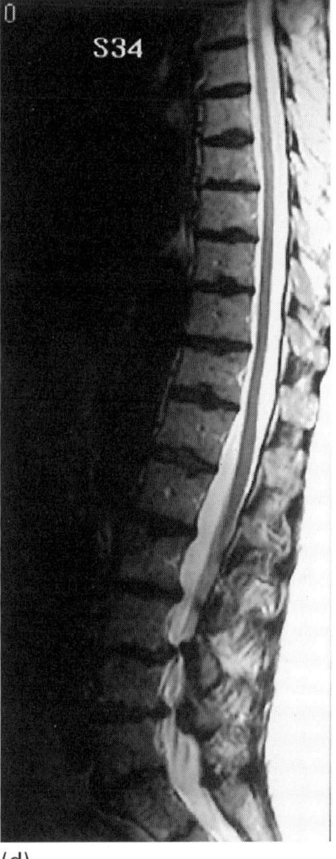



(d)

**Figure 10.30** (a) Phased array spinal coil; (b) patient positioned on phase array coil; (c,d) typical midline sagittal $T_2$ weighted images using a phased array spinal coil

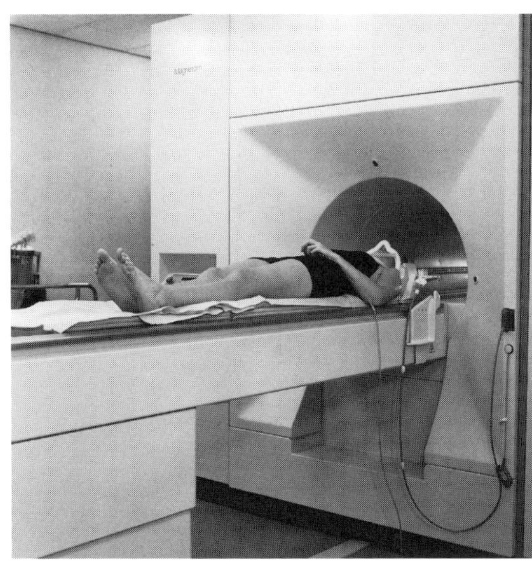

**Figure 10.31a** Patient positioned using a cervical spine surface coil

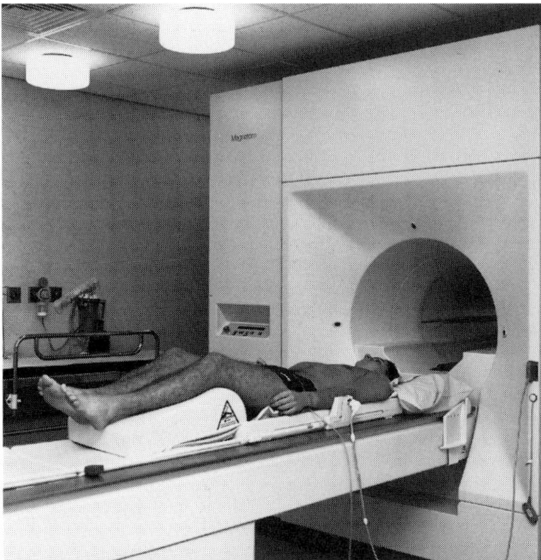

**Figure 10.31b** Patient positioned for lumbar spine imaging using a 'Bucky design' quadrature coil

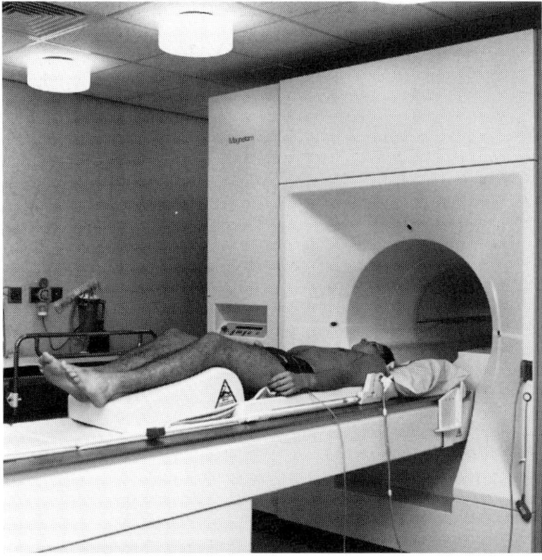

**Figure 10.31c** Patient positioned for thoracic spine imaging using a 'Bucky design' quadrature coil

### Method 2 – cervical spine

The patient lies supine, head first, with the median sagittal plane perpendicular to the imaging table. The head and neck are positioned over the surface coil and a band is placed across the forehead to minimise patient movement. Using the external alignment lights the table top is moved until the scan reference point is at the centre of the surface coil. The patient and surface coil are now advanced the fixed distance to the isocentre of the magnet.

### Method 2 – lumbar spine

The thoracolumbar surface coil is positioned on the scanner table. The patient lies supine, head first, over the surface coil with the median sagittal plane perpendicular to the surface coil. The head rests on a pillow and the knees are flexed to reduce lumbar curvature. This is often more comfortable for the patient and may also reduce patient movement. Using the external alignment lights the table top is moved to bring the scan reference point at the level of the iliac crests. The surface coil is now moved within the frame to position the centre of the coil at the level of the iliac crests. The patient and surface coil are now advanced the fixed distance to the isocentre of the magnet and localiser scans prescribed for the lumbar vertebrae.

### Method 2 – thoracic spine

To identify the thoracic vertebrae accurately, it is necessary to position the patient and perform the necessary localiser scans for lumbar imaging. After obtaining reference levels (L5/S1), move the surface coil to give image overlap. After obtaining these initial localiser scans, the patient and the surface coil are driven out of the magnet. The surface coil is moved cranially the required distance to allow the regions imaged to overlap, thus correctly identifying the vertebral levels. Using the external alignment lights, the table top is moved until the scan reference point is at the centre of the surface coil. Once more the patient and surface coil are advanced to the isocentre of the magnet.

# 10 Vertebral Column

## Magnet Resonance Imaging

### Imaging procedure

The imaging procedure is similar for all spinal regions. Initially, a coronal localiser scan is performed. From this image $T_1$ and $T_2$ weighted sagittal scans are prescribed through the spinal canal, ensuring that the scans start and end lateral to the spinal canal to demonstrate spinal nerve roots.

From the midline sagittal image, a transaxial series of images may be prescribed through any area of suspected abnormality.

In all cases, $T_1$ and $T_2$ weighted sequences are used to provide excellent anatomical and structural detail of both normal and abnormal areas. Further contrast-enhanced $T_1$ weighted images may be necessary to delineate tumours further, and in the case of postoperative recurrent prolapsed intervertebral disc, to differentiate fibrosis and remaining disc tissue. In complex spinal anomalies, such as dysraphic and/or scoliotic spines, 3D imaging may be useful.

*Contrast medium and injection data*

| *Volume* | *Concentration* | *Flow rate* |
|---|---|---|
| 0.2 ml/kg body weight | Gadolinium | Hand injection |

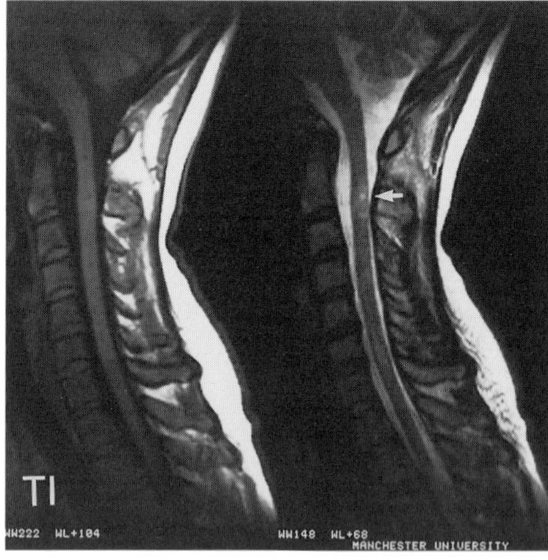


**Figure 10.32a** Sagittal $T_1$ and $T_2$ weighted images side by side, showing multiple sclerosis plaque of the cervical cord

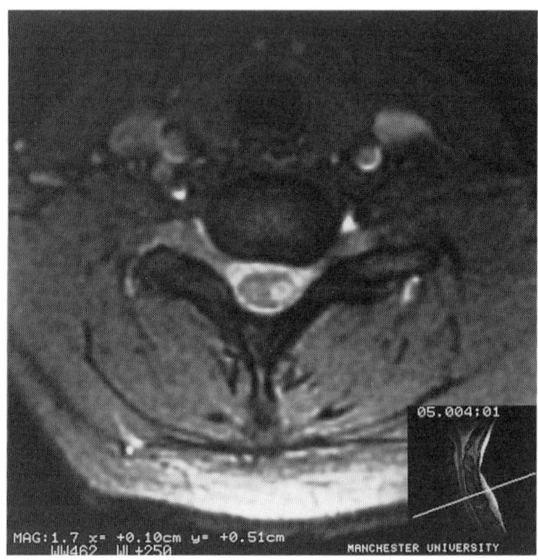


**Figure 10.32b** Transaxial $T_2$ weighted image of the cervical spine demonstrating plaque in the cord

**Table 10.4 Imaging parameters**

| *Imaging plane* | *Imaging sequence* | *TR* | *TE* | *Field of view* (cm) | *No. of NEX* | *Slice width/ gap* (mm) | *Matrix (horizontal – vertical)* |
|---|---|---|---|---|---|---|---|
| Sagittal | Spin-echo $T_1$ weighted | 500 | 25 | 25–30 | 4 | 3–5/1 (9 slices) | 128 × 256 |
| Sagittal | Fast spin-echo $T_2$ weighted (echo train length –12) | 3000 | 110 | 25–30 | 4 | 3–5/1–2 (9 slices) | 128 × 256 |
| **Lumbar spine** | | | | | | | |
| Transaxial or oblique | Spin-echo $T_1$ weighted | 500 | 25 | 20 | 4 | 5/1 | 224 × 160 |
| **Cervical spine** | | | | | | | |
| Transaxial or oblique | Gradient-echo $T_2$ weighted (flip angle 25°) | 600 | 25 | 20 | 4 | 5/1 | 224 × 160 |
| 3D volume (sagittal) with flip angle 45° | SPGR | 50 | 12 | 25–30 | 1 | 1.5 (no gap) 45 slices | 128 × 256 |

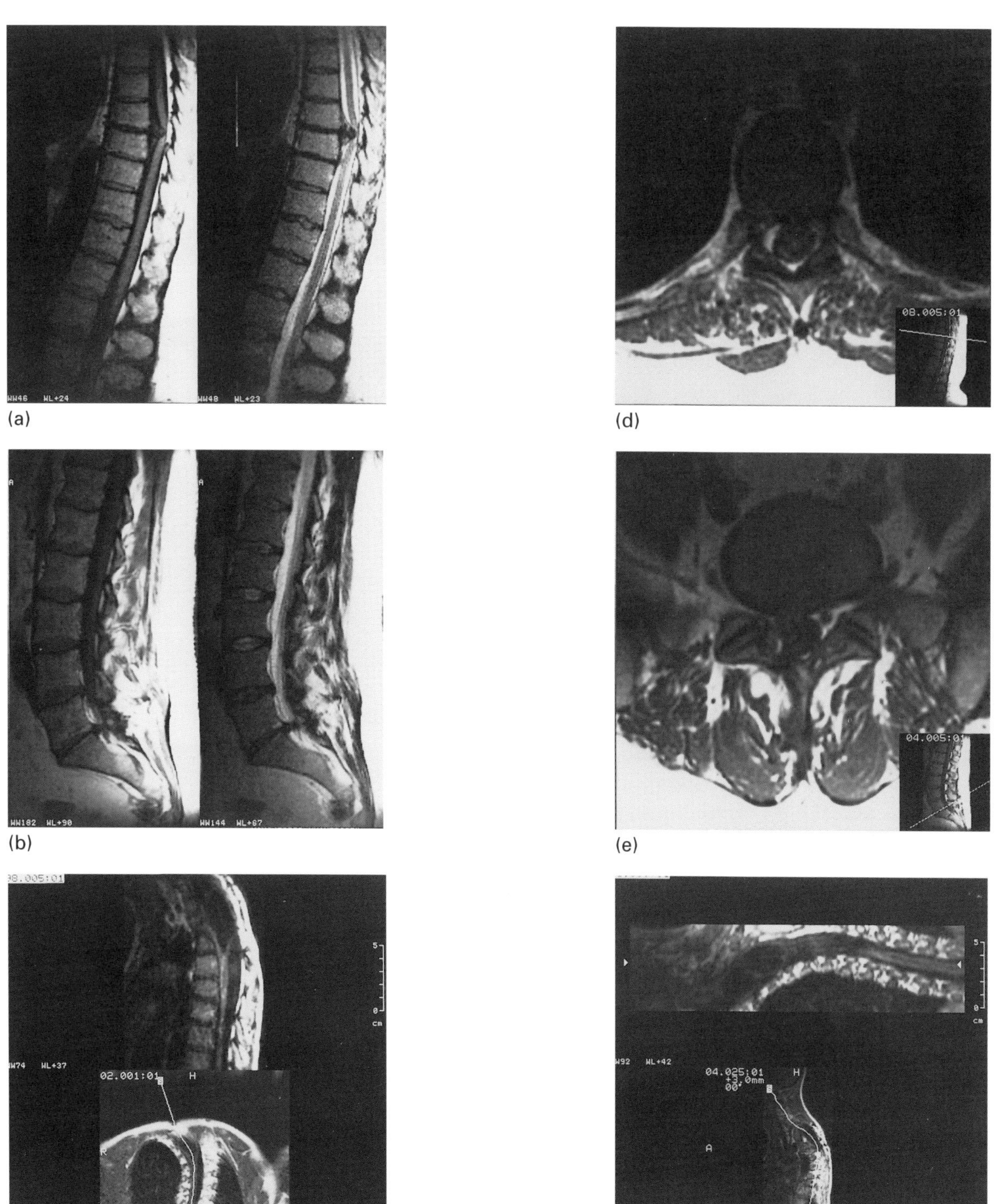

(a) (b) (c) (d) (e) (f)

**Figure 10.33** (a) $T_1$ and $T_2$ weighted sagittal images of the mid-thoracic spine showing cord compression; (b) $T_1$ and $T_2$ weighted sagittal images of the lumbar spine; (c,f) 3D reconstruction images showing a bizarre spinal anomaly. Note on the lower set of images oblique reference lines to produce (c) sagittal and (f) coronal images of the upper spinal cord. (d) Transaxial $T_2$ weighted image through the mid-thoracic spine; (e) transaxial $T_2$ weighted image through L5/S1 disc space showing a large prolapsed disc

# Vertebral Column

## Computed Tomography

Computed tomography produces high-quality transaxial images of the spine. It is used routinely in trauma, to assess destructive lesions and prolapsed intervertebral discs in the lumbar region. If MRI is unavailable it can be used in conjunction with myelography to identify prolapsed intervertebral discs in the cervical and thoracic region and the extent of space-occupying lesions in the spinal canal. Delayed sections, up to 24 h post-myelography, may be necessary in suspected syringomyelia to view pooling of contrast medium in any cavities within the spinal cord. Again this technique has been superseded by MRI.

Intravenous contrast medium may be used to delineate tumours further and, in the case of postoperative recurrent prolapsed intervertebral disc, to differentiate fibrosis and remaining disc tissue.

There are two scanning methods. Images can either be acquired in a block of contiguous sections through the abnormality or with the gantry angled parallel to each individual disc. The middle section is centred through the disc and the series should image the pedicle above and below. The former technique can be applied in all circumstances, whereas the latter is usually reserved for cases of suspected prolapsed intervertebral discs. Routinely 3–5 mm contiguous sections are acquired. However, overlapping sections with a slice width of 5 mm and a table increment of 4 mm may be advocated for selectively examining intervertebral discs. This technique does have a radiation dose penalty for the patient. In assessing disc disease it is necessary to scan the disc above and below the one clinically suspected.

To increase spatial resolution the sections may be targeted either prospectively or retrospectively and, in the case of bony abnormality, a high-resolution algorithm selected. Also the digital data may be reformatted to produce images in any other anatomical planes and in 3D.

### Indications

Tumour, prolapsed intervertebral disc, trauma and spinal anomalies.

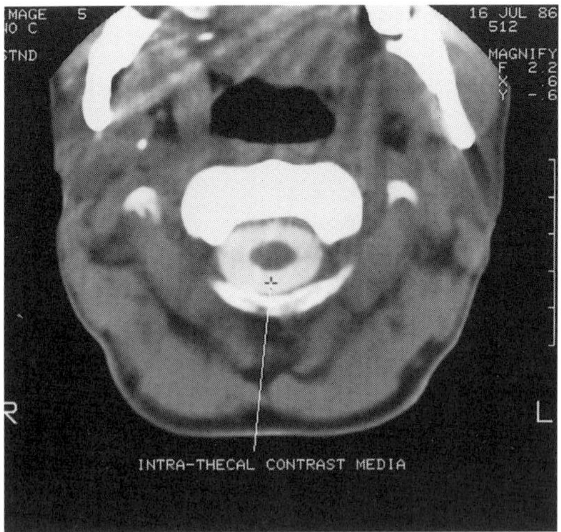


**Figure 10.34a** Example of a CT myelogram

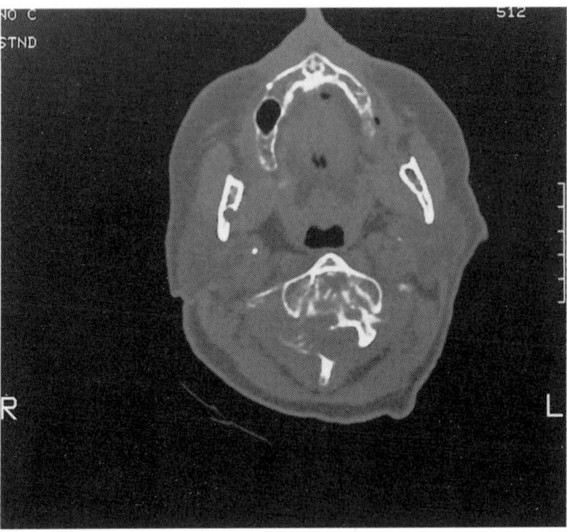


**Figure 10.34b** Transaxial image at the level of C2 showing erosion of bone due to tumour

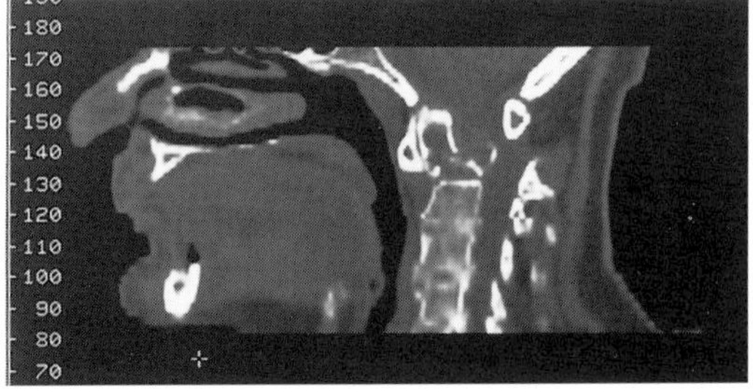


**Figure 10.34c** Midline sagittal reformatted image of (b)

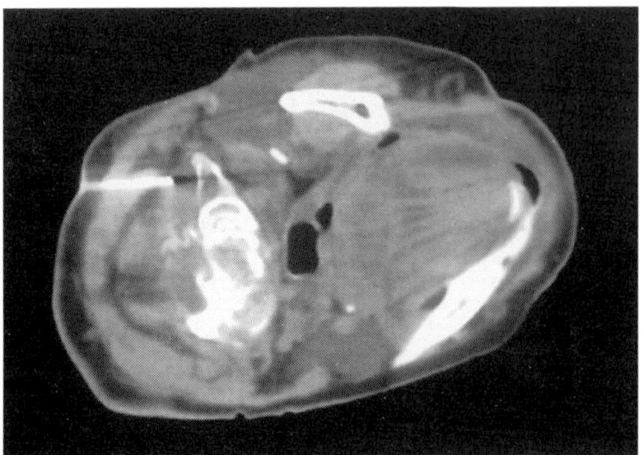

**Figure 10.34d** Example of a CT-guided bone biopsy procedure

## Computed Tomography

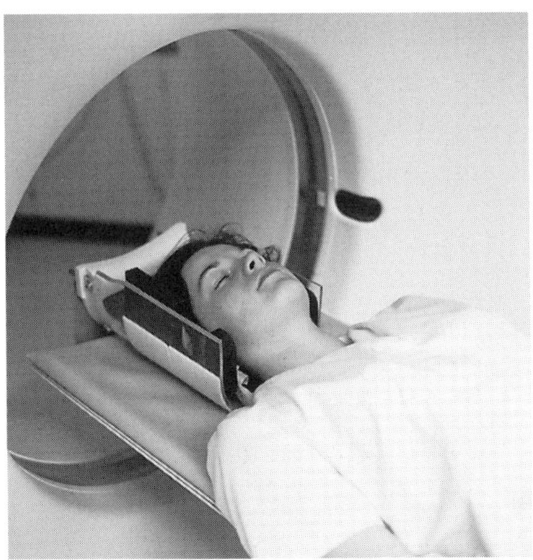

**Figure 10.35a** Patient positioned in CT scanner

### Cervical spine

*Position of patient and imaging modality*

The patient lies supine, head first on the scanner table, with the neck extended over a wedge pad and arms resting by the patient's side. The median sagittal plane is perpendicular to the table top and the head is held in position by a Velcro strap across the forehead. Using alignment lights to aid positioning, the table is moved until the scan reference point is at the level of the sternal notch. The scan table height is adjusted to bring the coronal alignment light at a level 2.5 cm behind the angle of the mandible.

*Imaging procedure*

A lateral scan projection radiograph is obtained, starting 20 cm above and ending 4 cm below the reference point. From this image 3–5 mm contiguous sections are prescribed through the area of abnormality.

If spiral scanning options are available, these images may be acquired with a volume acquisition, using a 5 mm slice thickness and 5 mm table increments, but with a 3 mm reconstruction index to give overlapping sections.

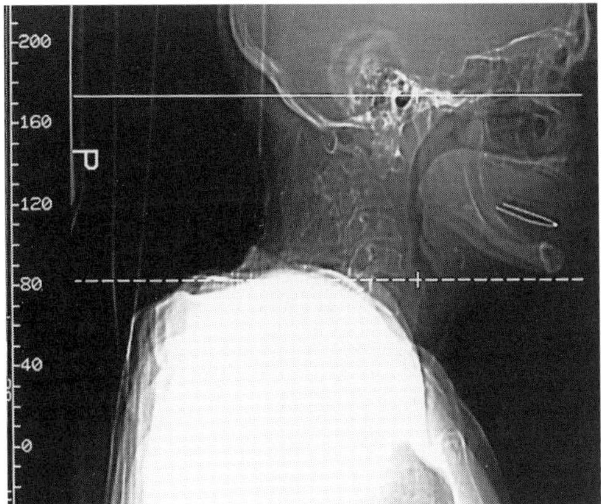


**Figure 10.35b** Scan projection radiograph showing start and end locations

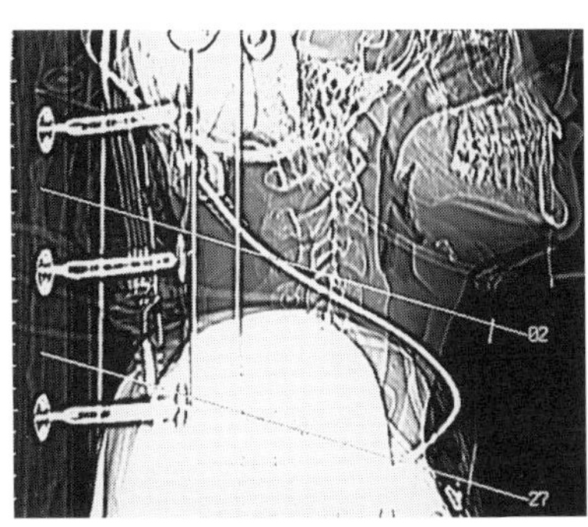


**Figure 10.35d** Scan projection radiograph of a patient in a Stryker frame showing start and end locations

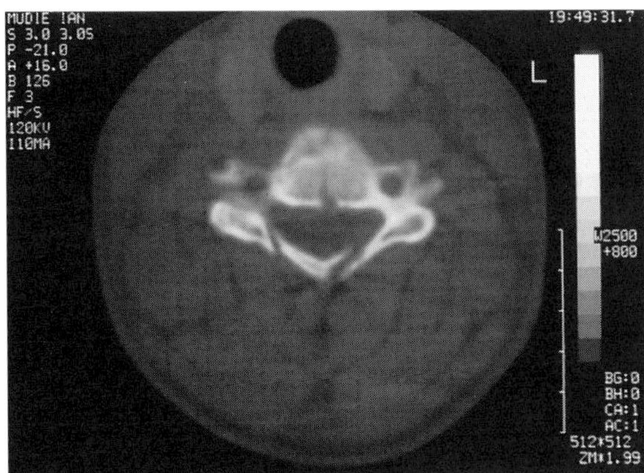


**Figure 10.35c** Transaxial image demonstrating a fracture of the fifth cervical vertebra

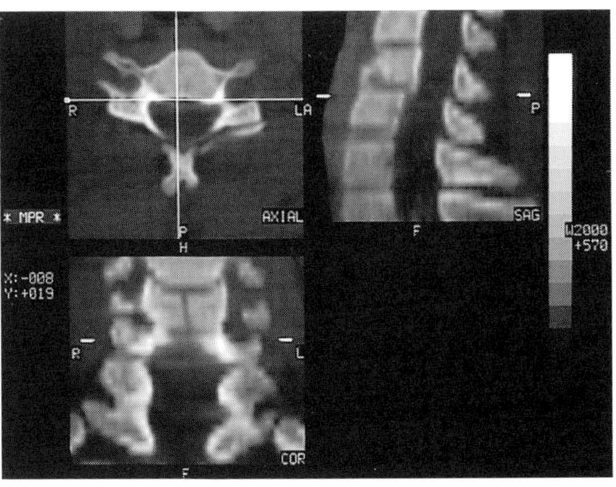


**Figure 10.35e** Composite image showing sagittal and coronal reformations of the fifth cervical vertebra

## Computed Tomography

### Thoracic spine

*Position of patient and imaging modality*

The patient is positioned as for the cervical spine but with the arms resting on the pillow beside the patient's head. Knees may be fixed over a pad for comfort. The scan reference point again is at the level of the sternal notch. The table height is adjusted to bring the coronal alignment light at the level of the mid-axillary line.

*Imaging procedure*

A lateral scan projection radiograph is obtained, starting 5 cm above and ending 40 cm below the scan reference point, to include one whole lumbar vertebra, enabling the vertebrae to be correctly identified. From this image, 3–5 mm contiguous sections are prescribed through the area of abnormality.

If spiral scanning options are available, these images may be acquired with a volume acquisition, using a 5 mm slice thickness and 5 mm table increments, but with a 3 mm reconstruction index to give overlapping sections.

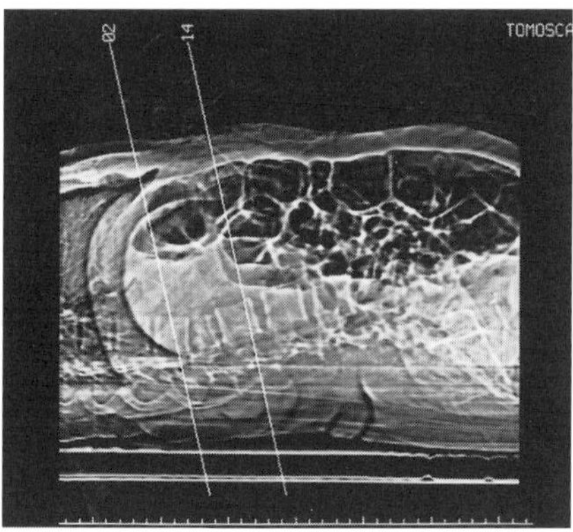

**Figure 10.36a** A localised scan projection radiograph of the lower thoracic spine showing a T12 fracture

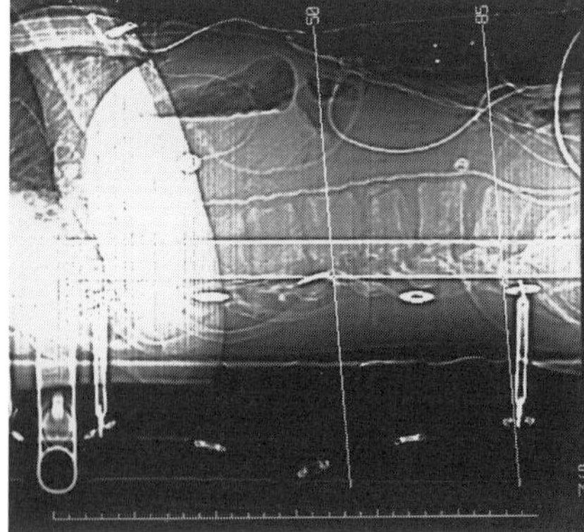

**Figure 10.36b** Scan projection radiograph showing start and end locations of a continuous block through L2–4 to show fracture of L3. Patient in a Stryker frame the metal clips of which are removed prior to scanning to avoid streak artefacts

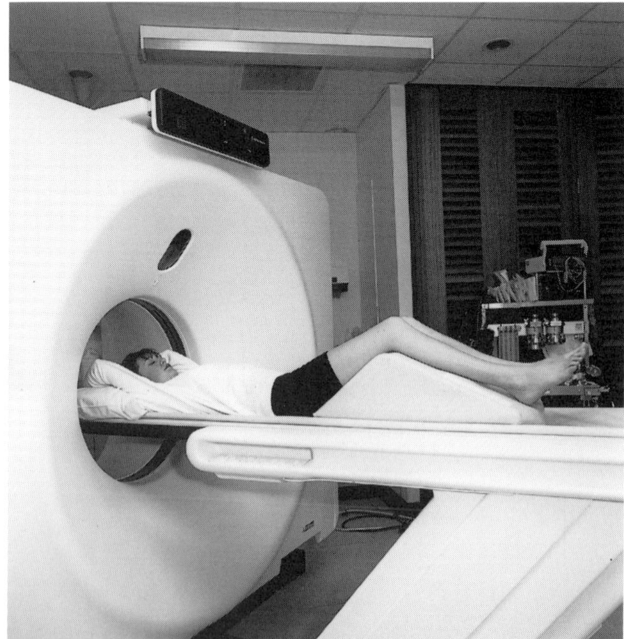

**Figure 10.36c** Patient and equipment

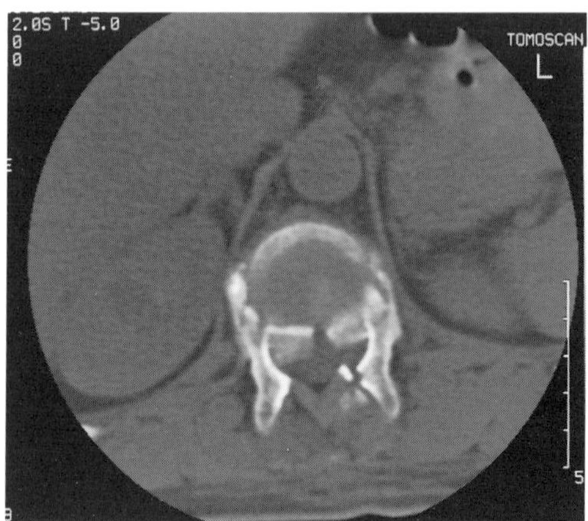


**Figure 10.36d** Transaxial image showing a fracture of T12

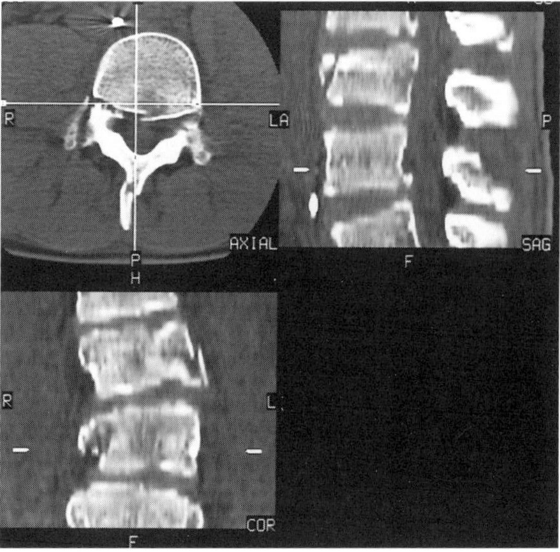


**Figure 10.36e** Composite image showing coronal and sagittal reformatted images of fractures involving L3 and L4

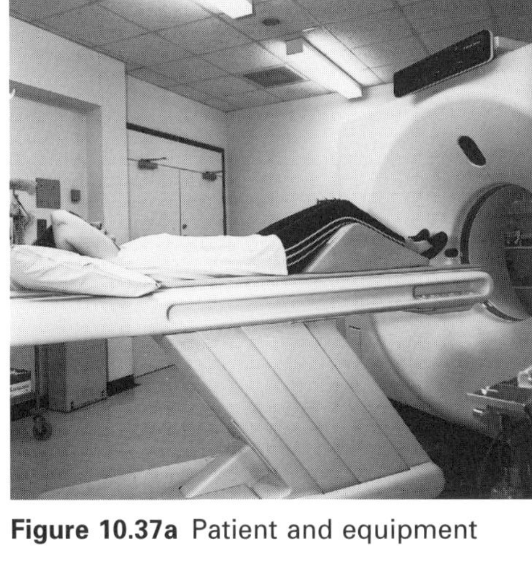

**Figure 10.37a** Patient and equipment

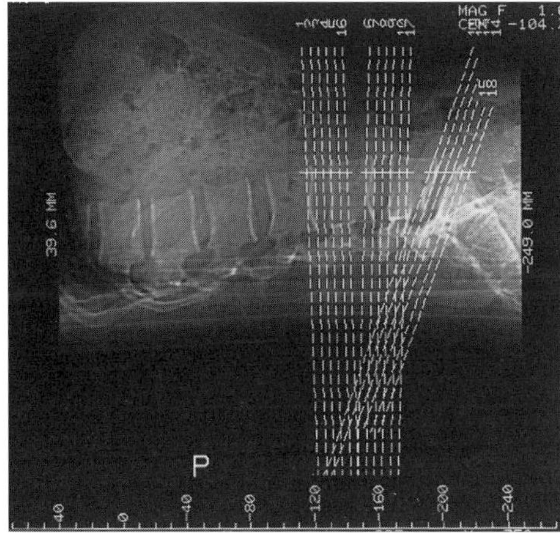


**Figure 10.37b** Scan projection radiograph showing scan levels and gantry angulations for the disc spaces, L3/4, L4/5 and L5/S1

## Lumbar spine

*Position of patient and imaging modality*
The patient lies supine, feet first on the scanner table, with the arms resting on the pillow beside the head and the knees flexed over an angled pad to reduce the lumbar curvature. The median sagittal plane is perpendicular to the table top. Using alignments to aid positioning the table is moved and the patient's position adjusted until the scan reference point is at the level of the xiphisternum.

The scanner table height is adjusted to bring the coronal alignment height at the level of the mid-axillary line.

*Imaging procedure*
A lateral scan projection radiograph is obtained, starting 5 cm above and ending 28 cm below the scan reference point to include the L5/S1 junction. From this image continuous 5 mm sections are prescribed through the relevant area, either in a block or parallel to the intervertebral disc.

If spiral scanning options are available, these images may be acquired with a volume acquisition, using a 5 mm slice thickness and 5 mm table increments, but with a 3 mm reconstruction index to give overlapping sections. The acquired data may be manipulated to produce planar reformations or 3D reconstructions.

*Contrast medium and injection data*
Intravenous contrast enhanced images may be required either to delineate a tumour mass further or to differentiate between fibrosis and remaining disc tissue in postoperative recurrent disc disease. In the former, scanning can commence after 60 ml of the contrast medium has been administered and in the latter after 80 ml has been administered. Contrast may be administered either by hand injection or more precisely by a pressure injector.

| *Volume* | *Concentration* | *Flow rate* |
|---|---|---|
| 100 ml | 300–370 mgI/ml | 2 ml/s or hand injection |

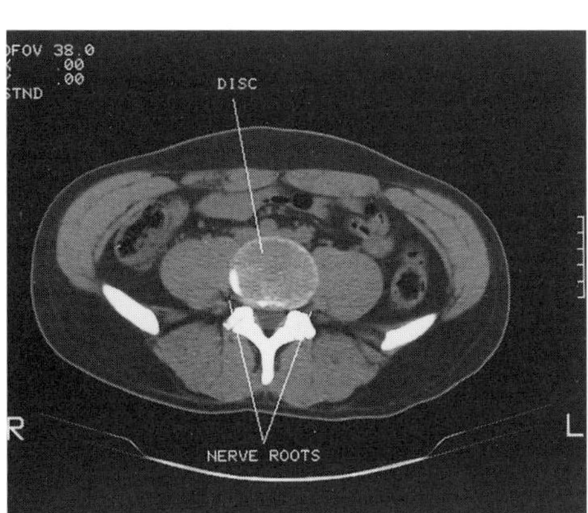


**Figure 10.37c** Transaxial image at the level of L4/5 showing intervertebral disc and nerve roots

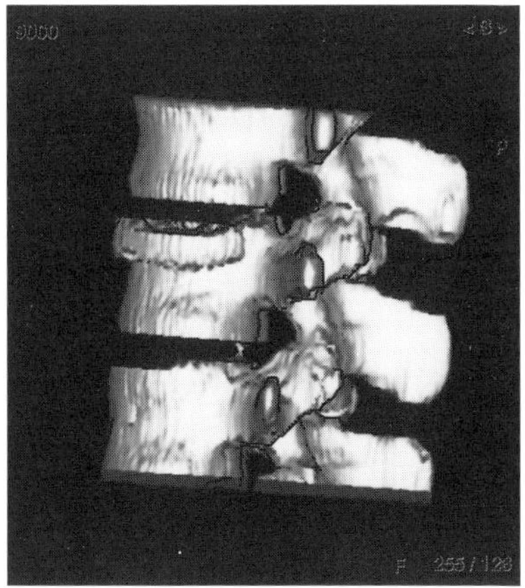

**Figure 10.37d** 3D reformatted image showing a fracture to the body of third lumbar vertebra

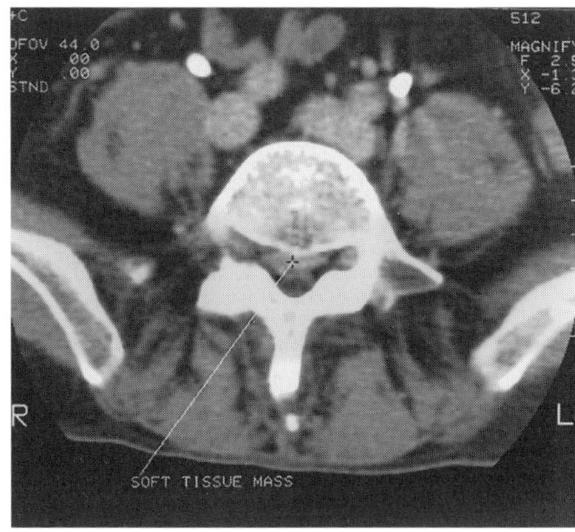


**Figure 10.37e** Post-contrast enhanced image showing a soft tissue mass in the spinal canal

# 10 Vertebral Column

## Myelography

Myelography is the radiographic investigation of the spinal canal. It requires the injection of a water-soluble, non-ionic contrast agent into the subarachnoid space, usually via a lumbar puncture (see page 51).

The contrast agent mixes with the cerebrospinal fluid as it flows along the subarachnoid spaces. By tilting the imaging table into the various positions, the full extent of the spinal cord and nerve roots can be examined. It is recommended that cervical and thoracic myelography be carried out at specialised neuroradiology centres with immediate access to CT and only if MRI is unavailable or contra-indicated (e.g. pacemaker in situ).

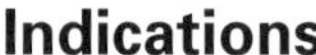

### Indications

Trauma, space-occupying lesions, syringomyelia, prolapsed intervertebral discs with associated nerve root entrapment.

### After-care of patient

Headache may occur up to 12 h after myelography. Patients are advised to sit upright for several hours after the procedure and to sleep on raised pillows. Fluids should not be restricted.

### Position of patient and imaging modality

The patient lies prone on the imaging table. A support pad is placed under the abdomen to reduce lumbar lordosis. This permits easy flow of the contrast medium up the subarachnoid space towards the cervical region as the table is slowly tilted downwards from the horizontal. To prevent the contrast medium running into the intracranial subarachnoid space, the neck is extended over a firm pad with the median sagittal plane still perpendicular to the table top.

In thoracic myelography it may be necessary to position the patient in the lateral position with the median plane parallel to the table top. This straightens the spine and will allow easier flow of the contrast medium into the dorsal region. Again care must be taken to support the patient's head and neck on a high firm pad.

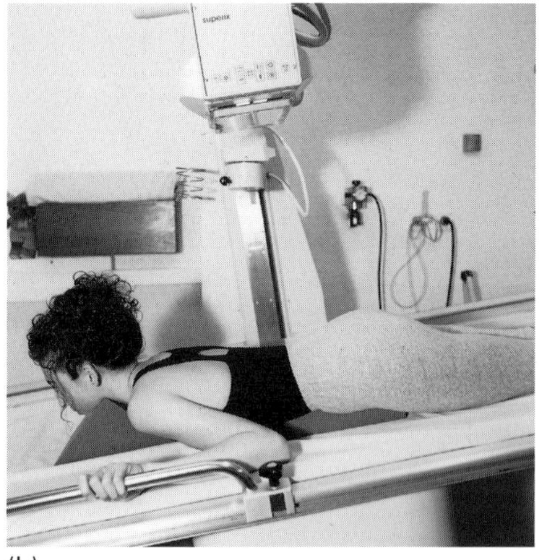

(b)

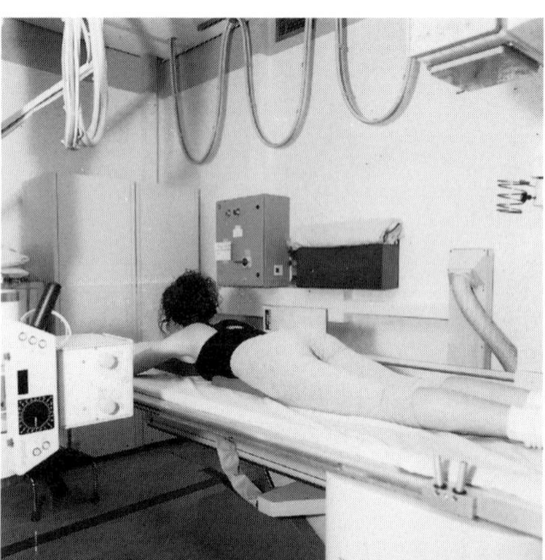

(c)

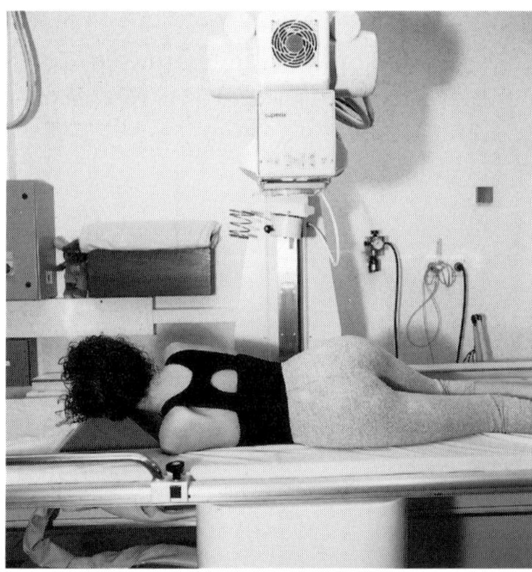

(d)

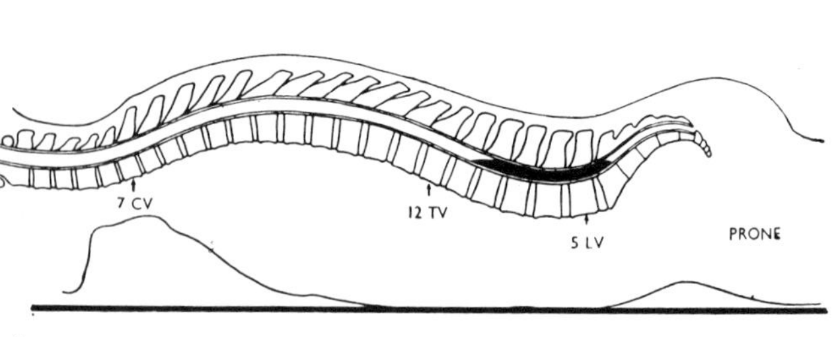


(a)

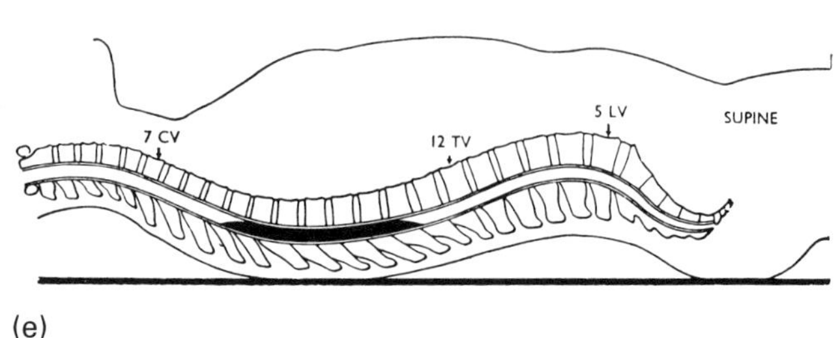


(e)



**Figure 10.38** (a) Opaque medium in subarachnoid space; (b–d) patient positioning; (e) opaque medium in subarachnoid space

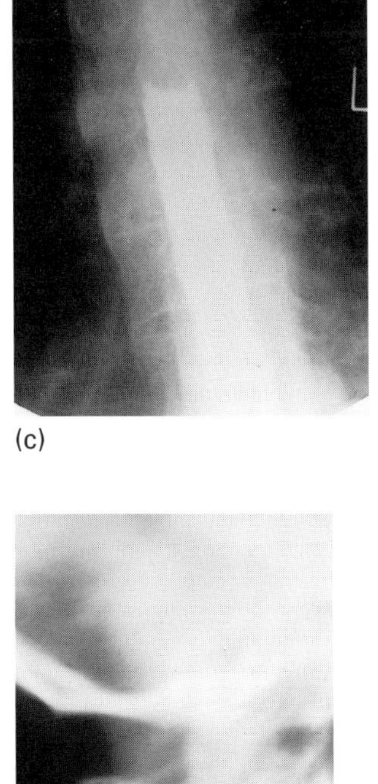

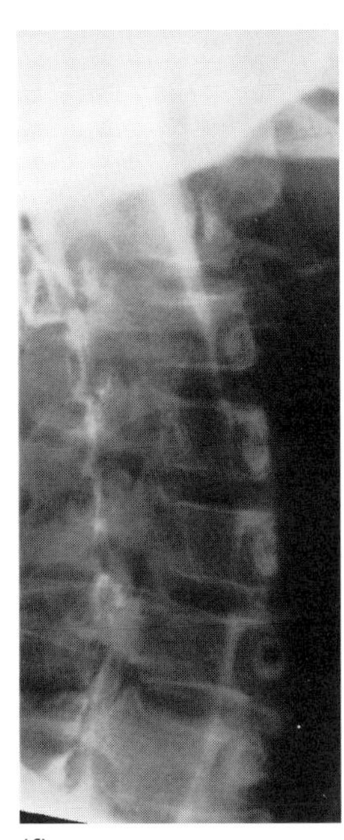

(a) (b) (c) (d) (e) (f)

## Imaging procedure

Contrast medium is introduced at the level of the intervertebral space immediately above the fourth lumbar vertebra. This is often done with the patient in position on the table or sitting erect and the spine flexed. Strict aseptic technique must be observed. The procedure described assumes the use of a remote control table with undercouch image intensification.

### Lumbar myelography

The table is raised approximately 45° from the horizontal to ensure complete filling of the thecal sac. Postero-anterior, 10–15° and 30–40° right and left anterior oblique projections are taken initially. Lateral radiographs are taken using a horizontal beam.

### Thoracic myelography

Once the contrast is within the thoracic region the patient is turned through 90° from the lateral into the supine position. The thoracic curvature of the spine acts as a reservoir, preventing the contrast medium from flowing back into the lumbar region or up into the cervical region. Anteroposterior and horizontal beam lateral images are recorded under fluoroscopic control.

### Cervical myelography

Because of the exaggerated neck extension and the associated risk of spinal cord compression this examination has to be performed as quickly as possible. By tilting the table 10–25° downwards from the horizontal, the contrast is allowed to run into the cervical region. The table is brought back to the horizontal plane and postero-anterior and anterior oblique images taken under fluoroscopic control. Horizontal beam lateral projections are required to show the foramen magnum and the thoracocervical junction.

*Contrast medium and injection data*

| *Volume* | *Concentration* | *Flow rate* |
|---|---|---|
| 10 ml | 300 mgI/ml | Lumbar puncture |

This is equivalent to 3 g of iodine and is the maximum recommended intrathecal dose.

**Figure 10.39** (a,b) PA and lateral lumbar images showing (a) L4/5 disc lesion, and (b) posterior disc; (c,d) PA and lateral thoracic spine images showing spinal block from a meningioma; (e,f) PA and oblique images of the cervical spine with expansion of the cord (syringomyelia)

# 10 Central Nervous System

## Orbits

### Bony orbit

The orbit is a pyramid-shaped bony cavity formed by 7 bones of the skull. It has four walls, a base (orbital margin) and an apex (optic canal). It contains the eyeball and associated muscles, vessels and nerves, together with part of the lacrimal apparatus. The orbital margin is formed by the frontal maxillary and zygomatic bones. The superior border is marked by the superior orbital foramen (notch) which transmits supraorbital vessels and nerves.

### Boundaries

The lateral wall is formed by parts of the zygomatic and sphenoid bones and is the thickest. The medial wall is formed by parts of the maxilla, lacrimal, ethmoid and sphenoid bones and is very thin. It is marked anteriorly by the lacrimal groove.

The inferior wall (floor) also forms the roof of the maxillary sinus. It is formed by parts of the maxilla, zygomatic and palatine bones. The superior wall of the orbit (roof) is formed by parts of the frontal and sphenoid bones.

### Foramen

The superior orbital fissure is situated posteriorly in the sphenoid bone between the lateral wall and roof of the orbit. It transmits the oculomotor, trochlear, abducent and ophthalmic branch of the trigeminal nerve and the ophthalmic veins.

The inferior orbital fissure is situated between the greater wing of sphenoid and the maxilla at the junction of the lateral wall and floor. It transmits the maxillary branch of the trigeminal nerve and the infraorbital artery.

The optic foramen or canal, which is situated at the apex of the orbit in the sphenoid bone, transmits the optic nerve and the ophthalmic artery. The optic nerves from both eyeballs intercommunicate at the optic chiasma which is situated in the middle cranial fossa anterior to the sella turcica. The optic tract then passes posteriorly through the lateral geniculate bodies to the visual cortex in the occipital lobe of the cerebrum.

### Muscles and movements

The six muscles which move the eyeball comprise the superior, inferior, medial and lateral rectus, together with the superior and inferior oblique muscles. Together they are responsible for elevation, depression, abduction, adduction and rotational movements of the eyeball.

This is pictured diagrammatically opposite.

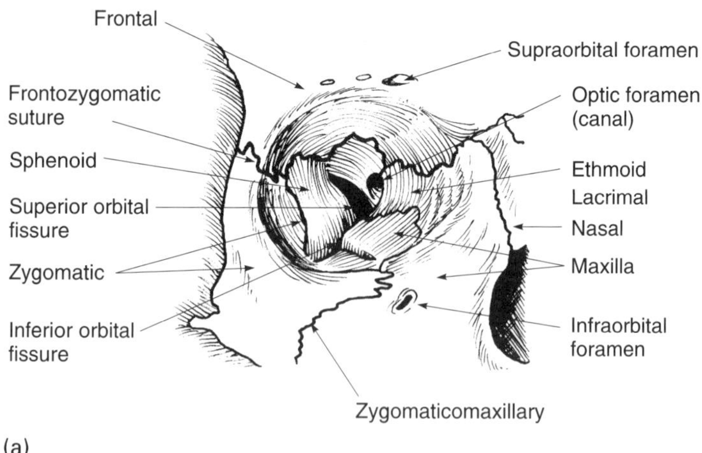


(a)

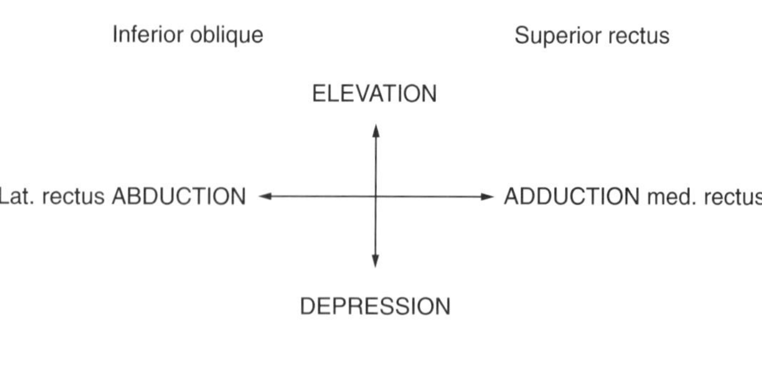


(b)

**Figure 10.40** (a) Right orbit anterior view; (b) muscles and movements of the eyeball

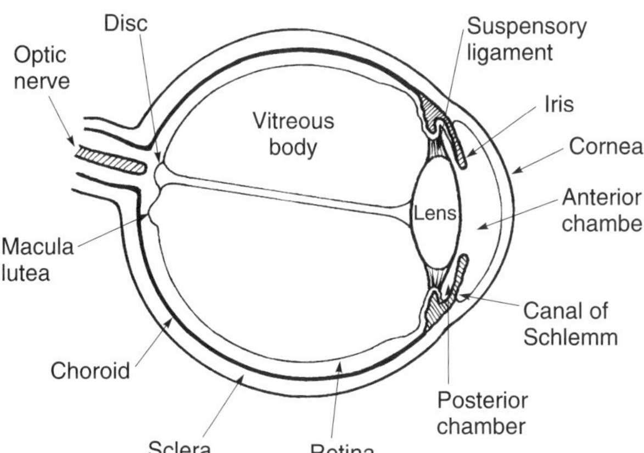


**Figure 10.41a** Schematic diagram of the eye

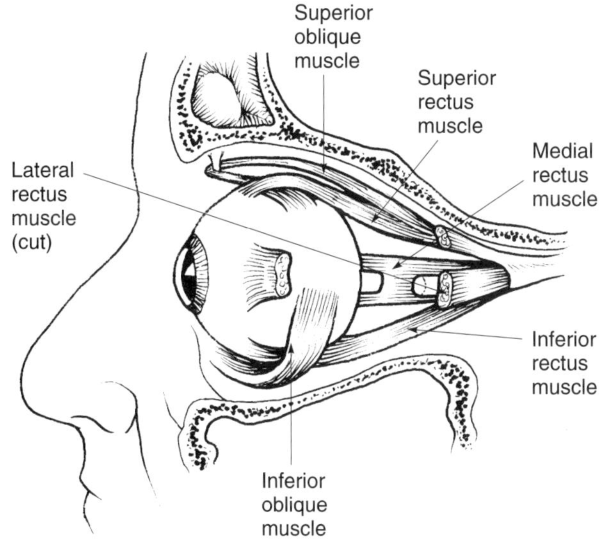


**Figure 10.41b** Extrinsic muscles of the eye

## The eye

The eye is the special sense organ of sight. It is situated in the orbital cavity, surrounded by adipose tissue which affords protection from trauma.

It is almost spherical with an anterior bulge, comprising three layers: an outer fibrous layer, a middle vascular layer and an inner nervous layer. It contains three substances: the aqueous humour, the lens and the vitreous humour.

The outer fibrous layer forms a complete sphere, the anterior one-sixth is known as the cornea and the posterior five-sixths the sclera. It has no blood supply but derives its nourishment from lymph.

The middle vascular layer forms nine-tenths of a sphere incomplete anteriorly. It comprises the choroid, ciliary body and the iris.

The innermost layer forms three quarters of a sphere (posteriorly) and is known as the retina. This has an outer pigmented layer and an inner nervous layer. It contains special cells designed for vision – rods and cones. The optic disc (or blind spot) is that part of the retina where the optic nerve enters the eyeball.

The aqueous humour is a clear watery fluid which fills the anterior chamber. The lens is a biconvex transparent structure assisting in the focusing of light onto the retina and separates the anterior and posterior chambers. The vitreous humour occupies the posterior chamber and together with the aqueous humour acts as a refractive medium, maintaining the shape of the eyeball, and helps to hold the retina in contact with the choroid.

The optic nerve is formed at the optic disc and leaves the orbital cavity via the optic foramen to the middle cranial fossa.

### Recommended imaging procedures

Many conventional radiographic procedures such as tomography have now been replaced by ultrasound, CT scanning and MRI.

Because of the superficial position of the eyeball within the orbital cavity, ultrasound is used routinely to detect both normal and pathological intraocular structures.

Both CT and MRI are used to examine the orbit and its contents. MRI has the major advantage of no radiation dose penalty, but is contraindicated in cases of suspected metallic intraocular foreign body. Computed tomography is the preferred technique to delineate fractures and may be complementary to MRI in demonstrating bony destruction due to tumour.

# 10 Orbits

## Computed Tomography

Computed tomographic sections may be obtained in either the coronal or transaxial planes. Coronal imaging shows the intraorbital structures in cross-section and may be the preferred method to evaluate the superior and inferior aspects of the cavity, including the bony roof and floor. The paranasal sinuses are also well demonstrated.

Transaxial imaging is used routinely in patients either unable to maintain the coronal position (paediatrics, geriatrics and trauma cases) or who possess a large number of dental fillings which would severely degrade the image. Positioning in the transaxial plane is critical. The scans obtained must be parallel to the anthropological baseline to produce a section showing the globe, the lens, the optic nerve, the medial and lateral recti muscles and the posterior clinoid processes of the sphenoid bone. This is achieved by either raising the chin 18–20° cranially or by angling the gantry accordingly. The digital data from the transaxial sections are normally reformatted to produce images in the coronal and paraxial plane.

In both techniques, 3 mm contiguous sections are prescribed to cover the entire orbital cavity. Further 5 mm sections may be necessary beyond the orbits to evaluate either intracranial tumour spread from an orbital lesion or conversely intraorbital spread from an intracranial lesion.

The presence of intraorbital fat provides inherent image contrast between the anatomical structures and may limit the use of contrast enhanced sections to those lesions with suspected intracranial extension.

### Indications

Trauma (including location of foreign bodies), exophthalmos, tumour, ocular lesions, orbital inflammatory disease, vascular anomalies, bony anomalies.

### Coronal plane imaging

**Position of patient and imaging modality**

*Method 1*

The patient lies prone on the scanner table. The neck is extended and the chin rests on the head support. Ideally the coronal plane is positioned parallel to the scan plane, with the median sagittal plane and the transaxial plane perpendicular to the scan plane. The patient is then moved into the scanner and positioned so that the scan reference point is at the level of the external auditory meatus. This position may be uncomfortable for some patients and it may be impossible to extend the neck adequately to obtain the optimum coronal plane. This can be compensated for by angulation of the gantry.

This position may be associated with respiratory movement artefact.

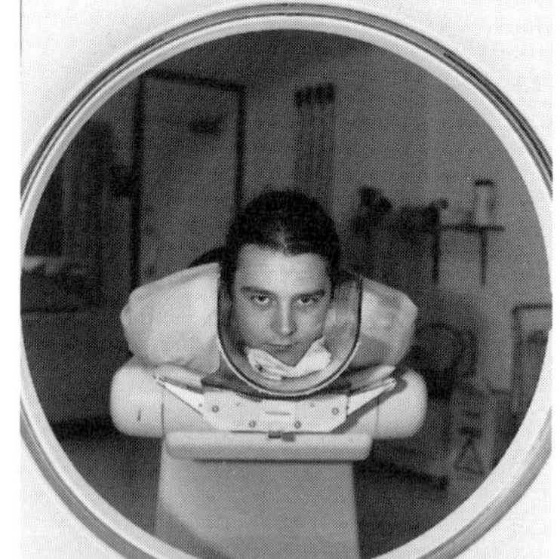

**Figure 10.42a** Method 1 – patient prone

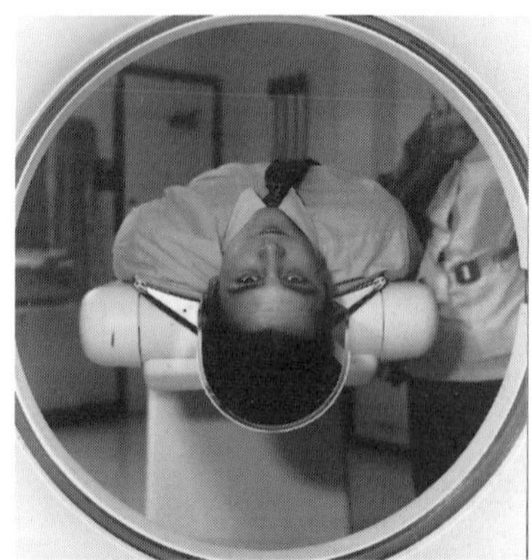

**Figure 10.42b** Method 2 – patient supine

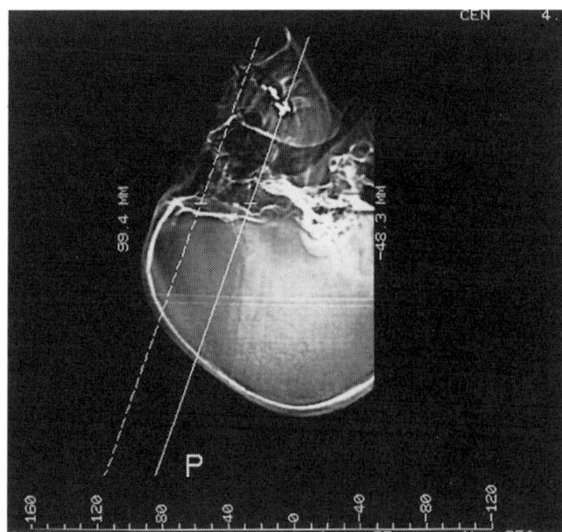


**Figure 10.42c** Scan projection radiograph showing start and end locations with gantry angled

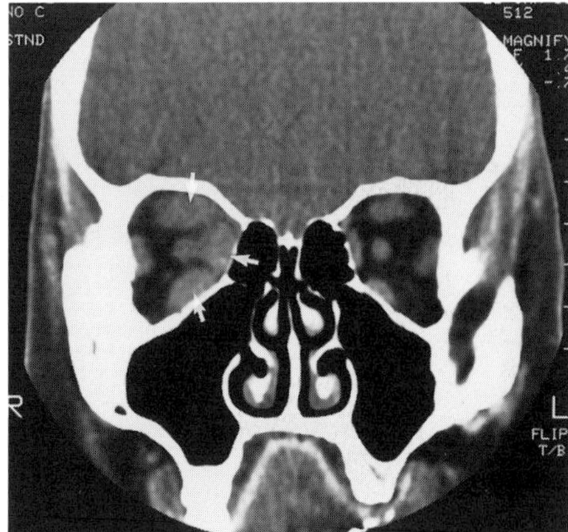


**Figure 10.42d** Coronal image on patient with dysthyroid eye disease (enlarged muscles)

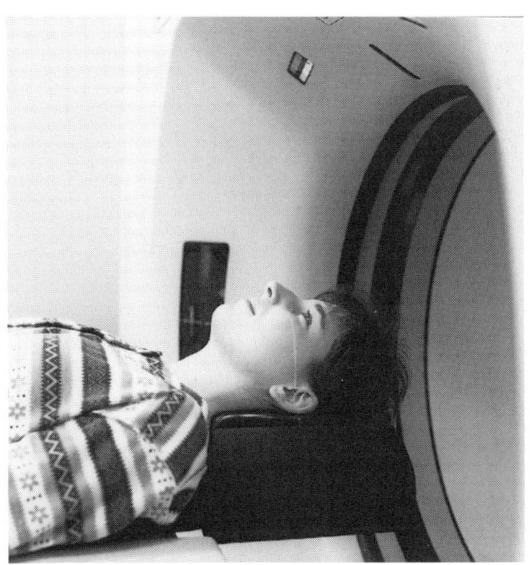

Figure 10.43a Transaxial method

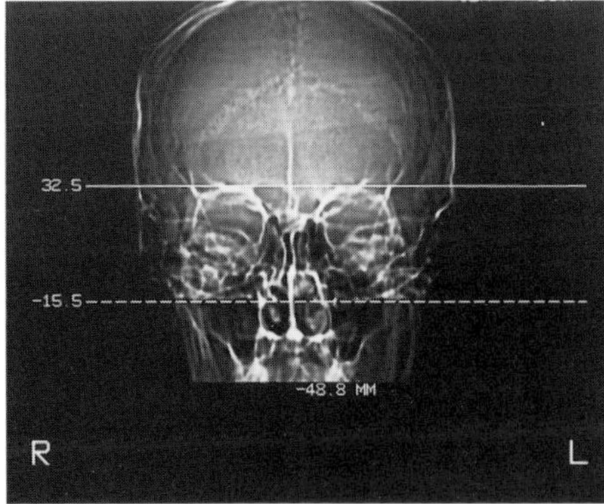


Figure 10.43b PA scan projection radiograph showing start and end locations

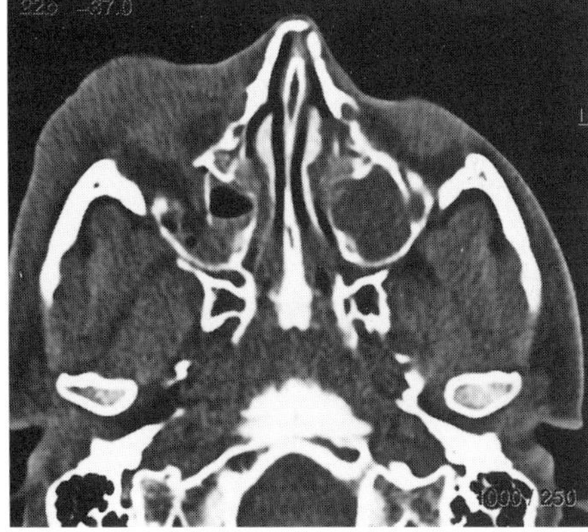

Figure 10.43c Transaxial image showing fracture through the bony orbits

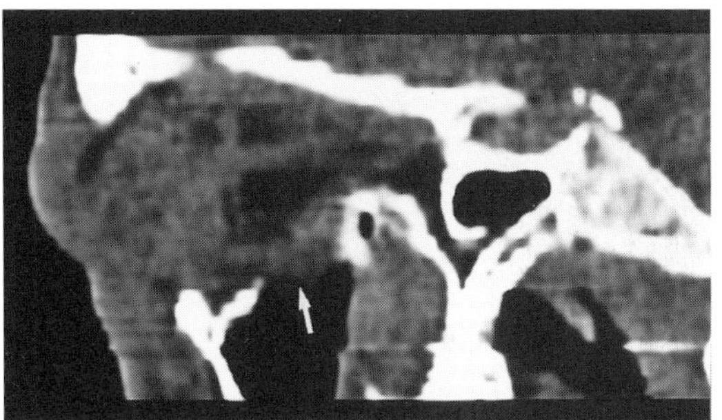

Figure 10.43d Reformatted image along the optic nerve showing a right-sided 'blow-out' fracture

*Method 2*
The patient lies supine on the scanner table. The neck is extended and the vertex of the skull supported on a coronal head rest. The coronal plane is positioned parallel to the scan plane and the gantry angled to compensate for any positioning difficulties. Although still uncomfortable for the patient, this position is tolerated better than method 1 and results in less movement artefact.

**Imaging procedure**
A lateral scan projection radiograph is obtained starting 10 cm anteriorly and ending 4 cm posterior to the external auditory meatus. From this image 3 mm contiguous sections are prescribed through the entire orbital cavity from the anterior aspect of the upper orbital margin to the orbital apex. If spiral scanning options are available, these images may be acquired with a volume acquisition, using a 3 mm slice thickness and 3 mm table increments, but with a 2 mm reconstruction index to give overlapping sections.

## Transaxial plane imaging

**Position of patient and imaging modality**
The patient lies supine on the scanning table, head resting in the transaxial head support. The anthropological baseline is positioned parallel to the transverse alignment light and the median sagittal plane is perpendicular to the table and coincident with the sagittal alignment light. To ensure that the skull is symmetrically positioned, the external auditory meati must be equidistant from the head support and the interorbital (interpuillary) line parallel to the scan plane. The head is secured in position using Velcro straps. The patient is moved into the scanner and the table is raised to bring the scan reference point to the level of the external auditory meatus.

**Imaging procedure**
A postero-anterior or lateral scan projection radiograph is obtained, starting 10 cm above and ending 10 cm below the baseline. From this image, 3 mm contiguous sections are prescribed through the entire orbit from the superior orbital margin to the maxillary sinuses. Spiral scanning may also be employed using the same parameters as that described for coronal plane imaging.

**Image analysis**
Using the digital data from the transaxial images, a set of coronal reformations through both orbits and a set of paraxial reformations along the optic nerve are obtained.

# 10 Orbits

## Magnetic Resonance Imaging

At the time of writing MRI in orbital imaging has yet to achieve its full potential. Routine imaging is done with a convential head coil. A combination of $T_1$ and $T_2$ weighted spin-echo sequences with a section width of 3–5 mm are prescribed in several anatomical planes. Small-diameter surface coils are currently being evaluated. These can be monocular or binocular in design, the latter having the advantage of imaging both orbits, enabling comparisons to be made. The surface coils give an increase in the signal-to-noise ratio, permitting narrower sections to be prescribed. This increases spatial resolution without an increase in scan time which would increase the risk of motion artefacts. However, there is always a signal drop-off proportional to the distance from the surface coil which may prevent either the orbital apex or intracranial lesions from being fully assessed. To overcome this, a series of $T_2$ weighted images are acquired using the conventional head coil.

Fat suppression techniques are also under review, an example of which is the short time inversion recovery (STIR) sequence. This sequence adds together $T_1$ and $T_2$ while suppressing the signal from orbital fat. Because pathology has long $T_1$ and $T_2$ relaxation times, the contrast between normal and abnormal tissues is greatly increased, leading to a greater sensitivity in detecting disease.

Gradient-echo sequences may be useful in assessing flow, but can also be used to produce high-resolution 3D images which can be reconstructed in different anatomical planes.

Most image degradation in MRI is related to patient movement. To minimise this in orbital scanning, the patient must be advised of the length of the investigation and the importance of keeping steady. It is usual practice to ask the patient to fix the gaze on a particular reference point during image acquisition. Other image artefacts can occur from tattoos along the eyelid and certain eye make-up, such as mascara, which should therefore be removed prior to scanning.

### Indications

Exophthalmos, ocular lesions, orbital inflammatory disease, orbital tumours, vascular anomalies.

### Contraindications

These centre on the presence of metallic objects. Patients with surgical aneurysmal clips must not be scanned. Torque forces on the clips from the magnetic field can result in movement of the clips and rupture of the vessel walls. New non-ferromagnetic clips are now available, but it is imperative that the operator ascertains which type of clip has been used before scanning a postoperative patient.

Foreign bodies in the eye either due to occupational injury, other trauma or surgery are also a contraindication, as are patients with cardiac pacemakers and cochlear implants.

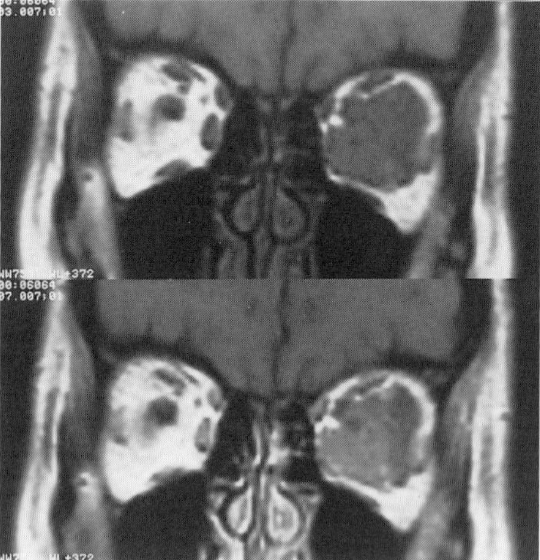

**Figure 10.44a** Coronal STIR fast spin-echo $T_2$ weighted image showing a large mass in the left orbit

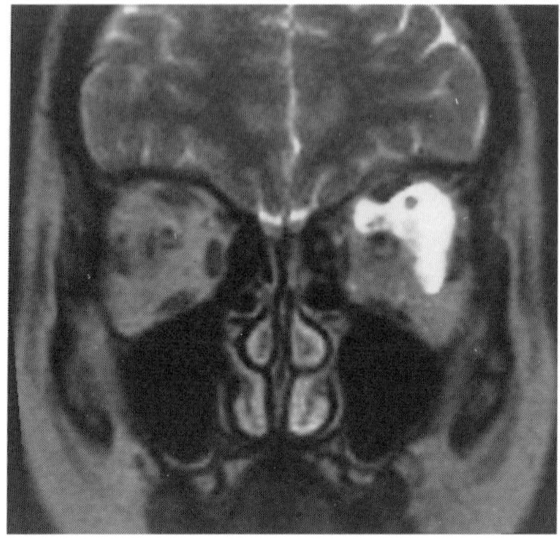

**Figure 10.44b** Pre- and post-contrast coronal images of the same patient in (a). An intermediate increase in signal in the left orbit in the post-contrast image is shown

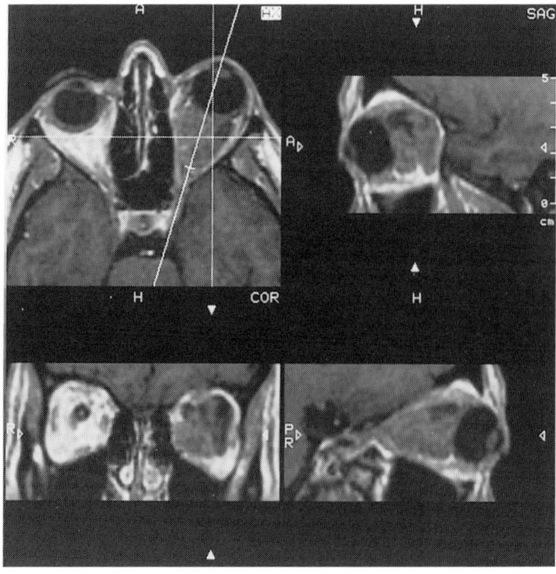


**Figure 10.44c** SPGR 3D image set showing sagittal and oblique images of the left orbit

## Magnetic Resonance Imaging

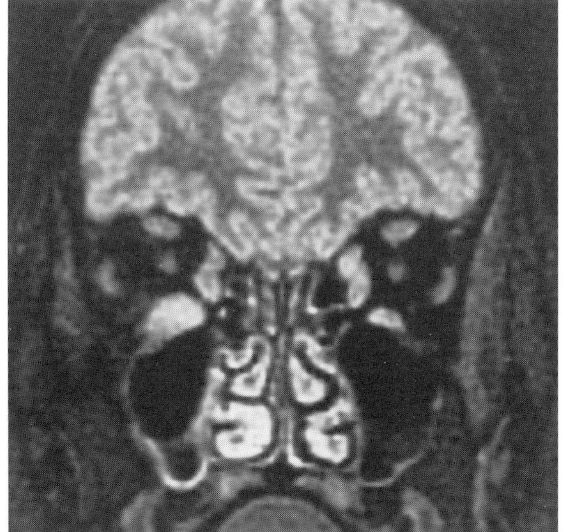

(a)

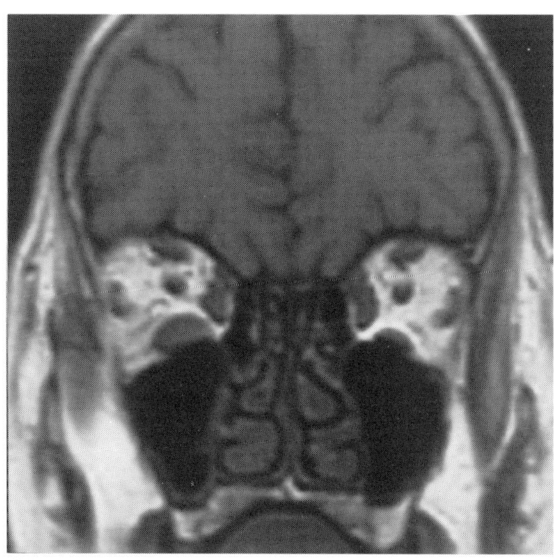

(b)

**Figure 10.45** Coronal images: (a) spin-echo $T_1$ weighted; (b) $T_2$ (STIR) showing increased muscle bulk in a patient with dysthyroid disease

### Position of patient and imaging modality

The patient lies supine on the scanner table, head resting in the head support of the head coil. Positioning is aided by external alignment lights. The median sagittal plane is parallel to the sagittal alignment light and the transaxial alignment light parallel to the anthropological baseline. The table is now adjusted until the external reference point is at the outer canthus of the eye. From this position the patient and head coil assembly are driven the fixed distance to the isocentre of the magnet.

### Imaging procedure

Initial localiser scans are obtained in the sagittal, coronal and transaxial planes. From these images there are two scanning methods of choice – either $T_1$ weighted images in the transaxial and coronal planes or a $T_1$ weighted 3D volume acquisition with subsequent reconstruction in any anatomical plane can be prescribed.

Additional images may include either a STIR sequence or a $T_2$ weighted sequence, with the fat saturation option in the appropriate anatomical plane.

Intravenous contrast enhancement may be necessary to delineate tumour extent further. A $T_1$ weighted sequence must be used, preferably with fat suppression if available.

To complete the examination, a further series of $T_2$ weighted sections may be required to exclude intracranial extension.

*Contrast medium and injector data*

| *Volume* | *Pharmaceutical* | *Flow rate* |
|---|---|---|
| 0.2 ml/kg body weight | Gadolinium DTPA | Hand injection |

**Table 10.5 Imaging parameters**

| *Imaging plane* | *Imaging sequence* | *TR* | *TE* | *Field of view* (cm) | *No. of NEX* | *Slice width/ gap* (mm) | *Matrix (horizontal – vertical)* |
|---|---|---|---|---|---|---|---|
| Transaxial or coronal | Spin-echo $T_1$ weighted | 500 | 20 | 25 | 4 | 3–5/1 | 160 × 256 |
| 3D volume (transaxial) with flip angle 45° | SPGR | 50 | 12 | 25 | 1 | 1.25 (no gap) | 160 × 256 |
| Coronal | STIR | 1500 | 25/114 | 25 | 2 | 5/1 | 160 × 256 |
| Coronal | Fast spin-echo $T_2$ weighted | 5000 | 102 | 25 | 4 | 5/1 | 160 × 256 |

## Ultrasound

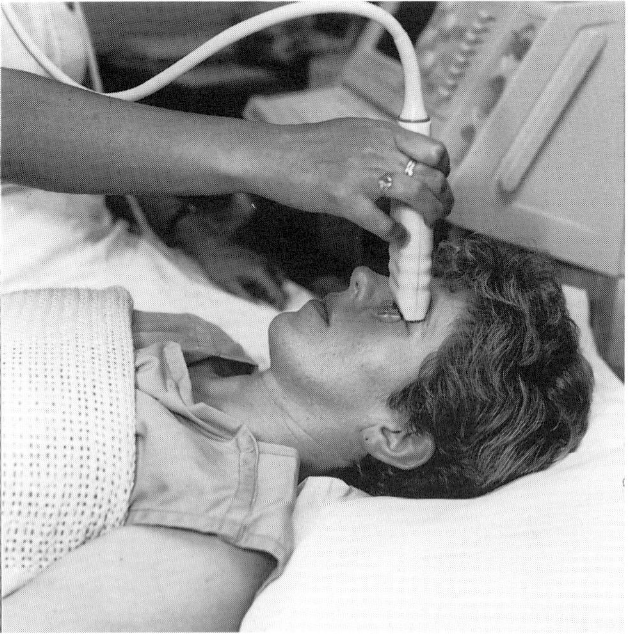
**Figure 10.46** Patient and ultrasound probe

Ultrasound is a fast non-invasive method of examining the soft tissue structures of the orbits using B-mode real-time scanning. It has no role, however, in the examination of the bony structures since bone does not act as a medium for the transference of ultrasound waves.

It is the examination of choice in investigating the eye for possible haemorrhage, retinal detachment or tumours. Because the eye is a superficial structure, an electronic linear array transducer should be used to give good skin contact and provide a wide field of view in the near field. A sector probe can, however, be used provided that a suitable stand-off material is applied across the eyes. A 7.5–10 MHz frequency is used to give good resolution with adequate penetration to the 4 cm depth that is needed in this examination. A broad bandwidth provides maximum resolution over a range of frequencies between 5 and 10 MHz. Apart from a hard copy facility, a video recording system is also required to record movement of the eye in real time for future viewing. Colour Doppler flow can also be performed in investigation of vascular disease and tumour blood supply (see Plates 17 and 18).

### Indications

Retinal detachment, localisation of foreign bodies, assessment of the eye when the lens and/or the aqueous and vitreous substances are opaque and do not permit direct examination with an ophthalmoscope, and suspicion of intraocular or extraocular tumours.

### Position of patient and imaging modality

The patient is examined supine, with the head resting on a low pillow. The patient is asked to keep the affected eye still and to focus on a fixed point on the ceiling. With a small amount of gel placed on the transducer face, the patient is asked to close both eyes and the transducer is then placed gently on the eyelid of the eye to demonstrate a mid-transverse section of the eye.

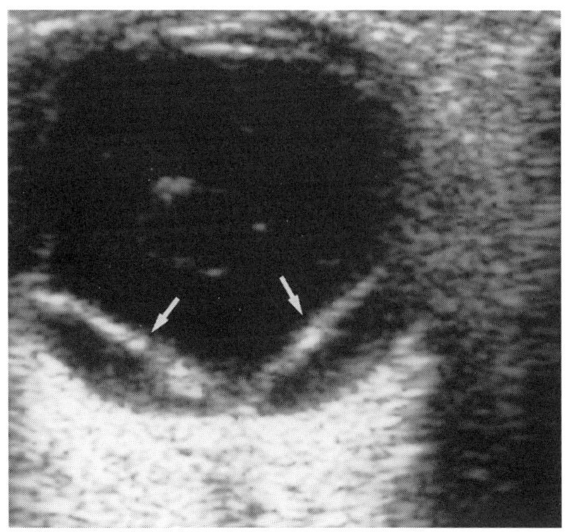

**Figure 10.47a** Chronic retinal detachment

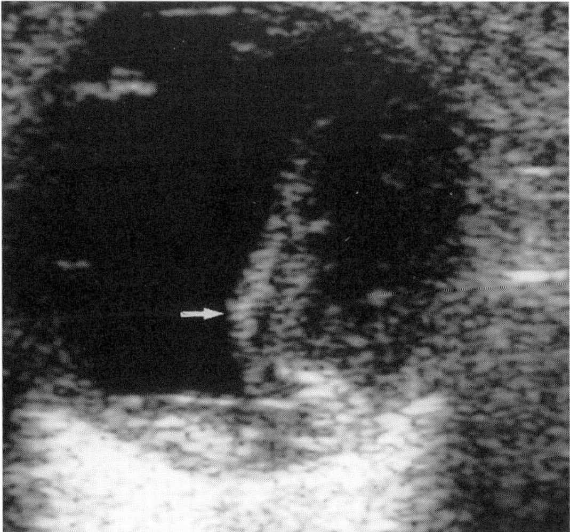

**Figure 10.47b** Intravitreal haemorrhage

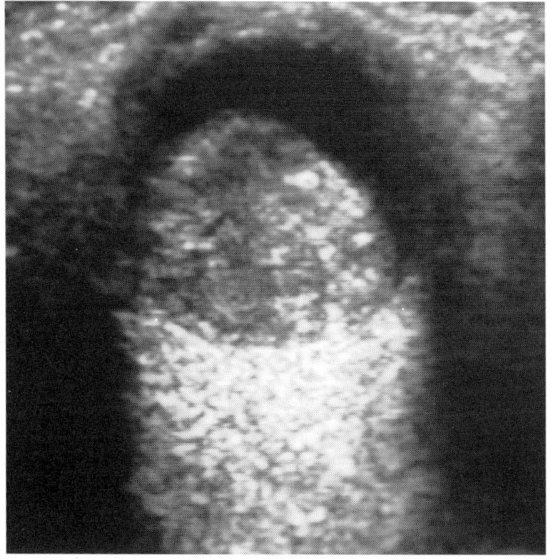

**Figure 10.47c** Intraglobal metastases from primary bronchial carcinoma

## Imaging procedure

During this procedure both eyes are examined for comparison. The imaging protocol consists of a series of static images demonstrating anatomy and pathology and a video recording of dynamic eye movements showing any detached membrane or floaters within the globe.

Initially, a series of transverse scans of the entire eye are acquired, demonstrating on each image both anterior and posterior borders of the eye and the area posterior to the eye. From the initial scanning position the probe is gently moved and angled both cranially and caudally, with the patient encouraged to keep the eye motionless during the procedure. If the patient has difficulty keeping the eye still, images can be acquired using a cine loop facility if this is available on the ultrasound machine.

When static image acquisition is completed the video recorder is switched to record mode for real-time dynamic image recording of eye movements. At the commencement of this procedure a mid-transverse scan is acquired, with the patient's affected eye held in a fixed position. With the transducer held in a static position the patient is then asked to move the eye gently as if looking first to the left and then to the right, in turn. On playback of this recording, movement in the interior of the eye is observed, with permanent images acquired of any of the frozen images in the dynamic recording.

## Image analysis

Demonstrated on a transverse section is the eyelid, cornea, anterior chamber, optic nerve and posterior part of the eye. Both eyes should be demonstrated as roughly spherical structures. Each optic nerve should be demonstrated as a hypoechoic structure approximately 2–3 mm thick, directed medially from the posterior aspect of the globe.

A detached retina is diagnosed if the membrane is firmly attached to the optic disc. Vitreous haemorrhage is demonstrated as an echogenic mass within the eyeball which is separate to the wall and moves as the eye moves. Tumours are echogenic masses attached to the wall of the eyeball which move with the eye as it moves.

## Dacrocystography

Dacrocystography is the radiographic examination of the lacrimal system following the introduction of a contrast agent.

The lacrimal system comprises the lacrimal gland, which secretes tears, the lacrimal sac and the ducts through which the tears pass into the nasal cavity.

The lacrimal gland lies anteriorly in the upper outer quadrant of the orbit and communicates with the lacrimal sac via the lacrimal canaliculi. Tears wash over the surface of the eye and drain through the lacrimal canaliculi into the lacrimal sac through two openings, the puncta lacrimalia, which are situated on the medial aspects of the upper and lower eyelids. The lacrimal sac drains into the nasolacrimal duct which runs vertically through the lateral nasal wall on the medial aspect of the maxillary antrum. The nasolacrimal duct opens into the nasal cavity below the inferior nasal conchus.

The examination is performed using undercouch image intensification, with digital imaging equipment to facilitate production of subtracted images. Alternatively, the examination may be performed using a dedicated skull unit, with a focal spot size 0.3 mm to facilitate macroradiography.

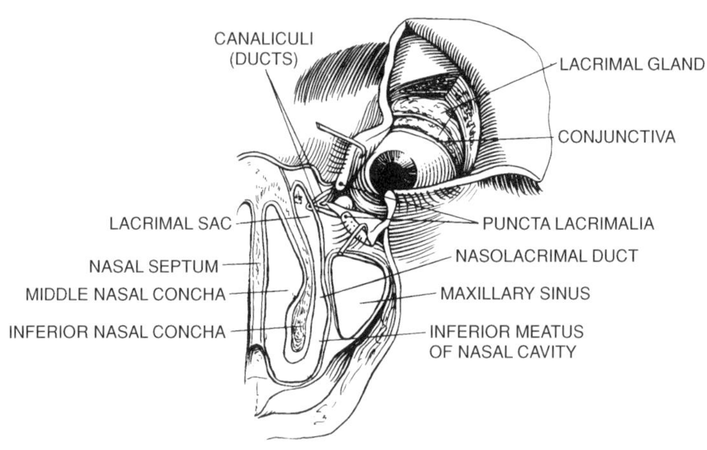


(a)

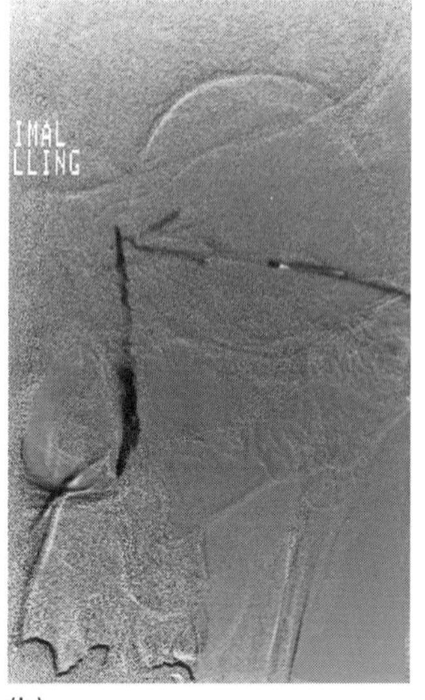

(b)

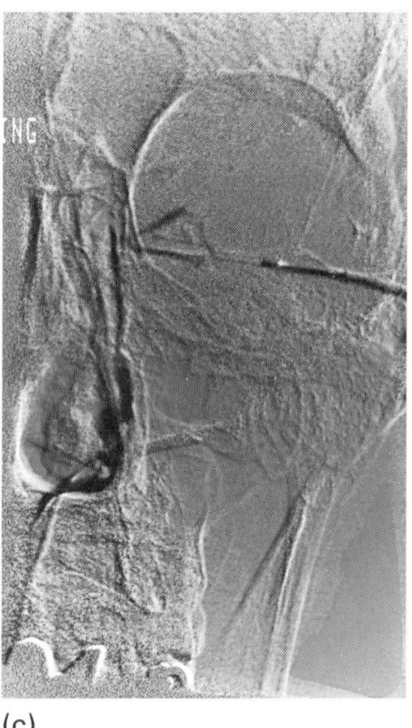

(c)

**Figure 10.48** (a) Lacrimal apparatus (left eye); (b,c) Normal examination showing (b) filling and (c) emptying of the left nasolacrimal duct

### Indications

Dacrocystography is performed in cases of epiphora to demonstrate the presence and extent of obstruction.

### Patient preparation

A small quantity of local anaesthetic is dropped into the inner canthus of the eye prior to cannulation of the punctum lacrimalia.

### Imaging procedure

The examination is performed with the patient supine on the imaging couch. The lower punctum is dilated using a dilator and the tip of a lacrimal cannula (or fine catheter) is inserted through the punctum into the lacrimal canaliculus. Using a 5 ml syringe, 1–2 ml of a non-ionic water-soluble contrast medium (350 mgI/ml) is introduced. The injection is terminated when the contrast agent is observed spilling into the nasopharynx or when obstruction is demonstrated. The contrast agent is usually kept in a refrigerator prior to the examination, in order to increase its viscosity. Images in the mento-occipital position are acquired, with the aid of fluoroscopy, immediately following the injection, to show filling and emptying of the nasolacrimal duct. A mask image is usually taken at the start of the procedure to allow real-time subtraction. Both sides may be examined simultaneously.

The eye is covered for approximately 1 h after conclusion of the examination to prevent the ingress of foreign material.

### Position of patient and imaging modality

The patient lies supine on the imaging couch. The chin is raised and the head adjusted so that the median sagittal plane is perpendicular to the couch top and the radiographic baseline is at 30° to bring the nasolacrimal duct parallel to the image intensifier face. The head is secured in this position with the aid of a head pad in order to eliminate patient movement and facilitate real-time subtraction.

When a skull unit is employed, a 24 × 40 cm cassette is positioned such that the focus–object distance is equal to the object–film distance. This produces a magnification factor of 2.

### Direction and centring of the X-ray beam

A vertical central ray is directed 2 cm below the inner canthus of the eye of the side under investigation.

# 11

# MISCELLANEOUS PROCEDURES

## CONTENTS

# 11 Miscellaneous Procedures

## Female Breast

The breast (mammary gland) is one of the accessory organs of the female reproductive system. The adult breasts comprise two rounded eminences situated on the anterior and lateral walls of the chest, lying superficially to the pectoral muscles and separated from them by areolar tissue and fascia. They extend from the second to the sixth rib and from the lateral border of the sternum to the mid-axillary line. The superolateral part is prolonged upwards and laterally towards the axilla to form the axillary tail. The nipple is a conical projection just below the centre of the breast, approximately corresponding to the fourth/fifth intercostal space.

The breast is composed of glandular, fibrous and fatty tissue. Its size, shape and consistency vary significantly, dependent upon patient size, shape and age. Each breast consists of a number of lobes (15–20), each of which is divided into several lobules. The lobules comprise large numbers of secretory alveoli which drain into a single lactiferous duct for each lobe, before converging towards the nipple into the ampullae before opening onto the surface. The blood supply is derived from branches of the axillary, intercostal and internal mammary arteries. The lymph drainage is shown diagrammatically opposite.

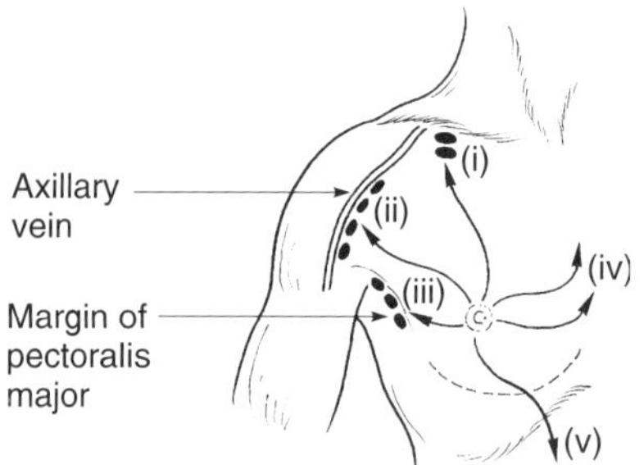


**Figure 11.1a** Schematic diagram of the lymph drainage of the breast: (i) apical axillary nodes; (ii) lateral axillary nodes; (iii) pectoral nodes; (iv) to anterior mediastinal nodes; (v) to abdominal wall

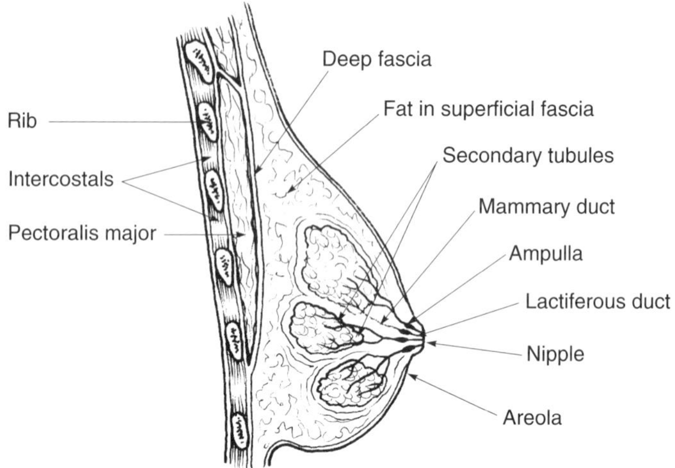


**Figure 11.1b** Profile of a breast (diagrammatic) lying against a pectoral muscle

### Recommended imaging procedures

The breasts may be examined by means of plain film radiography (mammography), ultrasound and MRI. X-ray examination of specimen breast tissue may also be employed during surgery to determine if a localised lesion has been successfully excised.

Mammography is used extensively as a primary diagnostic tool and as an effective screening method for early detection of breast cancer in the over-50 age group female population. Its sensitivity, however, is limited in dense tissue. To achieve optimum image quality the imaging system selected must provide excellent resolution at both high and low contrast, with a corresponding low radiation dose.

Ultrasound is used in preference to mammography in examining young breasts due to the amount of glandular tissue within them, which makes them too dense to be examined effectively with mammography, and as a follow-up to mammography to differentiate between a benign or malignant mass. It is also used in interventional procedures such as tissue biopsy and the drainage or aspiration of cysts. It is limited in the detection of lesions smaller than 1 cm.

The role of MRI is being developed and is used in combination with mammography to further define the nature and size of lesions and extent of disease.

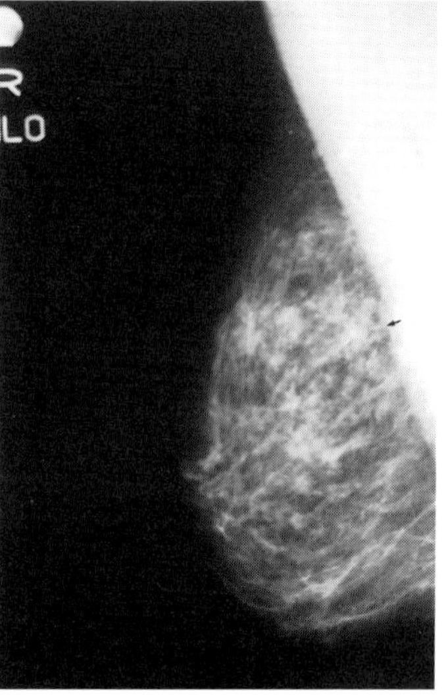


**Figure 11.1c** Example of mammogram showing a suspected lesion deep in the upper part of the breast

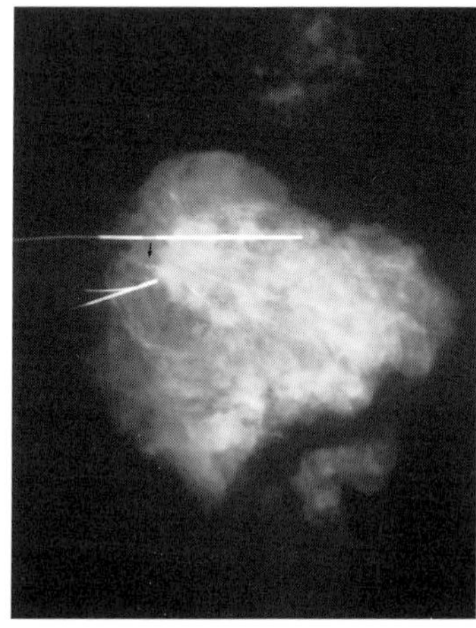

**Figure 11.1d** Radiograph of breast tissue specimen excised from suspected breast region shown in (c). Note microcalcifications consistent with intraductal carcinoma

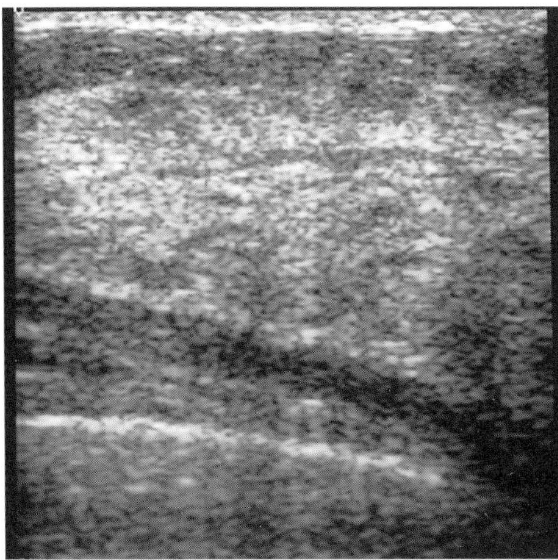

(a)

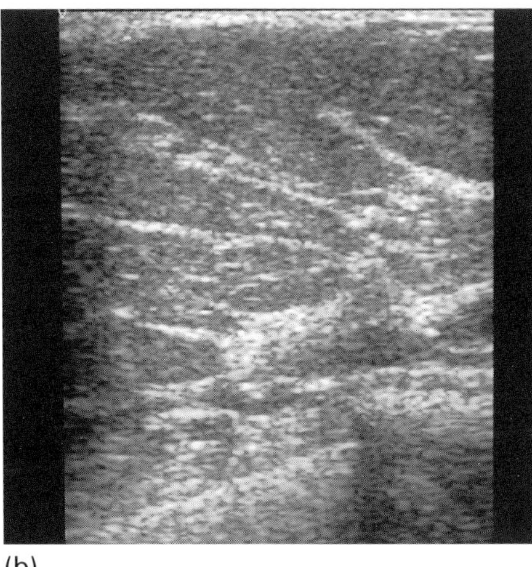

(b)

**Figure 11.2** (a,b) Typical echo patterns associated with (a) young and (b) older breast tissue. Note the younger glandular breast tissue with its often more homogeneous and bright appearance, compared with the older breast tissue which has undergone fatty replacement rendering the supporting ligaments more clearly visible

# Female Breast 11

## Ultrasound

Ultrasound is a quick non-invasive method of examining the breasts for the presence and nature of a mass, which has been found by palpation. It can determine whether a lesion has originated in the breast and whether it is cystic, solid or a mixture of cystic and solid components. It also has the advantage of being a non-ionizing investigation.

It is used in preference to mammography in examining young breasts due to the amount of glandular tissue within them. Older breasts with less glandular tissue and more fatty tissue are more easily examined with mammography than ultrasound.

With breasts differing widely in their sonographic appearance, the unaffected breast is usually examined first in order to ascertain normality for the patient.

The procedure is normally carried out using a real-time B-mode imaging with a 5–10 MHz linear array transducer. A linear transducer ensures good skin contact on the surface of the breasts compared to a curvilinear array transducer. It also provides a wider field of view in the near field, than a sector or phased array probe, in order to examine the superficial breast tissue. If a sector transducer is used, a stand-off material should be used which will enable more of the superficial tissue to be examined at one time.

The frequency chosen ensures good resolution with adequate penetration to the depth that is needed in this examination. The minimum power level is selected to reduce patient dose, while gaining adequate penetration, to examine the entire breast, back to the anterior chest wall muscles. The depth of field is set in order to demonstrate the entire breast at a reasonable magnification factor without loss of detail. The overall gain is set in order to demonstrate an even echodensity without over- or under-enhancement of echoes.

### Indications

Palpable masses which may present as cysts, fibroadenomas, abscesses, galactoceles, ductal carcinomas, invasive ductal carcinomas and medullary carcinomas. As a follow-up to mammography to differentiate between a benign or malignant mass. To assist in interventional procedures such as tissue biopsy and the drainage or aspiration of cysts.

# 11 Female Breast

## Ultrasound

### Position of patient and imaging modality

The patient is asked first to lie supine on the couch. The breast being scanned is exposed and paper tissue is tucked into the patient's skirt to protect her clothes. In order to provide a stable flat base for scanning, the patient is then asked to raise the side under investigation and to place the arm of the raised side above the head. A foam pad is positioned behind the patient for support. Coupling gel is applied to the entire breast and the transducer is gently placed in the upper outer quadrant.

### Imaging procedure

Each breast is examined in a systematic clockwise fashion, with the nipple as the centre of the clock. The axillary tail and each of the four quadrants of the breast are examined using a combination of longitudinal and transverse scanning techniques.

As stated above, scanning commences initially at the axillary tail of the breast with the transducer placed in the upper outer quadrant and angled towards the axilla so that the tail of the breast is seen. From this position, slow lateral movements using a continuous scanning action are carried out until the entire axillary tail is examined.

The transducer is then positioned relative to the upper inner quadrant to gain a longitudinal section of the breast. From this position, using gentle pressure, the transducer is moved medially to the medial border of the upper inner quadrant and then laterally to the upper border of the upper outer quadrant. This technique is repeated, moving the transducer slightly cranially or caudally to ensure that the entire breast tissue is examined. When completed, the transducer is rotated through 90° to gain a transverse section at the superior border of the upper outer quadrant from where it is moved caudally to the lower border of the lower outer quadrant, so that both the outer quadrants are examined entirely in transverse sections.

The transducer is then rotated 90° back into the longitudinal position and placed at the lateral border of the lower outer quadrant and moved medially to the medial border of the lower inner quadrant so that both lower quadrants are examined in longitudinal sections.

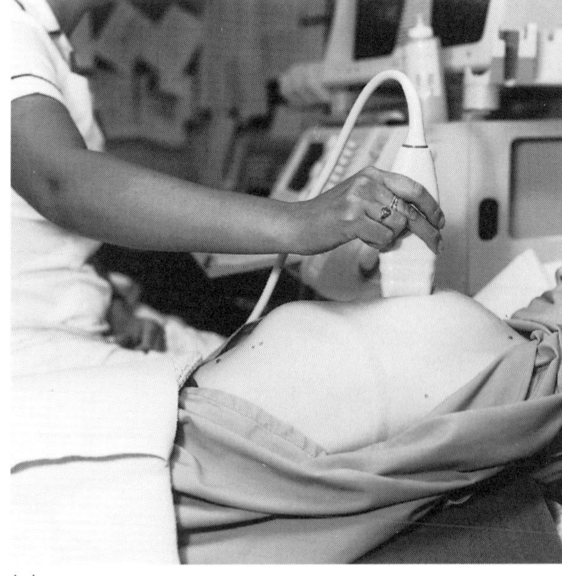

(a)

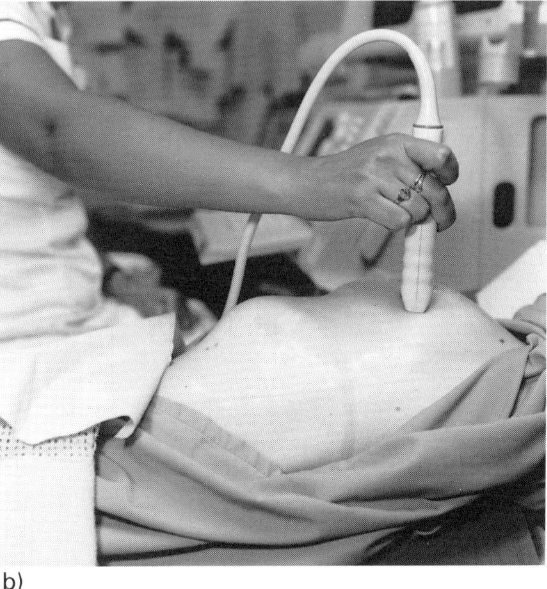

(b)

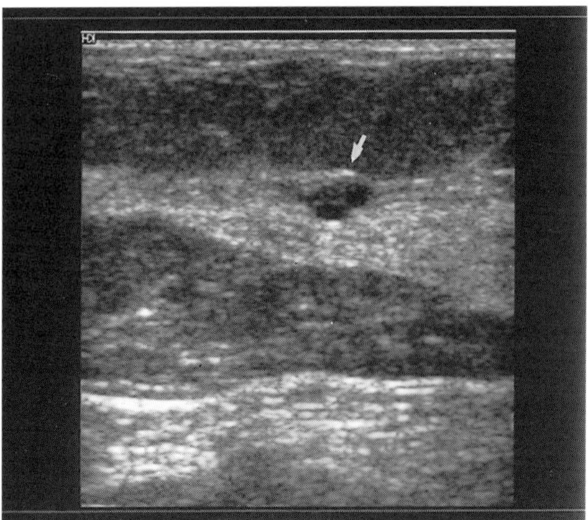

(c)

**Figure 11.3** (a,b) Patient and ultrasound transducer showing (a) longitudinal section and (b) transaxial section; (c) example of a fibroadenoma

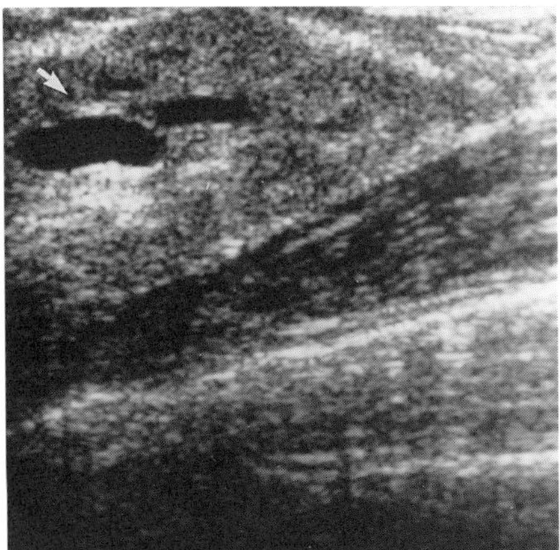

**Figure 11.4a** Example of breast cysts clustered together

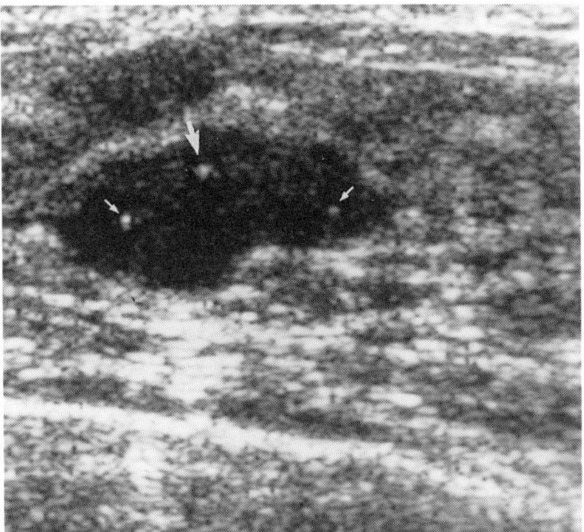

**Figure 11.4b** Example of microcalcifications

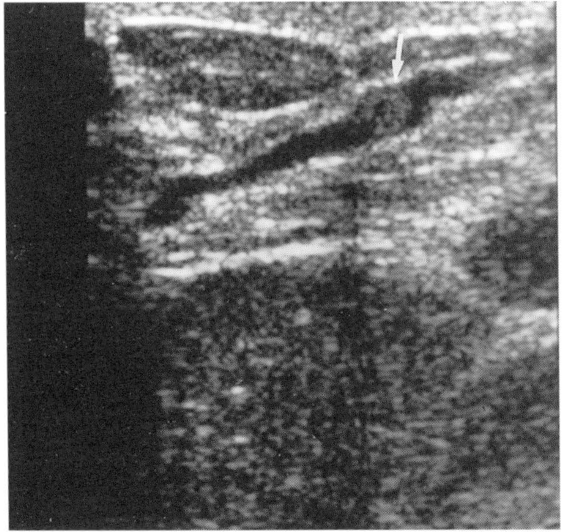

**Figure 11.4c** Intraductal papilloma

When the initial series is completed, the transducer is rotated 90° into the transverse position and placed at the lower border of lower inner quadrant and moved cranially to the superior of the upper inner border, so that both inner quadrants are examined in transverse sections.

The nipple is difficult to scan due to its shape. However, examination of the tissue posterior to it is made by first placing the transducer in a longitudinal direction immediately lateral to the nipple and then angling the transducer medially to scan the tissues posterior to it. When this examination is completed, the transducer is further rotated 90° to obtain a series of transverse images. The transducer is placed below the nipple and angled cranially.

During this imaging procedure, overall appearances of the breast is noted and hard-copy images made of any sections of notable interest.

**Image analysis**

The normal breast image appearance consists of a heterogeneous, echogenic glandular tissue, seen beneath hetrogenic, hypoechoic fatty tissue.

A cyst will appear with smooth well-defined walls surrounding an anechoic area. They may be multiple or contain septae.

Fibroadenomas are usually ovoid in shape, homogeneous in echo texture, with a regular border.

Abscesses are fluid filled and may contain some internal echoes. They have a thick, irregular border and usually occur around the nipple.

Galactoceles are cysts containing milk caused by a blocked lactiferous duct and are demonstrated as a poorly defined echo-free area.

Ductal carcinomas are demonstrated by dilated ducts proximal to the mass.

Invasive ductal carcinomas have an irregular border and a homogeneous echo texture. Thickening and indentation of the skin over the mass may also be seen.

Medullary carcinomas have a similar appearance to fibroadanomas, but are slightly more echogenic and have an irregular border (see Plate 19).

# 11 Female Breast

## Magnetic resonance imaging

Magnetic resonance imaging, using conventional spin-echo and gradient-echo sequences, has not proved to be sensitive or specific in the characterisation of breast masses. At the time of writing, however, research is being carried out at different centres to develop dynamic, contrast enhanced protocols which will assess tumour perfusion and hopefully distinguish between malignancy and benign disease. With this method the change in signal intensity after the administration of intravenous contrast is plotted as a function of time. It is hoped that by identifying characteristic patterns of contrast uptake from the blood plasma into tissues and its subsequent elimination back into the plasma, normal and malignant and benign tissues can be identified. This method is also successful in detecting small and pre-invasive carcinomas and identifying benign and post-therapeutic lesions. This protocol may prove effective in reducing the number of lesions that need to be biopsied for pathological testing.

Such protocols include 3D multi-slice fast-image sequences of the entire breast before and after intravenous administration of contrast, and 2D dynamic contrast medium studies of preselected slices. Conventional $T_1$ and $T_2$ weighted spin-echo sequences in the coronal plane may be used to examine the axilla in the post treatment patient for tumour recurrence.

**Indications**

Detection of non-palpable carcinomas, especially in the breast with dense tissue, when mammography is not as sensitive in detecting small lesions. To differentiate between malignant and benign or fibrotic scars and during a needle-guided tissue biopsy procedure.

*Contrast and injection data*

| *Volume* | *Pharmaceutical* | *Flow rate* |
|---|---|---|
| 0.1 mmol/kg body weight | Gadolinium DTPA | Hand injection |

A bolus hand injection technique is used with the contrast, followed by 20 ml bolus injection of saline.

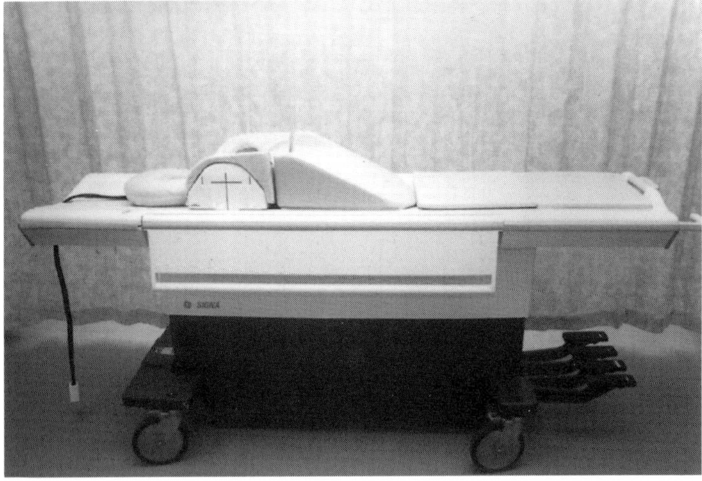

(a)

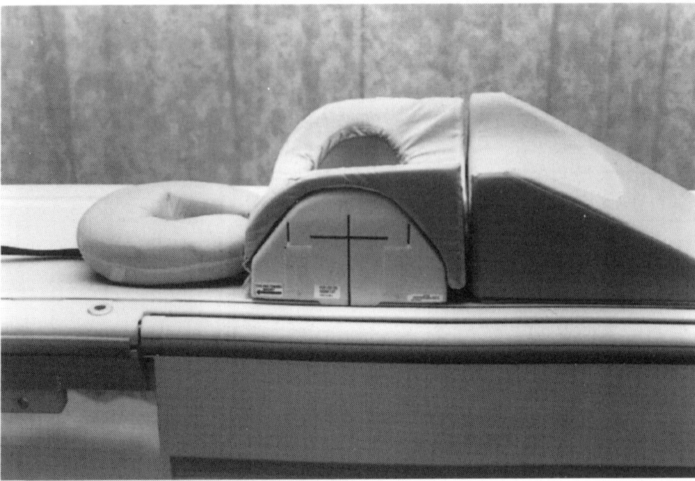

(b)

**Figure 11.5** (a,b) Imaging couch and breast coil

## Magnetic resonance imaging

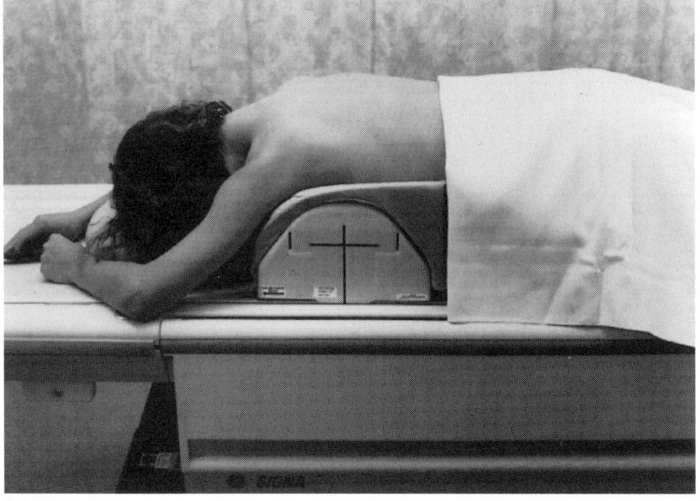

(a)

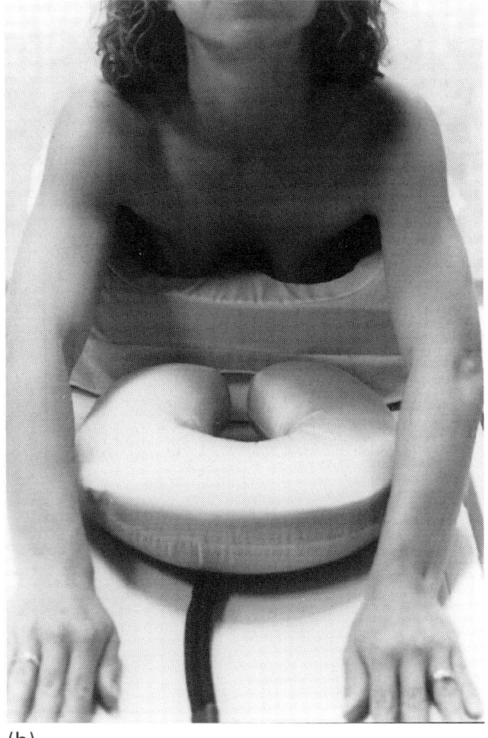

(b)

**Figure 11.6** (a,b) Patient positioned on breast coil at different angles

### Breast coil

For successful breast imaging a specially designed breast coil has to be used. A typical unit is seen in the photograph opposite. This device is so constructed that each breast is suspended freely in a cavity, while the patient is firmly supported lying in the prone position. The device is quickly attached to the scan table.

A number of designs are available. In one such design, within the firm enclosure are single coils on each side of the device, so oriented as to provide maximal cover of the breast and axillary tail. The coils may be used in 'surface coil mode' when a switched connector box permits scanning of the right, left or both breasts, in which case the signal-to-noise ratio (SNR) is reduced. Alternatively, the coil may be used in the 'phased array mode', whereby the signal from each coil is received by its own RF input channel before the two are combined. This permits both breasts to be scanned with the same SNR as the single breasts examined in the surface coil mode. Right, left or bilateral examinations may be selected at the operator's console.

A device with only one coil allows either bilateral or unilateral imaging of the breasts. In bilateral mode, however, the sensitive volume of the coil covers both breasts and axillae as well as the chest wall adjacent to both breasts with a lower SNR. In unilateral mode, the coil performance SNR is improved, but the sensitive volume of the coil will only cover the right or left breast, the right or left axilla and the chest wall adjacent to either the right or left breast.

### Position of patient and imaging modality

Using the specially designed breast coil the patient lies prone with the breasts lying freely within two cavities in an elevated chest wall support. Foam rubber supports are provided for the support of the nipple area to prevent motion artefacts. Padded supports are provided for the chin, chest, abdomen and lower legs to ensure comfort during the procedure. Positioning is aided by halogen positioning lights. Using the external alignment lights the table top is moved until the scan reference point is at the centre of the breast coil. The patient and breast coil are now advanced the fixed distance to the isocentre of the magnet.

# 11 Female Breast

## Magnetic resonance imaging

### Imaging procedure

The following is an example of a protocol for a symptomatic breast using a 1.5 T magnet.

*Initial axial localiser*
Up to 17 images are acquired of both breasts using a fast GRASS pulse sequence. One of these images is used to plan the subsequent sagittal sequences.

*Pre-contrast images*
From the axial localiser a series of 21 sagittal images of the entire breast are prescribed using both $T_1$ weighted spin-echo ($T_1$W SE) and $T_2$ weighted fast spin-echo ($T_2$W FSE) pulse sequences. The $T_2$W FSE images are fat saturated.

*Dynamic contrast study*
A dynamic gradient-echo contrast study using a fast spoiled grass pulse sequence (FSPGR), which ensures good temporal resolution, is prescribed at four preselected slice locations, usually 10 mm apart, to investigate suspected tissue abnormality seen on the pre-contrast images. Up to 25 scans are acquired per location, with a scan repetition rate of 1 scan per 12 s, using a multi-phase technique.

*Post-contrast fat-suppressed study*
To conclude the examination, a series of post-contrast sagittal images are acquired using $T_1$W SE with chemical-shift-selective fat-suppression (FS $T_1$W SE) through the same slice locations as the original $T_1$W SE images.

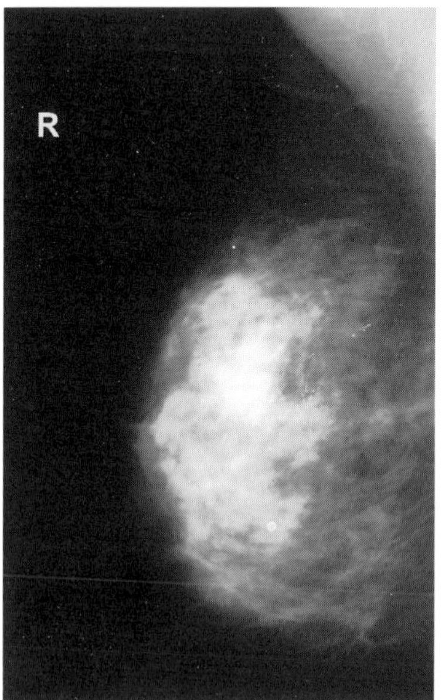


**Figure 11.7a** Mammogram showing suspected lesion

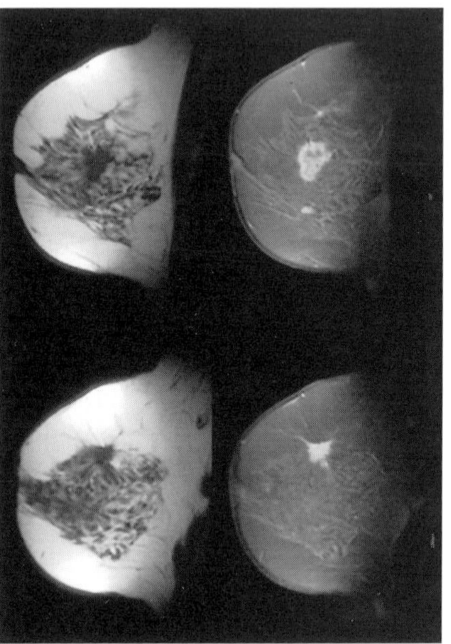

**Figure 11.7b** Selection of sagittal sections: pre-gadolinium $T_1$ weighted spin-echo (left images); post-gadolinium $T_1$ weighted with fat saturation (right images)

**Table 11.1 Imaging parameters**

| *Imaging plane* | *Imaging sequence* | *TR* | *TE* | *Field of view* (cm) | *No. of NEX* | *Slice width/ gap* (mm) | *Matrix* |
|---|---|---|---|---|---|---|---|
| Transaxial | Localiser fast grass | 7.9 | 2.9 | 36 | 1 | 5/2 | 128 |
| Sagittal | Spin-echo | 640 | 11 | 20–24 | 2 | 4/1 | 192 |
| Sagittal | Fast spin-echo | 4000 | 96–120 | 20–24 | 2 | 4/1 | 256 |
| Sagittal – dynamic uptake | FSPGR multi-phase | 11.1 | 4.2 | 20–24 | 2 | 5–7/1.5–3 | 128 |
| Sagittal | Fat-suppressed | 600 | 11 | 20–24 | 1 | 5 | 192 |

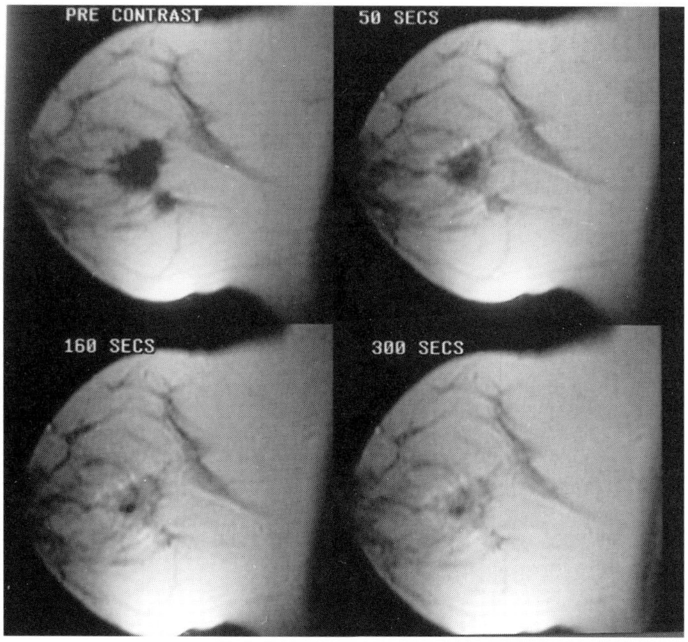

Figure 11.8a Selection of dynamic images showing increase in signal intensity in region of suspected lesion

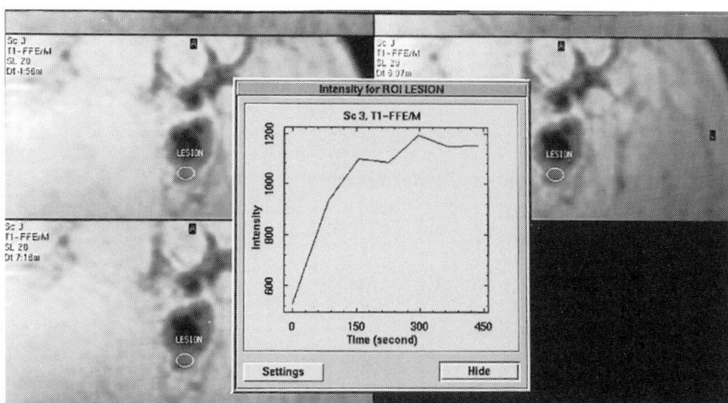


**Figure 11.8b** Computer-generated graph showing a rapid enhancing focal lesion (80% uptake within 1 min)

*Pre-contrast images*

On both non-enhanced $T_1W$ and $T_2W$ images, fat is bright and glandular breast tissue dark. Many tumours can readily be identified as focal lesions of abnormal architecture with low signal intensity on both $T_1W$ and $T_2W$ images, especially if large. Confident identification of tumours, however, is only possible on either the dynamic gradient-echo scans or fat-suppressed $T_1W$ images following the administration of contrast. Small additional foci of tumours are invariably not visible prior to contrast administration. Cysts are markedly hyperintense on $T_2W$ images, but breast carcinomas do not generally appear bright, unlike carcinomas elsewhere in the body.

*Dynamic contrast study*

Analysis of the dynamic data is performed by reviewing images from each section in a movie loop in order to identify those areas that show enhancement. User-defined regions-of-interest (ROIs) are then drawn in such areas and the mean pixel signal intensity for each area is recorded. Images of the ROIs and pixel values are made. ROIs are drawn in areas suspected of harbouring focal lesions as well as in ostensibly normal parenchyma. Up to 10 ROIs may be measured on each data set. The numerical data are then manually transferred into a spreadsheet running on a personal computer, corrections made for baseline values and time after injection of contrast, and the results plotted as an enhancement index versus time. Experience suggests that all carcinomas show uptake of contrast with varying rates. Some lesions achieve maximum signal intensity within 30 s following the end of injection, while others become brighter after more than 4 min. Signal intensity appears to decline at different rates, some within the first 30 s. It appears that the rate of reduction of signal is considerably slower than the rate of increase. Prominent enhancement of a tumour periphery is noted on some fat-saturated images, suggesting that the central lower signal intensity is due to 'wash-out' of contrast or to the presence of central areas of fat.

The actual mechanism for this peripheral enhancement is not as yet fully understood, but may be as a result of increased vascularity.

*Post-contrast fat-suppressed study*

Fat suppression is desirable to depict contrast enhancement in breasts which frequently contain abundant fat. It reduces chemical-shift artefacts and provides improved internal lesion characterisation and delineation of interfaces of fat- and water-containing tissues.

# 11 Miscellaneous Procedures

## Percutaneous Biopsy

Percutaneous biopsies are performed using ultrasound, CT or fluoroscopy, to enable the radiologist precisely to place a fine needle into an abnormal mass to obtain a core of tissue for cytology or histology.

Ultrasound is used in those lesions which vary significantly in echogeneity from surrounding anatomy. Many abdominal lesions can be well demonstrated and ultrasound offers the advantage of real-time imaging and needle manipulation without the penalty of ionising radiation. It is therefore often the first modality of choice. Either an attachable needle guide which directs the needle into the lesion located by the transducer can be used, or the position of the needle as it is advanced towards the lesion can be monitored by a transducer placed at approximately 90° to the needle path.

It may be inappropriate to use ultrasound if lesions are small, isoechoic, hidden by gas (e.g. bowel or lung) or if overlying structures are invisible to ultrasound and therefore at risk.

Fluoroscopy is used in lesions which vary in density from the surrounding structures, e.g. lesions in the lungs. This usually requires equipment which can easily be rotated through 90° during the procedure to judge the depth of the needle in relation to the lesion accurately. An isocentric C-arm imaging system such as used for angiography is ideal for this purpose.

Computed tomography is used to pinpoint accurately lesions which are difficult to locate by either ultrasound or fluoroscopy.

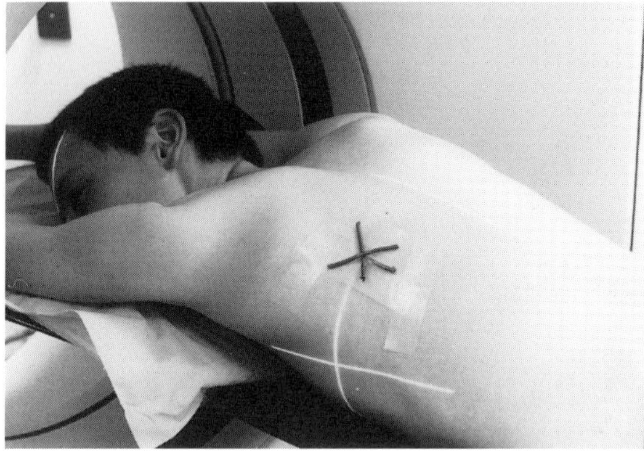
(a)

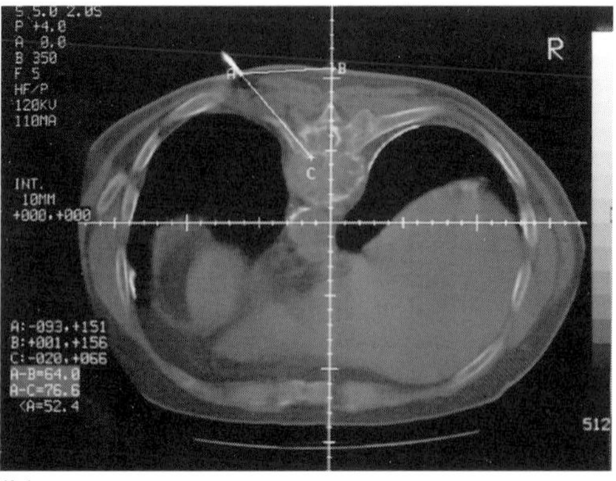

(b)

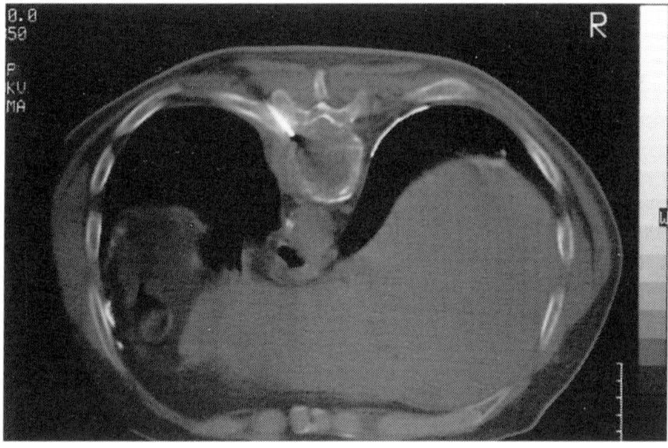

(c)

**Figure 11.9** (a) Patient positioned for CT localisation scan image; (b,c) CT images showing planned biopsy route (b) and needle in position with tip in a spinal mass (c)

### Patient preparation

Written consent must be obtained. Haemoglobin, prothrombin time and platelet count must be within normal limits. Premedication may be given to the anxious patient but is not routinely administered.

### Imaging procedure

The lesion is located by the imaging method chosen and the patient rotated into the optimum position for needle puncture. The point chosen for entry is marked on the skin surface which is then cleansed and surrounded by sterile drapes. A local anaesthetic agent is administered around the entry point of the needle and a small incision is made in the skin. The fine biopsy needle is then advanced towards the lesion under imaging guidance. For example, in CT scanning, the initial scans are taken to locate the lesion. The selected path is chosen from these images and the point of entry and depth of the lesion is measured from the midline. The selected point is then marked on the patient's skin and a radio-opaque marker is placed at the point and the scan repeated to verify the position. The procedure continues as described previously. Several repeat images at the chosen location are taken during the procedure to ensure that the needle is guided into the lesion. One final image is taken prior to the biopsy showing the needle in situ.

A post-procedure chest radiograph or a single CT section image is needed after a biopsy of a chest lesion to exclude a pneumothorax.

## Sinography and Fistulography

Sinuses are soft tissue channels extending from the skin surface into deeper tissues, frequently down to bone, and may be a result of a previous abscess. A fistula is a similar soft tissue channel but connecting the skin with an internal hollow viscus in the abdomen or a communication between two organs.

The examination may be performed under fluoroscopic control and may include full-size plain film radiography.

### Indications

The examination is required to demonstrate the extent of the sinus or fistula.

### Contraindications

The examination is not normally performed on patients suffering from severe pyrexia or severe localised infection.

### Patient preparation

The patient lies supine on the fluoroscopy table, with the opening of the sinus or fistula uppermost, and is made as comfortable as possible. The skin surrounding the area is prepared using a suitable antiseptic preparation and sterile towels are placed around the opening. A control radiograph may be undertaken to exclude the presence of a radio-opaque foreign body.

### Imaging procedure

If a drainage tube is in situ, the contrast agent may be introduced through this; if not, a fine catheter is inserted into the orifice and a gauze pad is placed around the site of entry to reduce reflux of the contrast agent.

A sufficient quantity of a water-soluble contrast agent (e.g. 280 mgI/ml) is introduced under fluoroscopic control to outline the extent of the lesion. Two images are normally taken at right angles to each other. Erect views using a horizontal beam may also be taken.

## Abscess Drainage

Abscess drainage can also be undertaken by radiological guidance. The techniques are similar to that used in percutaneous biopsies requiring an initial fine-needle puncture, using a sheathed needle, if no sinus tract is present. However, because of the size of the drainage catheters (8–24F) it is critical when planning the direction of needle puncture that no important structures lie between the abnormal fluid collection and the skin surface.

Once the needle or catheter is successfully positioned, some dilute contrast medium may be introduced to determine the size and the presence of any tract communicating with bowel. Fluid may then be aspirated.

If the catheter is to remain in place for prolonged drainage, a soft-tipped angiographic guide wire is advanced through the catheter part of the sheathed needle and the catheter further advanced over the guide wire.

To allow the needle tract to be dilated, the guide wire is exchanged and a stiff one introduced to facilitate dilatation of the tract, using a selection of dilators which are advanced over the stiff guide wire.

Once the tract has been sufficiently dilated, the drainage catheter is introduced, fixed to the skin surface and connected to a drainage bag.

The abscess cavity should be irrigated with saline at regular intervals, dependent on the thickness of the fluid within the abscess and the antibiotics prescribed.

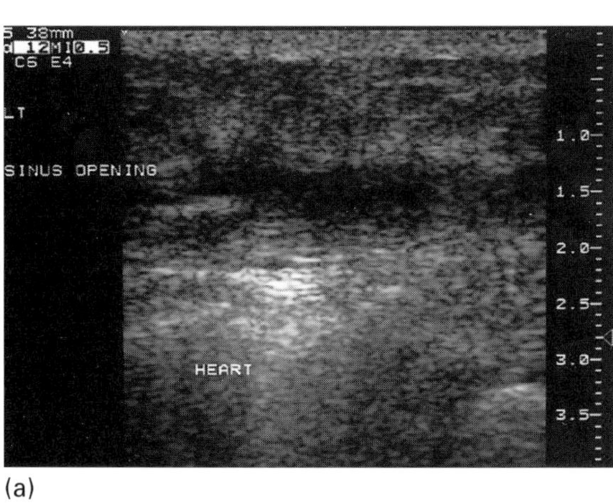

(a)

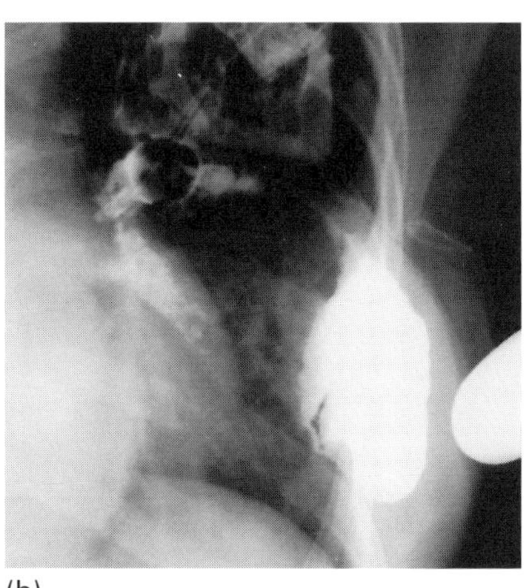
(b)

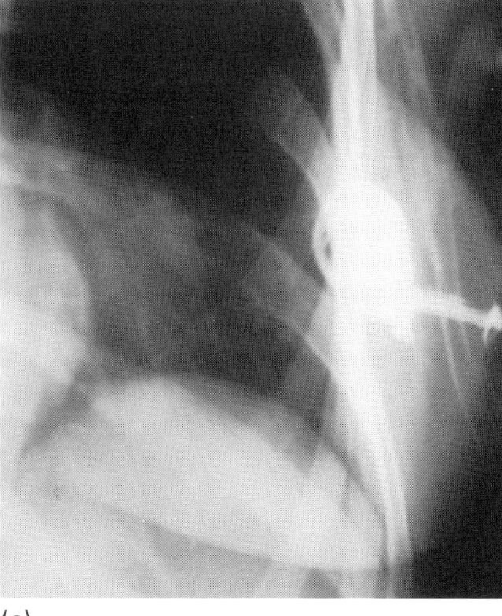
(c)

**Figure 11.10** (a–c) Study of a patient with a breast abscess: (a) ultrasound image showing sinus opening; (b) radiograph with a 10F Foley balloon catheter in sinus opening and contrast filling a sinus tract and abscess cavity; (c) follow-up radiograph showing shrinkage of abscess cavity

# 11 Inflammation and Infection Localisation

## Introduction – radionuclide imaging

Radionuclide imaging using radiolabelled leucocytes offers a sensitive and specific means of identifying sites of inflammation or infection within the body. The procedure, commonly referred to as 'labelled white blood cell imaging', is used in hospitals worldwide.

*In vitro* radioisotope labelling of the patient's leucocytes is carried out under strict controls to prevent cross-contamination. Once labelled, the cells are then reinjected into the patient.

This section will deal specifically with technetium-99m exametazime (Ceretec, Amersham International plc) as the agent of choice for *in vitro* $^{99m}$Tc leucocyte labelling. Other techniques use the isotope indium-111.

The actual labelling protocol is a multi-staged process involving centrifugation of the patient's blood to separate out the leucocytes in a cell-free plasma. A detailed protocol is provided in the manufacturer's literature and the reader is referred to this information and details of possible hypersensitivity reactions associated with the use of cell separation materials such as Hespan (Dupont).

### Basic principles

Leucocyte-labelled imaging exploits the natural migration of white cells towards areas of infection and inflammation. A patient's white cells are isolated from a sample of whole blood and labelled with a suitable gamma-emitting radioisotope. The radiolabelled white blood cells are then reinjected and their distribution imaged using a gamma camera. Their location will demonstrate active inflammatory disease or infected sites.

White cells are divided into three subtypes: granulocytes, lymphocytes and monocytes. The granulocyte fraction is the largest, representing 70% of the total number of cells. Granulocyte subtypes also exist. These are the eosinophils, basophils and neurtrophils. Granulocytes are the cells primarily involved in the body's response to infection and inflammation.

Agents such as $^{99m}$Tc exametazime and $^{111}$In-oxine are capable of labelling all cell types and therefore the leucocytes must be isolated.

$^{99m}$Tc exametazime labels the cells by crossing their intact cell membranes via passive diffusion and becoming trapped within the leucocyte. This trapping mechanism is thought to involve an interaction with glutathione.

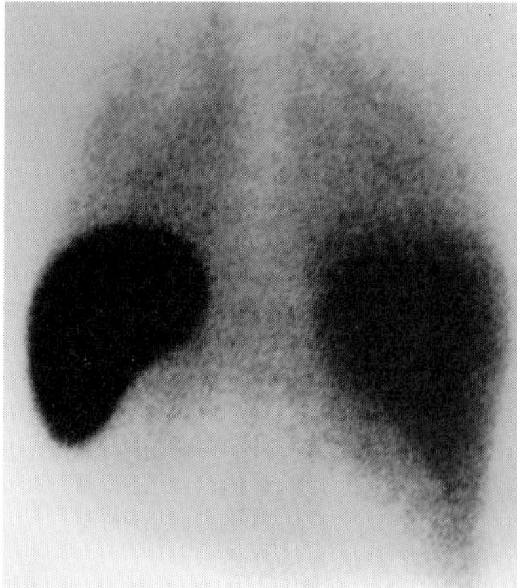

**Figure 11.11a** Normal scan showing labelled cells passing through the pulmonary vasculature and pooling in the liver and spleen at 5 min post-injection

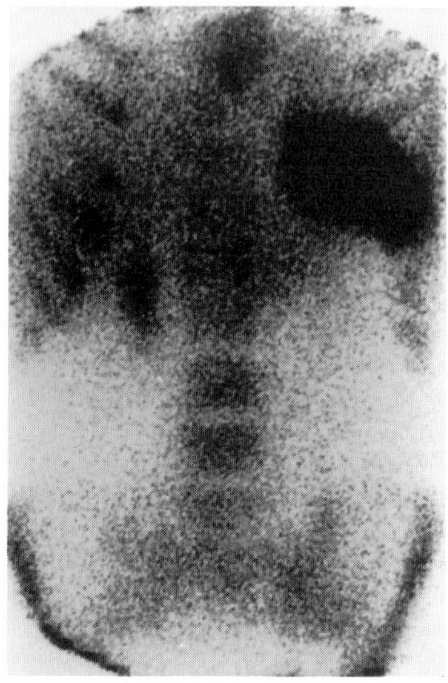

**Figure 11.11b** Normal anterior scan of the abdomen at 1 h post-injection showing uptake of cells in the liver, spleen and bone marrow

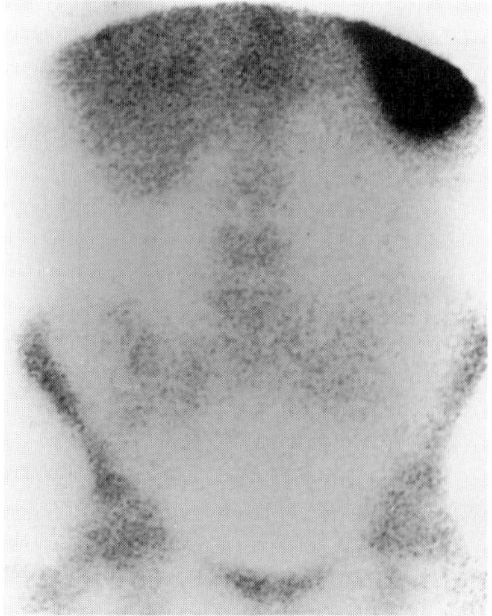

**Figure 11.11c** Normal anterior scan of the abdomen at 3 h post-injection showing gallbladder activity

## Radionuclide imaging

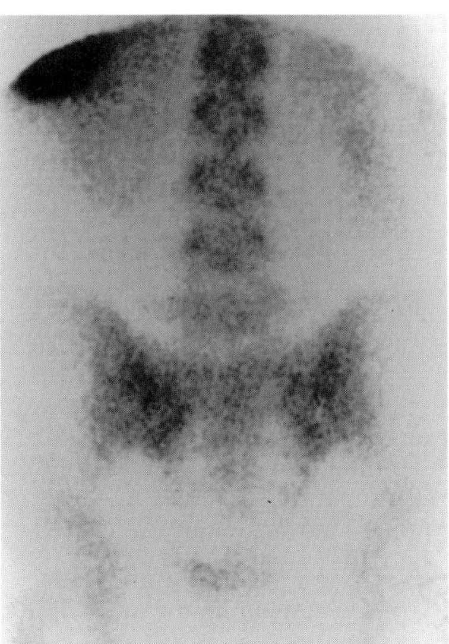

**Figure 11.12a** Normal abdominal posterior scan at 2 h post-injection showing bilateral parenchymal renal activity

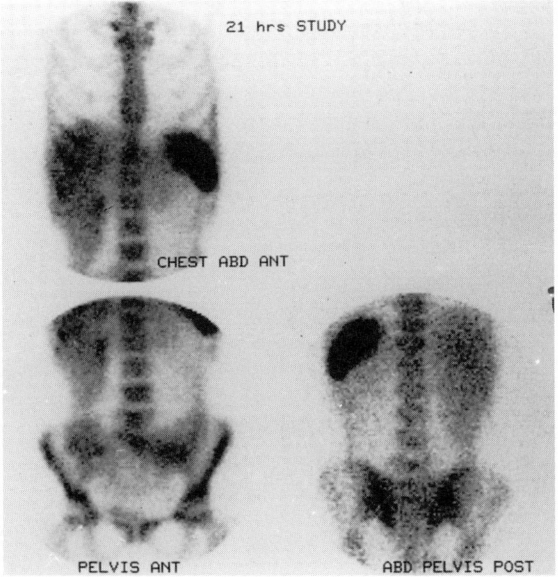


**Figure 11.12b** Selection of normal images at 21 h post-injection showing non-specific bowel activity

### Distribution of $^{99m}$Tc-labelled white cells

Studies show that labelled granulocytes are equally divided between the circulating granulocyte pool (CGP) and the migrating granulocyte pool (MCP), both together being the total blood granulocyte pool (TBGP).

The granulocytes in the CGP are circulating in the blood stream and are capable of going to sites of inflammation and infection. The granulocytes in the MGP are found in the spleen, liver, lungs and bone marrow.

The cells in the CGP and the MGP are in dynamic equilibrium. The cells leave the TBGP with a half-life of about 6 h and in the absence of inflammation are destroyed in the reticulo-endothelial system. Replacements are manufactured in the red bone marrow.

At 45 min post-injection, the normal distribution of labelled granulocytes is 40% blood pool, 20% liver, 20% spleen, with the remainder distributed in the lungs and bone marrow. This process reaches equilibrium at 45 min and therefore a normal scan image will show activity in the liver, spleen and bone marrow.

If cells have been damaged during the cell separation process, then at 30 min post-injection there will be high activity in the lungs where the cells get trapped. There will also be higher activity in the liver as the cells go to be destroyed earlier than expected.

#### Indications

- intra-abdominal sepsis and postoperative infection
- inflammatory bowel disease
- orthopaedic infection
- vascular graft infection.

#### Contraindications

The procedure is not recommended for children or in pregnancy. Breast-feeding mothers should discontinue breastfeeding for up to 24 h after the procedure.

#### Position of patient and imaging procedure

For all the investigations mentioned above, the patient will lie supine on the imaging couch. Anterior views will be acquired in the majority of cases with the gamma camera positioned parallel to the imaging couch and situated as close as possible to the anterior surface of the patient, over the patient's abdomen or bony extremities, etc., depending on the type of investigation. Posterior views, with the gamma camera positioned below the imaging couch, may also be necessary.

*Imaging and radiopharmaceutical parameters*

| *Type* | *Administered activity* | *Principal energy* |
|---|---|---|
| $^{99m}$Tc, exametazine leucocyte | 200 MBq | 140 keV |

| *Window width* | *Acquisition counts/time* |
|---|---|
| 20% | See separate text |

# 11 Inflammation and Infection Localisation

## Radionuclide imaging

### Intra-abdominal sepsis

Technetium-labelled white blood cell imaging can identify sepsis with a high level of specificity.

An abdominal abscess appears as an area of high abnormal activity which gradually becomes 'hotter' relative to spleen and liver. This represents the migration of cells into the abscess, with no redistribution of activity from it.

#### Indications

The procedure is especially recommended for postoperative fever and suspected acute abscess. Technetium-labelled white blood cell imaging is not suitable for chronic infection, urinary tract infections or pyrexia of unknown origin. For urinary tract infections, $^{111}$In is usually prescribed.

#### Imaging procedure

A high-resolution collimator is selected for static scanning. An intravenous injection of $^{99m}$Tc exametazime-labelled leucocytes is administered into the antecubital vein. Static anterior and lateral images are acquired at 1 and 3 h post-injection. An additional image may be acquired 18–24 h post-injection.

SPECT imaging can be employed and is helpful in detecting a cerebral abscess.

#### Image analysis

- The ease with which an abscess is detected depends on its location, size and its age. The rate of radiolabelled leucocyte accumulation depends on the leucocyte turnover in the abscess. As a result of this factor $^{99m}$Tc exametazime is not suitable for investigating chronic infection due to the relatively short half-life (6 h) of $^{99m}$Tc.
- If an abscess lies in an area of usual uptake, e.g. liver/spleen, three-phase scanning at 1, 3 and 18 h is needed.
- A communicating abscess may be difficult to detect where the septic fluid drains into the gastrointestinal tract.
- Redistribution of large quantities of intra-abdominal purulent fluid when the patient changes posture may cause difficulties in diagnosis.
- False positives may arise due to fresh haematoma, renal transplant, normal postoperative inflammation and granulocyte infiltrating tumours.

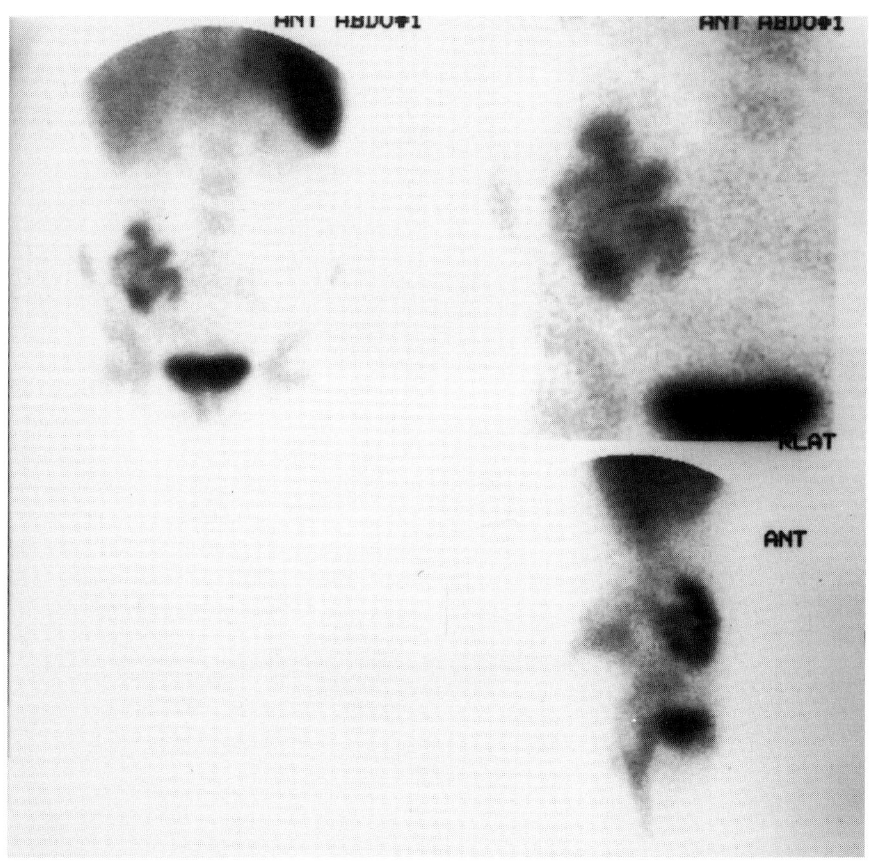


**Figure 11.13** Composite set of images at 3 h post-injection showing appendix abscess (anterior and right lateral images)

## Radionuclide imaging

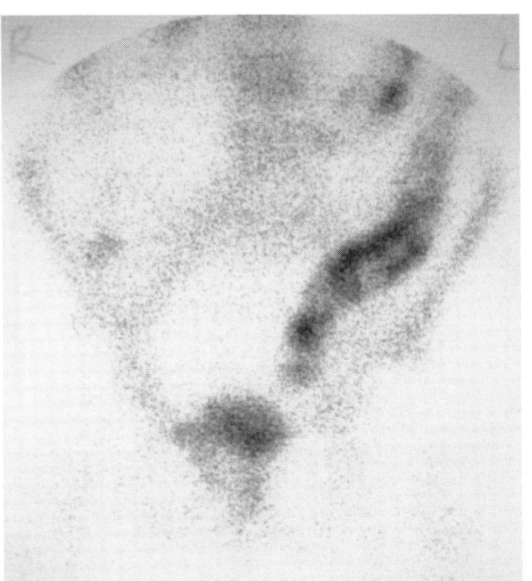

**Figure 11.14a** Abnormal anterior abdominal scan at 1 h post-injection confirming Crohn's disease

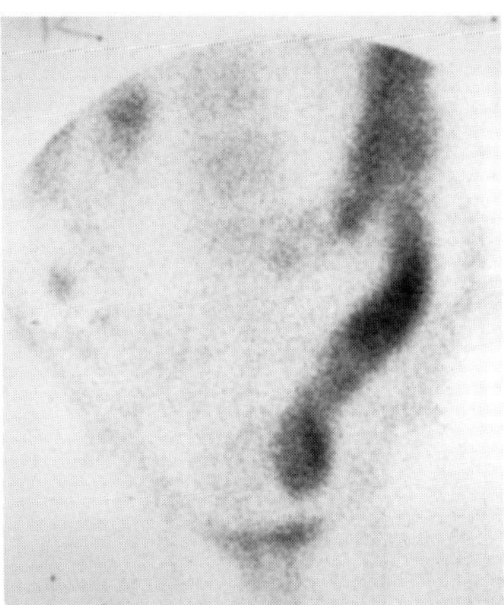

**Figure 11.14b** Abnormal abdominal scan at 3 h post-injection on same patient as (a) with Crohn's disease and similar distribution of activity

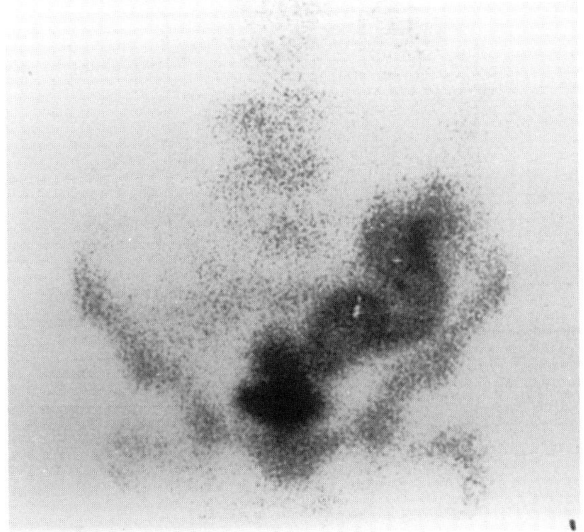

**Figure 11.14c** Abnormal anterior abdominal scan at 3 h post-injection confirming ulcerative colitis

### Inflammatory bowel disease

$^{99m}$Tc-labelled leucocyte scanning visualises the extent and location of active disease in the large and small bowel simultaneously.

No special preparation of the bowel is needed and the procedure is well tolerated.

From approximately 4 h post-injection the labelled cells migrate through the bowel wall into the lumen and are excreted in the faeces.

#### Indications

Diagnosis of ulcerative colitis and Crohn's disease. The procedure is useful in determining the extent of active disease and distinguishing between scarring and active disease. It is also useful for monitoring disease, detecting relapse and in presurgical planning.

It is also used in other related inflammatory bowel disorders such as diverticulitis and enteric vasculitis and in cases of radiation enteritis and bowel ischaemia.

#### Imaging procedure

A high-resolution collimator is selected for static scanning. An intravenous injection of $^{99m}$Tc exametazime-labelled leucocytes is administered into the antecubital vein. Static images are acquired at 1 and 3 h post-injection.

#### Image analysis

- An abnormality will be demonstrated in the majority of cases 1 h post-injection.
- At 3 h any lesion will be shown with increased intensity.
- Later scans will not show the true disease distribution, but may be helpful in confirming diagnosis and in locating the colon.
- A communicating abscess, where septic fluid drains into the gut, may give rise to a false positive.

# 11 Inflammation and Infection Localisation

## Radionuclide imaging

### Orthopaedic infections

$^{99m}$Tc-labelled leucocyte scanning is extensively employed for the detection of orthopaedic infections.

The labelled cells migrate to a source of infection associated with bones and joints.

**Indications**

Diagnosis of acute postoperative infections and osteomyelitis, also to monitor disease activity in cases of rheumatoid arthritis. Information about the location and extent of an infection can be used in determining either a conservative or surgical approach to patient management.

**Imaging procedure**

A high-resolution collimator is selected for static scanning. An intravenous injection of $^{99m}$Tc exametazime-labelled leucocytes is administered into the antecubital vein. Static images are acquired 4, 6 and possibly 18–24 h post-injection.

The use of external point-marker sources may be helpful in pinpointing sites of infections for planning surgery.

**Image analysis**

- Infected bone will be demonstrated as an area of abnormal activity within 3–4 h post-injection.
- A chronic prosthetic infection or osteomyelitis may give rise to a false-negative result due to low leucocyte turnover.
- Normal postoperative inflammation may give rise to a false-positive result soon after an operation.
- Unexpected sites of bone marrow uptake may also give rise to false-positive results. Consequently the use of $^{99m}$Tc colloid scanning is recommended, in order to define the bone marrow distribution and allow this to be subtracted from the radionuclide leucocyte scan.

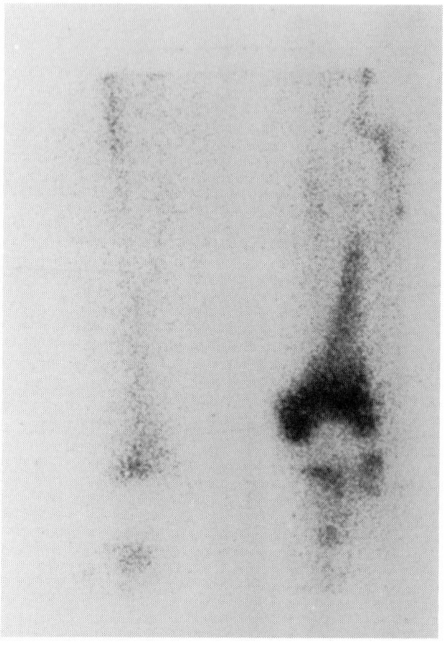
(a)

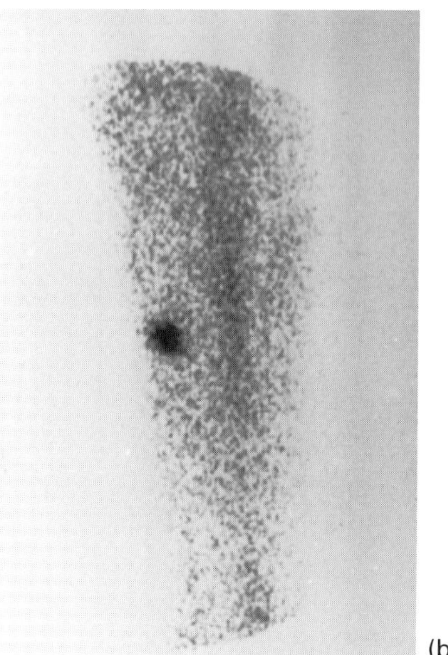
(b)

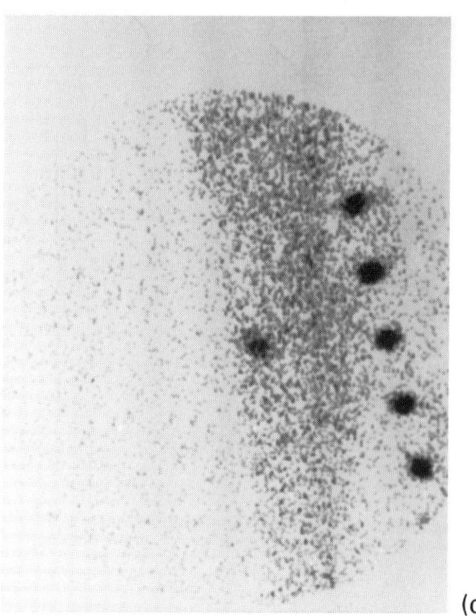
(c)

**Figure 11.15** (a) Abnormal anterior scan of knee at 3 h post-injection confirming osteomyelitis; (b,c) abnormal anterior (b) and right lateral (c) images with markers, at 5 h post-injection showing a subcutaneous abscess at the site of a bone graft

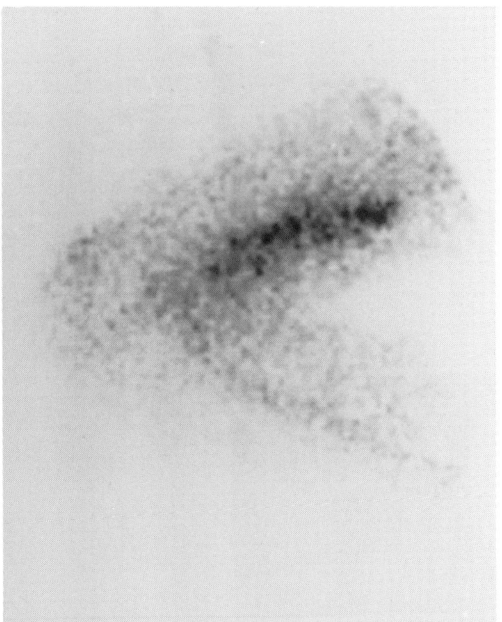

(a)

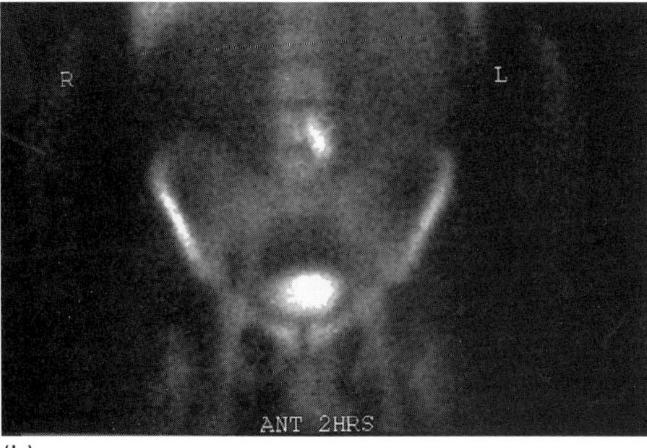


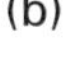

(b)

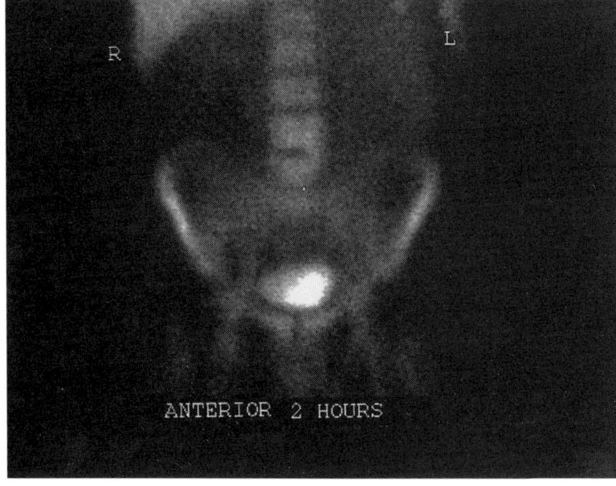


(c)

**Figure 11.16** (a) Abnormal scan at 3 h post-injection confirming infection of the lower end of a femoral popliteal bypass graft; (b,c) abnormal anterior scans of the abdominal aorta at 2 h post-injection confirming infection at the site of an aortic bypass graft (b), and at 2 h post-injection 5 months later following treatment, showing good resolution of the infection (c)

## Vascular graft infection

$^{99m}$Tc-labelled leucocyte scanning offers a highly sensitive and specific method of imaging the location and extent of vascular graft infection.

The procedure also has the benefit of detecting unexpected sites of sepsis.

In most cases the intensity of activity will exceed residual blood pool activity at 1 h post-injection. In all cases the graft activity should exceed or be equal to bone marrow activity at 3 h post-injection. Late images 18–24 h post-injection should show marked graft activity at a time when blood pool activity has reduced.

### Indications

Suspected vascular graft infection from a few days onwards after the initial operation. Vascular graft infection may occur many years after surgery.

### Imaging procedure

A high-resolution collimator is selected for static scanning. An intravenous injection of $^{99m}$Tc exametazime-labelled leucocytes is administered into the antecubital vein. Static images are acquired 1 and 3 h post-injection. Images at 18–24 h post-injection may be helpful in providing confirmation of diagnosis.

### Image analysis

- Infected bypass grafts are demonstrated as an accumulation of abnormal activity along the length of the infected area.
- An aortic graft infection may be difficult to detect due to the overlying normal uptake of labelled cells in the bone marrow of the spine.
- Normal postoperative inflammation may give rise to a false-positive result within the first few days of initial surgery.

# 11 Miscellaneous Procedures

## Lymphatic System

The lymphatic system is an extensive network of fine capillaries which drain interstitial fluid from all organs in the body except those in the central nervous system. The fine capillaries join to form long fine vessels which have valves at intervals which give them a knotted or beaded appearance. Lymph nodes are situated at various intervals along the course of lymphatic vessels. The lymph nodes produce lymphocytes and also act as a filter to remove bacteria and foreign particles entering them. Their size varies according to location and type of disease process.

The lymph vessels demonstrated by lymphangiography are usually the subcutaneous vessels of the leg, corresponding to the saphenous vein and then accompanying the iliac vessels and the aorta until they drain into the cisterna chyli. The cisterna chyli in turn drains into the thoracic duct which lies on the spine behind the aorta and eventually drains into the left subclavian vein.

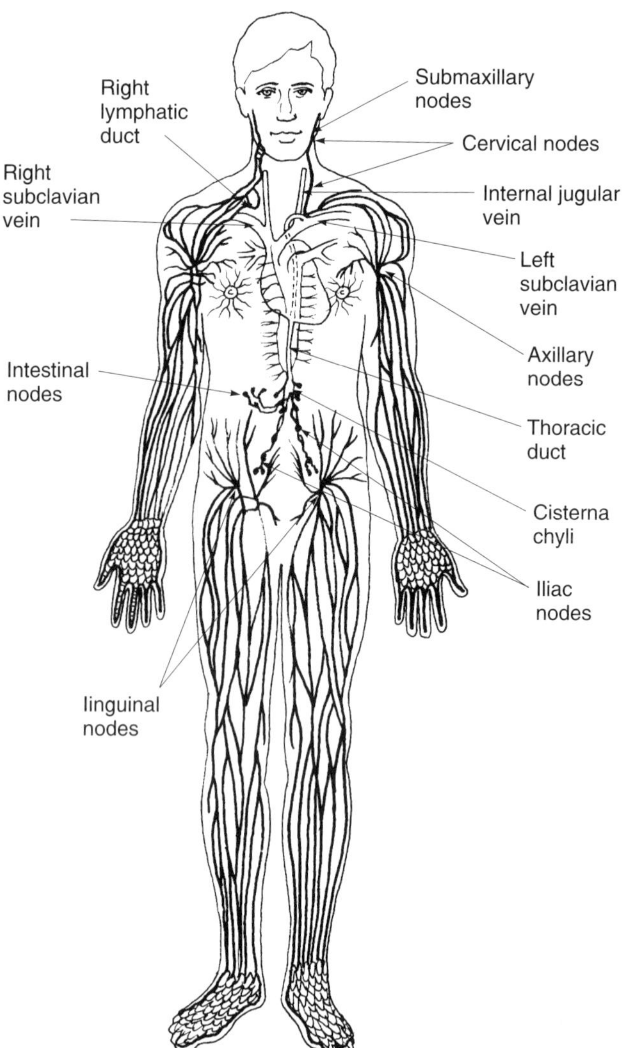


**Figure 11.17** Lymphatic system

### Recommended imaging procedures

Investigation of the lymphatic system is mainly confined to examination of the lymph nodes.

Computed tomography, because of its accessibility and ability to assess the lymphatic chain as a whole, is used extensively in the staging of many cancers for lymph node involvement and to aid biopsy of a nodal mass. It is also used routinely in patients with Hodgkin's disease and non-Hodgkin's lymphoma prior to and during treatment, to assess response to treatment.

Ultrasound has a limited role and is used mainly to investigate a specific region of the body where nodes are readily visualised. Magnetic resonance imaging also has a role in node evaluation. Radionuclide imaging, using gallium, may also be employed to show foci of occult disease in the mediastinum and, using a $^{99m}$Tc-labelled tin colloid injected into the interstitial tissues, may be used to demonstrate the lymphatics of the limbs.

Plain radiography is of little value in the investigation of lymph nodes but in certain cases, however, can demonstrate calcification in the nodes and the effect of extensive lymph node enlargement.

Lymphography can also be employed to evaluate the lymphatic system (nodes and vessels), but is a technique which is no longer a routine investigation.

### Computed tomography

A routine staging protocol consisting of transaxial scans of the chest, abdomen and pelvis is described. Contrast enhanced scans using a non-ionic contrast medium may be necessary to evaluate equivocal areas of lymph node disease. It is also necessary to opacify the small bowel, using dilute Gastrografin or barium sulphate prior to the procedure.

## Computed tomography

(a)

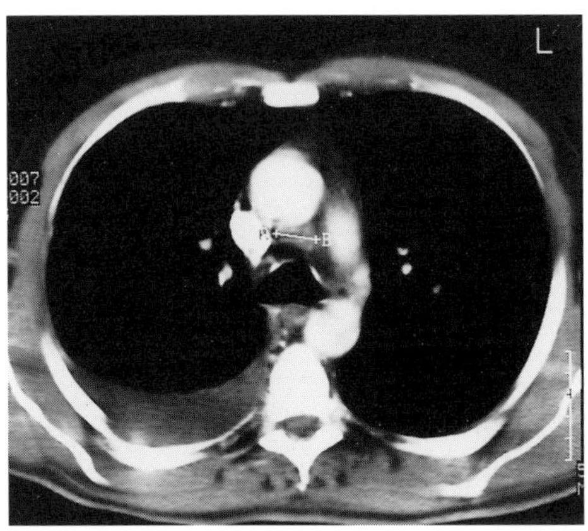

(b)

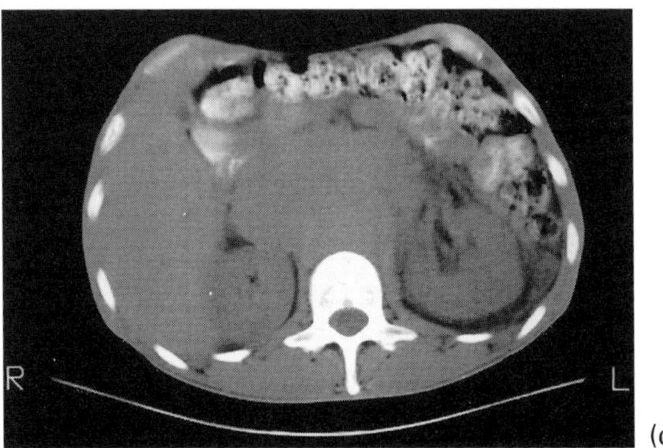

(c)

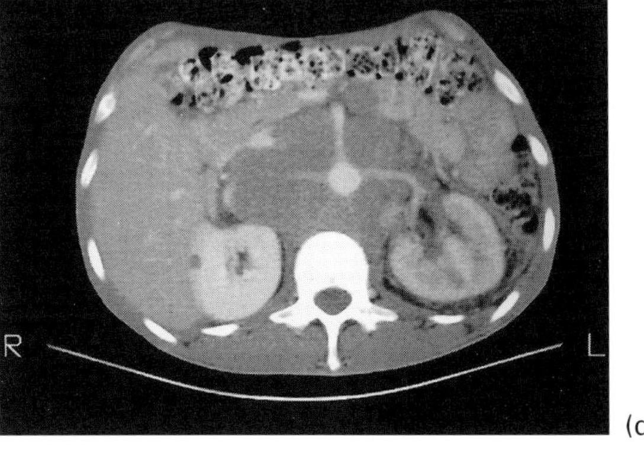

(d)

**Figure 11.18** (a) Patient and scanner; (b) post-contrast section through the mediastinum showing contrast enhancement of the ascending and descending aorta and a large non-enhanced mediastinal lymph node; (c,d) pre- and post-contrast enhanced scans of the abdomen showing enlarged para-aortic lymph nodes

### Indications

Staging of all nodes associated with Hodgkin's and non-Hodgkin's disease and the staging of lymph node involvement linked to specific organ tumours.

### Position of patient and imaging modality

The patient lies supine, head first on the scanner table, with the knees bent over an angle pad for comfort. Arms are raised and placed behind the patient's head, out of the scan plane. Positioning is aided by external alignment lights. The median sagittal plane is perpendicular and the coronal plane is parallel to the scanner table. The scan plane is now perpendicular to the long axis of the body to enable transaxial cross-sectional imaging to be undertaken. The scanner table height is adjusted to ensure that the coronal plane alignment light is at the level of the mid-axillary line. The patient is then moved into the scanner so that the scan reference point is at the level of the sternal notch.

### Imaging procedure

A full-length anteroposterior scan projection radiograph is performed, starting at the reference point and ending at the symphysis pubis. This will usually correspond to the maximum table travel, e.g. 48 cm.

From this image, for Hodgkin's disease, 10 mm contiguous sections are prescribed from the sternal notch to the symphysis pubis. For non-Hodgkin's disease, because of the relatively larger diseased nodes, a protocol using 10 mm sections with a 15 mm table increment is prescribed.

These images are reviewed and if necessary an area may be rescanned during the infusion of a non-ionic contrast agent to provide further assessment of the disease.

For the abdomen and pelvis, 100 ml of 300 mgI/ml strength contrast is selected using a 40 s scan delay, while for the chest, 100 ml of 240 mgI/ml contrast with a 30 s delay is employed.

If spiral scanning options are available, these images may be acquired with a volume acquisition, using a 10 mm slice thickness and 10 mm table increments, but with a 5 mm reconstruction index to give overlapping sections.

### Image analysis

Lymph nodes are assessed for their size relative to their anatomical location, the number of enlarged nodes present, their relationship with surrounding structures and the presence of any venous anomalies. For staging purposes in Hodgkin's disease, progression of the malignancy is classified using the Ann Arbor staging classification. For non-Hodgkin's lymphoma extranodal involvement and spread to other organs is assessed. When assessing lymphatic spread of malignancy, the adjacent and distant lymph nodes are evaluated for their size and the nature of any structural changes.

# 11 Lymphatic System

## Lymphography

Lymphography is the radiographic examination of the lymphatic system following the introduction of a radio-opaque contrast agent. The examination has been largely superseded by the introduction of CT, but does have the advantage of demonstrating the lymphatic vessels to detect structural changes in normal sized nodes.

**Patient preparation**

If a recent chest radiograph is not available, this should be performed prior to the examination.

Oedematous legs should be elevated for 24 h prior to the examination or in severe cases it may be necessary to bind the limbs with crepe bandages.

The dorsum of the foot should be shaved if necessary and the patient should be warned that the skin may turn a blue/green colour for 24 h following the procedure. Similarly, they should be warned that their urine is likely to appear blue.

The patient should be informed that the examination is a lengthy procedure and that they should micturate immediately prior to commencement.

**Imaging procedure**

The first two web spaces of each foot are anaesthetised using a local anaesthetic. One millilitre of blue dye is injected into the web spaces and the patient is encouraged to walk around until the dye is taken up by the lymphatics of the dorsum of the foot.

The patient lies supine on a fluoroscopy table and local anaesthetic is introduced around the site of a visible lymphatic vessel.

The lymphatic vessel is then dissected out through a small incision and cannulated with a small needle–catheter arrangement which is tied in position and strapped to the dorsum of the foot.

The contrast agent is introduced slowly using a pump to prevent damage to the fragile vessel and extravasation of the contrast agent.

The progress of the contrast agent through the lymphatic system is monitored either fluoroscopically or radiographically until it is observed to reach the level of the second lumbar vertebra.

With the patient supine the following series of radiographs are taken:

- anteroposterior of both tibia and fibula
- anteroposterior of both femora
- anteroposterior pelvis
- anteroposterior abdomen
- anteroposterior (penetrated chest).

The heightened awareness of radiation hazards may well result in a modification of this protocol.

Delayed radiographs taken 24 h later will demonstrate the lymph nodes without overlying vessels. A typical series may include:

- anteroposterior pelvis
- right and left posterior oblique pelvis
- lateral abdomen/pelvis
- lateral chest.

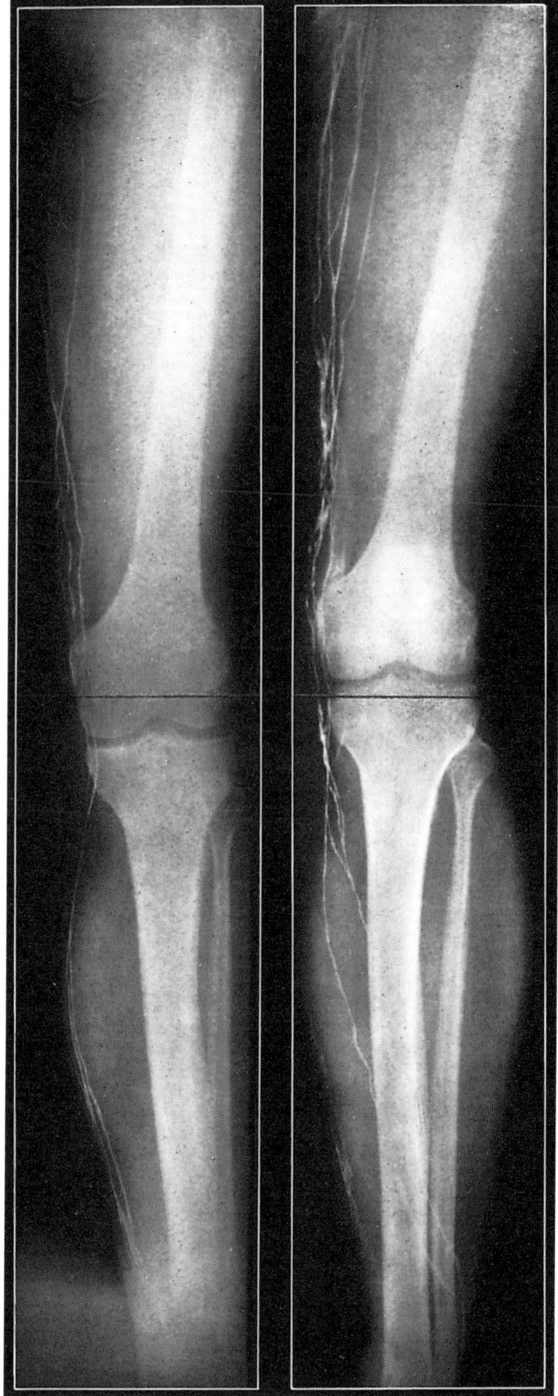

**Figure 11.19** Normal lymphatics of the lower limb on the day of injection

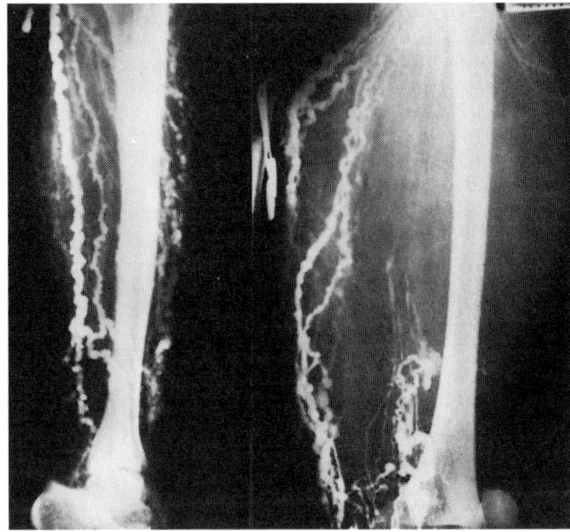

**Figure 11.20a** Markedly dilated lymphatics in the leg and thigh

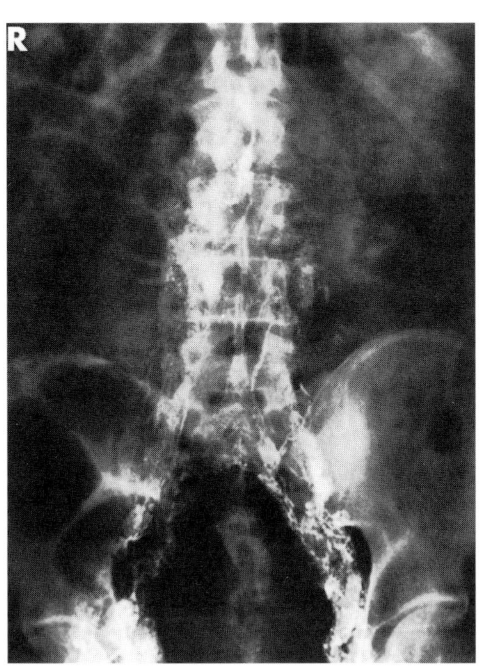


**Figure 11.20b** Lymphatic vessels are shown in between lymph nodes up to the level of the cisterna chyli overlying L1/2

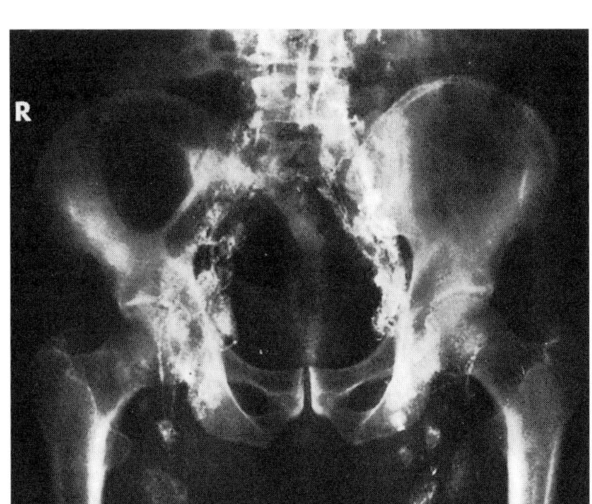


**Figure 11.20c** Lymph nodes with intervening vessels at the femoral, external iliac and common iliac regions

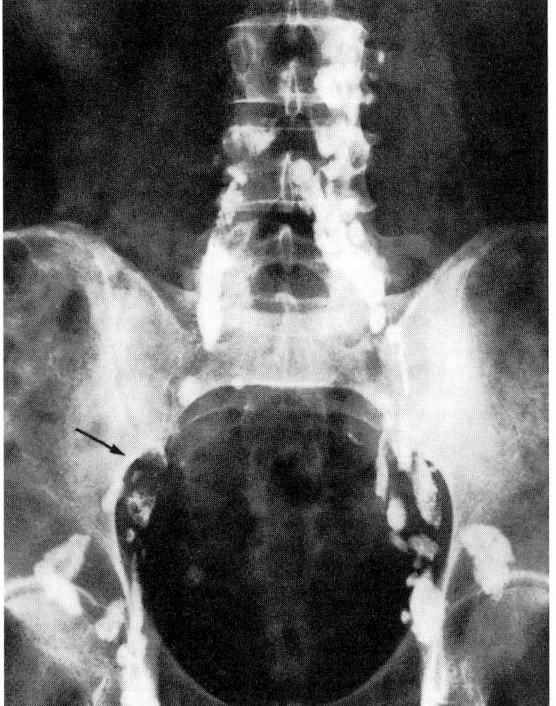

**Figure 11.20d** Lymphogram at 24 h post-injection showing a filling defect in a lymph node (arrow)

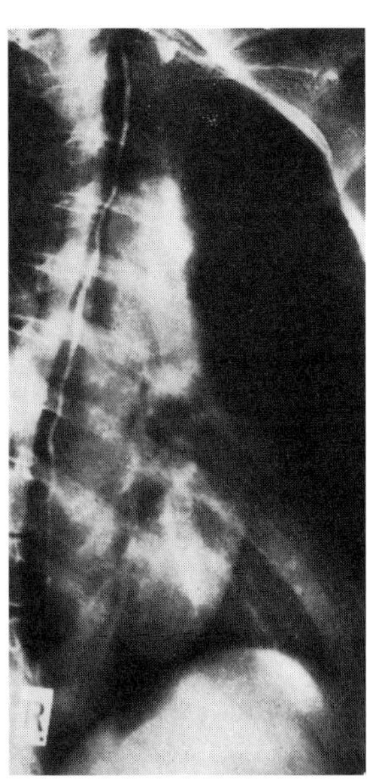

**Figure 11.20e** Cisterna chyli

# REFERENCES AND SUGGESTED READING


## Magnetic resonance imaging

Anderson, C.M., Edelman, R.R. and Turski, P.A. (1993) *Clinical Magnetic Resonance Angiography*, Raven Press, New York

Andrew, R.E. (1990) *Clinical Magnetic Resonance: Imaging and Spectroscopy*, Wiley, New York

Atlas, S.W. (1996) *Magnetic Resonance Imaging of the Brain and Spine*, 2nd edn, Lippincott Raven, Philadelphia

Ballinger, P.W. (1995) *Merrill's Atlas of Radiographic Positions and Radiologic Procedures*, 8th edn, Mosby, St. Louis

Berquist, T.H. (1996) *MRI of the Musculoskeletal System*, 3rd edn, Lippincott Raven, Philadelphia

Bushong, S. (1996) *Magnetic Resonance Imaging: Physical and Biological Principles*, Mosby, St. Louis

Cordoza, J. and Herfkens, R. (1994) *MRI Survival Guide*, Lippincott Raven, Philadelphia

Curry, T., Dowdey, J. and Murry, R. (1990) *Christensen's Physics of Diagnostic Radiology*, 4th edn, Lea and Febiger, Philadelphia

Elster, A.D. (1994) *Questions and Answers in Magnetic Resonance Imaging*, Mosby, St. Louis

English, P.T. and Moore, C. (1995) *MRI for Radiographers*, Springer Verlag, Berlin

Grainger, R.G. and Allison, R.G. (1996) *Diagnostic Radiology*, Churchill Livingstone, Edinburgh

Hashemi, R.H. and Bradley, W.G. Jr. (1997) *MRI: The Basics*, Williams and Wilkins, Baltimore

Hendrick, R.E., Russ, P.D. and Simon, J.H. (1993) *MRI: Principles and Artefacts* (Raven MRI teaching file), Raven Press, New York

Heywang and Brunner, K.U. (1990) *Contrast – Enhanced MRI of the Breast*, Schering, Burgess Hill

Horowitz, A. (1987) *MRI Physics for Physicians*, Springer Verlag, Berlin

Hricak, H., Carrington, B.M. (1991) *MRI of the Pelvis – A Text Atlas*, Duwitz, London

Moller, T.B. (1993) *MRI Atlas of the Musculoskeletal System*, Blackwell Scientific, Oxford

Ness Aiver, M. (1996) *All You Really Need to Know About MRI Physics*, University of Maryland, Baltimore

Newhouse, J. and Wienner, J. (1991) *Understanding MRI*, Little, Brown, Boston

Poho, G.N. (1993) *Cardiovascular Applications of Magnetic Resonance*, Futura, London

Powell, M.C. (1994) *Magnetic Resonance Imaging in Obstetrics and Gynaecology*, Butterworth-Heinemann, Oxford

Schild, H.H. (1990) *MRI Made Easy*, Schering, Burgess Hill

Shelloch, F. and Kanal, E. (1996) *Magnetic Resonance Imaging Bioeffects. Safety and Patient Management*, Lippincott Raven, Philadelphia

Smith, H.J. and Ranallo, F.N. (eds.) (1989) *A Non-Mathematical Approach to Basic MRI*, Medical Physics Publishing,

Stark, D.D. and Bradley, W.G. (1992) *Magnetic Resonance Imaging*, 2nd edn, Mosby, St. Louis

Wehrli, F.W. (1991) *Fast Scan Magnetic Resonance: Principles and Applications*, Raven Press, New York

Westbrook, C. (1994) *Handbook of MRI Technique*, Blackwell, Oxford

Westbrook, C. and Kaut, C. (1993) *MRI in Practice*, Blackwell, Oxford

Wheeler, G. and Withers, K. (1996) *Lippincott Magnetic Resonance Imaging Review*, Lippincott Raven, Philadelphia

## Radionuclide imaging

1990 *Medical Radiation Protection within the EEC*,

1990 *Recommendations of the International Commission on Radiological Protection*, ICRP No. 60, Pergamon Press, Oxford

1991 *Advances in Radiation Protection*, Kluwer Academic, Kingston-upon-Thames

1991 *Statistics of Human Exposure to Ionizing Radiation*, Nuclear Technology Publishing,

1992 *Dosimetry of Diagnostic Radiology*, Nuclear Technology Publishing,

1992 *Quality Standards in Nuclear Medicine*, The Institute of Physical Sciences in Medicine,

1992 *Radiation Protection – A Guide for Scientists and Physicians*, Butterworth-Heinemann, Oxford

1992 *Radiation Protection in Nuclear Medicine and Pathology*, Report No. 60, The Institute of Physical Sciences in Medicine, York

Beller, G. (1995) *Clinical Nuclear Cardiology*, Saunders, Washington

Bernier, D. (1997) *Nuclear Medicine: Technology and Techniques*, 4th edn, Mosby, St. Louis

Bernier, D.R., Christian, P.E. and Langan, J.K. (1994) *Nuclear Medicine Techniques and Technology*, Mosby, St. Louis

Cerqueira, M.D. (1994) *Nuclear Cardiology*, Blackwell, Oxford

Datz, F.L. and Taylor, A. (1991) *Clinical Practice of Nuclear Medicine*, Churchill Livingstone, Edinburgh

Davidson, A.J. and Hartman, D.S. (1994) *Radiology of the Kidney and Urinary Tract*, 2nd edn, W.B. Saunders, Philadelphia

Fogelman, I., Maisey, M.N. and Clarke, S.E.M. (1993) *An Atlas of Clinical Nuclear Medicine*, 2nd edn, Martin Dunitz, London

Frier, M. (1988) *Hospital Radiopharmacy Principles and Practices*, Institute of Physical Sciences in Medicine, York

Goldberg, H.I. (1993) *Contemporary Imaging: Magnetic Resonance Imaging, Computed Tomography and Interventional Radiology*, Mosby, St. Louis

Hart, and Smith, (1992) *Quality Assurance Standards in Nuclear Medicine*, Institute of Physical Sciences in Medicine, York

Lisle, D. (1996) *Imaging for Students*, Arnold, London

Maisey, M., Britton, K. and Gilday, D. (1991) *Clinical Nuclear Medicine*, Chapman and Hall, New York

Markisz, J.A. (1991) *Musculoskeletal Imaging: MRI, CT, Nuclear Medicine and Ultrasound in Clinical Practice*, Little, Brown, Boston

Pennell, D.J. (1992) *Thallium Myocardial Perfusïon Tomography in Clinical Cardiology*, Springer Verlag, Berlin

Sampson, C. (1993) *Textbook of Radiopharmacy*, Gordon and Breach, New York

Smith, Gemmell, and Sharpe, (1989) *Practical Nuclear Medicine*, IRL Press,

Sutton, D. (1993) *A Textbook of Radiology and Imaging*, 5th edn, Churchill Livingstone, Edinburgh

Whitehouse, G.H. and Worthington, B.S. (1990) *Techniques in Diagnostic Imaging*, 2nd edn, Blackwell, Oxford

## Computed tomography

Gedgaudes-McClees, R.K. and Torres, W.E. (1990) *Essentials of Body Computed Tomography*, W.B. Saunders, Philadelphia

Goldberg, H.I. (1993) *Contemporary Imaging: Magnetic Resonance Imaging, Computed Tomography and Interventional Radiology*, Mosby, St. Louis

Gillespie, J.E. and Gholkar, A. (1994) *Magnetic Resonance Imaging and Computed Tomography of the Head and Neck*, Chapman and Hall, London

Grainger, R.G. and Allison, D.J. (1992) *Diagnostic Radiology: An Anglo-American Textbook of Imaging*, 2nd edn, Churchill Livingstone, Edinburgh

Hendee, W.R. (1993) *The Principles of Computed Tomography*, Little, Brown, Boston

Logan, B.M., Dixon, A.K. and Ellis, H. (1991) *Human Cross-sectional Anatomy: Atlas of Body Sections and CT Images*, Butterworth-Heinemann, Oxford

Merran, S., Hureau, J. and Dixon, A. (1991) *CT & MRI Radiological Anatomy*, Butterworth-Heinemann, Oxford

Seeram, E. (1994) *Computed Tomography*, W.B. Saunders, Philadelphia

Wastie, M.L. and Armstrong, P. (1992) *Diagnostic Imaging*, 2nd edn, Blackwell Scientific, Oxford

Webb, W.R., Brant, W.E. and Helms, C.A. (1991) *Fundamentals of Body CT*, W.B. Saunders, Philadelphia

Wegener, O.H., Fassel, R. and Welger, D. (1992) *Whole-Body Computed Tomography*, 2nd edn, Blackwell, Oxford

Weir, J. and Abrahams, P.H. (1992) *An Imaging Atlas of Human Anatomy*, Wolfe, London

## Ultrasound

Altman, D.G. and Chitty, L.S. (1994) New charts for ultrasound dating of pregnancy. *Ultrasound in Obstetrics and Gynaecology* **10**(3): 174–91

Bismuth, H., Kunstlinger, F. and Castaing, D. (1991) *Liver Ultrasound: An Illustrated Guide:6*, Chapman and Hall, London

Bismuth, H., Kunstlinger, F. and Castaing, D. (1991) *A Text and Atlas of Liver Ultrasound*, Chapman and Hall, London

Callen, P. (1994) *Ultrasound in Obstetrics and Gynaecology*, 3rd edn, W.B. Saunders, Philadelphia

Chitty, L.S. and Altman, D.G. (1994) *British Medical Ultrasound Society Bulletin* **2**(4): 9–19

Chudleigh, P. and Pearce, J.M. (1992) *Obstetric Ultrasound*, 2nd edn, Churchill Livingstone, Edinburgh

Cosgrove, D., Meire, K. and Dewbury, H. (1993) *Clinical Ultrasound: A Comprehensive Text*, Vols 1 and 2 (*Ultrasound in Obstetrics and Gynaecology* and *Abdominal and General Ultrasound*), Churchill Livingstone, Edinburgh

Evans, D.H., McDicken, W.N., Skidmore, R. and Woodcock, J.P. (1989) *Doppler Ultrasound – Physics, Instrumentation and Clinical Applications*, Wiley, New York

Evans, J.A. (ed.) (1986) *Physics in Medical Ultrasound*, Institution of Physics and Engineering in Medicine and Biology,

Fish, P. (1990) *Physics and Instrumentation of Medical Ultrasound*, Wiley, New York

Fleicher, A.C., Romero, R., Manning, F. and Jeanty, P. (1995) *The Principles and Practice of Ultrasound in Obstetrics and Gynaecology*, 5th edn, Appleton & Lange,

Hill, (1998) *Physical Principles of Medical Ultrasound*, 2nd edn, Wiley, New York

Institute of Physical Sciences in Medicine (1995) *Routine Quality Assurance of Ultrasound Imaging Systems No. 71*, Institute of Physical Sciences in Medicine,

Kremkau, F. (1993) *Diagnostic Ultrasound – Principles and Instruments*, 4th edn, W.B. Saunders, Philadelphia

Proud, J. (1994) *Ultrasound for Midwives: A Guide for Midwives and other Health Professionals*, Books for Midwives Press, Cheshire

Robinson and Fleming (1990) *Clinical applications of ultrasonic fetal measurements* (from the British Medical Ultrasound Society Fetal Measurements Working Party Report), British Institute of Radiology

Royal College of Radiologists (1997) *Guidance for the Training in Ultrasound of Medical Non-Radiologists*, Royal College of Radiologists, London

Wilde, P. (1993) *Clinical Ultrasound – A Comprehensive Text – Cardiac Ultrasound*, Churchill Livingstone, Edinburgh

## Journals

American Journal of Roentgenology

British Journal of Radiology

British Medical Journal

Clinical MRI

Clinical Radiology

Diagnostic Imaging

Journal of Computer Assisted Tomography (contains MRI Literature)

Journal of Magnetic Resonance Imaging

Magnetic Resonance Quarterly

Radiology

Radiography

## Journal articles

Cheesman, A.D., Knight, J., McIvor, J. and Perry, A. (1986) Tracheo-oesophageal 'puncture speech': an assessment technique for failed oesophageal speakers. *Journal of Laryngology and Otology*, **C** (2): 191–199.

McIvor, J., Evans, P.F., Perry, A. and Cheesman, A.D. (1990) Radiological assessment of post laryngectomy speech. *Clinical Radiology* **41**: 312–316

Wylie, J., Dodds, E., Stewart, T. and Logemann, J.A. (1990) Physiology and radiology of the normal oral and pharyngeal phases of swallowing. *American Journal of Roentgenology* **154**: 953–963

# INDEX